MW01030341

ESSENTIALS OF

HOSPITAL MEDICINE

A Practical Guide for Clinicians

ESSENTIALS OF HOSPITAL MEDICINE

A Practical Guide for Clinicians

Editors

Andrew Dunn

Mount Sinai School of Medicine, New York, USA

Navneet Kathuria

Paul Klotman

Baylor College of Medicine, Texas, USA

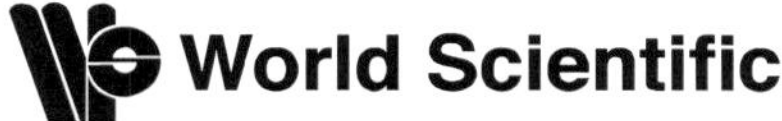

NEW JERSEY • LONDON • SINGAPORE • BEIJING • SHANGHAI • HONG KONG • TAIPEI • CHENNAI

Published by

World Scientific Publishing Co. Pte. Ltd.
5 Toh Tuck Link, Singapore 596224
USA office: 27 Warren Street, Suite 401-402, Hackensack, NJ 07601
UK office: 57 Shelton Street, Covent Garden, London WC2H 9HE

Library of Congress Cataloging-in-Publication Data
Essentials of hospital medicine : a practical guide for clinicians / [edited by] Andrew Dunn, Navneet Kathuria & Paul Klotman.
p. ; cm.
Includes bibliographical references and index.
ISBN 978-9814354905 (hardcover : alk. paper)
I. Dunn, Andrew (Andrew S.) II. Kathuria, Navneet. III. Klotman, Paul.
[DNLM: 1. Hospitals. 2. Patient Care. 3. Hospitalists. 4. Hospitalization. WX 162]
362.11--dc23
2012034420

British Library Cataloguing-in-Publication Data
A catalogue record for this book is available from the British Library.

Typeset by Stallion Press
Email: enquiries@stallionpress.com

Printed in Singapore.

Contents

List of Contributors

Amir Abadir
University of Toronto
Toronto, ON
Canada

Evaristo O. Akerele
Mount Sinai School of Medicine
New York, NY
USA

Reza Akhtar
Mount Sinai School of Medicine
New York, NY
USA

Louis Aledort
Mount Sinai School of Medicine
New York, NY
USA

Yousaf Ali
Mount Sinai School of Medicine
New York, NY
USA

Sridhar R. Allam
Mount Sinai School of Medicine
New York, NY
USA

Zygimantas C. Alsauskas
University of Louisville
Louisville, KY
USA

Imuetinyan Asuen
Mount Sinai School of Medicine
New York, NY
USA

Uma S. Ayyala
Mount Sinai School of Medicine
New York, NY
USA

Eric Barna
Mount Sinai School of Medicine
New York, NY
USA

Joseph Betancourt
The Disparities Solutions Center
Massachusetts General Hospital
Boston, MA
USA

Kabir Bhasin
Mount Sinai Medical Center
New York, NY
USA

Catherine Bigelow
Mount Sinai School of Medicine
New York, NY
USA

Noa Biran
Mount Sinai School of Medicine
New York, NY
USA

Nicole M. Bouvier
Mount Sinai Medical Center
New York, NY
USA

Elise M. Brett
Mount Sinai School of Medicine
New York, NY
USA

Alan S. Briones
Mount Sinai School of Medicine
New York, NY
USA

Andrew Burke
McMaster University
Hamilton, ON
Canada

David P. Calfee
Weill Cornell Medicial College
New York, NY
USA

Daniel Caplivski
Mount Sinai School of Medicine
New York, NY
USA

Joseph M. Cerimele
Mount Sinai School of Medicine
New York, NY
USA

Emily Chai
Mount Sinai School of Medicine
New York, NY
USA

Dennis Chang
Mount Sinai School of Medicine
New York, NY
USA

Sita Chokhavatia
Mount Sinai School of Medicine
New York, NY
USA

Salvatore Cilmi
New York Presbyterian Hospital-Weill Cornell Medical Center
New York, NY
USA

Lisa Coplit
Quinnipiac University School of Medicine
Hamden, CT
USA

Caroline Cromwell
Mount Sinai School of Medicine
New York, NY
USA

Kelly Cunningham
Mount Sinai School of Medicine
New York, NY
USA

Anuj K. Dalal
Birgham and Women's Hospital
Boston, MA
USA

Bruce J. Darrow
Mount Sinai School of Medicine
New York, NY
USA

Douglas T. Dieterich
Mount Sinai School of Medicine
New York, NY
USA

Anca Dinescu
Washington VA Medical Center
Washington DC
USA

Celia M. Divino
The Mount Sinai Hospital
New York, NY
USA

Sakshi Dua
Mount Sinai Medical Center
New York, NY
USA

Andrew Dunn
Mount Sinai School of Medicine
New York, NY
USA

Kevin G. Dunsky
Mount Sinai School of Medicine
New York, NY
USA

Erin DuPree
Mount Sinai Medical Center
New York, NY
USA

Alejandra Durango
Mount Sinai School of Medicine
New York, NY
USA

Lane Duvall
Mount Sinai Medical Center
New York, NY
USA

Kerri E. B. El-Sabrout
The Mount Sinai Hospital
New York, NY
USA

Phillip A. Erwin
Mount Sinai School of Medicine
New York, NY
USA

George Farag
McMaster University
Hamilton, ON
Canada

Jeffrey I. Farber
Mount Sinai School of Medicine
New York, NY
USA

Madeline C. Fields
Mount Sinai School of Medicine
New York, NY
USA

Avi Fischer
Mount Sinai School of Medicine
New York, NY
USA

Eva Flores
New York Presbyterian Hospital-Weill Cornell Medical Center
New York, NY
USA

Beverly Forsyth
Mount Sinai School of Medicine
New York, NY
USA

Jeffrey Glassberg
Mount Sinai School of Medicine
New York, NY
USA

Jill D. Goldenberg
Mount Sinai School of Medicine
New York, NY
USA

Peter D. Gorevic
Mount Sinai Medical Center
New York, NY
USA

Alexander Green
The Disparities Solutions Center
Massachusetts General Hospital
Boston, MA
USA

Richard S. Haber
Mount Sinai School of Medicine
New York, NY
USA

Jonathan L. Halperin
Mount Sinai Medical Center
New York, NY
USA

Timothy J. Harkin
Mount Sinai School of Medicine
New York, NY
USA

Adam Harris
Stony Brook School of Medicine
Stony Brook, NY
USA

Mark Harrison
The Hudson Valley Heart Center
Poughkeepsie, NY
USA

Lisa Hayes
North Shore-Long Island Jewish Health System
Lake Success, NY
NY

Ira M. Helenius
Mount Sinai School of Medicine
New York, NY
USA

Anne Holbrook
McMaster University
Hamilton, ON
Canada

Carol R. Horowitz
Mount Sinai School of Medicine
New York, NY
USA

Jay R. Horton
Mount Sinai School of Medicine
New York, NY
USA

Dan V. Iosifescu
Mount Sinai Medical Center
New York, NY
USA

Amir K. Jaffer
University of Miami School of Medicine
Miami, Fl
USA

Ruchi Jain
Montefiore Medical Center
Bronx, NY
USA

Ramiro Jervis
Mount Sinai School of Medicine
New York, NY
USA

Scott Kaatz
Henry Ford Hospital
Wayne State University School of Medicine
Detroit, MI
USA

Susan Kahane
Mount Sinai School of Medicine
New York, NY
USA

Thomas H. Kalb
Feinstein Institute
Hofstra School of Medicine
New York, NY
USA

Surinder Kaul
Baylor College of Medicine
Houston, TX
USA

Leslie Dubin Kerr
Mount Sinai School of Medicine
New York, NY
USA

Sarah Kharkhanechi
McMaster University
Hamilton, ON
Canada

June Kim
Mount Sinai School of Medicine
New York, NY
USA

Michael C. Kim
Mount Sinai Medical Center
New York, NY
USA

Tonia K. Kim
Mount Sinai School of Medicine
New York, NY
USA

Deborah R. Korenstein
Mount Sinai School of Medicine
New York, NY
USA

Maria E. Lamothe
Mount Sinai School of Medicine
New York, NY
USA

Kyle Lapidus
Mount Sinai Medical Center
New York, NY
USA

Mikyung Lee
Mount Sinai School of Medicine
New York, NY
USA

Alice C. Levine
Mount Sinai School of Medicine
New York, NY
USA

Teresa Lim
Mount Sinai School of Medicine
New York, NY
USA

Evgenia Litrivis
Mount Sinai School of Medicine
New York, NY
USA

Richard MacKay
Mount Sinai School of Medicine
New York, NY
USA

Charles E. Mahan
New Mexico Heart Institute
Albuquerque, New Mexcio
USA;
University of New Mexico College of Pharmacy
Albuquerque, New Mexcio
USA

Lara V. Marcuse
Mount Sinai School of Medicine
New York, NY
USA

Deborah B. Marin
Mount Sinai School of Medicine
New York, NY
USA

Brian A. Markoff
Mount Sinai School of Medicine
New York, NY
USA

Joseph R. Masci
Elmhurst Hospital Center
Elmhurst, New York
USA

Jeffrey I. Mechanick
Mount Sinai School of Medicine
New York, NY
USA

Raj K. Medapalli
Mount Sinai School of Medicine
New York, NY
USA

Marc Miller
Mount Sinai School of Medicine
New York, NY
USA

Noga C. Minsky
Mount Sinai School of Medicine
New York, NY
USA

Somnath Mookherjee
University of California
San Francisco, CA
USA

Adam S. Morgenthau
Mount Sinai School of Medicine
New York, NY 10029
USA

Thanu Nadarajah
McMaster University
Hamilton, ON
Canada

Niru S. Nahar
Haslem Hospital Center
New York, NY
USA

Ajith P. Nair
Mount Sinai School of Medicine
New York, NY
USA

Rajeev L. Narayan
Mount Sinai School of Medicine
New York, NY
USA

Ira S. Nash
Mount Sinai Medical Center
New York, NY
USA

Kathy Navid
Mount Sinai Queens Hospital
Long Island City, NY
USA

Sofia Novak
North Shore-Long Island Jewish
Health System
Lake Success, NY
USA

Vladan Novakovic
Mount Sinai School of Medicine
New York, NY
USA;
James J. Peters Veterans Affairs
Hospital
Bronx, NY
USA

Kevin J. O'Leary
Northwestern University Feinberg
School of Medicine
Chicago, IL
USA

William K. Oh
Mount Sinai School of Medicine
New York, NY
USA

Okey Justin Oparanaku
Mount Sinai School of Medicine
New York, NY
USA

Keren Osman
Mount Sinai School of Medicine
New York, NY
USA

Maria L. Padilla
Mount Sinai Medical Center
New York, NY
USA

David G. Paje
Henry Ford Hospital
Wayne State University School of
Medicine
Detroit, MI
USA

Tuhin Pankaj
Office of the President
Baylor College of Medicine
Houston, TX
USA

Gopi Patel
Mount Sinai School of Medicine
New York, NY
USA

Kalpesh K. Patel
Baylor College of Medicine
Division of Gastroenterology and Hepatology
Houston, TX
USA

Sanjay H. Patel
Mount Sinai School of Medicine
New York, NY
USA

Tony Philip
Hofstra North Shore-Long Island Jewish Hospital System
Lake Success, NY
USA

Sean P. Pinney
Mount Sinai School of Medicine
New York, NY
USA

Maurice Policar
Elmhurst Hospital Center
Elmhurst, NY
USA

Jonathan Potack
Mount Sinai School of Medicine
New York, NY
USA

Brian D. Radbill
Mount Sinai School of Medicine
New York, NY
USA

Meenakshi M. Rana
Mount Sinai School of Medicine
New York, NY
USA

Anand C. Reddy
Mount Sinai School of Medicine
New York, NY
USA

Maria A. A. Reyna
Mount Sinai School of Medicine
New York, NY
USA

Kendall Rogers
University of New Mexico School of Medicine
Albuquerque, NM
USA

Michael J. Ross
Mount Sinai School of Medicine
New York, NY
USA

Erin Rule
Mount Sinai School of Medicine
New York, NY
USA

Gabriel Sayer
Massachusetts General Hospital
Boston, MA
USA

Neil Schachter
Mount Sinai Medicial Center
New York, NY
USA

Laura Schimming
Mount Sinai School of Medicine
New York, NY
USA

Niraj L. Sehgal
University of California
San Francisco, CA
USA

Sonia M. Seng
Southcoast Centers for Cancer Care
Fall River, MA
USA

Chirayu J. Shah
Baylor College of Medicine
Houston, TX
USA

Abhinav Sharma
McMaster University
Hamilton, ON
Canada

Brad A. Sharpe
University of California at
San Francisco Medical Center
San Francisco, CA
USA

Patricia Shi
Mount Sinai School of Medicine
New York, NY
USA

Keith Sigel
Mount Sinai School of Medicine
New York, NY
USA

Steve K. Sigworth
Mount Sinai School of Medicine
New York, NY
USA

Maria Skamagas
Mount Sinai School of Medicine
New York, NY
USA

Gwen S. Skloot
Mount Sinai School of Medicine
New York, NY
USA

Ekaterina Sokolova
Mount Sinai Hospital of Queens
Long Island City, NY
USA

Laili Soleimani
Mount Sinai Medical Center
New York, NY
USA

Alex C. Spyropoulos
University of Rochester Medical Center
Rochester, New York
USA

Carmen M. Stanca
Brooklyn Hospital Center
Brooklyn, NY
USA

Sarah Steinberg
Mount Sinai School of Medicine
New York, NY
USA

James K. Stulman
Mount Sinai School of Medicine
New York, NY
USA

Che-Kai Tsao
Mount Sinai School of Medicine
New York, NY
USA

Stanley Tuhrim
Mount Sinai Hospital
New York, NY
USA

Thomas A. Ullman
Mount Sinai Medical Center
New York, NY
USA

Jaime Uribarri
Mount Sinai School of Medicine
New York, NY
USA

Prashant Vaishnava
Mount Sinai School of Medicine
New York, NY
USA

Tomas Villanueva
Baptist Hospital of Miami
Baptist Health South Florida
Miami, Fl
USA

Qingliang T. Wang
Mount Sinai Hospital
New York, NY
USA

Robert Yanagisawa
Mount Sinai School of Medicine
New York, NY
USA

Hospitalists as Leaders

Chapter 1

Hospitalists as Hospital Leaders

*Andrew S. Dunn**

Key Pearls

- Hospitalist leadership in quality improvement and patient safety was spurred on by the Institute of Medicine report, "To Err is Human: Building A Safer Health System," which estimated that 44,000–98,000 patients die each year in US hospitals due to medical errors.
- The co-management model shows promise as a means of enhancing the quality of care for patients with conditions normally cared for by subspecialists.
- The recognition that hospitals are prone to error and harm has made it increasingly important for physicians-in-training to become knowledgable in quality improvement methods. Hospitalists will need to be involved in leading innovative efforts to incorporate new material in residency training.
- Hospitalist leaders need to understand the risk of burnout and address this issue directly by paying close attention to work hours and schedules, allowing flexibility and hospitalist input in their schedule wherever possible, promoting engagement and ownership of group policies and performance, and fostering participation in the quality improvement and other activies that many hospitalists find stimulating.

* Mount Sinai School of Medicine, New York, NY, USA.

- New models of delivery of care and reimbursement, such as value-based purchasing and Accountable Care Organizations, will require leadership of hospitalists to ensure these initiatives are implemented in a manner which both enhances efficiency and patient care.

Introduction

The revolution is over and the evolutionary process has begun. Hospitalists are now at the center of clinical care for inpatients and the movement to enhance hospital quality and patient safety. This book has been developed in recognition of the motivation of hospitalists to become masters of their craft and be able to improve hospital processes and systems. The primary goal is to provide a practical, easily accessible reference to help busy clinicians deliver outstanding patient care. Additional sections address other vital aspects of the hospitalist role, including principles of hospital quality and patient safety, the essential elements of the business of medicine, pearls for teaching in the hospital setting, and the hospitalist as a researcher.

The Path to Leadership

The field of hospital medicine began modestly after recognition that many physicians were devoting most of their time to inpatient work. A major advantage was quickly noted in the ability to provide a continuous presence for hospitalized patients and for hospital administrators to have a core group providing inpatient care. Primary care physicians also noted the benefits of the efficiency of focusing on their outpatient practice. The momentum grew as many hospitals found they needed inpatient clinicians to help them meet the increasing demands of implementing process improvement initiatives and at teaching institutions to meet compliance with new work duty hour limitations for housestaff. Researchers have since demonstrated the advantages, primarily consisting of decreased length of stay and cost and improvement in some quality measures.[1,2]

The next step in the evolution of hospital medicine has been to focus on efforts to enhance hospital quality and decrease medical errors. The emphasis on quality and patient safety was markedly spurred on by the 1999 Institute of Medicine report, "To Err is Human: Building A Safer Health System," which estimated that 44,000–98,000 patients die each year in US hospitals due to medical errors.[3] The maturing hospitalist movement and the abrupt public recognition of the need to address the quality of care in our hospitals had intersected. As many in the medical field took note of the call to arms, hospitalists were already primed to seize opportunities and lead change.

Over the past decade hospitalists have become local and national leaders in numerous initiatives. Advances include the development of new models of care (e.g. surgical co-management); initiatives in patient safety (e.g. decreasing risk of catheter-related bloodstream infections); enhanced hospital quality (e.g. improved glycemic control); and efforts to enhance efficiency and communication (e.g. transitions of care). Though work in each of these areas is far from over, the accomplishments and lessons learned are invaluable as clinicans look to implement best practices at their local sites.

Leading in Care Delivery

The advantages of the hospitalist model have led to extraordinary growth in hospitalist programs and hospitalists. It has been estimated that there were 30,000 hospitalists in the United States as of 2010, up from 5,000 in 2002 and from 1,000 in the mid-1990s when Wachter and Goldman first described the movement and coined the term "hospitalist."[4] The rate of growth has been extraordinary and has resulted in hospitalists providing direct care to many patients who would have normally been seen by a primary care provider or a subspecialist. This includes patients beyond the scope of traditional "general medicine" practice, such as patients with acute stroke, acute myocardial infarction, critical illness, and patients at the end of life receiving palliative care. The breadth and the acuity of these conditions challenge hospitalists to master many aspects of medicine. Clearly a "jack of all trades, master of none" approach is inadequate in the hospital setting.

Hospitalists have also been involved in developing new systems of care delivery. Specifically, the co-management model (Chapter 84) has shown promise as a means of enhancing the quality of care for patients with conditions normally cared for by subspecialists. One area where this model has become prominent is in orthopedic surgery. Patients with hip fracture and total hip replacement are typically older and have multiple comorbidities, and assigning a hospitalist attending as the primary physician or as co-attending in a co-management model can allow for comorbid conditions to be fully addressed and care to be coordinated while the specialist focuses on the surgical issue.

Leading in Hospital Quality and Patient Safety

Change is difficult in large organizations, and can be particularly challenging within hospitals. Hospitals are inherently complex systems with multiple stakeholders, various agendas, and competing goals. In addition, each hospital has a cultural norm that has developed over many years. "That's just the way we do it" is a common reason why inadequate processes are not addressed. Hospitalists are uniquely positioned within hospitals to identify errors and vulnerable processes where the risk for future error is high. This opportunity has allowed many hospitalists to lead and implement change (Chapters 6–7). Leadership efforts may also be formalized in key roles for the institution, such as membership on the Pharmaceutical and Therapeutics Committee, Chief Medical Officer, and Director of Quality for a section, division, or department.

Leadership in quality and safety also extends beyond individual hospital walls to the national arena. The Society of Hospital Medicine (SHM) is the field's main specialty organization in the US, and has grown dramatically in size and influence. SHM has been involved in the development of tools to address crucial hospital processes and outcomes, including medication reconciliation, care transitions, prevention of complications, and reduced readmissions. In addition, hospitalist advocacy helps influence policy decisions at the governmental level on a regional or national stage.

Leading in Education

Many hospitalists now have a major presence on teaching wards, and have direct exposure to medical students, housestaff and fellows (Chapters 16–17). Teaching skill has taken on greater importance given the movement of medical education away from a memorization model towards developing clinicians who can integrate and incorporate large amounts of data into an appropriate assessment and plan of care. Developing skills in "systems-based learning" has been increasingly emphasized, as the ability to navigate hospital, governmental, and commercial aspects of the health-care system has become essential. Also, it has become increasingly important for physicians in training to be knowledgable in quality improvement terminology and techniques. The recognition that hospitals are prone to error and harm and that careful physician oversight can help ameliorate many of these issues has led to greater recognition of the need for training in the relevant skills. However, traditional medical education has ignored this aspect of hospital care. It is now important for hospitalists to become expert teachers as they develop the next generations of hospitalists who will advance current gains and address future problems.

Challenges

The benefits achieved through broad implementation of hospitalist programs have come with recognition of inherent difficulties with the model. Most notably, replacement of the outpatient primary care provider with a hospitalist during hospitalization inserts a minimum of two handoff points. Given that the hospitalist model is responsible for a portion of the discontinuity that plagues a fragmented system, it becomes incumbent on hospitalists to address and overcome these hazardous transition periods. Though much work has been done in this area, the gap persists and needs to be closed.

A second challenge faced by the hospitalist movement is the lack of formal training on clinical topics that are not emphasized in traditional internal medicine residencies, such as hip fracture and stroke, and non-clinical topics, including quality improvement and the business of medicine. Many hospitalists are eager to work in these areas and train future hospitalists on these topics, but most are unprepared based on being products of the current model of medical education. Hospitalists can address these deficiences by pursuing additional training (e.g. Six Sigma certification or Masters courses); attending CME (e.g. SHM's annual meeting); learning by doing (i.e. the "see one, do one, teach one" model); using web-based materials (e.g. the Institute for Healthcare Improvement's open school); and reviewing easily digested texts (e.g. this textbook).

Another concern is that the intensity of patient care will lead to hospitalist burnout, poor retention, and high tunover at hospitals. A study of 266 academic hospitalists found that 67% experienced high levels of stress and 23% reported some degree of burnout.[5] Factors associated with burnout include lack of control of their work schedule and low satisfaction with the amount of time at home or with family. This issue is particularly important given the data showing that many of the benefits of a hospitalist model are seen in the 2nd year of practice and beyond, indicating the importance of retention in any successful hospitalist service.[6,7] Hospitalist services need to address this issue directly by paying close attention to work hours and schedules, allowing flexibility and hospitalist input in their schedule wherever possible, promoting a sense of ownership in group policies and performance, and fostering participation in the quality improvement and other activities that hospitalists find stimulating.

The Future

Several factors continue to spur on the growth of hospitalist programs, many of which are likely to become more prominent over time. These include:

- Financial pressure on primary care practices to maximize the number of patients seen in the outpatient setting.
- Increasing acuity and complexity of hospitalized patients.
- The need for expertise in the navigation of healthcare sytems to provide timely dispositions for patients.

- The need to maximize subspecialists' focus on their field by having hospitalists coordinate care for complex patients.
- Introduction of electronic medical records within hospitals, which will likely encourage some physicians who infrequently admit patients to refer their patients to hospitalist services rather than learn new systems.
- Governmental and commercial initiatives to reduce or eliminate payment for preventable complications.
- Public reporting of quality indicators.
- Emphasis on patient satisfaction, which is likely to be linked to hospital reimbursement.

In addition to continued expansion of clinical care, it is likely that hospitalists will become increasingly vital to efforts to reduce healthcare costs and increase standardization for hospitalized patients. In the US and for many nations, costs are spiraling out of control and the delivery of safe and effective care remains inconsistent across hospitals and regions. Relying on disparate clinicians whose primary clinical focus is in the outpatient arena to systematically address issues related to resource utilization or the structured application of evidence-based recommendations for hospitalized patients is unrealistic. For these issues to be remedied, hospitalists will need to take an even greater role in the delivery of care and its coordination with physicians in ambulatory settings.

Healthcare reform initiatives in the US will spur hospitals to provide higher quality care in a more efficient manner. These include incentives for previously independent entities to collaborate, such as through formation of Accountable Care Organizations (ACOs), in order take a broader view of patient care to achieve overall cost savings. Also, value-based purchasing (VBP) is a model where the traditional fee-for-service system based on the quantity of care is replaced with payment based largely on the quality of care. A VBP formula reduces compensation for hospitals with lower quality scores and provides enhanced compensation for those performing at a high level. Though these sweeping initiatives have the potential to shift the cost curve, patient care may suffer if implemented locally without the input and leadership of hospitalists. For example, an initiative to deliver antibiotics promptly to all patients with pneumonia to increase a hospital's VBP score may result in overuse of antibiotics in patients without infection if not designed in a thoughtful manner.

Rigorous analyses of different management options that include assessment of the benefits, harms, and costs, termed *comparative effectiveness research*, has become a vital tool to inform clinicians, patients, payors, and policy makers on the relative benefits of various interventions. Hospitalists will need to become increasingly involved in these real-world investigations to identify those interventions that are indicated for specific groups, those which should not be implemented due to the harms, and those unlikely to be cost-effective. Many hospitalists are prepared to design, implement, and participate in these crucial studies.

The hospitalist movement will continue to grow and be spurred on by increasing regulatory and financial pressures on physician practices, hospitals, and healthcare systems. Whether these changes result in better outcomes, more uniform implementation of best practices, and more cost-effective care will be up to today's hospitalists.

References

1. Peterson MC. (2009) A systematic review of outcome and quality measures in adult patients cared for by hospitalists vs nonhospitalists. *Mayo Clin Proc* **84**: 248–254.
2. Lindenauer PK, Rothberg MB, Pekow PS, *et al*. (2007) Outcomes of care by hospitalists, general internists, and family physicians. *New Engl J Med* **357**: 2589–2600.
3. Institute of Medicine Report. (2000) To Err is Human: Building A Safer Health System. National Academy of Sciences.
4. Wachter RM, Goldman L. (1996) The emerging role of hospitalists in the American health care system. *New Engl J Med* **335**: 514–517.
5. Glasheen JJ, Misky GJ, Reid MB, *et al*. (2011) Career satisfaction and burnout in academic hospital medicine. *Arch Intern Med* **171**: 782–785.

6. Auerbach AD, Wachter RM, Katz P, *et al.* (2002) Implementation of a voluntary hospitalist service at a community teaching hospital: Improved clinical efficiency and patient outcomes. *Ann Intern Med* **137**: 859–865.
7. Meltzer D, Manning WG, Morrison J, *et al.* (2002) Effect of physician experience on costs and outcomes on an academic general medicine service: Results of a trial of hospitalists. *Ann Intern Med* **137**: 866–874.

Key Clinical Pearls

Chapter 2

Evidence-based Medicine Primer

Sarah Kharkhanechi, Amir Abadir†, Abhinav Sharma‡, Andrew Burke‡, George Farag‡, Thanu Nadarajah‡ and Anne Holbrook‡,§*

Introduction

Clinicians who specialize in hospital medicine face numerous information challenges in the course of every working day; there are likely to be at least two important but unanswered clinical questions per patient seen per day. Most clinicians are experienced information gatherers, but many find it challenging to sort high quality "wheat" from the lower quality "chaff" of literature found. We have two choices — either we must limit ourselves to information sources already critically appraised, of which at least one outstanding example exists (MacPlus, available via http://plus.mcmaster.ca/macplusfs), or learn how to critically appraise relevant literature ourselves. Fortunately, a systematic and well-tested approach to the latter is available. This chapter describes such an approach to four key types of questions that are routinely encountered: Diagnosis, therapy, prognosis and economics/resource utilization. Each is presented using an example relevant to hospital medicine practice.

*Department of Radiology, McMaster University;
†Department of Medicine, University of Toronto, Canada;
‡Department of Medicine, McMaster University;
§Division of Clinical Pharmacology & Therapeutics, McMaster University, Canada

Diagnosis

Assessing the value of a diagnostic test is a crucial part of every clinician's practice. It is important to consider the limits and applicability of these tests and understand their role in clarifying the diagnosis.

Clinical Scenario

Mrs. Green is a healthy 45-year-old woman who presents to your clinic with a swollen left calf. There are no significant risk factors for venous thromboembolism (VTE). Are there any tests that can aid you in ruling out a deep venous thrombosis (DVT)?

Diagnosis Study

A study evaluating the use of a latex agglutination quantitative D-Dimer assay in outpatient clinics of four hospitals retrospectively examined 595 unselected patients with a follow-up period of three months.[1] The sensitivities, specificities, predictive values, and likelihood ratios of the assay were calculated for all patients using objective testing and eventual clinical diagnosis as the gold standard.

Diagnosis Criteria[2–3]

a) Availability: Is this test available in your institution? Do you have a well-trained person to perform the test? Are you sufficiently knowledgeable or do you have an expert available to interpret the results? Can the test be completed and reported in the necessary timeframe? If your answer is NO to any of the above practical questions, then there is likely not much point in ordering the test no matter how valid it may be.
b) Validity: This term refers to the accuracy and the ability of the test to rule in or rule out the diagnosis in question, and thus help you make your clinical decision.
c) Conclusiveness: How much do the results of this test help you in making a diagnosis? Will you need another test to confirm the diagnosis? This depends on the answers to the questions presented below in Table 1.

Table 1. Criteria for Evaluating a Study on a Diagnostic Test

Was there truly uncertainty about the diagnosis in the sample used in the study?	A diagnostic test is useful if it is able to distinguish between disorders when they have overlapping clinical presentations. For example, pulmonary embolism is difficult to diagnose clinically due to variability in presentation and overlap of its symptoms with other diseases.
Was the test being evaluated compared to a gold (reference) standard? Was the gold standard applied to ALL *of the patients?*	Many diseases do not have a high quality diagnostic standard (gold standard) test. However, to avoid bias, the new test and the diagnostic standard test should be performed on everyone in the study.
Were the results of the gold standard interpreted without knowledge of the new test result and vice versa?	Blinding of the test interpreters is crucial to ensure no bias is introduced in the analysis of the results.
What is the "sensitivity" (% patients with condition who have positive results — true positives) of the test?	A highly sensitive test helps to rule out the condition (SNout — sensitive rules out). Sensitivity = true positive/(true positive + false negative).
What is the "specificity" (% patients who do not have the condition who have negative results — true negatives) of the test?	A highly specific test helps to rule in the condition (SPin — Specific rules in). Specificity = true negative/(true negative+ false positive).
What is the "likelihood ratio" (LR) associated with the test?	The probability of getting this test result in those with the condition divided by those without the condition. Positive likelihood ratio (LR+) = Sensitivity/(1– Specificity), while negative likelihood ratio (LR-) = (1– Sensitivity/Specificity). A test with a LR+ more than 10 or a LR- less than 0.1 will provide a considerable change from pre-test to post-test probability.
Have the results of the diagnostic accuracy study been confirmed in a prospective management study?	Results of retrospective studies determining Sn, Sp, and LR should be confirmed with a prospective management study where the results of the diagnostic test are incorporated into patient management decisions.

d) Applicability: Generally, diagnostic tests are only worth considering if they will change your management decisions. In addition to good diagnostic properties, a test must also be safe to use and provide acceptable cost-effectiveness.

Discussion

The study mentioned above included patients with suspected VTE presenting to an outpatient hospital setting.[1] Patients were categorized according to their pretest probability of VTE as "low," "intermediate" or "high." All patients underwent further testing, for example with compression ultrasound or V/Q scan, except for a portion of patients who had both a low pretest probability and a negative SimpliRED D-Dimer. Patients with no objective evidence of VTE were followed for three months. This differential application of the "gold standard" is a minor methodologic flaw in the study, but is a well-validated clinical approach to VTE. The sensitivity and specificity of the latex agglutination quantitative D-dimer test using a cut-off point of 0.5 μg FEU/mL, were found to be 96 and 45%, respectively. The PPV and NPV of the test were 29 and 98%, with LR+ and LR− at 1.4 and 0.09, respectively. These results indicate that for patients with low or moderate pre-test probability of VTE, a negative quantitative latex D-Dimer assay can rule out VTE due to its high sensitivity and good negative likelihood ratio. However, the test is not very helpful when it is positive. A subsequent prospective cohort management study confirmed that a negative D-dimer result safely eliminated the need for further testing in patients with low or moderate pre-test probability of DVT.[4]

Mrs. Green, meanwhile, has a low pre-test probability of having a DVT given her history, so a quantitative latex D-Dimer was conducted and its result was negative. She was reassured and sent home.

Prognosis

An estimate of prognosis is essential to guide treatment and inform patients about clinically relevant outcomes.

Clinical Scenario

Mr. Bing, 65 years of age, is brought to the ER with right-sided facial droop and mild hemiparesis. His symptoms resolve within 60 min of onset. After blood tests and a CT scan, you explain that he has likely suffered a transient ischemic attack (TIA). He asks you what his chances are of having a major debilitating stroke.

Prognosis Study

A recent trial looked at the ABCD2 score for determining risk of recurrent TIA, minor stroke or major stroke after presentation with a TIA.[5] This was a prospective sub-study of all consecutive individuals with identified TIA or stroke in the region of Oxfordshire, England. A consecutive sample of 500 patients diagnosed with a TIA were identified and followed-up in person at 30 days.

Prognosis Criteria[6]

Table 2. Criteria for Evaluating a Study on Prognosis

a) Are the results valid (worth reading)?	
Does the population in the study include a spectrum of patients with the disease, and were they entered in the study at a similar stage of disease?	An inception cohort (everyone entered at the same stage of their disease, preferably early) has the potential to provide the best prognosis information.
Was the duration of follow-up sufficient to capture development of the outcome? Was follow-up complete?	The study's validity may be compromised if there are a large number of patients lost to follow-up relative to those who have suffered an event or if the follow-up period is too short.
Were the outcomes of interest defined and determined in an objective and unbiased manner?	There should be a clear definition of outcomes of interest before study commences. Detailed adjudication rules may be required for subjective outcomes such as disability.

(*Continued*)

Table 2. (*Continued*)

Were there adjustments for other important prognostic factors?	Prognostic characteristics, including treatments provided, other than those being studied, will need to be considered.
b) What are the results?	
How large was the likelihood of the outcome event in a specified period of time?	The quantitative results from studies of prognosis are the number of outcome events that occur over time.
How precise was the estimate of likelihood?	The precision of this outcome can be evaluated based on the confidence interval (CI). The smaller the CI, the greater the precision.
c) How can I apply the results to my patient care?	
Were the study patients similar to my patient?	Consider whether your patient would meet the inclusion and exclusion criteria of the study.
Will the results lead directly to selecting or avoiding therapy?	Useful prognosis markers will help guide treatment selection.
Are the results useful for reassuring or counseling patients?	Giving patients an estimate of outcomes will allow them to make informed decisions regarding treatment options.

Discussion

The ABCD2 score (age, blood pressure, clinical findings, duration of symptoms, diabetes) is a tool developed to predict individual risk of stroke at seven days and thus meant to affect the triaging of patients with TIA symptoms.[5] The ABCD2 score in these patients presenting initially with TIA, was highly predictive of the 7-day risk of major stroke — 12.8% in patients with ABCD2 scores of 5 or more versus 1.3% in patients with a score 4 or less ($P < 0.001$).

Going back to Mr. Bing, he scores 5 on the ABCD2 scoring system (age $\geq 60 = 1$ point, unilateral weakness $= 2$ and duration of symptoms ≥ 60 min $= 2$), giving a 7-day risk of stroke of 12.8%. This ABCD2 score would suggest that the patient should be counseled on the high risk of early major stroke and should potentially be hospitalized to facilitate further diagnostic testing and to optimize preventive treatment quickly.

Therapy

As the number of therapeutic options increase, clinicians must be able to identify treatments that will minimize patient morbidity and mortality without undue harm of the treatment itself.

Clinical Scenario

Mrs. Geller is a 65-year-old woman with hypertension who presents to the ER with a non-ST elevation myocardial infarction (NSTEMI). Her troponin T is 0.8 μg/L and her EKG shows inferior ST depression. She has already received 160 mg of aspirin, 25 mg of metoprolol, 5000 units of subcutaneous heparin and 40 mg of atorvastatin. The Emergency physician asks you to decide about clopidogrel.

Therapy Trial

The CURE trial was a large, randomized, placebo-controlled trial that studied the effect of clopidogrel added to aspirin versus placebo plus aspirin, on the composite outcome of cardiovascular (CV) death, non-fatal myocardial infarction (MI) or stroke in patients with acute coronary syndromes without ST-segment elevation.[7]

Therapy Criteria[8]

Table 3A. Criteria for Evaluating a Study on Therapy

a) Are the results valid (worth reading)?	
Were the patients randomized?	Randomization is the key to minimizing bias — it balances factors that predict outcome, both those known and unknown, between the groups.

(*Continued*)

Table 3A. (*Continued*)

Was randomization allocation concealed?	Concealment ensures that those enrolling patients in the study cannot influence the arm to which patients are allocated (and thus bias the results).
Were all participants blinded?	Patients, caregivers, data collectors, adjudicators, and data analysts should be blinded to group allocation throughout the study.
How complete was the follow-up to the end of the study?	Ideally, every patient's study outcome would be known. If many patients drop out and are lost to follow-up, the study results may be unreliable even with imputation techniques.
Was intention to treat analysis utilized?	Intention to treat analysis (participant outcomes are assigned to the group that the participant was randomized, no matter whether they stayed in that group or not) is the most conservative method of analyzing a typical randomized trial (non-inferiority trials are different, but are beyond the discussion in this chapter)
Did all of the groups receive similar co-interventions?	Similar co-intervention helps ensure that the treatment versus control comparison is the only cause of any difference in outcome.
b) What are the results of the study?	
How large was the treatment effect?	The treatment effect is determined by a number of variables, including the absolute risk, relative risk, relative risk reduction, number needed to treat, and number needed to harm. These are defined below in Table 3B.
How precise was the estimate of the treatment effect?	The precision of the effect of a treatment is based on the confidence interval. A 95% confidence interval tells you how widely the true result might vary from the actual result found — the smaller the confidence interval, the greater the precision of the treatment.

(*Continued*)

Table 3A. (*Continued*)

c) Can I apply the results of this study to my patient?	
Is there reasonable similarity between my patient and the study patients?	Consider whether your patient would meet the inclusion and exclusion criteria of the study. If not, consider whether there is a compelling reason why your patient would not be similar.
Were all patient-important outcomes considered?	Ensure that the investigators have chosen outcomes that would be considered important by patients. Also ensure that all important adverse effects of the intervention have been documented.
Is treating my patient worth the potential harms and costs?	The NNT must be weighed against the adverse effects (see NNH below) as well as the cost of treatment. (see Economics)

Table 3B. Definitions of Terms to Measure Treatment Effect

Treatment Effect	Calculation
Control event rate (CER)	Number of events in control (placebo, for example) arm/Total patients in control arm
Experimental event rate (EER)	Number of events treatment arm/Total patients in treatment arm
Absolute risk reduction (ARR): The decrease in risk of a experimental treatment in relation to a control treatment.	CER — EER
Relative risk (RR): Probability of the event occurring in the treated group versus the non-treated group.	EER/CER. Relative risk reduction (RRR) = 1-RR
Number needed to treat (NNT): The number of people needed to be treated in order to prevent one bad outcome.	1/ARR. The same calculation can be applied to harmful outcomes; this is termed number needed to harm (NNH).

Discussion

The CURE trial meets all of the validity criteria, so is worth attending to the results. The ARR with clopidogrel added to ASA versus placebo, was 2.1% using the composite outcome, at a mean follow-up of nine months. The relative risk reduction was 20%.[6] Overall, approximately 50 people need to be treated to avoid one outcome of CV death, non-fatal MI or stroke, as compared with one major *bleed* caused for every 100 people treated with this combination antiplatelet regimen.

Going back to our patient, Mrs. Geller fits well the inclusion criteria of the CURE trial, has no increased bleeding risk, and is not going immediately for cardiac catheterization. You therefore order 300 mg of clopidogrel loading dose followed by 75 mg daily.

Economics

Health economics analyses inform policy-makers and clinicians by explicitly measuring and comparing the health outcomes value and costs associated with healthcare strategies. Health economics is essential to determining the most equitable access to shared healthcare resources by optimizing health outcomes per money spent. Individuals who pay for their own healthcare are usually even more concerned about economics, as an expensive test or treatment may mean difficult choices involving their budget for housing, education, etc.

Clinical Scenario

Mr. Singh, a 54-year-old gentleman with hypertension, dyslipidemia, obesity (BMI = 38.4) and new onset diabetes mellitus type II, presents to your office. He has been diligently attempting to lose weight for two years with little to no success. You consider whether to enroll him in a multi-disciplinary weight loss program or refer him for bariatric surgery. You know that bariatric surgery is very expensive but you have heard that it is also very effective in helping patients lose weight and maintain weight loss.

Economics Study

A recent economic analysis carried out as part of a randomized trial was performed on 60 subjects comparing outcomes and costs at two years of laparoscopic adjustable gastric band plus conventional therapy with conventional therapy alone.[9]

Economics Criteria

Table 4. Criteria for Evaluating a Study on Health Economics[10]

a) Are the results valid (worth reading)?	
Was the perspective of all relevant parties included?	Data on costs and outcomes should include all of the relevant groups impacted — including the patient, provider, institution, healthcare plan, and society-at-large.
Were both costs and outcomes considered?	Full economic analysis requires patient-important outcomes in addition to resource utilization.
Were all relevant clinical strategies compared?	The strategies of interest should be compared to the relevant current standard therapy.
Was clinical effectiveness established?	No intervention or strategy will be cost-effective if it is not effective. Economic analyses generated within randomized controlled trials benefit from high internal validity but need to be scrutinized to see if the results are generalizable to usual clinical practice.
Were costs measured accurately?	Costs often differ from charges; costs and charges may vary dramatically across jurisdictions. Likewise, idiosyncrasies in clinical practice across jurisdictions for the same condition can generate resource utilization different from that measured in the study.

(*Continued*)

Table 4. (*Continued*)

Was appropriate allowance made for uncertainties in the analysis?	Given that costs are often more uncertain than effectiveness, sensitivity analyses are very important in economic analyses to ensure that the range in possible cost-effectiveness is captured.
b) What are the results?	
What were the incremental costs and outcomes of each strategy?	Costs should include all materials and healthcare work hours. Outcomes are usually summarized as cost per life year saved or cost per quality-adjusted life year gained (QALYs).
Do the incremental costs and outcomes differ between subgroups?	As for any study, subgroup analyses should be minimized, be specified *a priori* and be considered as hypothesis-generating.
How much does allowance for uncertainty change the results?	Sensitivity analyses which reveal a wide range of cost-effectiveness will reduce confidence in the results.
c) How can I apply the results to patient care?	
Are the treatment benefits worth the harms and costs?	When a treatment is both more effective and more expensive, incremental cost-effectiveness estimates and range of sensitivity analyses are key to informing decisions regarding adoption.
Could we expect similar outcomes and costs with our patients?	Generalizability of outcomes is assessed as described in the "Therapy" section. Costs may differ depending on the local price of materials and clinical practice patterns.

Discussion

Bariatric surgery is clinically effective in causing remission of diabetes mellitus[11] but its cost-effectiveness has been unclear. A 2009 study tackled this question by investigating the cost-effectiveness of laparoscopic gastric band surgery for patients with Type 2 diabetes who had failed lifestyle management. A healthcare sector viewpoint was used.[9] Effectiveness was based on results of a two-year randomized trial, so it is likely that testing and follow-up was more intensive (and therefore more costly) than would occur in usual practice. Uncertainty in costs was accounted for with appropriate modeling but the study is based on only 60 patients, thus raising concerns about the adequacy of the cost-effectiveness estimates. Surgical therapy resulted in remission of diabetes more frequently than conventional therapy alone, with an incremental cost-effectiveness ratio of US $12,300 per case of diabetes remitted. Expressing the outcome in terms of diabetes remitted, *while a relevant clinical outcome*, is less helpful than the more global patient-important outcome of quality-adjusted life year gained.

Going back to the case, Mr. Singh is similar to those in the study, so the treating physician might expect a similar clinical outcome. Costs, however, would likely not be similar as the study was performed in Australia, where healthcare costs are generally lower than in the United States or Canada. In addition, quality of life was not measured. Overall, although this cost-effectiveness ratio is attractive, you are unsure of its generalizability to your patient. After discussion with Mr. Singh, you decide to investigate the extent of his insurance coverage for this procedure and meet again to discuss. You also ask Mr. Singh to read the "plain language" summary of the Cochrane systematic review,[11] which is meant to provide patients with the key results.

References

1. Bates SM, Grand'Maison A, Johnston M, *et al.* (2001) A latex D-dimer reliably excludes venous thromboembolism. *Arch Intern Med* **161**(3): 447–453.
2. Richardson WS, Wilson MC. (2008) The process of diagnosis — Chapter 14. In: Guyatt G, Rennie D, Meade MO, Cook DJ (eds), *User's Guide to the Medical Literature: A Manual for Evidence-Based Clinical Practice*, 2nd ed. American Medical Association, New York, pp. 399–406.

3. Richardson WS, Wilson MC, McGinn TG. (2008) Differential diagnosis — Chapter 15. In: Guyatt G, Rennie D, Meade MO, Cook DJ, (eds) *User's Guide to the Medical Literature: A Manual for Evidence-Based Clinical Practice*, 2nd ed. American Medical Association, New York, pp. 407–417.
4. Bates SM, Kearon C, Crowther M, *et al.* (2003) A diagnostic strategy involving a quantitative latex D-Dimer assay reliably excludes deep venous thrombosis. *Ann Intern Med* **138**: 787–794.
5. Chandratheva A, Geraghty O, Luengo-Fernandez R, *et al.* (2010) ABCD2 score predicts severity rather than risk of early recurrent events after transient ischemic attack. *Stroke* **41**(5): 851–856.
6. Randolph A, Cook DJ and Guyatt G. (2008) Prognosis — Chapter 18. In: Guyatt G, Rennie D, Meade MO, Cook DJ, (eds), *Users' Guides to the Medical Literature: A Manual for Evidence-Based Clinical Practice*, 2nd ed. American Medical Association, New York, pp. 509–520.
7. CURE Study Investigators. (2001) Effects of clopidogrel in addition to aspirin in patients with acute coronary syndromes without ST-segment elevation. *N Engl J Med* **345**: 494–502.
8. Guyatt G, Straus S, Meade MO, *et al.* (2008) Therapy (randomized trials) Chapter 6. In: Guyatt G, Rennie D, Meade MO, Cook DJ, (eds). *User's Guide to the Medical Literature: A Manual for Evidence-Based Clinical Practice*, 2nd ed. American Medical Association, New York, pp. 67–86.
9. Keating CL, Dixon JB, Moodie ML, *et al.* (2009) Cost-efficacy of surgically induced weight loss for the management of type 2 diabetes: A randomized controlled trial. *Diabetes Care* **32**(4): 580–584.
10. Drummond MF, Sculpher MJ, Torrance GW, *et al.* (2005) *Methods for the Economic Evaluation of Health Care Programmes*, 3rd ed. Oxford University Press, Oxford, England.
11. Colquitt JL, Picot J, Loveman E, Clegg AJ. (2009) Surgery for obesity. Cochrane Database of Systematic Reviews, Issue 2.

Chapter 3

On the Fly: Using Electronic Resources to Enhance Evidence-based Practice

Deborah R. Korenstein and Laura Schimming**

Key Pearls

- Asking frequent questions is the key to evidence-based practice.
- Hospitalists can use pre-appraised electronic resources to quickly find evidence-based answers to clinical questions.
- For general questions about disease pathophysiology and treatment ("background questions"), topic summaries are most helpful.
- For specific questions about particular treatments or diagnostic tests ("foreground questions"), systematic reviews or summaries of systematic reviews are often most helpful.
- Practitioners should try various resources to find the most helpful ones.

Introduction

The rise of hospital medicine as an independent discipline over the last decade has coincided with an explosion in Internet-based electronic resources. At the same time, the nature of hospital stays has evolved so that patients are sicker, length of stay is shorter and physicians are busier with admitting and discharging responsibilities.[1,2] Hospitalists are under pressure to provide high quality evidence-based care but there are many challenges to this task, including an exponential rise in the volume of

*Mount Sinai School of Medicine, New York, NY, USA.

medical literature, time, and lack of expertise in evidence-based medicine (EBM).[3] The purpose of this chapter is to help hospitalists access and master the information resource tools they need to become efficient real-time practitioners of EBM, particularly pre-appraised resources, and to provide a summary of useful resources.

In recent years, experts in EBM have shifted their emphasis from the critical appraisal of individual studies to the mastery of pre-appraised resources.[4] Pre-appraised resources are produced by evidence experts and are designed to be easily utilized by clinicians. The best pre-appraised resources are current, undergoing nearly constant updating, "filtered" in that they select for the best available evidence related to the issue at hand, and processed so that the evidence is presented in a manner which is helpful to a busy clinician. Incorporating pre-appraised resources into practice can help hospitalists and others become master evidence-based practitioners.

A New Paradigm: The Evidence Hierarchy

The new paradigm for practicing EBM incorporates a hierarchy of evidence. In the model posed by Haynes and others,[4] these resources form a pyramid with increasing levels of information filtering. Individual studies form the base of the pyramid, followed by study summaries, systematic reviews, summaries of systematic reviews, evidence-based topic reviews (such as review articles or textbook chapters) and finally, computerized decision support systems at the top. Different types of questions are best answered by resources at different points on the pyramid.

There are many widely available electronic resources which can be utilized in real time to facilitate patient care, though their reliability and usefulness vary. In general, when evaluating a new resource, clinicians should look for ratings of evidence quality, sometimes presented as levels of evidence in support of each statement or recommendation. Resources which provide consistent evidence ratings for all clinical recommendations are generally more reliable than those without, since they are transparent about the basis of each statement. When searching resources which are higher in the pyramid, such as a summary of systematic reviews on a topic, it is better to use fewer and simpler terms and then navigate within the site until an answer is found. These databases tend to be smaller, so complex searches may miss relevant entries, and they often have well-designed internal navigation tools. When searching near the base of the pyramid, such as Medline®, which is a very large database, it is best to use more specific search terms. Table 1 summarizes a number of useful resources, including many pre-appraised resources, and indicates the type of information contained, the presence of consistent quality ratings, the Internet address and other details about access and usability. Many of these resources require subscriptions, which are often held by medical libraries.

Becoming an Evidence-based Practitioner

To become an evidence based practitioner and utilize the evidence hierarchy, clinicians should begin by asking questions, since good questions prompt searches for high quality answers. In general, clinicians should ask questions of themselves, questioning even common practice and of consultants, demanding evidence in support of recommendations. They can then begin looking for answers at the highest possible point on the evidence pyramid and move down if no evidence is found. The starting point to answer a given question depends upon the nature of the question. For *Background* questions, which relate to basic information about a topic, it is best to go first to evidence-based topic summaries. An example of a background question is "How is thrombotic thrombocytopenic purpura (TTP) treated?" *Foreground* questions are specific, concerning, for example, the impact of a certain treatment on a particular outcome in a specific patient population. Answers to foreground questions might be found in topic summaries if they relate to an issue which has been addressed by many studies, but if the issue is less well studied it might be better to start with systematic reviews or summaries of individual studies. An example of a foreground question is, "In young women with TTP, does plasma exchange improve mortality as compared with treatment with steroids?"

Table 1. EBM Resources

Resource	Ease of Use	Frequency of Updates[1]	Quality Ratings	Clinical Topic Summaries	Summaries of Systematic Reviews	Systematic Reviews	Single Study Summaries	Individual Studies	Comments
ACP Journal Club http://www.acpjc.org	😐	Monthly	None		✓		✓		Browse by issue or search using keywords. Limit by article type. Search engine will expand search with synonyms from a custom thesaurus.
Clinical Evidence http://clinical-evidence.bmj.com	😐	Daily	Systematic	✓					Browse alphabetically or by section. Search using keywords. Use horizontal menu at top of page to select each topic section. Outline format.

(*Continued*)

[1] Based on claims from each website.

Table 1. *(Continued)*

Resource	Ease of Use	Frequency of Updates[1]	Quality Ratings	Clinical Topic Summaries	Summaries of Systematic Reviews	Systematic Reviews	Single Study Summaries	Individual Studies	Comments
Cochrane Database of Systematic Reviews (CDSR) http://www.thecochranelibrary.com	😐	Monthly	None		✓	✓			Somewhat easy to use. Browse for topics using several criteria. Advanced search page allows Medical Subject Heading (MeSH) searching and full-text searching.
Cochrane Database of Abstracts of Reviews of Effects (DARE) http://www.thecochranelibrary.com	😐	Monthly	None		✓	✓			Select DARE from under "Browse Other Resources" on the Cochrane Library home page. Or, do a keyword search and select "Other Reviews" from the top of the results page to limit to DARE reviews.

(Continued)

Table 1. *(Continued)*

Resource	Ease of Use	Frequency of Updates[1]	Quality Ratings	Clinical Topic Summaries	Summaries of Systematic Reviews	Systematic Reviews	Single Study Summaries	Individual Studies	Comments
Dynamed http://www.ebscohost.com/dynamed	☺	Daily	Systematic	✓					A single search box, left side-bar and collapsible sections provide easy navigation. Outline format.
Epocrates Essentials http://online.epocrates.com	😐	Daily	Some	✓					Search by keywords. Use horizontal menu at the top of page to select each topic section.
eMedicine http://www.imedicine.com	😐	Quarterly	None	✓					Browse by specialty or search using keywords. Must scroll through entire topic; no way to select a section. Paragraph format.

(Continued)

Table 1. *(Continued)*

Resource	Ease of Use	Frequency of Updates[1]	Quality Ratings	Clinical Topic Summaries	Summaries of Systematic Reviews	Systematic Reviews	Single Study Summaries	Individual Studies	Comments
National Guideline Clearinghouse http://www.guideline.gov Free!	☹	Daily	Some					✓	Difficult to use. No way to rank or sort guidelines.
Essential Evidence Plus http://www.essentialevidenceplus.com	😐	Daily	Systematic	✓					Search by keywords or browse frequently searched topics. Use table of contents to select each section. Outline format.
First Consult http://www.mdconsult.com	😐	Daily	Some	✓					Browse alphabetically or search by keyword. Scroll through entire document or use left side-bar to select a section. Outline format.
PIER http://pier.acponline.com	😐	Quarterly	Systematic	✓					Browse by topic type or enter keywords in combination with a drop-down menu. Outline format.

Answering Questions

Resources to Answer Background Questions

In general, background questions are answered by evidence-based topic summaries, which incorporate several different types of resources. First, *guidelines* can be extremely helpful in directing care, but are only as reliable as their methodology. When reading guidelines, clinicians should look for the following:

- A transparent development process.
- Lack of bias or conflicts of interest among the committee members or in the umbrella organization.
- Quality ratings of the evidence.
- Strength ratings for the recommendations themselves.

One US-based electronic resource is dedicated to presenting guidelines. *The National Guideline Clearinghouse* (*NGC*) is produced by the Agency for Healthcare Research and Quality (AHRQ), the US Department of Health and Human Services, the American Medical Association and the American Association of Health Plans-Health Insurance Association of America. It is a comprehensive database of practice guidelines, and is quite complete, although the included guidelines are of varying quality and there are no ratings of the quality of the evidence.

The second type of resource to answer background questions is a collection of topic summaries, such as a textbook. When considering topic summaries, clinicians should look for an explicit process for inclusion of evidence and complete referencing (Table 1). Many textbooks will provide links to relevant guidelines. Some useful resources include:

Clinical Evidence. Produced by the BMJ Group, *Clinical Evidence* produces evidence summaries which include levels of effectiveness and provides links to relevant guidelines.

Dynamed. *Dynamed* performs daily systematic literature surveillance to incorporate new evidence, and presents the date of most recent update to each topic and the content that was updated. Evidence quality is provided for each recommendation and the site is quite user-friendly.

eMedicine. *eMedicine* provides clinical topic summaries in a traditional textbook format and does not systematically grade evidence in support of recommendations. It can be accessed via its own interface or through the TRIP database (described under Resources to Answer Foreground Questions).

Epocrates Essentials. *Epocrates Essentials* contains disease summaries written by the BMJ Group and includes evidence grades for most recommendations. It contains a well-known and widely utilized database of drug information.

Essential Evidence Plus. *Essential Evidence Plus* is made up of topic summaries, with key bullet points provided. It contains consistent strength of evidence ratings, but the interface is less sophisticated and more difficult to navigate than some other resources. There is a PDA option.

First Consult. Integrated with MDConsult, *First Consult* is an online textbook which provides inconsistent evidence grading, and evidence grades are not incorporated into the main text.

PIER. *The Physician's Information and Education Resource* (*PIER*) is produced by the American College of Physicians (ACP) and is updated quarterly. It contains clinical recommendations for many diseases, and provides standardized evidence ratings.

UpToDate. *UpToDate* is a well-written and user-friendly online textbook. It is well-referenced, but crafted much like a traditional textbook, with no explicit process for evidence selection. Age of chapters is variable and evidence quality ratings are available for a very small number of topic reviews. References are linked to abstracts and full text articles.

Resources to Answer Foreground Questions

Foreground questions are usually best answered by systematic reviews of individual studies or in summaries of those systematic reviews. The optimal database in which to begin searching for answers to these types of questions is determined by the specific question. For questions with a large amount of relevant data, it is best to first look for summaries of systematic reviews, or for systematic reviews themselves. For more obscure issues which are less well studied, it may be better to begin with single study summaries or even individual studies themselves. Useful resources for answering foreground questions include:

ACP Journal Club: *ACP Journal Club* is published by the ACP as part of the *Annals of Internal Medicine*, and is available free on-line to ACP members. It contains summaries of relevant high-quality original articles, including systematic reviews.

The Cochrane Database of Systematic Reviews (CDSR): *CDSR* contains systematic reviews completed by the Cochrane Review groups. These reviews are very complete and of uniformly outstanding quality and concern only issues of treatment and screening. A brief summary of the findings is provided on a first page. CDSR can be searched simultaneously with DARE (described below) within the Cochrane Library.

The Database of Abstracts of Reviews and Effects (DARE): *DARE* is published by the Cochrane Collaboration and contains summaries of systematic reviews (regarding diagnosis, treatment or screening) from a variety of sources which have been assessed for quality. It can be searched simultaneously with CDSR within the Cochrane Library.

PubMed Clinical Queries: *PubMed* is the Medline interface provided by the US National Library of Medicine and is available free on the Internet (although many links to full text articles require subscriptions). One of its features, "Clinical Queries," is a useful tool for finding individual high-quality articles. Clinical Queries performs one simultaneous search in three clinical research areas: "Clinical Study Categories," "Systematic Reviews" and "Medical Genetics." The user enters search terms in a central search box and selects the "Clinical Study Category" (therapy, diagnosis, prognosis). The search engine adds additional words to the search, resulting in the selection of high quality articles of the chosen type. For example, when "therapy" is selected, the system adds the words "randomized controlled trial" to the search. At the same time PubMed utilizes the same terms to simultaneously identify systematic reviews and medical genetics results, displayed in separate columns. Clinical Queries allows the user to find a variety of foreground studies using a single search and can be an excellent starting point when searching for individual articles.

TRIP Database: The *TRIP Database* provides searches of multiple free-access databases simultaneously, including a textbook (eMedicine) and foreground resources (the Cochrane Library and ACP Journal Club). Its results will vary in quality based on the source, but it allows the user to perform the search in multiple databases at once to maximize yield.

Summary

In summary, there are many useful resources to help hospitalists become expert evidence-based practitioners. Table 1 provides a summary of the resources discussed in this chapter. With a little practice any clinician can become an expert. Mastering the evidence is possible and even fun if you use the right tools.

References

1. Kalra A, Fisher R, Axelrod P. (2010) Decreased length of stay and cumulative hospitalized days despite increased patient admissions and readmissions in an area of urban poverty. *JGIM 25. published online April 29.*
2. Fry A, Shay D, Holman R, Curns A, Anderson L. (2005) Trends in hospitalizations for pneumonia among persons aged 65 years or older in the United States, 1988–2002. *JAMA* **294**: 2712–2719.
3. Oliveri R, Gluud C, Wille-Jorgensen P. (2004) Hospital doctors' self-rated skills in and use of evidence-based medicine — A questionnaire survey. *J Eval in Clin Pract* **10**: 219–226.
4. DiCenso A, Bayley L, Haynes RB. (2009) Accessing preappraised evidence: Fine-tuning the 5S model into a 6S model. *ACP J Club* **151**: 2–3.

Chapter 4

The Physical Exam: An Evidence Based Approach to Common Abnormal Findings

James K. Stulman, Catherine Bigelow* and Susan Kahane**

Key Pearls

- A postural pulse increment of ≥30/min is the most predictive vital sign for detecting hypovolemia.
- The presence of apical-carotid delay is highly confirmatory in patients with suspected aortic stenosis. Increased murmur intensity with transient arterial occlusion confirms both mitral regurgitation and aortic insufficiency.
- The presence of a fluid wave and shifting dullness helps rule-in ascites.
- The abdominojugular reflex has a low sensitivity but high specificity for diagnosing congestive heart failure.
- The presence of dullness to percussion and decreased vocal tactile fremitus are useful in detecting the presence of a pleural effusion.

Introduction

This goal of this chapter is to identify components of the physical exam which are most useful for ruling-in and ruling-out specific medical conditions. We do not attempt a complete head-to-toe review but focus on

*Mount Sinai School of Medicine, New York, NY, USA.

abnormalities that are commonly found among hospitalized patients and areas where strong evidence is available. The discussion focuses on the accuracy of common physical maneuvers and how best to perform them.

The Clinical Exam as Diagnostic Test

Clinicians frequently discuss the sensitivity or specificity when describing the accuracy of a physical exam maneuver. These terms, however, apply only when we already know if the patient does or does not have the target disorder.

The mathematical expression, likelihood ratio, combines sensitivity and specificity into a single function and can be utilized in diagnostic reasoning before we know if the disorder is present or absent. The likelihood ratio for a positive test result (LR+) = sensitivity/ 1- specificity. Similarly, the likelihood ratio for a negative test result (LR-) = 1-sensitivity/specificity. We will use the likelihood ratio as an expression of the clinical utility of a physical exam maneuver.

Physical exam maneuvers associated with likelihood ratios of >5.0 or <0.2 are generally the most clinically useful.

Assessing Volume Status

Hypovolemia is defined as an abnormal decrease in blood volume. Physical exam findings may help detect and assess the degree of hypovolemia in patients with hemorrhage, GI fluid loss, diuresis, or dehydration. The clinical reference standard for detecting hypovolemia is a combination of laboratory findings (e.g. BUN/creatinine ratio, fractional excretion of sodium) and the response to hydration.

Acute Blood Loss

Hematocrit correlates poorly with degree of blood loss because a fall in hematocrit is often delayed 24–72 hours.

A postural pulse increment of ≥30/min or the inability of the patient to stand for vital signs because of dizziness are the most useful physical exam findings. After moderate blood loss (450–650 ml), only 20% of patients demonstrate these findings (sensitivity 20%; specificity 98%). Sensitivity increases to 97% after large blood loss (630–1150 mL). If a patient sits rather than stands from supine, the sensitivity of a 30/min pulse increment decreases significantly. Sensitivity may also be lower in elderly patients or those taking as medications such as beta-blockers.

Postural hypotension has little additional predictive value for moderate blood loss after excluding those unable to stand for vital signs (LR+ 1). Supine hypotension is a specific but insensitive measure of blood loss, as is supine tachycardia. Bradycardia occurs frequently after significant blood loss.

A complaint of postural dizziness, not severe enough to prevent standing, and accompanied by a pulse increment <30/min, has little predictive value.

Non-Blood Loss Causes of Hypovolemia

Severe postural dizziness or a 30/min postural pulse increase is predictive of non-blood loss causes of hypovolemia. A dry axilla has an LR+ of 8. A moist axilla decreases the probability of hypovolemia only slightly (LR– 0.6). Confusion, extremity weakness, non-fluent speech, dry mucous membranes, dry tongue, furrowed tongue, and sunken eyes are useful in combinations but the isolated presence of any has an LR+ near 1.

How to Perform Postural Vital Signs

Accuracy is the highest when vital signs are measured with patient supine and then standing. Wait 2 minutes before measuring supine vital signs and 1 minute before measuring standing vital signs. Accuracy is also increased by counting pulse for 30 seconds and doubling, compared with counting for 15 seconds.

Cardiac Murmurs

This section will focus on three common left-sided heart murmurs for which the physical exam has good evidence: the systolic murmurs of aortic stenosis (AS) and mitral regurgitation (MR) and the diastolic murmur of aortic insufficiency (AI).

Systolic Murmurs

The presence of a systolic murmur during cardiac auscultation can be classified as functional or pathologic (and related to underlying cardiac structural defects). Aortic stenosis and mitral regurgitation are the two most common pathologic reasons for systolic murmurs. Aortic stenosis affects up to 25% of the population over the age of 65. Significant mitral regurgitation affects up to 2% of the population. Other structural causes of systolic murmurs (such as hypertrophic cardiomyopathy, tricuspid regurgitation, or mitral valve prolapse) and non-structural causes (such as anemia, thyrotoxicosis, or sepsis) must also be considered in the patient with a systolic murmur.

Most of the studies evaluating the utility of the clinical exam for distinguishing systolic murmurs were performed by cardiologists. There is very little data on the accuracy and precision of non-cardiologists for evaluating cardiac murmurs. The following likelihood ratios reflect cardiologist examinations.

Aortic Stenosis

Historical findings in patients with aortic stenosis (AS) are often nonspecific — many patients are asymptomatic. Patients with more advanced disease, however, may have any of the triad of shortness of breath, angina or syncope in varying degrees. The presence of effort syncope (transient loss of consciousness during effort or exertion) is the only historical finding that is consistently associated with AS. In a patient with a systolic murmur, the LR+ of a history of effort syncope approaches infinity and therefore, is diagnostic for the presence aortic stenosis.

The most useful physical exam findings for detecting AS include:

- slow rise in carotid upstroke (LR+ 2.8–130)
- peak murmur intensity in late or midsystole (LR+ 8–101)
- reduced (or absent) S2 (LR+ 3.1–50)
- apical-carotid delay (LR+ ∞)
- brachioradial delay (LR+ 6.8)

Absence of a systolic murmur (LR – 0) or lack of radiation to the right carotid (LR – 0.05–0.10) significantly decrease the likelihood of AS. A multivariable decision rule incorporating these findings for suspected aortic stenosis has been described.[8]

How to Perform the Useful Physical Exam for Aortic Stenosis

Ausculatation: Area of maximal intensity is over the second right intercostal space. Listen for radiation to the right carotid and right clavicle.

Apical-Carotid Delay: Simultaneously palpate the precordial apex at the point of maximal impulse and the right carotid artery. Any palpable delay between the pulsation of the apex and the carotid is abnormal.

Brachioradial Delay: Simultaneously palpate the patient's right brachial artery with your right thumb and his right radial artery with your left index and middle finger. Use light pressure on the brachial artery — this avoids diminishing the waveform. Any palpable delay between the pulses of these two arteries is considered abnormal.

Mitral Regurgitation

Patients with chronic mitral regurgitation (MR) are often asymptomatic. Some may complain of symptoms consistent with congestive heart failure and these patients are very prone to volume overload. Acute MR will cause acute decompensated congestive heart failure and signs/symptoms of cardiogenic shock.

On physical exam, the presence of a murmur in the 5th intercostal space with radiation to the axilla slightly increases the likelihood of MR (LR+ 3.6–3.9). Absence of a murmur, however, more significantly rules out MR (LR– 0.12–0.34). Increased murmur intensity significantly correlates with severity of regurgitation (Murmur grades 4–5 LR+ 14, grade 3 LR+ 3.5). Increased murmur intensity with transient arterial occlusion helps to rule in MR (LR+ 7.5, LR– 0.28). Studies in non-cardiologists showed lower accuracy in diagnosing MR than studies performed with cardiologists.

How to Examine the Useful Physical Exam for Mitral Regurgitation

Auscultation: Location of maximal intensity is over the 5th or 6th intercostal space, mid left thorax with radiation to left axilla.

Transient Arterial Occlusion: Sphygmomanometers are placed on the patient's arms and inflated to 20–40 mmHg above the patient's current systolic blood pressure. The murmur is auscultated 20 seconds after cuff inflation and changes in murmur intensity are noted. The murmur of mitral regurgitation will intensify due to increased systemic arterial resistance and backflow across the valve. This maneuver will increase the intensity of other left-sided regurgitant murmurs as well. (See section on "Aortic Insufficiency.")

Diastolic Murmurs

Aortic Insufficiency

Aortic insufficiency, characterized by incompetence of the aortic valve leaflets or inability to approximate due to aortic root dilatation, is a valvular abnormality associated with a variety of serious underlying cardiac pathologies. Detection of aortic insufficiency from the history and physical exam can help clarify which patients require more definitive cardiac imaging, such as echocardiography or cardiac catheterization with angiography.

Patients with aortic regurgitation are often asymptomatic. The Framingham heart study detected a prevalence of some degree of aortic insufficiency in 13% of men and 8.5% of women in their cohort. Some patients may report a sensation of pounding in the chest or awareness of the heartbeat, especially when lying supine or on the left side. Others may describe atypical chest pain or palpitations.

There are a variety of eponymous physical exam findings described for aortic insufficiency along with the characteristic early diastolic decrescendo murmur best appreciated at the right upper sternal border. Many of the peripheral hemodynamic signs (such as de Musset's head bobbing, widened pulse pressure, and Duroziez's femoral murmur) have been evaluated but have little predictive value for diagnosing aortic insufficiency. Other signs have not been evaluated, such as Mueller's pulsatile uvula and Quincke's capillary pulsation.

The most useful physical exam findings are the typical early diastolic murmur of aortic insufficiency (LR+ 4–8.3; LR– 0.1–0.3), increased murmur intensity with transient arterial occlusion (LR+ 8.4; LR– 0.3), and the presence of an S3 on cardiac auscultation (LR+ 5.9).

How to Perform the Useful Physical Exam for Aortic Insufficiency

Auscultation: The murmur of AI will be best heard at the right upper sternal border or the lower left sternal border and may be accentuated by the patient leaning forward or lying in the left lateral decubitus position. Place the diaphragm of the stethoscope firmly on the chest wall to hear this high pitched, early-diastolic, decrescendo blowing murmur. S2 may be obscured.

Transient Arterial Occlusion: (See section on "Mitral Regurgitation"). The murmur of aortic insufficiency will intensify due to increased systemic arterial resistance and backflow across the aortic valve — inter-examiner.

Hepatomegaly

The reference standard for hepatomegaly, the enlargment of the liver beyond its normal size, is ultrasonography or nuclear scintigraphy. Although there is normal variation in liver size with gender and height, 95% of normal adult livers have a sonographic span at the mid-clavicular line of ≤12.5 cm. A span of more than 12 or 13 cm measured on physical exam increases the probability of hepatomegaly. Inaccuracies of the physical exam for measuring liver span include a tendency to underestimate span as well as interexaminer variability. Formulas have been developed which take into account gender, body weight and height in determining expected normal span but are cumbersome for the clinical setting.

Palpating a liver edge below the costal margin moderately increases the likelihood that the patient has hepatomegaly (LR+ 2.5); however, over half of palpable livers are not enlarged. Similarly, failure to identify a liver edge does reduce the probability of a hepatomegaly but does not rule it out (LR− 0.41). Palpation specifically to assess the quality of the liver edge is recommended only if there are other signs of liver disease.

How to Perform the Useful Physical Exam to Assess Hepatomegaly

Start with gentle pressure in the RLQ; have the patient breathe in gently to bring the liver edge down to the examining fingertips. At each exhalation, move the fingers up about 2 cm. If a lower edge is palpated, mark the lower edge at the mid-clavicular line (MCL). To measure the vertical span, percuss down from about the level of the 3rd rib at the MCL until the tone changes. To confirm increasing dullness, spread two or three fingers over the adjacent rib spaces and percuss quickly a number of times from greater to lesser resonance. If doubts persist, have the patient take a deeper breath and hold it; then percuss to confirm an unequivocal increase in resonance at that rib space. The upper and lower borders should be marked either in quiet respiration or the same phase of respiration.

In patients with an unpalpable liver edge, and a high probability of liver disease, span may be measured by percussion alone, although it is less accurate in detecting hepatomegaly than when a palpated lower edge can be used for the lower border. Attempt to locate the lower edge by gentle percussion in the RUQ at the MCL.

Ascites

Ascites, the presence of free fluid within the abdomen is easily detected when it is present in large volumes. When small amounts of fluid are present, the diagnosis is less certain. The reference standard for detecting ascites is paracentesis or fluid visualization with imaging studies. Ultrasonography is most commonly used and can detect as a little as 100 mL of abdominal fluid which is much smaller than can be detected by physical exam.

Patients with ascites may report increased abdominal girth, recent weight gain and ankle swelling. The patient's history is most useful when ruling out ascites. An absence of recent ankle swelling (LR– 0.10) or increased abdominal girth (LR– 0.17) are helpful findings.

Common physical exam findings include bulging flanks, flank dullness, shifting dullness, fluid wave and Puddle sign. The most useful physical exam findings are the presence of a fluid wave (LR+ 5.3) and shifting dullness (LR+ 2.1).

How to Perform the Useful Physical Exam to Assess for Ascites

Fluid wave: A second examiner (or the patient) places a hand, pressing firmly down on the midline of the abdomen. This pressure will stop the transmission of an impulse through adipose tissue. The examiner then taps one flank of the patient's abdomen while palpating for a transmitted fluid wave on the other flank.

Shifting dullness**:** Percuss the abdomen, marking the borders of tympany and dullness. Ask the patient to turn on one side. In the presence of ascites the border between tympany and dullness will rise.

Central Venous Pressure

Central venous pressure, the pressure of blood in the thoracic vena cavae, is useful in assessing intravascular volume status, ventricular function, and obstruction to right ventricular inflow or outflow. Bedside evaluation of jugular venous pressure can facilitate the estimation of CVP. CVP can be approximated as JVP measured from the sternal angle + 5 cm, as 5 cm is the estimated distance between the sternal angle and the zero point at the mid-right atrium.

This approach has been challenged because the distance between the sternal angle and mid-right atrium varies considerably. Another approach to CVP estimation is to look for venous pulsation above the clavicle in a seated patient. If any pulsation above the clavicle is seen, the CVP can be assumed to be elevated, since the clavicle is at least 10 cm above the mid-atrium.

Despite the variation in mid-right atrial location, bedside JVP measurement can help qualify CVP as low normal or high. A JVP ≥3 cm above the sternal angle, or a sustained increase in JVP of ≥4 cm with abdominal compression, suggests a 3–4-fold increase in the likelihood that the CVP is abnormally elevated. When JVP is 0–2 cm above the sternal angle, this does not help rule out high or low CVP.

Evaluation of JVP

The head is supported to relax the neck muscles; the trunk is inclined at an angle (35–45°) which brings the meniscus of the right internal jugular venous pulse above the clavicle but below the jaw. Patients with low CVP may need an angle of 0–30°. In patients with an elevated CVP, the angle may be > 45°; patients with severe congestion may have to stand and inspire to bring the meniscus down into view. A penlight directed away from examiners eyes is often helpful. JVP is the vertical distance measured from the sternal angle to the meniscus of the right internal jugular pulse.

Abdominojugular Reflux Test

The patient is instructed to relax and breathe normally through an open mouth (to avoid false-positive increase in JVP from Valsalva maneuver.)

Firm pressure is applied with the palm to the mid-abdomen for 15–30 seconds. Positive test occurs when abdominal compression causes a sustained increase in JVP ≥4 cm. The abdominojugular reflux test is not sensitive for diagnosing CHF but has a high specificity (LR+ 6.4).

Kussmaul Sign

The Kussmaul sign is the paradoxic increase in JVP during inspiration, and can be seen when the heart cannot accommodate the increased venous return during inspiration, such as in constrictive pericarditis or severe right-sided heart failure.

Pleural Effusion

Pleural effusion is common in patients presenting with respiratory complaints. The most common symptoms of pleural effusion, chest pain and dyspnea are however, nonspecific. The accuracy of specific physical exam maneuvers in detecting pleural effusion is an important consideration in determining which patients should receive confirmatory imaging studies.

A systematic review of studies compared eight physical exam maneuvers (conventional percussion, auscultory percussion, breath sounds, chest expansion, tactile vocal fremitus, vocal resonance, crackles, and pleural friction rub) with radiographic confirmation of pleural effusions. Dullness to conventional percussion (LR+ 8.7) and asymmetric chest expansion (LR+ 8.1) were the most accurate for diagnosing pleural effusion, while the absence of reduced tactile vocal fremitus made pleural effusion less likely (LR– 0.21). Absence of dullness to percussion cannot be used to rule out pleural effusion in patients with moderate or high pretest probability (LR– 0.31).

How to Perform the Useful Physical Exam

Conventional Percussion

The clinician should firmly place the second or third finger of the non-dominant hand horizontally between the ribs on the patient's posterior chest wall. The second or third finger of the dominant hand should be slightly flexed, and using the fingertip, the clinician should tap the distal interphalangeal joint of the firmly placed finger. Starting at the apices and progressing down to the bases, the left and right hemithoraces should be compared at equal horizontal planes.

Chest Expansion

Inspect the posterior chest for symmetric movement during inspiration. Place the hands firmly on the lateral aspect of the thorax to best visualize movement of the hemithoraces in relation to one another. As the patient breathes, the physician should watch for equal movements of his/her hands.

Tactile Fremitus

The patient is asked to repeat a phrase such as "ninety-nine" or "toy boat" while the examiner places the ulnar surface of the hand on the chest assessing vibrations. Vocal tactile fremitus can also be assessed by firmly placing the palmar aspect of the hands and fingertips on the patient's posterior chest. The intensity of the vibration over all lung fields should be noted. Decreased tactile fremitus is consistent with pleural effusion.

References

1. Simel D, Rennie D (eds). (2009) *The Rational Clinical Examination.* McGraw Hill, NY.
2. Bickley L, Szilagyi P (eds). (2003) Bate's Guide to Physical Examination, 8th ed. Lippincott Philadelphia.
3. Castell DO, O'Brien KD, Muench H, Chalmers TC. (1969) Estimate of liver size by percussion in normal individuals. *Ann Intern Med* **70**: 1183–1189.

4. Light RW, Lee YCG (eds.) (2003) *Textbook of Pleural Diseases*, 2nd ed. Oxford, England: Oxford University Press (Arnold Publication).
5. Meidl EJ, Ende J. (1993) Evaluation of liver size by physical examination. *J Gen Inter Med* **8**(11): 635–637, DOI: 10.1007/BF02599724.
6. Rolston D, Diaz-Guzman E, Budev MM. (2008) Accuracy of the physical examination in evaluating pleural effusion. *Cleve Clin J Med* **75**(4): 297–303.
7. Wong CL, Holroyd-Leduc J, Straus SE. (2009) Does this patient have a pleural effusion? *JAMA* **301**(3): 309–317.
8. Hoagland PM, Cook EF, Wynne J, Goldman L. (1986) Value of non-invasive testing in adults with suspected aortic stenosis. *AM J Med* **60**(4): 399–401.

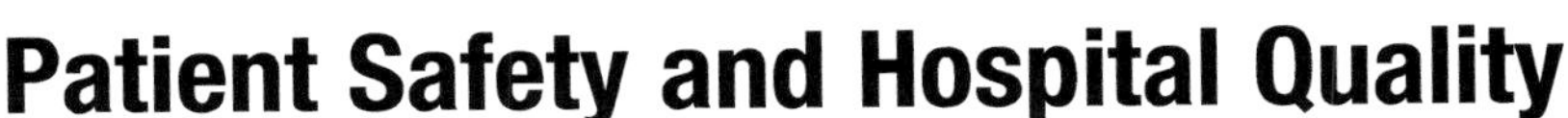
Patient Safety and Hospital Quality

Chapter 5

Doctor to Doctor Communication

*Brian A. Markoff**

Key Pearls

- The transition between the inpatient and outpatient venues puts patients at risk for adverse events.
- Communication between inpatient and outpatient physicians is poor despite the known risk of transition errors.
- Barriers to communication include lack of time, lack of perceived benefit, and inability to identify primary care physicians (PCPs).
- Key principles of communication include accountability, timeliness, inclusion of patient and family wishes, identification of and respect for the patient's medical home, and clear delineation of responsibility of care at each step of the care continuum.
- Hospitalists need to be diligent and creative to improve communication with PCPs.

Background

Transitions of care entail inherent risks and jeopardize patient outcomes. Poor transitions can affect patient safety, compliance with treatment, and outcomes. As more and more primary care physicians (PCP) rely on hospitalists to care for their patients when they are hospitalized, the need for excellent communication at times of transitions has never been more

*Mount Sinai School of Medicine, New York, NY, USA.

critical. Unfortunately, the known need for high-quality transitions has not improved communication between inpatient and outpatient providers.[1]

Multiple studies have shown that patients are at increased risk for adverse events in the immediate period after discharge from the hospital. One in five experiences an adverse event related to medical management.[2] In addition, 40% of patients have test results pending at the time of discharge, 9% of which require action by a provider; and 45% of outpatient physicians are not aware of these results.[3]

Medication discrepancies are common and lead to increased readmissions.[4] Overall, almost half of all patients experience an error in test follow-up, diagnostic workup, and medication continuity.[5] A study using patient interviews two weeks post-discharge found 42% of elderly patients had at least one problem during this time frame. The most common problem was with obtaining follow-up tests and follow-up appointments. Also common was difficulty obtaining medications and treatments. Many patients also felt ill-prepared for discharge. In the same study, patients whose primary physicians were unaware of their hospitalization, were two times more likely to report post-discharge issues.[6]

Communication Standards

The discharge summary is one standard way for inpatient and outpatient providers to communicate. However, numerous studies have shown that these summaries are less then ideal, either because of a lack of timeliness or a lack of key information.[1] Chapter 10 discusses the essential elements of discharge summaries in detail.

Communication directly from inpatient to outpatient physician may ameliorate much of the risk during the transition period. However, direct communication is poor, with only 23% of PCPs receiving any direct communication from an inpatient physician during a given hospitalization,[7] and 20% or less being notified about discharges.[8] These studies and many others suggest that poor communication between inpatient and outpatient physicians is the standard of care for many patients.

Why are inpatient physicians so poor at communication with outpatient physicians? Three barriers have been identified — perceived lack of benefit, lack of time, and inability to identify who to contact.[9] A lack of understanding of the importance of transitions in patient care is a significant barrier, as physicians will not invest the time and effort to ensure satisfactory communication when they are unconvinced or unaware of the benefit to their patents. Technology has the potential to improve communication through the use of electronic health records, email, text messaging, facsimiles, and cell phones. Though none of these methods will alter the lack of importance many hospital physicians place on communication with the outpatient provider, they may change behavior by making communication easier and more seamlessly integrated into the workflow.

In light of the above realities, six national physician groups came together for the Transitions of Care Consensus Conference (TOCCC). The TOCCC led to a consensus statement on how to improve communication across the continuum of care.[10] The basic principles highlighted include:

- Accountability
- Communication
- Timeliness
- Inclusion of patient and family
- Identification of and respect for the patient's medical home
- Clear delineation of responsibility of care at each step of the care continuum

The statement sets standards for multiple aspects of transitions of care (see Table 1).

Studies have shown that improving the quality of transitions can improve outcomes, though these studies typically involved comprehensive interventions utilizing multifaceted transition teams.[11] A structured discharge toolkit was also shown to decrease emergency department visits and 30-day readmissions in elderly patients.[13] To date, there is limited data on whether simple, direct physician to physician communication alone can improve outcomes. Bell *et al.* looked at a composite outcome of 30-day

Table 1. Standards for Safe Transitions form the Transitions of Care Consensus Conference

Standard	Key Elements
Care Plans/Transition Record Data	• Principle diagnosis/Problem list • Medication list • Medical home with contact information • Cognitive status • Test results/pending results
Communication Infrastructure	• Secure/HIPPA compliant • Two way with opportunity for clarification/ feedback • Include core dataset • Updateable database • Available prior to arrival • Medication list for patients
Standard Communication Formats	• Standard data transfer forms • Medical history accessible and modifiable • Patient/family accessible • Include patients' preferences, goals, and values (code status, etc.)
Transition Responsibility	• Sending provider/institution responsible until transfer of responsibility is confirmed • Sending provider available for clarification • Patient should be able to identify responsible provider • Hospital provider will not be required to assume responsibility after discharge for patients without a medical home
Timeliness	• Timeliness of information contingent on setting, circumstances, acuity, and responsibility • Information available at time of patient encounter
Community Standards	• Medical communities/institutions must be accountable for the quality of transitions
Measurement	• Standardized metrics should be monitored • Continuing transitions improvement based on metrics

mortality, readmission rate, and emergency department use and tried to correlate these with inpatient to primary care physician communication. In their study, 77% of PCPs were aware of the index admission but only 23% had direct communication with the medicine service. Only 42% of PCPs received a discharge summary within two weeks of discharge. The composite outcome was similar in both groups (22% when the PCP was aware of the hospitalization and 20% when unaware).[7] This suggests that the quality of communication may be a more important factor than simply whether communication took place.

Systematic Approaches

Innovative and aggressive approaches to facilitate and foster communication are needed. Audits, feedback, and incentives for timely and complete discharge summaries can be implemented. Documentation of communication with PCPs may also be beneficial. Periodic surveys of outpatient physicians on the communication practices of individual hospitalists and the hospitalist group as a whole can be done and physicians made aware of their own performance relative to the group. Another approach is to use administrative staff as physician liaisons, which may include sending outpatient physicians the name and contact information of the treating hospitalist or alternatively, providing the hospitalist with contact information for the outpatient physician. Improving direct availability and access to inpatient physicians by PCPs, such as via Internet access and dissemination of cell phone numbers, can be helpful. Maximizing the use of electronic communication and electronic medical records to facilitate communication across venues is needed. Lastly, emphasizing the benefit and added value of direct communication to all physicians is essential.

Conclusions

The growing use of hospitalists is one cause of the discontinuity in patient care. Though current systems make communication difficult, the burden is on hospitalists to ensure communication is suitable at all transition points.

Hospitalist groups should seek out ways to facilitate quality communication for every patient, including enhanced use of advanced electronic solutions and producing a culture that recognizes the value of a simple telephone call.

References

1. Kripalani S, LeFevre F, Phillips CO, *et al*. (2007) Deficits in communication and information transfer between hospital-based and primary care physicians. *JAMA* **297**: 831–841.
2. Forster AJ, Murff HJ, Peterson JF, *et al*. (2003) The incidence and severity of adverse events affecting patients after discharge from the hospital. *Ann Intern Med* **138**: 161–167.
3. Roy CL, Poon EG, Karson AS, *et al*. (2005) Improving patient care: patient safety concerns arising from test results that return after hospital discharge. *Ann Intern Med* **143**: 121–128.
4. Coleman EA, Smith JD, Raha D, Min SJ. (2005) Posthospital medication discrepancies: Prevalence and contributing factors. *Arch Intern Med* **165**: 1842–1847.
5. Moore C, Wisnivesky J, Williams S, McGinn T. (2003) Medical errors related to discontinuity of care from an inpatient to an outpatient setting. *J Gen Intern Med* **18**: 646–651.
6. Arora VM, Prochaska ML, Farnan JM, *et al*. (2010) Problems after discharge and understanding of communication with their primary care physicians among hospitalized seniors: a mixed methods study. *J Hosp Med* **5**: 385–391.
7. Bell CM, Schnipper JL, Auerbach AD, *et al*. (2009) Association of communication between hospital-based physicians and primary care providers with patient outcomes. *J Gen Intern Med* **24**: 381–386.
8. Pantilat SZ, Lindenauer PK, Katz PP, Wachter RM. (2001) Primary care physician attitudes regarding communication with hospitalists. *Am J Med* **111**: 15S–20S.
9. Roy CL, Kachalia A, Woolf S, *et al*. (2009) Hospital readmissions: Physician awareness and communication practices. *J Gen Intern Med* **24**: 374–380.

10. Snow V, Beck D, Budnitz T, *et al.* (2009) Transitions of Care Consensus Policy Statement American College of Physicians–Society of General Internal Medicine-Society of Hospital Medicine-American Geriatrics Society–American College of Emergency Physicians-Society of Academic Emergency Medicine. *J Gen Intern Med* **24**: 971–976.
11. Coleman EA, Parry C, Chalmers S, Min SJ. (2006) The care transitions intervention: Results of a randomized controlled trial. *Arch Intern Med* **166**: 1822–1828.
12. Jack BW, Chetty VK, Anthony D, *et al.* (2009) A reengineered hospital discharge program to decrease rehospitalization: A randomized trial. *Ann Intern Med* **150**: 178–187.
13. Dedhia P, Kravet S, Bulger J, *et al.* (2009) A quality improvement intervention to facilitate the transition of older adults from three hospitals back to their homes. *J Am Geriatr Soc* **57**: 1540–1546.

Chapter 6

Approach to the Analysis of Medical Errors

*Erin DuPree**

Key Pearls

- A just culture is critical to developing an organization that relies on front line workers (nurses and physicians) to report errors.
- The Swiss cheese model illustrates how a series of weaknesses in organizational defenses leads to adverse outcomes.
- Root cause analysis is a performance improvement tool that can be used to systematically look at organizational weaknesses that contribute to an adverse outcome.
- Patient disclosure is an important aspect of medical errors that requires planning and effective communication skills.

In the 21st century, healthcare is a complex endeavor. The processes of healthcare can and should be designed to anticipate and mitigate human errors, and ensure that they occur in the way they are intended. In 2000, The Institute of Medicine report "To Err Is Human," asserted that the problem with medical errors is not bad people in healthcare — it is that good people are working in bad systems that need to be made safer. The report

*Mount Sinai Medical Center, New York, NY, USA.

concluded that 44,000–98,000 people die from medical errors in inpatient settings each year.[1]

Dr. James Reason, a Professor of Psychology who has published extensively on the nature of human error, describes error as *circumstances in which planned actions fail to achieve the desired outcome.*[2] Providing healthcare will always involve humans in the decision-making and care delivery, yet as humans, we will make errors. Systems must be created to prevent or catch the inevitable human errors before they result in harm.

There is no universally agreed upon definition of error and thus there are many ways in which errors may be classified. Rasmussen defines levels of human performance,[3] which Reason used to develop an intentional taxonomy for errors.[2] This approach looks at the underlying psychology leading to the error by asking,

1. " Was there a prior intention to act?"
2. If intended, did the actions go as planned? If the actions did not go as intended, then these are **slips** or **skill-based errors.** Slips tend to occur in automatic skill-based activities like grabbing ointment instead of toothpaste when one intends to brush his teeth. In healthcare, an example is an experienced nurse administering the wrong medication by picking up the wrong syringe.
3. Were the actions intended and did they achieve the desired outcome? If not, then this is a failure in planning. This is a more complex error than making slips. These are **mistakes** and are either **rule- or knowledge-based**. Rules are attained through training and experience and lead to expertise. A rule-based activity would be following a treatment protocol. If a person is time-constrained and working in the service of production, the person may simply forget a step. This is a lapse, or a rule-based error, which is typically not visible. Knowledge-based mistakes occur when clinicians encounter a new situation and have to think on their feet. This requires laborious conscious effort and is highly error prone and subject to biases. These turn up in complex processes, such as prescribing the wrong medication because of inadequate knowledge about the drug of choice and are also seen in diagnostic errors.

Errors can also be classified in other ways, such as through the actions (e.g. omissions); the task at hand (e.g. surgery); context (e.g. fatigue, distraction); and outcomes (e.g. near-misses, risky behaviors, incidents, accidents).

Accountability

A **just culture**, a key component of a safety culture, has fairness as the backbone for understanding errors, with a balance between individual accountability and systems thinking.[4] The *person model* is based on the assumption that the person who makes an error has certain characteristics under his or her control and therefore is to blame for the errors made. From this perspective, error reduction is focused on "doing better," retraining, discipline, and suspension. The legal perspective on error and medical negligence are built on personal responsibility. This is a narrow view that does not incorporate the vast systems in which healthcare workers perform. The *systems model* looks at the interplay between individuals and systems when analyzing errors and human behavior.[5] Errors in this light are not as much individual fallibility as they are consequences of the working environment. The United Kingdom Decision Error Tree is a useful tool for assessing individual accountability when analyzing errors in an incident (see Fig. 1).[6]

1. Was there malicious intent? Did the individual intentionally cause harm?
2. Was the person knowingly impaired?
3. Were safe operating procedures knowingly violated?
4. Did the individual make a mistake someone of similar training and experience would make?
5. Is there a history of unsafe acts with this individual?

Fig. 1. Error accountability questions. (Adapted from *Reason J*, 1997.[6])

Causal Factors of Error (Swiss cheese model)

James Reason distinguishes **active failures** which are errors and violations by people at the front lines and **latent conditions** which are the organizational processes that are hidden and become obvious only when they combine with other failures to breach the defenses that typically prevent an adverse event. He developed the "Swiss cheese model" to illustrate how organizational accidents are a compilation of multiple, smaller failures leading up to the actual event (see Fig. 2).[2,5] Each slice of Swiss cheese represents a defense, or barrier, against a particular hazard in the system. The defenses in healthcare can include effective hiring protocols, training, adequate supervision, communication, equipment maintenance, staffing ratios and proper working environments. When there are weaknesses in a defense, such as inadequate supervision of trainees, then that failure can line up with other weaknesses and active failures at the front lines to lead to an adverse event. Organizations need to be able to identify the "holes" or weaknesses in accident investigations (e.g. root cause analyses) or ideally, before such incidents occur.

Reporting

Safety reporting systems in healthcare are based on systems in other industries such as aviation, and is often referred to as incident reporting.

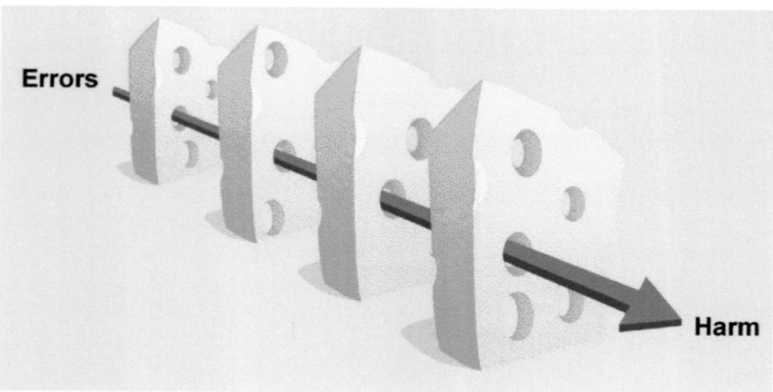

Fig. 2. Swiss cheese model: How defenses, barriers and safeguards may be penetrated by an accident trajectory. (Adapted from *Reason J*, 2000.[5])

Anything that worries frontline healthcare workers about the care provided should be reported. Near miss reporting gives warnings of potential catastrophes and enables a preventative approach. The key components of an effective event reporting system include:

- A supportive environment for reporting that protects the privacy of staff who reports.
- The ability to report by a broad range of personnel.
- Summaries that are dispersed in a timely manner.
- A structured mechanism to review reports and develop action plans.

Reporting systems do not have to be limited to a single organization; for instance, the United Kingdom's National Patient Safety Agency and the MEDMARX system in the US maintain national reporting systems.

Event reports are a passive form of surveillance for unsafe conditions, in contrast to active methods such as direct observation, and typically only capture a small percentage of events. Event reporting systems are underutilized by providers due to concerns about their own performance reports, lack of feedback, time involved in submitting a report, and lack of understanding about what to report.[7] Therefore, event reports typically provide only a snapshot of organizational vulnerabilities. It is important for an organization to have an infrastructure in place to deal with the analysis and follow up of events rather than encouraging reporting for its own sake.

Root Cause Analysis

Root cause analysis (RCA) is an invaluable and powerful performance improvement tool to evaluate the underlying causes in adverse events and prevent future harm by eliminating latent errors. It is typically conducted reactively, in response to an adverse event. It identifies changes that could be made in organizational systems and processes through redesign in order to improve the reliability of the process, for achieving the intended result.[8] The product of a root causes analysis is an improvement plan that identifies risk reduction strategies along with plans for measuring the effectiveness of those strategies.

To conduct a root causes analysis, a team must be organized that includes:

- Front line staff familiar with the processes.
- Subject matter experts.
- Representatives from departments under review.
- Organizational leaders.
- Others familiar with the RCA process.

The team defines what happened by creating a detailed timeline. The next step is to identify how the event occurred (through identification of active errors at the front line) and then why it occurred (through systematic identification and analysis of latent errors). The team can use brainstorming; cause-and-effect diagrams (see "Process Improvement" chapter for more details); and literature review to determine why the event occurred. This requires repeatedly digging deeper by asking " why?" and when answered, asking "why?" again.

The root causes of the event are identified and a *corrective action plan* is developed to reduce the risk of the event occurring again. Quick fix interim changes are put in place to protect patients. The corrective action plan must identify the strategies that an organization intends to implement to reduce the risk of recurrence and the measurement that will be undertaken to assess the effectiveness of those strategies. People closely involved in the processes should participate in developing the improvement strategies to ensure that the plan is realistic and possible to implement. Oversight and responsibility for implementation and monitoring of each specific improvement item should be assigned to an individual. If incorporating system-wide changes, pilot-testing the changes prior to widespread implementation are advisable. Report the results of implementation and monitoring to institutional quality committees and ultimately to the governing board of the hospital.

Disclosure

Patient disclosure is important in the medical error process as patients have specific information needs after an adverse event, including:

- Acknowledgement
- Information about why it happened
- How it will be prevented
- An apology

Since 2001, The Joint Commission patient safety standards require the disclosure of certain "unanticipated outcomes of care." Healthcare professionals worry about the risks of disclosure, including litigation. A clinician's disclosure of an error may be admissible in a malpractice lawsuit. In 2008, only eight US states explicitly prohibited "admissions of fault" from being used as evidence at trial, although the majority of states exclude "expressions of sympathy" from being used as evidence.[9]

Effective disclosure can be facilitated by planning ahead (review the record, determine who will speak with the patient/family, be mindful of cultural and language differences); factual documentation of the conversation in the medical record; arranging for next steps (e.g. future discussions as necessary); and understanding what to expect from patients and families (the need to express their feelings and strong emotions). When disclosing, defend the actions of the staff and institution when care was reasonable and appropriate, and accept responsibility on behalf of the institution when the hospital was clearly at fault. It is important to do so after discussion with risk management personnel. Explain clearly the known facts in layperson's language and invite questions and participation. The patient's reaction will often depend on how the information is disclosed. Effective disclosure communication can lead to improved patient outcomes and ultimately improved patient satisfaction which in some cases can reduce the cost associated with medical malpractice claims.

References

1. Kohn LT, Corrigan JM, Donaldson MS (Institute of Medicine). (2005) *To Err is Human: Building a Safer Health System.* National Academy Press, Washington, DC.
2. Reason J. (1990) *Human error.* Cambridge University Press, New York.
3. Rasmussen J. (1983) Skill, rules and knowledge; signals, signs, and symbols and other distinctions in human performance models. *IEEE Trans Syst Man Cyberneti* **13**(3): 257–266.
4. Marx D. (1999) *Maintenance Error Causation.* Federal Aviation Authority Office of Aviation Medicine, Washington, DC.
5. Reason J. (2002) Human error: Models and management. *BMJ.* **320**: 768–770.
6. Reason J. (1997) *Managing the Risk of Organizational Accidents.* Ashgate, Aldershot, Hampshire, England.
7. Evans SM, Berry JG, *et al.* (2006) Attitudes and barriers to incident reporting: A collaborative hospital study. *Qual Saf Health Care* **15**: 39–43
8. The Joint Commission Sentinel Event Policy and Procedures (updated July 2007). Available at http://www.jointcommission.org/NR/rdonlyres/F84F9DC6-A5DA-490F-A91F-A9FCE26347C4/0/SE_chapter_july07.pdf
9. Agency for Healthcare Research and Quality (AHRQ). Accessed at: http://psnet.ahrq.gov/primer.aspx?primerID=2.

Chapter 7

Process Improvement Tools

*Ira S. Nash**

Key Pearls

- Measuring the quality of care is a necessary prerequisite for improving it.
- Quality can be assessed by evaluating structure, process and outcome.
- Improving outcomes requires changing processes.
- Successful process improvement requires a methodical data-driven approach.
- Process maps, Pareto charts, and fishbone diagrams are specific tools that facilitate understanding of processes.

Introduction

One of the most important developments in medicine over the last decade has been the emergence of the "quality movement" — the focus on assessing and improving the quality of healthcare. The 2000 publication of the Institute of Medicine report, *To Err is Human*,[1] exposed the quality deficiencies in medical care in the United States, and transformed the understanding of the public and medical professionals alike. The follow-up report, *Crossing the Quality Chasm*,[2] laid out a path for fixing these deficiencies. This chapter reviews methods and tools for making progress along that path.

*Mount Sinai Medical Center, New York, NY, USA.

Quality

Evaluating the quality of care is a necessary prerequisite for improving it. In earlier eras, when medicine had few effective treatments to offer, evaluating the quality of care was most often a subjective assessment of the strength of the doctor-patient relationship. In the context of the contemporary armamentarium, evaluating the quality of care should assess objectively the extent to which appropriate diagnostic and therapeutic interventions are used to advance the health of individuals and populations, or "increase the likelihood of desired health outcomes."[3]

Donabedian[4] pointed out that one could assess three different aspects of quality:

- Structure — the environment in which care is delivered.
- Process — the steps taken in the delivery of care.
- Outcome — the impact of care on patients.

While it is important to assess outcomes — since the ultimate goal of care is to have a positive impact on patients — efforts at improving those outcomes necessarily involve making changes to structure and process. For example, it is important to track the mortality of patients admitted with acute myocardial infarction (AMI) (now publicly reported by the Center for Medicare and Medicaid Services for all acute care hospitals), but lowering mortality requires examining and improving how care for AMI patients is delivered. Successful process improvement involves the systematic selection of the right questions and the application of effective techniques for improving performance.

Choosing Performance Improvement Targets

Choosing which elements of care to address is a critical first step in effective performance improvement. The focus should be on elements:

- That can be measured (and, preferably, measured without expending considerable resources).
- That are under the control of the organization.

- On which the institution currently performs poorly.
- That have a clear causal relationship with the outcome of interest.

For many contemporary performance improvement efforts, the selection of performance improvement targets is driven by external organizations, such as the Joint Commission or The Center for Medicare and Medicaid Services (CMS) in the United States. These agencies have established "core measures" of hospital performance,[5] which are process measures chosen based on criteria similar to those stated. These process measures are also used in public report cards on hospital performance, and as elements of "pay for performance" formulas, which link hospital payment to quality measures — two strong reasons why they have become the central focus for many institutional quality improvement efforts. Indeed, there is concern that so much attention has been paid to these measures that may be driving out other valuable efforts aimed at improving patient care.[6]

For many important areas of care, there are no clearly prescribed processes to address, or the stated process is itself too complex to tackle directly. For example, the drive for quality improvement may start with an observation about poor performance on an outcome, such as higher than expected mortality for a particular procedure or diagnosis, or the recognition that an important process, such as the assignment of inpatient care teams to patients admitted from the emergency department, does not work as well as it should. What next?

Do Your Homework — Gather Baseline Data

The first step should be to verify the impression that performance is not what it should or could be. Gather preliminary data. Try to define best practice through the use of public reports on hospital performance, published scholarly work, contacts at other institutions, or the use of comparative data from hospital cooperatives to which your institution may belong, such as the University HealthSystem Consortium (UHC)[7] or the Association of American Medical Colleges (AAMC).[8] This may also require reviewing clinical records to verify that data generated from administrative (e.g. billing) systems, which are generally most readily available and often the source of the initial observation or concern, reflect the actual care and outcomes.

Form the Right Team

Successful process improvement, especially in complex organizations such as hospitals, is always a "team sport." Administrators control resources, but lack clinical expertise; front line clerical staff understand many processes at "the ground level," but may lack perspective on how their work impacts other areas of the institution; physicians have the most sophisticated medical knowledge, but often lack understanding of nursing workflows; nurses understand how care is delivered at the bedside, but are not necessarily clinical content experts. Pulling together the right combination of participants is the next step in successful process improvement. Seek a balance of individuals — clinical experts as well as experts on the current practice. Whenever possible, engage the physician and nursing leadership in the unit or department where the care is provided, so that solutions and improvements come "from within" and are therefore more likely to be embraced than those designed and "imposed" by outsiders. Although it may seem obvious to recruit participants who are enthusiastic and invested in improving the status quo, this important consideration is often overlooked.

Define Goals

Specify the level of performance you hope to achieve. Sometimes a particular level of future performance will be demanded by others, such as the Board of Trustees or senior institutional leadership. Very often, however, it will be up to those engaged in a project to define "success." Avoid the temptation to leave the goal vague, such as "improved patient satisfaction" or "lower rates of central line associated bacteremia." Directional change does not motivate participants as much as hitting a target does, and only a specified endpoint allows progress to be tracked in a meaningful way. When the ultimate goal may be quite distant, or even perhaps unattainable with the best medical practice (e.g. "*no* central line infections"), it is important to specify intermediate levels of improvement (e.g. "a 50% decline in central line infections by the second quarter of next year"), or the achievement of rates comparable with the best reported (e.g. "lowest decile of infection rates in the state").

Break Down the Problem — Process Maps

Improving a complex process or a specific clinical outcome ultimately comes down to changing one or more specific steps in care. A very useful tool for determining what those steps are is a flow chart or process map. A process map has directionality (a beginning and an end) and is a graphic representation of the specific actions and decisions that are embedded in a larger process (Fig. 1). The typical convention uses rectangles for actions and diamonds for branch points. Breaking down a complex process this way allows team members to come to a consensus on how a particular process is currently working, helps point out complexity and redundancy that can often be eliminated, and allows for the selection of specific points in the process to collect data and target interventions.

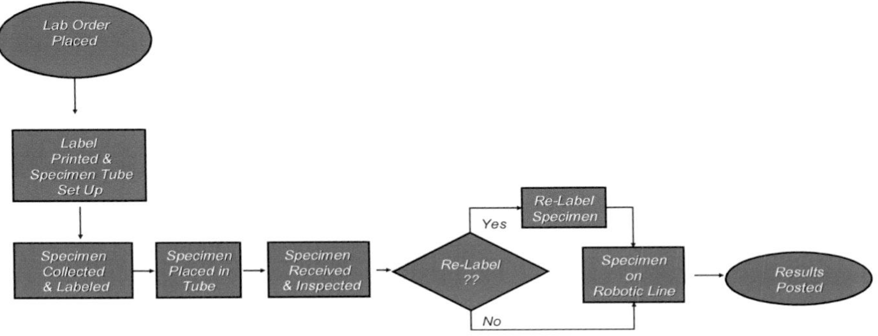

Fig. 1. An example of a process map for ordering lab tests and reporting on the results.

Collect Data

Once the process map is established, collect data about the specific steps that your group believes may be most problematic, based on familiarity with the current state. Note that the data you collect may prove your beliefs wrong. For instance, suppose that you were trying to reduce lab turnaround time, and had created the process map in Fig. 1. You would then select steps, such as "specimen collected," "specimen labeled" and "specimen placed on robotic line" to see which of these steps (or others) is contributing the most to the overall delay in getting from the beginning of the process to the end. A powerful graphical tool for assisting with this is a Pareto chart (Fig. 2). A Pareto chart is created by plotting, in rank order, the contributions of each step in a process (typically as vertical bars), and then displaying the cumulative total contribution (as a line) on the same axes. The simple "80/20" rule often becomes apparent — 80% of the problem (e.g. the accumulated turnaround time) is attributable to 20% of the steps in the process. This,

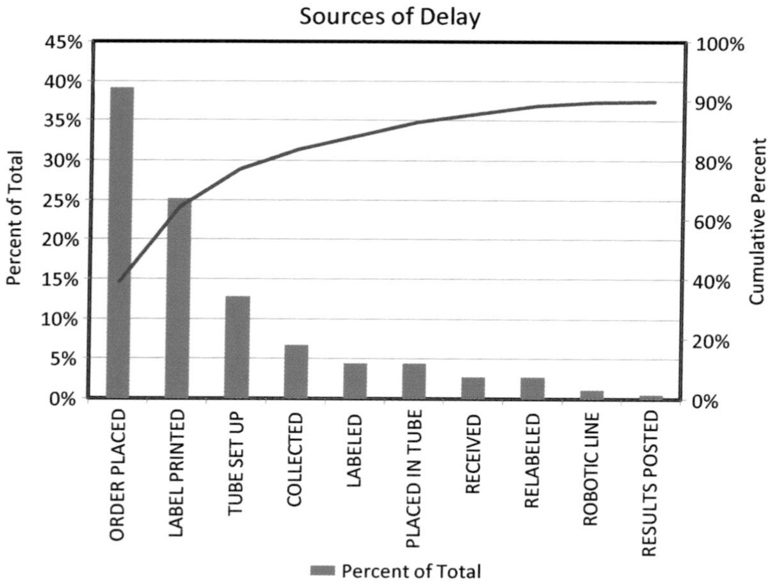

Fig. 2. Pareto Chart.

in turn, will allow you to prioritize your efforts, by focusing on those specific steps.

Analyze the Findings

Once a specific step is targeted for improvement, it is important to understand why it is not working as expected. A "fishbone" diagram, also called an Ishikawa or cause-and-effect diagram can be used for this purpose (Fig. 3). Major categories of potentially contributing factors are identified with successive "layers" of causes for each one. In this example, the factors contributing to delays in admitting a patient to the medical intensive care unit are detailed. This allows for a deeper understanding of the problem.

Implement Change

Ultimately, something must be done differently in order to create the new, desired outcome. It can often be difficult to select which step to change, or what change to implement. One way to organize your team's approach is to make a simple 2 × 2 table and segregate possible interventions into the four quadrants, defined by whether the intervention/change is

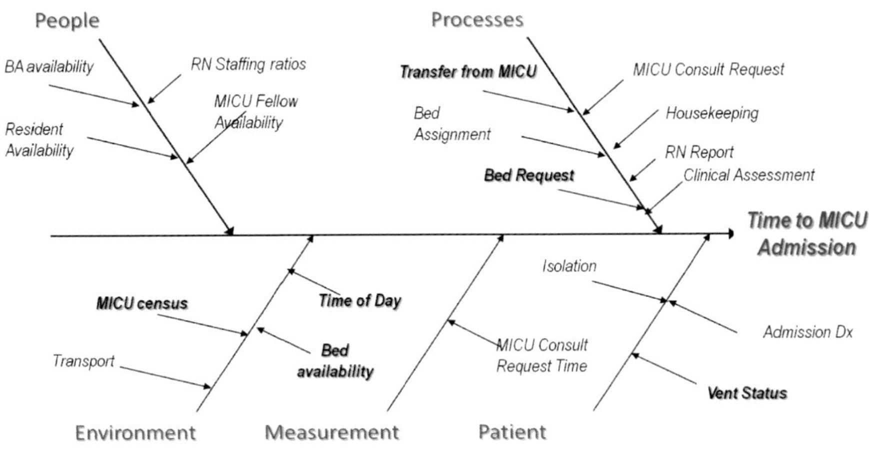

Fig. 3. Fishbone Diagram.

hard or easy (based on required resources and training, or on the anticipated resistance or consequences for other activities) and whether is it likely to have a large or small impact. Clearly, those changes that can have the biggest potential positive impact at the lowest anticipated cost (in resources and effort) ought to be tried first. This is often referred to as "picking the low hanging fruit."

Measure, Track and Repeat

The final step in any successful quality improvement effort is to measure the impact of the intervention and track it over time. A graph of the value of key measures over time ("run charts") is a useful tool; one can plot either the overall outcome that sparked the improvement project (e.g. AMI mortality) or the specific process that was changed. These charts should be updated frequently so that positive trends can be celebrated, and deteriorating performance can be addressed. Ideally, the measurements made to track the impact of an intervention should serve as the baseline for further interventions, following the same steps outlined above, so that performance can be continuously improved. A "control chart" is a specific form of a run chart, which includes the upper and lower bounds of expected performance, and allows one to assess whether the process being assessed is functioning as expected.

Summary

High quality healthcare improves patients' outcomes. A methodical, data-driven approach to process improvement is the best way to achieve it.

References

1. Kohn LT, Corrigan JM, Donaldson MS (Institute of Medicine). (2000) *To Err is Human: Building a Safer Health System.* National Academy Press, Washington, DC.

2. Committee on Quality of Health Care in America (Institute of Medicine). (2001) *Crossing the Quality Chasm: A New Health System for the 21st Century*. National Academy Press, Washington, DC.
3. Institute of Medicine. (1990) *Medicare: A Strategy for Quality Assurance*. National Academy Press, Washington, DC.
4. Donabedian A. (1988) The quality of care: How can it be assessed? *JAMA* **260**: 1743–1748.
5. Chassin M, Loeb JM, Schmaltz SP, Wachter RM. (2010) Accountability measures — Using measurement to promote quality improvement. *N Engl J Med* **363**(7): 683–688.
6. Bardach NS, Cabana. (2009) The unintended consequences of quality improvement. *Curr Opin Pediatr* **21**(6): 777–782.
7. http://www.uhc.edu
8. http://www.aamc.org

Chapter 8

Teamwork in Hospital Medicine

Kevin J. O'Leary and Niraj L. Sehgal†*

Key Pearls

- Teamwork and communication failures are a known threat to patient safety.
- Challenges include large teams with membership that is dynamic and often dispersed.
- Measurement of teamwork is essential to understand baseline performance, evaluate the effectiveness of interventions, and demonstrate the utility of resources invested.
- Successful interventions include formal teamwork training, daily goals of care forms, interdisciplinary rounds, and nurse-physician unit co-leadership.
- The optimal approach is implementation of one or more interventions with adaptations to fit unique clinical settings and local culture.

Background and Essential Elements of Teamwork

Teamwork and communication failures are a known threat to patient safety and cited by the Joint Commission as the most frequent root cause

*Northwestern University Feinberg School of Medicine, Chicago, IL, USA.
†University of California, San Francisco, CA, USA.

in reported sentinel events.[1–3] Contributing factors include a failure to acknowledge human fallibility, communication barriers across hierarchies and disciplines, and an increasingly complex hospital environment. Within inpatient medical settings, nurses and physicians often differ in their ratings of collaboration, and these discrepancies further highlight opportunities for improving teamwork.[4]

A team is defined as two or more individuals with specified roles interacting adaptively, interdependently, and dynamically toward a shared and common goal.[5] Elements of effective teamwork have been identified through research conducted in aviation, the military, and more recently, healthcare. Salas and colleagues have synthesized this research into five core components: team leadership, mutual performance monitoring, backup behavior, adaptability, and team orientation (see Table 1).[5]

Table 1. Core Components and Coordinating Mechanisms of Teamwork*

Teamwork	Definition	Behavioral Examples
Team leadership	Direction and coordination of team members activities	• Facilitate team problem solving • Provide performance expectations • Clarify team member roles • Assist in conflict resolution
Mutual performance monitoring	Team members are able to monitor one another's performance	• Identify mistakes and lapses in other team member actions • Provide feedback to fellow team members to facilitate self-correction
Backup behavior	Team members anticipate and respond to one another's needs	• Recognition of workload distribution problem • Shift work responsibilities to underutilized members
Adaptability	The team adjusts strategies based on new information	• Identify cues that changes have occurred and develop plan to deal with changes • Remain vigilant to changes in internal and external environment

(*Continued*)

Table 1. *(Continued)*

Teamwork	Definition	Behavioral Examples
Team orientation	Team goals are prioritized above individual goals	• Take into account alternate solutions by teammates • Increase task involvement, information sharing, and participatory goal setting
Shared mental model	An organizing knowledge of the task of the team and how members will interact to achieve their goal	• Anticipating and predicting one another's needs • Identify changes in team, task, or teammates
Closed-loop communication	Acknowledgement and confirmation of information received	• Following up with team members to ensure message received • Acknowledging that message was received • Clarifying information received
Mutual trust	Shared belief that team members will perform their roles	• Information sharing • Willingness to admit mistakes and accept feedback

*Adapted from Salas *et al.*[38]

Additionally, three supporting and coordinating mechanisms are essential for effective teamwork: A shared mental model, closed-loop communication, and mutual trust (see Table 1).[5] Successful teams use these elements to develop a culture for "speaking up" and *situational awareness* among team members. Situational awareness refers to a person's perception and understanding of their dynamic environment. Human errors often result from a lack of such awareness.[6]

Challenges to Improving Teamwork

There are several important barriers to effective teamwork and communication in the hospital setting. Teams are large, formed in an ad hoc fashion, and membership is dynamic and often dispersed. Team members in their respective disciplines care for multiple patients at the same time and usually work in shifts, or rotations, resulting in team membership variability (few patients will have identical team membership) and instability (each team has members joining and departing from the team). Furthermore, while nurses and other hospital staff usually work on specific patient care units, physicians often care for patients on multiple units and floors. Research has shown that nurses and physicians do not communicate consistently and often disagree on the plan of care for their patients.[7] When communication does occur, clinicians may overestimate how well their messages are understood by other team members, reflecting a phenomenon well-known in communication psychology related to egocentric thought processes.[8,9] Ineffective communication and incomplete understanding of patients' care creates and reinforces a culture of low expectations and an environment unable to prevent and/or intercept medical errors before they reach the patient.

Technology may serve as an additional barrier to effective communication despite the common notion that it serves to do the opposite. With increasing use of electronic health records and the exchange of text-messages delivered via pager or email, we move to asynchronous modes of communication which lack important face-to-face communication elements (tone of voice, expression, gesture, eye contact).[10,11]

Assessment of Teamwork

Another major challenge in improving teamwork is the difficulty in measuring it. Assessment of teamwork entails measurement of knowledge, skills and attitudes of teams composed of multiple individuals. Approaches to evaluate interventions to improve teamwork include:

- self-assessment
- peer assessment
- direct observation
- survey of teamwork climate or culture
- measurement of clinical outcomes

While self-report tools are easy to administer and can capture affective components influencing team performance, they may not reflect actual skills or team performance. Peer assessment includes the use of 360-degree evaluations or multisource feedback, and provides evaluation of individual performance. Direct observation offers a more accurate assessment of team-related behaviors using trained observers. Observers use checklists and behaviorally anchored rating scales (BARS) to evaluate individual and team performance. Checklists and BARS include specific, observable behaviors reflective of optimal team performance. Teamwork may also be assessed using survey tools to assess attitudes and teamwork climate.[12–14] Higher ratings of collaboration and teamwork have been associated with better patient outcomes in observational studies.[15–17] The ultimate goal of teamwork efforts is to improve patient outcomes. However, it is often difficult to clearly link improved outcomes with teamwork interventions because patient outcomes are affected by a number of factors and because hospitals frequently engage in multiple, simultaneous efforts to improve care.

Examples of Successful Interventions

Team Training

Formal teamwork training programs have been implemented in several clinical environments, including emergency departments, operating rooms, labor and delivery suites, and intensive care units.[18–21] These "closed" environments provide the advantage of having all providers identify with a unit-based setting, whereas most medical units have the added challenge of having nurses who are unit-based and physicians (and others) who are often service-based with patients housed on several different units.

The effectiveness of these teamwork training programs is mixed. While many demonstrate increased knowledge of teamwork principles, attitudes about the importance of teamwork, and overall safety climate, evidence for the ability to improve patient outcomes or reduce errors is less compelling.[22] In the hospital medicine setting, a multifaceted teamwork training program improved provider safety knowledge and attitudes and patient perceptions of teamwork and communication.[23–25]

Daily Goals of Care

In intensive care unit (ICU) settings, physicians and nurses work in proximity, allowing interdisciplinary discussions to occur at the bedside. The finding that professionals in operating rooms and ICUs have widely discrepant views on the quality of collaboration[10, 11] indicates that proximity, alone, is not sufficient for effective communication. Researchers have used daily goals of care forms for bedside ICU rounds in an effort to standardize communication about the daily plan of care.[26, 27] The forms define essential goals of care for patients and their use has resulted in significant improvements in teams' understanding of those daily goals. The daily goals forms provide structure to the interdisciplinary conversations during rounds in order to enhance collaboration and create a shared understanding of patients' plans of care (i.e. shared mental model).

Interdisciplinary Rounds

Interdisciplinary Rounds (IDRs) have been used for many years as a means to assemble team members in a single location[28–31] and the use of IDR has been associated with lower mortality among ICU patients.[32] IDR may be particularly useful for clinical settings in which team members are traditionally dispersed in time and place. Early research demonstrated improved ratings of collaboration on the part of physicians.[30,31] Recently, O'Leary and colleagues studied the effect of Structured Inter-Disciplinary Rounds (SIDRs).[33,34] SIDR combines a structured format for communication, similar to a daily goals of care form, with a forum for regular interdisciplinary meetings. The use of SIDR resulted in significantly higher ratings of the quality of collaboration and teamwork climate on both a non-teaching hospitalist unit and a resident teaching unit. The majority of clinicians in the studies agreed that SIDR improved patient care, improved the efficiency of their work day, and that SIDR should continue indefinitely.

Nurse-Physician Unit Co-Leadership

Leadership plays a key role in shaping team culture and norms.[35] Nurse-physician co-leadership is one recommended strategy for a model to improve the quality and safety of care on hospital units.[36,37] The model includes a new role, a physician unit leader, who partners with the nurse manager to collaboratively take ownership for and accountability of care delivery on that unit. At the University of Pennsylvania Health System, the model is known as Unit Based Clinical Leadership.[36] Nurse managers and unit physician leaders co-lead weekly IDR, operations meetings, orientation of housestaff, and ongoing performance improvement projects.

Conclusions

In summary, teamwork is critically important to provide safe and effective care. Despite the noted challenges in implementation and evaluation, a number of interventions demonstrate promise for improving teamwork. Future efforts must carefully measure the impact of efforts to assess their effectiveness on patient care and also to demonstrate the utility of resources invested. The optimal approach is implementation of one or more interventions with adaptations to fit unique clinical settings and local culture.

References

1. Joint Commission on Accreditation of Healthcare Organizations. Sentinel Event Statistics. http://www.jointcommission.org/SentinelEvents/Statistics/. Accessed March 31, 2008.
2. Sutcliffe KM, Lewton E, Rosenthal MM. (2004) Communication failures: An insidious contributor to medical mishaps. *Acad Med* **79**(2): 186–194.
3. Gawande AA, Zinner MJ, Studdert DM, Brennan TA. (2003) Analysis of errors reported by surgeons at three teaching hospitals. *Surgery* **133**(6): 614–621.

4. O'Leary KJ, Ritter CD, Wheeler H, *et al.* (2010) Teamwork on inpatient medical units: Assessing attitudes and barriers. *Qual Saf Health Care* **19**(2): 117–121.
5. Salas E, Sims DE, Burke CS. (2005) Is there a "big five" in teamwork? *Small Group Res* **36**: 555–599.
6. Wright MC, Taekman JM, Endsley MR. (2004) Objective measures of situation awareness in a simulated medical environment. *Qual Saf Health Care* **13**(Suppl 1): i65–71.
7. O'Leary KJ, Thompson JA, Landler MP, *et al.* (2010) Patterns of nurse-physician communication and agreement on the plan of care. *Qual Saf Health Care* **19**(3): 195–199.
8. Chang VY, Arora VM, Lev-Ari S, *et al.* () Interns overestimate the effectiveness of their hand-off communication. *Pediatrics* **125**(3): 491–496.
9. Keysar B, Henly AS. (2002) Speakers' overestimation of their effectiveness. *Psychol Sci* **13**(3): 207–212.
10. Daft RL, Lengel RH. (1986) Orgnaizational information requirements, media richness, and structural design. *Man Sci* **32**(5): 554–571.
11. Mehrabian A, Wiener M. (1967) Decoding of inconsistent communications of personality and social psychology. *J Pers Soc Psychol* **6**(1): 109–114.
12. Sexton JB, Helmreich RL, Neilands TB, *et al.* (2006) The Safety Attitudes Questionnaire: Psychometric properties, benchmarking data, and emerging research. *BMC Health Serv Res* **6**: 44.
13. Baggs JG. (1994) Development of an instrument to measure collaboration and satisfaction about care decisions. *J Adv Nurs* **20**(1): 176–182.
14. Hojat M, Fields SK, Veloski JJ, *et al.* (1999) Psychometric properties of an attitude scale measuring physician-nurse collaboration. *Eval Health Prof* **22**(2): 208–220.
15. Baggs JG, Schmitt MH, Mushlin AI, *et al.* (1999) Association between nurse-physician collaboration and patient outcomes in three intensive care units. *Crit Care Med* **27**(9): 1991–1998.

16. Davenport DL, Henderson WG, Mosca CL, *et al.* (2007) Risk-adjusted morbidity in teaching hospitals correlates with reported levels of communication and collaboration on surgical teams but not with scale measures of teamwork climate, safety climate, or working conditions. *J Am Coll Surg* **205**(6): 778–784.
17. Wheelan SA, Burchill CN, Tilin F. (2003) The link between teamwork and patients' outcomes in intensive care units. *Am J Crit Care* **12**(6): 527–534.
18. Awad SS, Fagan SP, Bellows C, *et al.* (2005) Bridging the communication gap in the operating room with medical team training. *Am J Surg* **190**(5): 770–774.
19. Morey JC, Simon R, Jay GD, *et al.* (2002) Error reduction and performance improvement in the emergency department through formal teamwork training: Evaluation results of the MedTeams project. *Health Serv Res* **37**(6): 1553–1581.
20. Nielsen PE, Goldman MB, Mann S, *et al.* (2007) Effects of teamwork training on adverse outcomes and process of care in labor and delivery: A randomized controlled trial. *Obstet Gynecol* **109**(1): 48–55.
21. Sherwood G, Thomas E, Bennett DS, Lewis P. (2002) A teamwork model to promote patient safety in critical care. *Crit Care Nurs Clin North Am* **14**(4): 333–340.
22. Salas E, Wilson KA, Burke CS, Wightman DC. (2006) Does crew resource management training work? An update, an extension, and some critical needs. *Hum Factors* **48**(2): 392–412.
23. Auerbach AA, Sehgal NL, Blegen MA, *et al.* (2012) Effects of a multicenter teamwork and communication program on patient outcomes: results from the Triad for Optimal Patient Safety (TOPS) project. *BMJ Qual Saf* **21**(2): 118–126.
24. Blegen MA, Sehgal NL, Alldredge BK, *et al.* (2010) Improving safety culture on adult medical units through multidisciplinary teamwork and communication interventions: The TOPS Project. *Qual Saf Health Care* **19**(4): 346–350.
25. Sehgal NL, Fox M, Vidyarthi AR, *et al.* (2008) A multidisciplinary teamwork training program: The Triad for Optimal Patient Safety (TOPS) experience. *J Gen Intern Med* **23**(12): 2053–2057.

26. Pronovost P, Berenholtz S, Dorman T, *et al.* (2003) Improving communication in the ICU using daily goals. *J Crit Care* **18**(2): 71–75.
27. Narasimhan M, Eisen LA, Mahoney CD, *et al.* (2006) Improving nurse-physician communication and satisfaction in the intensive care unit with a daily goals worksheet. *Am J Crit Care* **15**(2): 217–222.
28. Cowan MJ, Shapiro M, Hays RD, *et al.* (2006) The effect of a multidisciplinary hospitalist/physician and advanced practice nurse collaboration on hospital costs. *J Nurs Adm* **36**(2): 79–85.
29. Curley C, McEachern JE, Speroff T, *et al.* (1998) A firm trial of interdisciplinary rounds on the inpatient medical wards: An intervention designed using continuous quality improvement. *Med Care* **36**(Suppl 8): AS4–A12.
30. O'Mahony S, Mazur E, Charney P, *et al.* (2007) Use of multidisciplinary rounds to simultaneously improve quality outcomes, enhance resident education, and shorten length of stay. *J Gen Intern Med* **22**(8): 1073–1079.
31. Vazirani S, Hays RD, Shapiro MF, Cowan M. (2005) Effect of a multidisciplinary intervention on communication and collaboration among physicians and nurses. *Am J Crit Care* **14**(1): 71–77.
32. Kim MM, Barnato AE, Angus DC, *et al.* (2010). The effect of multidisciplinary care teams on intensive care unit mortality. *Arch Intern Med* **170**(4): 369–376.
33. O'Leary KJ, Haviley C, Slade ME, *et al.* (2010) Impact of structured interdisciplinary rounds on teamwork on a hospitalist unit. *J Hosp Med* 6(2): 88–93.
34. O'Leary KJ, Wayne DB, Haviley C, *et al.* (2010) Improving teamwork: Impact of structured interdisciplinary rounds on a medical teaching unit. *J Gen Intern Med* **25**(8): 826–832.
35. Lemieux-Charles L, McGuire WL. (2006) What do we know about health care team effectiveness? A review of the literature. *Med Care Res Rev* **63**(3): 263–300.
36. Buckley M, Laursen J, Otarola V. (2009) Strengthening physician-nurse partnerships to improve quality and patient safety. *Physician Exec* **35**(6): 24–28.

37. Ponte PR. (2004) Nurse-physician co-leadership: A model of interdisciplinary practice governance. *J Nurs Adm* **34**(11): 481–484.
38. Baker DP, Salas E, King H, *et al*. (2005) The role of teamwork in the professional education of physicians: Current status and assessment recommendations. *Jt Comm J Qual Patient Saf* **31**(4): 185–202.

Chapter 9

Medication Reconciliation

Kelly Cunningham and Jill D. Goldenberg**[†]

Key Pearls

- Medication reconciliation is the process of compiling an accurate list of all medications a patient is taking at the time of admission; comparing that list to all hospital admission, transfer and discharge orders; resolving any discrepancies; and communicating the updated list to the patient and follow-up provider at the time of hospital discharge.
- Regulatory organizations, including the Joint Commission in the US, recognize medication reconciliation as a key strategy to decrease medication errors during transitions of care.
- One effective model of medication reconciliation utilizes pharmacists to take medication histories, partner with physicians to clarify discrepancies, and communicate medication changes to patients and outpatient providers at hospital discharge.
- Recommended practices include adopting a standardized reconciliation tool; clearly defining responsibility and accountability for each step of the process; specifying a time frame for completion of admission medication reconciliation; making the pre-admission medication list easily accessible in the chart; targeting high risk patients for more intensive interventions and empowering patients to actively maintain a medication list.

*Mount Sinai School of Medicine, New York, NY, USA.

- Hospitalists can contribute to medication reconciliation efforts by serving as physician champions; modeling effective teamwork; helping integrate processes into provider workflow; leveraging information technology; and measuring the impact on clinically relevant outcomes.

Background

Medication errors are common and often preventable causes of patient harm. Patients are most vulnerable to medication errors during transitions of care, such as hospital admission, transfers of service, location or level of care during hospitalization, and at hospital discharge.[1] Studies have shown that up to 67% of admitted patients have at least one discrepancy between the prescription medication list obtained by the admitting provider and the patient's actual pre-admission medication regimen.[2] Furthermore, in up to 59% of cases, discrepancies occurring at the time of admission have the potential to cause harm, particularly if the errors persist beyond discharge.[3] Discharge medication reconciliation errors are also prevalent, with as many as 70% of patients having an unintentional medication discrepancy at discharge, and nearly one-third of those discrepancies having the potential to cause harm.[4] The implications of these errors are significant, resulting in post-discharge adverse drug events that may lead to emergency room visits, hospital readmissions, and utilization of other healthcare resources.[5,6]

Medication reconciliation is a strategy to reduce the risk of potential adverse drug events among patients transitioning across different care settings. Medication reconciliation is defined as the process by which a patient's medication list is obtained, compared, and clarified across different sites of care.[1] Specific steps in the process are detailed in Fig.1. The process typically includes the following:

- Developing a list of medications that the patient is currently taking
- Generating a list of medications to be ordered
- Comparing these two lists

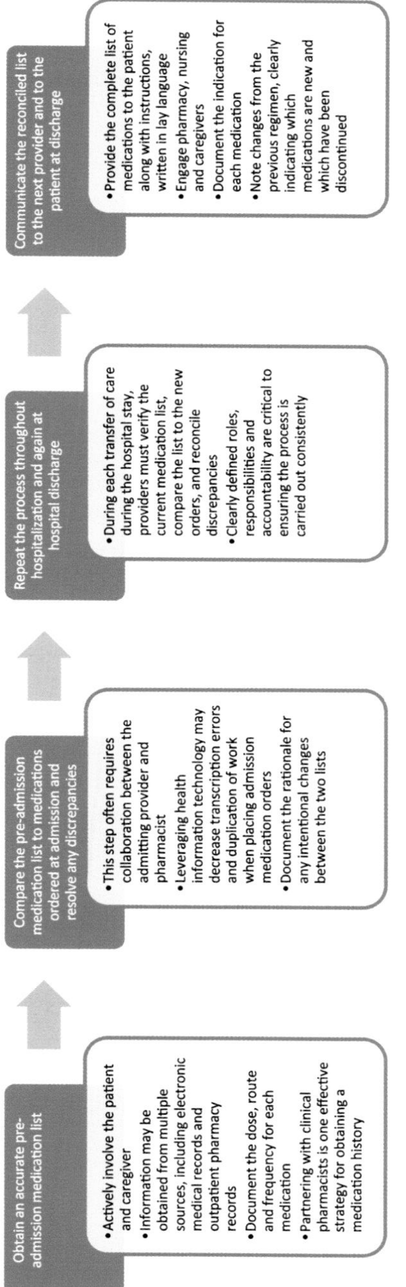

Fig. 1. Steps of medication reconciliation.

- Resolving any discrepancies
- Communicating the new, reconciled list to the patient, appropriate caregivers, and receiving provider

Evidence has supported the concept of medication reconciliation. In a study of a pharmacist-based medication reconciliation program involving hospital admission and discharge, Vira and colleagues found that 18% of patients had at least one clinically important medication error, none of which had been detected by usual clinical practice before medication reconciliation was conducted.[7] Other groups have demonstrated significant decreases in medication errors by implementing comprehensive, multidisciplinary medication reconciliation programs.[1,8] Though these findings are encouraging, most published studies have been limited by small sample sizes, single study sites, lack of randomization, and a paucity of clinically relevant outcomes.

Recognizing that minimizing medication errors is a fundamental part of patient safety, several organizations have emphasized medication reconciliation as a priority. The Institute for Healthcare Improvement highlighted medication reconciliation as a key intervention for its 100,000 and 5 Million Lives Campaigns.[9,10] In 2005, the Joint Commission added medication reconciliation to its list of National Patient Safety Goals (NPSG), setting the expectation that hospitals "accurately and completely reconcile medications across the continuum of care".[11] This NPSG requires healthcare organizations to develop and implement a process for obtaining and documenting the full list of medications a patient is taking at the time of admission, comparing that list to medications ordered for the patient while under the care of the hospital, and communicating the complete list to the next provider of care. In addition, a standard was added for institutions to provide the reconciled list of medications to the patient and/or family at the time the patient leaves the organization's care.[12]

Barriers

The process of medication reconciliation is complex and, as a result, can be challenging for organizations to put into practice. Numerous barriers to implementation have been identified, comprising patient, provider and system factors. For instance, admission history taking can be compromised by the providers' lack of time and knowledge required to perform an accurate medication history; unclear expectations of who is responsible for taking the history; patients' lack of knowledge of their medications; and multiple, often conflicting, sources of medication information. In addition, many medication reconciliation programs lack the integration of history taking and medication ordering or fail to incorporate these processes into providers' workflow. Pervasive issues such as increasing numbers of handoffs, low health literacy, and limited resources for staffing and information technology further complicate the effective implementation of medication reconciliation practices.

Successful Strategies

Institutions have taken varied approaches to operationalizing medication reconciliation. Successful programs have engaged different types of healthcare providers and have built processes around both paper-based and electronic interventions, depending on available resources. One effective strategy is to leverage the skills of pharmacists. A randomized controlled trial conducted by Schnipper and colleagues evaluated an intervention using pharmacists to compare discharge medications to pre-admission medications, reconcile discrepancies with the assistance of the physician, and perform discharge medication counseling. The authors found a significant decrease in the occurrence of preventable adverse drug events and preventable medication-related emergency room visits and hospital readmissions 30 days post-discharge as compared with usual care.[14]

Programs can also take advantage of health information technology to help automate processes and streamline workflow. In one study, the use of a computerized medication reconciliation tool that facilitated the creation of a pre-admission medication list and the reconciliation of admission and discharge medication regimens significantly decreased the number of potential adverse drug events as compared with usual care, when used in the setting of redesigned provider roles and workflows.[15]

Successful programs share common features, such as having buy-in of frontline staff, clearly defined roles and procedures, executive sponsorship, involvement of multidisciplinary teams, and mechanisms for assessing process and outcome measures. Based on the available evidence, hospital medicine and patient safety organizations recommend specific practices, including:[10,16]

- Adopting a standardized tool for use in reconciling medications
- Ensuring that the pre-admission medication list is readily accessible in the chart
- Specifying a time frame for completion of admission medication reconciliation
- Identifying the highest risk patients (i.e. the elderly, low health literacy, on many medications)
- Empowering each patient to maintain a medication list and/or personal health record

Remaining Challenges

Despite the progress that has been made in the arena of medication safety, numerous challenges remain. Basic concepts such as standardized definitions of what constitutes a medication and designating responsibility and accountability for completing each step in the process must be clarified. The need for an accurate medication history remains paramount, as evidence suggests that most errors originate during the admission medication history; therefore, resources must be invested in providing the knowledge, time and information sources to aid providers in accurately completing this critical initial step.[17] Furthermore, efficient and sustainable medication reconciliation processes will require better integration of different stages to minimize duplication of work and transcription errors. Institutions must take advantage of health information technology, where available, to facilitate order entry, prescription writing and maintenance of correct medication lists, to offer timely decision support, and to make possible the sharing of information among different institutions. Lastly, and perhaps most importantly, hospitals must focus on the process of medication reconciliation with the goal of patient safety rather than simply satisfying accreditation requirements.

Hospitalists have been instrumental in developing and implementing medication reconciliation in their institutions and in conducting studies to measure the impact of these processes. In their roles as clinicians, researchers, administrators and patient safety leaders, hospitalists are well positioned to address these challenges and further advance the field by developing best practices and collaborating on multi-center studies with relevant clinical outcomes.

References

1. Rozich JD, Resar RK. (2001) Medication safety: One organization's approach to the challenge. *J Clin Outcomes Manage* **8**: 27–34.
2. Lau HS, Florax C, Porsius AJ, *et al.* (2000) The completeness of medication histories in hospital medical records of patients admitted to general internal medicine wards. *Br J Clin Pharmacol* **49**: 597–603.
3. Gleason KM, Groszek JM, Sullivan C, *et al.* (2004) Reconciliation of discrepancies in medication histories and admission orders of newly hospitalized patients. *Am J Health Syst Pharm* **61**: 1689–95.
4. Wong JD, Bajcar JM, Wong GG, *et al.* (2008) Medication reconciliation at hospital discharge: Evaluating discrepancies. *Ann Pharmacother* **42**: 1373–9.
5. Johnson JA, Bootman JL. (1995) Drug-related morbidity and mortality: A cost of illness model. *Arch Intern Med* **155**: 1949–56.
6. Forster AJ, Murff HJ, Peterson JF, *et al.* (2005) Adverse drug events occurring following hospital discharge. *J Gen Intern Med* **20**: 317–23.
7. Vira T, Colquhoun M, Etchells E. (2006) Reconcilable differences: Correcting medication errors at hospital admission and discharge. *Qual Saf Health Care* **15**: 122–6.
8. Murphy EM, Oxencis CJ, Kaluck JA, Meyer DA, Zimmerman JM. (2009) Medication reconciliation at an academic medical center: Implementation of a comprehensive program from admission to discharge. *Am J Health-Syst Pharm* **66**: 2126–31.

9. Berwick DM, Calkins DR, McCannon CJ, Hackbarth AD. (2006) The 100 000 Lives Campaign: Setting a goal and a deadline for improving healthcare quality. *JAMA* **295**: 324–7.
10. Institute for Healthcare Improvement. (2008) 5 Million Lives Campaign. Getting started kit: Prevent adverse drug events (medication reconciliation) how-to guide. Cambridge, MA. Available at www.ihi.org.
11. The Joint Commission. (2006) Using medication reconciliation to prevent errors. Sentinel Event Alert. Available at: http://www.jointcommission.org/SentinelEvents/SentinelEventAlert/sea_35.htm Accessed May 20, 2010.
12. Joint Commission on Accreditation of Healthcare Organizations. (2007) 2008 National Patient Safety Goals. *Joint Commission Perspectives* **27**: 10–22.
13. The Joint Commission. (2010) Medication reconciliation National Patient Safety Goal to be reviewed, refined. Available at: http://www.jointcommission.org/PatientSafety/NationalPatientSafetyGoals/nspg8_review.htmAccessed May **20**, 2010.
14. Schnipper JL, Kirwin JL, Cotugno MC, *et al.* (2006) Role of pharmacist counseling in preventing adverse drug events after hospitalization. *Arch Intern Med* **166**: 565–71.
15. Schnipper JL, Hamann C, Ndumele CD, *et al.* (2009) Effect of an electronic medication reconciliation application and process redesign on potential adverse drug events: A cluster-randomized trial. *Arch Intern Med* **169**: 771–80.
16. Greenwald JL, Halasyamani L, Greene J, *et al.* (2010) Making inpatient medication reconciliation patient centered, clinically relevant and implementable: A consensus statement on key principles and necessary first steps. *J Hosp Med* **5**: 477–85.
17. Pippins JR, Gandhi TK, Hamann C, *et al.* (2008) Classifying and predicting errors of inpatient medication reconciliation. *J Gen Intern Med* **23**: 1414–22.

Chapter 10

Transitions of Care: The Hospital Discharge

Jill D. Goldenberg, Ramiro Jervis and Kelly Cunningham*

Key Pearls

- The transition from hospital to home is complex, error prone and can result in post-discharge adverse events if poorly executed.
- The discharge process requires a team approach using the expertise of physicians, nurses, pharmacists, and social workers.
- At discharge, special attention should be given to medication management, close follow-up post-discharge, and anticipatory guidance.
- Patients should receive clear verbal and written discharge instructions tailored to their needs, literacy and native language.
- Communication with the receiving outpatient provider should occur in the form of a verbal handoff and discharge summary or letter.
- Transitional care workers can facilitate the discharge process by assisting with discharge medication management, scheduling of follow-up appointments, patient education, communication to the next provider, follow-up phone calls and home visits.

Background

Adverse events have been linked to poor transitions and handoffs.[1] Moreover, these transitions have become increasingly common as patients

*Mount Sinai School of Medicine, New York, NY, USA.

are transferred from one provider to another within hospital walls and at the time of discharge. Work hour restrictions for house staff and the increased use of hospitalists may be contributing to this trend. In fact, in one teaching institution, residents alone had 300 signouts per month and 4,000 handoffs occurred per day among all providers.[2] In response to this, the Joint Commission has implemented several National Patient Safety Goals relating to handoffs, medication reconciliation at transition points, and discharge communication to better standardize care.[3] While all transitions of care and handoffs are problematic, the process of discharging a patient from an acute setting to home or another care facility can lead to a host of problems, including medication errors, patient dissatisfaction, increased healthcare costs, patient confusion and misunderstanding, and readmission.

The discharge process requires the careful coordination of a multidisciplinary team to optimally arrange the needed resources for patients. As patients transition from the hospital to the next level of care, medications are altered, follow-up testing and procedures may be needed, and additional follow-up care involving appointments and therapy is often required. This process takes adequate preparation and coordination to ensure success, and when poorly executed, frequently results in errors. For example, one in five patients experience an adverse event upon discharge, the most common of which is an adverse drug events.[5] With system improvements, as many as two-thirds of these adverse events could be avoided or mitigated.[5] Additionally, over 40% of patients have test results return after they leave the acute setting, with as many as 9% of these returned tests considered actionable.[7] Perhaps more concerning is that outpatient physicians are unaware of these tests 62% of the time.[7] Physician communication between the inpatient provider and outpatient provider is poor, occurring only 3 to 20% of the time.[8] Similarly, discharge summaries are only available at first follow-up 12 to 24% of the time.[8] Moreover, patients with an error in their work-up post-discharge are 6.2 times more likely to be readmitted in the following three months.[6] The fact that almost 20% of Medicare recipients are readmitted within 30 days of hospital discharge suggests that focusing on the discharge transition may be high yield.[4]

This chapter will review the components needed to transition a patient from the hospital to home, first reviewing the required key features and secondly discussing those interventions considered optional given the intensive resources needed for implementation.

Required Components of the Discharge Process

The ideal discharge process should be a team approach using the combined efforts of physicians, nurses, pharmacists and social workers. The team should pay extra attention to the psychosocial aspects of the patient's care, the acuity of disease, and any barriers to care. The discharge process starts at the time of admission and should include thoughtful planning and teaching on a daily basis until discharge is carried out.

The discharge transition is complex and has many critical components, as listed in Table 1. The discharge process should always include a careful review of home medications and hospital medications and the generation of a discharge medication list. Follow-up arrangements should be made ideally within seven to 14 days after discharge.[9] Patients given scheduled appointments are more likely to show up for their appointments than patients asked to call to arrange follow-up.[10] Patients with high risk diagnoses (i.e. congestive heart failure) or those patients taking medications that require close monitoring (i.e. warfarin) should be seen in less than one week.[9]

Anticipatory guidance in the form of directions to patients, caregivers and providers on which symptoms and signs may occur post-discharge and how to respond should be clearly outlined. Instructions to the patient and next provider should detail any needed tests, studies, or referrals.[6] Any pending labs at the time of discharge should be explicitly indicated.[6] Patients should receive both clear verbal and written instructions. Written material should be at a 6th grade reading level and should be reinforced by the multidisciplinary team.[11] These instructions should be tailored to the patient's or care giver's cognitive level and native language. The technique of teach-back should be employed whenever possible.[12] To perform teach-back, the teacher asks the learner to repeat back the information they have

Table 1. Key Components of the Discharge Transition

Key Components	Details/Comments
Medication Management[11]	• Reconcile home and hospital medications to compile one accurate list of discharge medications. • Clearly identify new medications, changed medications and stopped medications; add indications and explanation for changes whenever possible. • Use a pharmacist when available to assist with process.
Follow-up[9]	• Schedule within 7–14 days. • High risk diagnoses and medications will require follow-up in less than 7 days.
Pending Data; Follow-up Tests and Procedures[6]	• Alert patient and next provider about needed follow-up tests, procedures, and pending data and provide. anticipatory guidance based on results.
Patient Education[12]	• Provide clear and simple verbal and written instructions to patient and caregiver. • Tailor to patient's literacy level and native language whenever possible. • Employ techniques of teach-back to verify understanding.
Emergency Contact Information	• Provide patients with instructions about who to call with questions and which scenarios require medical attention.
Verbal Communication to Next Provider[13]	• Verbally hand over care at the time of discharge.
Discharge Letter or Summary[8]	• Complete on the day of discharge and forward to the next provider before first follow-up visit. • Include: o Problem that led to hospitalization. o Discharge diagnosis. o Condition at discharge. o Key findings and test results. o Brief problem-based hospital course. o Recommendations and contact information of subspecialty consultants. o Comprehensive and reconciled discharge medication list. o Follow-up appointments with names, dates and times and contact information. o Pending lab work and tests. o Contact information for hospitalist.

just learned to confirm understanding.[12] The patient's paperwork at discharge should be clear, simple, legible, and contain:

- Details about the reason for hospital admission
- Discharge diagnosis
- Relevant tests and procedures
- Discharge medications
- Follow-up appointments
- Anticipatory guidance
- Red flags
- Emergency contact information

Any transportation needs and other home services (i.e. physical therapy, nursing services) should be carefully considered and arranged. A standard verbal communication in the form of a phone call should be considered mandatory to the receiving provider to highlight any special discharge needs or instructions.[13]

Discharge summaries are an important target for improving the discharge process, as they are frequently difficult to read, tardy, and lacking in important information regarding the hospitalization. For example, most physicians (between 66% and 88%) do not receive a copy of the discharge summary in time for the patient's follow up appointment.[8] A quarter of physicians never receive a discharge summary at all.[8] These discharge summaries are often lacking the primary diagnosis (17.5%), a list of discharge medications (21%) and pending test results (65%).[8]

Most importantly, a discharge summary must be timely, as a thorough discharge summary is of little value if the patient has contact with a healthcare setting before the discharge summary is made available. Ideally, discharge summaries should be completed the day that the patient is discharged. Handing the discharge summary to the patient may facilitate the transfer of the discharge summary to the outpatient physician, but this should be done in addition to a more formal transfer of information with the receiving physician. An electronic facsimile or other delivery service to the accepting physician is usually preferred and the mode of delivery should be confirmed during a verbal exchange.

The required components of a discharge summary are listed in Table 1. A structured template rather than a free form narrative is the best strategy to produce discharge summaries in an accurate and efficient manner.[14] In one study, structured discharge summaries were shorter (302 versus 619 words) and were rated as having more clinically relevant information.[14] Electronic summaries should be used when available to increase efficiency and decrease the delay imposed by transcription services.[15]

Optional Components of the Discharge Process

While every discharge should contain the above key components, additional interventions can be useful and should be considered for high risk patients (i.e. multiple co-morbidities, elderly, congestive heart failure). Optional components of the discharge process are listed in Table 2. These interventions often require increased staffing and organizational support. One such intervention includes follow-up phone calls to patients. These phone calls can help inpatient providers collect information on the discharge process and more importantly serve as a venue to field patient questions, clarify medication changes, and understand patient compliance.[16]

Table 2. Optional Components of the Discharge Transition

Optional Components	Details/Comments

Follow-up Phone Calls[16]	• Can assist in:
	  ○ Fielding patient questions
	  ○ Resolving medication discrepancies
	  ○ Identifying medication side effects
	  ○ Ensuring compliance with therapy and follow-up

Home Visits with an Enhanced Discharge Process[17–20]	• Initial in hospital visit made by transitional worker followed by continued home visits and telephone contact for extended period of time post-discharge. • Emphasis on early response to status changes that could precipitate readmission. • Has been shown to lower health care costs, improve patient satisfaction and reduce hospital readmission.

Another optional intervention is a comprehensive discharge process followed by home visits and telephone contact with the help of a transitional care provider. This approach allows for early identification of problems with medications and symptom control and allows for active participation with patients and families.[17–20] The Care Transitions Intervention is a program that uses a "transition coach" to guide patients from the hospital to home.[20] The program starts when the patient is still inpatient and the "transition coach" follows the patient out into community with both home visits and phone calls. The goals of the intervention include patient (and caregiver) understanding of medications, a self directed and compiled personal health record, scheduled and made follow-up appointments, and an understanding of "red flags" and how to respond. These four pillars are emphasized in the hospital, at home visits and by telephone.[20] The authors of this study found that patients in the intervention group had lower 30 and 90 day rehospitalization rates as compared with the control group and lower rehospitalization rates for same condition that precipitated index hospitalization at 90 and 180 days.[20] Another example of success was noted in the Reengineered Discharge Study, known as Project Red. Their intervention uses a nurse "discharge advocate" who assists patients in arranging follow-up, confirmation of medication reconciliation, and assists with providing discharge information to the next provider.[19] A pharmacist is responsible for a post-discharge follow-up call at two to four days.[19] The authors found a 30% lower rate of hospital utilization in the intervention group as compared with usual care.[19] These two interventions along with a few other similar approaches have demonstrated reduced hospital readmission rates, decreased health care costs, and increased patient satisfaction.[18–20]

Conclusions

The transition from hospital to home is a complex and time-intensive multidisciplinary process. Hospitalists are key players in improving the way this transition occurs. Hospitalists can lead efforts to improve and standardize the transition. Every discharge should contain the discussed key features, highlights of which include medication reconciliation, follow-up arrangements, and communication with the receiving provider. When staffing allows, organizations should consider a more comprehensive interventions that may include follow-up phone calls, transitional workers, and home visits.

References

1. Horwitz LI, Moin T, Krumholz HM, *et al.* (2008) Consequences of inadequate sign-out for patient care. *Arch Intern Med* **168**(16): 1755–1760.
2. Triple Handoff, Arpana R. Vidyarthi. AHRQ WebM&M [serial online]. September 2006. Available at: http://webmm.ahrq.gov/case.aspx?caseID=134. Accessed Sept 2010.
3. National Patient Safety Goals. Joint Commission on Accreditation of Healthcare Organizations. Available at: http://www.jointcommission.org/PatientSafety/NationalPatientSafetyGoals. Accessed Sept 2010.
4. Jencks SF, Williams MV, Coleman EA. (2009) Rehospitalizations among patients in the medicare fee-for-service program. *New Eng J Med* **360**(14): 1418–1428.
5. Forster AJ, Murff HJ, Peterson JF, *et al.* (2003) The incidence and severity of adverse events affecting patients after discharge from the hospital. *Ann Intern Med* **138**: 161–167.
6. Moore C, Wisnivesky J, Williams S, McGinn T. (2003) Medical errors related to discontinuity of care from an inpatient to an outpatient setting. *J Gen Intern Med* **18**: 646–651.
7. Roy CL, Poon EG, Karson AS, *et al.* (2005) Improving patient care: Patient safety concerns arising from test results that return after hospital discharge. *Ann Intern Med* **143**: 121–128.
8. Kripalani S, LeFevre F, Phillips CO, *et al.* (2007) Deficits in communication and information transfer between hospital-based and primary care physicians. *JAMA* **297**: 831–841.
9. Kripalani S, Jackson AT, Schnipper JL, Coleman EA. (2007) Promoting effective transitions of care at hospital discharge: A review of key issues for hospitalists. *J Hosp Med* **2**: 314–323.

10. Lowenthal G. (2006) The best way to improve emergency department follow-up is actually to give the patient a specific appointment. *J Gen Intern Med* **21**: 398.
11. Ideal Discharge for the Elderly Patient: A Hospitalist checklist. Available at: http://www.hospitalmedicine.org/AM/Template.cfm?Section=QI_Clinical_Tools&Template=/CM/ContentDisplay.cfm&ContentID=10303. Accessed Sept 2010.
12. Shojania KG, Duncan BW, McDonald KM, Wachter RM, (eds). *Making Healthcare Safer: A Critical Analysis of Patient Safety Practices*. Evidence Report No. 43 from the Agency for Healthcare Research and Quality. AHRQ Publication No. 01-E058 2001.
13. Pantilist SZ, Lindenauer PK, Katz PP, Wachter RM. (2001) Primary care physician attitudes regarding communication with hospitalists. *Am J Med* **111**: 15S–20S.
14. van Walraven C, Duke SM, Weinberg AL, Wells PS. (1998) Standardized or narrative discharge summaries. Which do family physicians prefer? *Can Fam Physician* **44**: 62–69.
15. Bolton P. (1999) A review of the role of information technology in discharge communications in Australia. *Aust Health Rev* **22**: 56–64.
16. Nelson JR. (2001) The importance of postdischarge telephone follow-up for hospitalists: A view from the trenches. *Am J Med* **111**: 43S–44S.
17. Naylor MD, Brooten DA, Campell RL, *et al*. (2004) Transitional care of older adults hospitalized with heart failure: A randomized, controlled trial. *J Am Geriatr Soc* **52**: 675–684.
18. Naylor MD, Brooten D, Campbell R, *et al*. (1999) Comprehensive discharge planning and home follow-up of hospitalized elders: A randomized clinical trial. *JAMA* **281**: 613–620.
19. Jack BW, Veerappa KC, Anthony D, *et al*. (2009) A reengineered hospital discharge program to decrease rehospitalization. *Ann Intern Med* **150**: 178–187.
20. Coleman EA, Smith JD, Frank JC, Min S, Parry C, Kramer AM. (2004) Preparing patients and caregivers to participate in care delivered across settings: The care transitions intervention. *J Am Geriatr Soc* **52**(11): 1817–1825.

Chapter 11

Health Informatics for Hospitalists

Anuj K. Dalal and Kendall Rogers*[†]

Key Pearls

- Health information technology (HIT) can dramatically improve health-care quality and safety when effectively designed and implemented.
- As a function of the electronic health record (EHR), computerized physician order entry (CPOE) with clinical decision support (CDS) reduces errors and improves the delivery of evidenced-based medical care.
- The importance of EHR functionality to improve patient safety and quality of care often competes with the need for efficient system design for pharmacy, central supply and administrative services.
- Hospitalists should understand the benefits and risks to patient safety offered by the EHR at their institution.
- Hospitalists are uniquely qualified to drive EHR design and implementation to improve patient safety and quality of care.

Introduction

Practicing hospitalists have first-hand experience with the benefits, pitfalls, and challenges of health information technology (HIT). Most clinicians agree that current technology often does not meet patient's and provider's

*Birgham and Women's Hospital, Boston, MA, USA.
[†]University of New Mexico School of Medicine, Albuquerque, NM, USA.

desires for high quality care in the hospital. When designed or implemented improperly, HIT can frustrate providers and potentially harm patients. Nevertheless, the true potential of HIT has yet to be realized. Hospitalists are ideally positioned to lead efforts to implement and improve systems with a vision of delivering safe, efficient, reliable and quality healthcare.

Health informatics involves understanding and promoting the effective organization, analysis, management and use of information in healthcare.[1] Health informatics tools include not only hardware, software, networks and devices, but also clinical guidelines, medical terminologies, information and communication systems as well as methods required to optimize information acquisition, storage, retrieval and use. Hospitalists should possess a fundamental understanding of health informatics that goes beyond simply using the technology. This chapter provides an introduction to the field of health informatics as it pertains to hospital medicine.

Drivers for Health Information Technology

HIT is increasingly viewed as the most promising tool for improving the quality, safety and efficiency of our health care delivery system.[2] Broad and consistent utilization of effective HIT can:

- Prevent medical errors
- Reduce healthcare costs
- Improve healthcare quality
- Improve administrative efficiency
- Improve utilization of evidenced-based practices
- Expand access to affordable care

However, HIT is not a panacea and users must be aware of unintended consequences.[3]

Beyond well publicized cost and privacy issues, HIT adoption has been slow primarily because HIT products and applications are difficult to implement and use effectively. Moreover, because healthcare delivery is highly complex, developing ideal informatics solutions has proven to be challenging and costly as a consequence of individual variations among providers and hospitals, incomplete evidence of benefit, and many undefined processes. Nevertheless, to meet clinical needs, HIT must surpass the sophistication of information technology in other industries.

The ARRA and the HITECH Act of 2010 established HIT adoption as a major national initiative in the United States. Currently, hospitals are working towards "meaningful use of a certified EHR" and will likely engage hospitalists to achieve this goal. The federal government established objectives for "meaningful use" of certified EHRs and will provide payment incentives to physicians, clinics, and hospitals who realize significant improvements in care through effective use of the EHR. Core objectives include utilization of essential features (e.g. entry of basic demographic and medical data) and functions that improve the safety, quality, and efficiency of care (e.g. computerized physician order entry (CPOE), clinical decision support, and quality measure reporting).[4] On an individual provider level, the ABIM now requires an understanding of "meaningful use" in its Maintenance of Certification (MOC) evaluations.

The Electronic Health Record

The Electronic Health Record (EHR) is defined as "a longitudinal electronic record of patient health information generated by one or more encounters in any care delivery setting."[5] The EHR is the primary HIT tool used by hospitalists. Its functionality extends beyond point-of-care applications by integrating clinical, administrative, financial, and increasingly, quality and population health functions.

Most EHR systems were initially developed to facilitate administrative functions such as registration, billing, coding and scheduling. Clinical functions, such as storing and retrieving clinical data, were added over time. These functions now include other aspects of data management such as picture archiving and communication software (PACS), documentation, and analysis of trends in care. Although sharing of patient information is currently limited across different EHR platforms, interoperability will facilitate point-of-care access for clinicians caring for patients across hospitals and healthcare networks, thereby reducing redundancy and costs.

Sophisticated EHR systems can integrate almost every aspect of patient care and are becoming an essential part of the healthcare delivery process. EHRs provide clinicians with tools for robust results and data viewing, medication management, communication, CPOE and CDS. Adoption of these advanced tools has been markedly low: Less than 10% of hospitals utilize CPOE and less than 1% of hospitals have achieved high levels of adoption per Health Level 7.[6]

The EHR's potential for aggregating and sharing data will provide nationwide access to de-identified patient data for population health analysis. Although enhancing patient care and monitoring quality are the primary drivers for promoting interoperability of EHRs, an interconnected health information network will also facilitate real-time disease detection, epidemiological surveillance, drug resistance monitoring, and sophisticated outcomes and comparative effectiveness research.

Clinical Decision Support (CDS)

Evidenced-based CDS is one of the most valuable features of the EHR. CDS encompasses a wide variety of tools and interventions that aid in therapeutic and diagnostic decision making. Well-designed CDS is integrated within daily workflow and facilitates evidence-based care. Examples of CDS extend far beyond unsolicited alerts (e.g. drug–drug interaction) and include order sets promoting best practices, documentation templates helping with diagnosis, data displays showing real-time patient parameters, and dashboards showing quality outcomes. (See Table 1.)

To be successful, CDS tools should follow the "CDS 5 Rights": Provide the *right information* (pertinent evidenced-based guidelines) to the *right person*, in the *right format* (i.e. an alert, order set, reference info-button), through the *right channel* (i.e. the clinical information system, Internet, mobile-device), at the *right time* (i.e. the time in the workflow when action is needed).[7] Speed, delivery, and integration within clinical work-flow can have a tremendous impact on user acceptance. Understanding the patterns

Table 1. Examples of CDS Interventions

A. CDS during data-entry tasks
 1. Smart documentation forms
 2. Order sets, care plans and protocols
 3. Parameter guidance
 4. Critiques and warning — "immediate alerts"

B. CDS during data-review tasks
 5. Relevant data summaries (single-patient)
 6. Multi-patient monitors
 7. Predictive and retrospective analytics

C. CDS during assessment and understanding tasks
 8. Filtered reference information and knowledge resources
 9. Expert workup and management advisors

D. CDS not triggered by a user task
 10. Event-driven alerts (data-triggered) and reminders (time-triggered)

Reprinted with permission from Osheroff J, *et al.* (2012) *Improving Outcomes with Clinical Decision Support: An Implementers Guide*, 2nd ed. HIMSS: Chicago.

of physician resistance, providing simple interventions, monitoring impact, requesting feedback, and maintaining the knowledge-based system are key strategies for managing clinical decision support systems.[8]

The Risks and Benefits of HIT

To effectively advocate for EHRs that enhance patient safety and quality of care, hospitalists should understand the risks and benefits of EHR systems. When implemented and used effectively, HIT can facilitate safe and efficient delivery of care. This has been convincingly shown for CPOE with CDS and medication management. When developed, implemented and locally adapted at institutions with adequate infrastructure support, CPOE with CDS can reduce the rate of serious medication errors by 55% and all medication errors by 88%.[9,10] However, a report showed that 33% of fatal medication errors were still missed by CPOE systems,[11] demonstrating an ongoing need to optimize the configuration of existing systems. It has been estimated that CPOE could prevent 3 million adverse drug events each year in non-rural hospitals.[12] Much of medication error reduction has been attributed to CDS systems that provide alerts for drug interactions and drug allergies at the time of order entry.

In recent years, electronic medication reconciliation applications and bar-coding electronic medication administration systems have demonstrated a reduction of medication errors and potential adverse drug events.[13–15] HIT has the potential to impact other areas as well. For example, automated test result alerting systems have been shown to reduce the time until appropriate treatments are ordered for patients with critical laboratory results.[16] Computerized test result management applications may improve the coordinated hand-off of the results of tests pending at discharge. Although few studies have rigorously evaluated the impact of HIT on sign-outs, discharge modules, and diagnosis errors to date, HIT holds much promise in these areas.

Implementing or adopting HIT may have many untoward and unanticipated effects (Table 2). Some studies of CPOE implementations have demonstrated problems with organizational adaptation and change,[17] speed of order entry, alert fatigue, increased medication error risk,[18] and an increase in mortality.[19] It is important to recognize that errors may occur with either the design or local implementation of a system; both aspects must be considered to ensure safe and effective adoption.

Roles for Hospitalists in Health Informatics

Hospitalists are ideal candidates for certain hospital-based informatics roles and are naturally poised for advancement in these areas. Examples of typical roles include:

- A physician champion that works with the informatics department to develop order sets,
- A participating member on IT-oriented committees (e.g. pharmacy and therapeutics, EHR, CPOE committees, etc.),
- A physician liaison to the Chief Medical Information Officer (CMIO).

Training in quality improvement and acquisition of management skills are important in such roles. Increasingly, a number of professional societies are providing this training, including the Health Information Management Systems Society, the American Medical Informatics Association, the Association of Medical Director of Information Systems, and the American College of Physician Executives.

Even without formal informatics training, hospitalists should learn to navigate their local EHR system and know their institution's organizational

Table 2. Unintended Consequences of HIT[20]

Unintended Consequence (UC)	Description
More/New work issues	Physicians find that CPOE adds to their workload by forcing them to enter required information, respond to alerts, deal with multiple passwords, and expend extra time.
Workflow issues	Many UCs result from mismatches between the clinical information systems (CIS) and workflow, including issues related to process, policy/procedure, human-computer interaction, clinical personnel, and situation awareness.
Never-ending demands	Because CPOE requires hardware technically advanced enough to support the clinical software, there is a continuous need for new hardware, more space in which to put this hardware, and more space on the screen to display information. In addition, maintenance of the knowledge base for decision support and training demands are ongoing requirements.
Paper persistence	It has long been hoped that CIS will reduce the amount of paper used to communicate and store information, but that is not necessarily the case since it is useful as a temporary display interface.
Communication issues	The CIS changes communication patterns among care providers and departments, creating an "illusion of communication." A user may feel that the right person will see and act on information appropriately because the information was sent electronically.

(Continued)

Table 2. (*Continued*)

Unintended Consequence (UC)	Description
Emotions	CIS causes intense emotions in users, many which are negative and often result in reduced efficacy of system use initially.
New kinds of errors	CPOE generates new kinds of errors. For example, juxtaposition errors occur when clinicians click on the adjacent patient name or medication from a list and inadvertently enter the wrong order.
Changes in the power structure	The presence of a system that enforces specific clinical practices through mandatory data entry fields may change the power structure of organizations. Often the power or autonomy of physicians is reduced in an effort to standardize, while the power of the nursing staff, information technology specialists, and administration is increased.
Over-dependence on technology	As hospitals become more dependent on CIS, system failures can spread havoc when paper backup systems are not readily available.

Adapted with permission from Ash, Sitting *et al.* (2009) The unintended consequences of computerized provider order entry: Findings from a moved methods exploration. *Int J Meth Inform* **78**(Suppl1): S69–S76.

structure. Because they are well-positioned to recognize potential errors and identify needed enhancements in their institution's existing EHR, they should possess a basic understanding of how such systems operate and how to provide feedback and suggestions for improvement. As per Berwick's "Soldiers of Quality," hospitalists are one of the last lines of defense for patients. As such, hospitalists should be vocal advocates for improved HIT tools to provide efficient, high quality care.

Conclusion

The field of health informatics is in its infancy and in the future we will look back at current conditions as untenable. Advancement will require not only significant improvement in HIT design and implementation strategies, but also active involvement by the users of these technologies. Hospitalists will play a vital role at the local and national levels to ensure that HIT achieves its potential to revolutionize the quality and safety of healthcare.

References

1. About Informatics|AMIA <https://www.amia.org/informatics>. Accessed 9/20/2010.
2. Chaudhry B, Wang J, Wu S, *et al.* (2006) Systematic review: Impact of health information technology on quality, efficiency and costs of medical care. *Ann Intern Med* **144**(10): 742–752.
3. Ash JS, Berg M, Coiera E. (2004) Some unintended consequences of information technology in health care: The nature of patient care information system-related errors. *J Am Med Inform Assoc* **11**(2): 104–112.
4. Blumenthal D, Tavenner M. (2010) The "meaningful use" regulation for electronic health records. *N Engl J Med* **363**(6): 501–504.
5. HIMSS — Electronic Health Record (EHR) <http://www.himss.org/ASP/topics_ehr.asp>. Accessed 9/20/2010.
6. The Leapfrog Group. New CPOE Evaluation Tool Results Report. <http://www.leapfroggroup.org/media/file/NewCPOEEvaluationToolResultsReport.pdf>. Accessed 9/29/2010.
7. Osheroff JA, Teich JM, Middleton B, *et al.* (2007) A roadmap for national action on clinical decision support. *J Am Med Inform Assoc* **14**(2): 141–145.
8. Bates DW, Kuperman GJ, Wang S, *et al.* (2003) Ten commandments for effective clinical decision support: Making the practice of evidence-based medicine a reality. *J Am Med Inform Assoc* **10**(6): 523–530.
9. King WJ, Paice N, Rangrej J, Forestell GJ, Swartz R. (2003) The effect of computerized physician order entry on medication errors and adverse drug events in pediatric inpatients. *Pediatrics* **112**(3): 506–509.
10. Bates DW, Leape LL, Cullen DJ, *et al.* (1998) Effect of computerized physician order entry and a team intervention on prevention of serious medication errors. *JAMA* **280**(15): 1311–1316.

11. The Leapfrog Group. <http://www.leapfroggroup.org/>. Accessed 9/21/2010.
12. Lwin A, Shepard D. Lives Saved Leapfrog Report <http://www.leapfroggroup.org/media/file/Lives_Saved_Leapfrog_Report_2008-Final_(2).pdf>. Accessed 9/29/2010.
13. Schnipper JL, Hamann C, Ndumele CD. (2009) Effects of a medication reconciliation application and process redesign on potential adverse drug events: A cluster-randomized trial. *Arch Intern Med*, In Press.
14. Poon EG, Blumenfeld B, Hamann C, *et al.* (2006) Design and implementation of an application and associated services to support interdisciplinary medication reconciliation efforts at an integrated healthcare delivery network. *J Am Med Inform Assoc* **13**(6): 581–592.
15. Poon EG, Keohane CA, Yoon CS, *et al.* (2010) Effect of bar-code technology on the safety of medication administration. *N Engl J Med* **362**(18): 1698–1707.
16. Kuperman GJ, Teich JM, Tanasijevic MJ, *et al.* (1999) Improving response to critical laboratory results with automation: Results of a randomized controlled trial. *J Am Med Inform Assoc* **6**(6): 512–522.
17. Massaro TA. (1993) Introducing physician order entry at a major academic medical center: I. Impact on organizational culture and behavior. *Acad Med* **68**(1): 20–25.
18. Koppel R, Metlay JP, Cohen A, *et al.* (2005) Role of computerized physician order entry systems in facilitating medication errors. *JAMA* **293**(10): 1197–1203.
19. Han YY, Carcillo JA, Venkataraman ST, *et al.* (2005) Unexpected increased mortality after implementation of a commercially sold computerized physician order entry system. *Pediatrics* **116**(6): 1506–1512.
20. Ash JS, Sittig DF, Dykstra R, *et al.* (2009) The unintended consequences of computerized provider order entry: Findings from a mixed methods exploration. *Int J Med Inform* **78**(Suppl 1): S69–S76.

Business of Hospital Medicine

Chapter 12

Financial Planning for a Hospitalist Program

*Chirayu J. Shah**, *Tuhin Pankaj*† *and Surinder Kaul*‡

Key Pearls

- Clearly state the primary purpose of the program (education, hospital efficiency)
- Define your Hospitalist model (shift work, night float, etc.)?
- Know your payer-mix
- Define the support services for your program (IT, Physician Assistants, Nurse Practioners)
- Will you need hospital support and how much?

Introduction

Healthcare systems in the US are complex adaptive systems.[1] The healthcare industry in the US is growing at an alarming rate. As per CMS annual report of January, 2011,[2] US healthcare spending decelerated in 2009, increasing 4.0% as compared with 4.7% in 2008. The total health expenditures reached $2.5 trillion, which translates to $8,086 per person

*Internal Medicine Residency Program, Baylor College of Medicine, Houston, TX, USA.
†Office of the President, Baylor College of Medicine, Houston, TX, USA.
‡Section of General Internal Medicine Director, Hospitalist Program, Baylor College of Medicine, Houston, TX, USA.

or 17.6% of the nation's gross domestic product (GDP), the largest one-year increase in the last 50 years. About 21% ($506 billion) of healthcare spending is accounted for by physicians. The breakup of physician share — private insurance accounted for 240 billion; public funding (Medicare — 113 billion and Medicaid — 40 billion and others — 35 billion), $188 billion; out of pocket $50 billion; and other private fund, $28 billion. There are many causes that contribute to the escalation of healthcare spending and the major cause can be attributed to the technological advancement in diagnostics and therapeutics and availability of new treatment options which are more effective and expensive as well. Better care has resulted in prolonged survival with secondary increase in complication rates which add to the consumption of healthcare resources. Compounding these is an ageing population with increased prevalence of multiple chronic diseases such as diabetes, hypertension, stroke, ischemic heart disease, dementia and many other diseases.

Hospitalist Movement a Way Out to Provide Cost Effective Treatment

The major drivers of the development of hospital medicine are: care fragmentation arising from specialization; dependence on technology; rise in chronic complex diseases due to ageing populations; and escalation of healthcare costs. The significant changes in medical practice also contributed to its growth. The changes that have occurred are:

1. Limitations on house staff duty hours which has resulted in overall reduction of inpatient coverage by 10–25%.
2. Most primary care physicians involved in traditional practice in inpatient and outpatient settings are confining themselves to exclusive outpatient practice, and require hospitals to make arrangements to provide comprehensive inpatient care to their patients.

Presently in nearly 70% of US hospitals, hospitalist programs are becoming an increasingly important mode of care. Since 1996, the specialty has grown to more than 31,000 practicing hospitalists today, according to the Society of Hospital Medicine.

Multiple studies, prospective and retrospective, have supported the notion that the use of hospitalists lowered both length of hospital stay and overall cost of inpatient care. Hospitalist programs have also gained favor amongst the nursing and other ancillary staff of the hospital in view of the quick availability of physicians when needed. Preliminary studies have revealed that hospitals with hospitalist programs have done well, with **cost reduction** owing to decreasing **direct variable cost (DVC)**; increased **revenue generation** resulting from decreasing average length of stay (LOS) which increases patient flow and limit ED diversions; and **cost avoidance** by adhering to the hospital policies to decrease medical–legal liability cases and decrease in re-admission rates.

Business Plan for a Hospitalist Program

Establishing a hospitalist program requires a viable business plan.

Initial Phase of Financial Planning: This is perhaps the most important phase which will lead to overall success of the program and should include the following considerations:

a) A thorough evaluation of the purpose of the program — is the purpose to increase the volume of patients (as in private hospitals), to manage ER throughput, (as in academic hospitals), etc.
b) The mix of the hospital — ratio of patients who are having private insurance, Medicare, Medicaid, and uninsured.
c) Structure of the hospital — whether an academic hospital, private hospital, community hospital, rural hospital.
d) How much a hospital is going to support the program.
e) An estimate of how busy the hospital is by way of total annual admissions and what proportion of admissions the hospital needs help with.
f) Which model of hospitalist — coverage 365/24 days, nights included or weekdays only.

g) Use of allied health workers (Nurse Practioners, Physician Assistants or nurses).
h) Availability of hospitalists and other allied health providers in the community.

Developing a Business Plan: Hospital administrators will closely scrutinize the business plan to integrate a new hospitalist program. As further detailed below, the value of a hospitalist program to the overall patient flow of the hospital needs to be highlighted.

Staffing Structure of the Program

Staffing needs vary widely depending on the hospitalist model implemented. Most hospitalist groups utilize three groups of employees: physicians, clinical support staff (physician assistants, nurse practitioners, case managers, etc.), and nonclinical support staff (secretary, billing and collections). Another option would be to use a third-party company to offload some of the nonclinical support staff activities, such as billing and collections. An example of a staffing model is shown below in Table 1.

Cost Projection

Costs vary widely across the country, so some research into the local environment will be necessary. An example of expenses is shown below in Tables 2 and 3.

Revenue Generation

Revenue generation is directly related to the compensation for professional services provided. Identical physician services are compensated at different rates depending on the payer. Understanding the payer mix for the hospitalized patients will be essential for accurate revenue estimates. This information is not publicly available, but hospitals generally track

Table 1. Hospitalist Group Staffing Model

Physicians	
4 FTE Physicians	Responsibilities include admitting new patients from the ER and from PCPs, daily patient care, and inpatient consultation. Shifts are 12 hr 7 am–7 pm on a 7 days on/7 days off schedule.
1 FTE Night Hospitalist	Responsibilities include cross coverage of acute patient care issues between 7 pm–7 am, admitting new patients from the ER.
Clinical Support Staff	
2 Physician Assistants	Responsibilities include daily rounding on the established inpatients. Schedule 7 am–5 pm Monday through Friday.
Nonclinical Support Staff	
1 Secretary	Responsibilities include coordinating of administrative activities (providing support to physicians, communications by fax, phone, email).
1 Business Operations	Responsibilities include coordinating billing/collections process and office management.

Table 2. Staff Expenses (Annual)

4 FTE Hospitalists	4 × \$220,000 = \$880,000
1 FTE Night Hospitalist	1 × \$350,000 = \$350,000
2 Clinical staff	2 × \$65,000 = \$130,000
2 Nonclinical Staff	2 × \$45,000 = \$90,000
Staff Benefits (estimated 15%)	15% of \$1,450,000 = \$217,500
TOTAL STAFF EXPENSES	\$1,667,500

Table 3. Operational Expenses (Annual)

Information Technology (pagers, computer hardware, Internet, phones, etc.)	\$20,000
Centralized pager/call answering service for group	\$10,000
Office space	\$20,000
Recruitment/Advertising	\$5,000
Legal Consulting Fees	\$10,000
Misc. Other Expenses	\$5,000
TOTAL OPERATIONAL EXPENSES	\$70,000

this data. Based on recent hospitalist productivity surveys in 2011, the median work relative value unit (wRVU) for each FTE hospitalist is approximately 4200 wRVU/year. In addition to work RVU, Medicare compensation takes into account practice expense RVU, professional liability insurance RVU, and adjustments based on the geographical practice cost index. Each piece of this formula is available on the CMS website. The sum of the work, practice expense, and professional liability insurance RVU forms the total RVU. This number is then multiplied by the Conversion Factor set by Congress. Fee schedule calculators are available on the Internet to assist with these calculations.

In our example, each FTE hospitalist generates 5480 total RVUs (4200 wRVU + 1080 PE-RVU + 200 PLI-RVU). The 2011 Medicare conversion factor is set at $33.9764. FTE Hospitalist Revenue = 5480 total RVUs × $33.9764 = $186,190. For the 5 FTE Hospitalists in our example, the total revenue would be estimated at $930,953.

Revenue generation continues to evolve with a movement towards increased payments based on achieving quality measures. This "pay for performance" model is already impacting primary care physician and hospital facility compensations.

Based on the example presented here, the costs exceed the revenue generation. This occurs for 90% of hospitalist groups across the nation. Additional funding sources need to be identified, and partnering with the hospital becomes very important. On average, each hospitalist receives $135,000 per year of support from the hospital. The business plan should emphasize the value added to the hospital by partnering with a hospitalist group. Employing a hospitalist group can provide the hospital with significant benefits that cannot directly be included in the cost/revenue analysis. These include decreased patient length of stay (which corresponds to better hospital payments); reduced resource utilization; and increased throughput including reducing ER congestion and earlier discharges. In addition, hospitalists often lead quality and patient safety initiatives which become more important as health agencies increasingly scrutinize core clinical quality measures. These measures are now being made public in efforts to provide customers objective information to possibly attract them to a better scoring hospital.

Business Plan Outline and Factors

Developing a Business Plan: Hospital administrators will closely scrutinize the business plan to integrate a new hospitalist program. As further detailed below, the value of a hospitalist program should be outlined using the following structure:

- **Expected volumes** — The analysis around volume projections from the Emergency Department, private physician referrals, and managed care referrals will be critical in driving the economics relating to the hospitalists programs viability and profitability. Two major categories that should be identified are payer mix and sources of referrals.
- **Revenue Projections** — Once volume projections have been established, revenue projections can be calculated using the same volume projections along with payer mix and reimbursement rates specific to levels of care and/or procedures. There are available resources, such as your local Medicare carrier and also private insurance carriers, to tap into and to acquire your local area's typical reimbursement rates. In addition, you need to determine how the mix of capitation and fee-for-service in your area will affect the revenue analysis.
- **Staffing Matrix** — The first step in determining your staffing ratios is to make a decision on whether the hospitalist program will be a 24/7 program or will there only be a need for rounding on weekdays, weekends, days or nights? Once this is determined, a staffing grid which outlines daytime and nighttime coverage should be developed with costs associated with staffing. One final step in this process is to determine sources of staffing, i.e. will there be significant recruitment from the community to staff the hospitalist positions or will there be an internal network developed. Expenses associated with recruitment and development have also to be considered.
- **Expense Projections** — When identifying total expenses to operate the hospitalist group, it is critical to include all expenses sources so

that a calculated estimate can be established. Below are some of the regular ongoing expenses that should be considered:

- o Hospitalist Salary
- o Hospitalist Benefits
- o Administrative Support
- o Clinical Support
- o SSO (Staff, Student, Other)
- o Equipment
- o Marketing / Promotional
- o Malpractice

- **Projected First Year Profit / Loss Statement** — A profit / loss statement will bring the aforementioned categories together for a full view of the program to better understand the profitability of the practice. It is important for the key stakeholders and investors to know, from a projections standpoint, how long it will take for the practice to breakeven and in turn begin returning a profit (ROI).

References

1. State of Hospital Medicine: 2010 Report Based on 2009 Data. Society of Hospital Medicine and Medical Group Management Association, September 2010.
2. Centers for Medicare and Medicaid Services: Physician Fee Schedule Overview. (Accessed August 1, 2011 at https://www.cms.gov/physicianfeesched/)
3. Establishing a Hospitalist Program: Society of Hospital Medicine. (Accessed August 1, 2011 at http://www.hospitalmedicine.org/AM/Template.cfm?Section=Practice_Resources&Template=/CM/HTMLDisplay.cfm&ContentID=4505)

Chapter 13

Metrics and Dashboards

*Jeffrey I. Farber**

Key Pearls

- Understanding key metrics is critical to a hospitalist program's success.
- Physician dashboards are powerful tools to manage a program, drive improvements, and demonstrate effectiveness.
- Increasing financial pressures require greater attention to clinical documentation and a deeper understanding of the revenue cycle, coding, billing, and publicly-reported quality data.
- Medical necessity drives utilization management and is the backbone for audits and payment denials.
- Hospitalists should leverage their unique skill sets to assume leadership positions and drive care quality improvements.

Metrics

Hospital Medicine has a vital role to play in healthcare quality and successful hospitalist programs need to have a firm understanding of healthcare finances and hospital reimbursement to best leverage their positions with administration and effect improvements in value. Hospitalists must appreciate the commonly used metrics in hospital operations, including volume and growth, length of stay (LOS), avoidable readmissions, patient satisfaction, and clinical documentation.

* Mount Sinai School of Medicine, New York, NY, USA.

Volume

Hospitals generally operate under very thin margins (0–3% range)[1] and so constant growth in volume is critical in maintaining solvency. Thus, volume is the basic metric for hospitalist programs and strategies should be based on ways to increase the number of medically necessary discharges.

Length of Stay

Hospitals are primarily paid by both government and commercial payers on an inpatient prospective payment system, which means they receive a lump-sum payment for each discharge, regardless of the specific resources consumed by caring for the patient. In this DRG (Diagnosis-related Group) system, therefore, the hospital gets paid the same when caring for a patient admitted for pneumonia, for example, who is discharged in five days as for one who stays for 14 days. This is the main reason why LOS is such an important metric. Each DRG has an expected LOS, based upon the reason for admission and the severity of illness during the hospitalization, and so LOS is typically looked at as the ratio of actual or observed to expected (A/E), with the goal being < 1.0.

Patient Protection and Affordable Care Act (PPACA)

A key piece of legislation impacting healthcare in the United States was enacted in 2010. Half of the $1.2 trillion cost for the Patient Protection and Affordable Care Act (PPACA) was projected to come from cuts in Medicare and Medicaid, with roughly one-quarter of that ($157 billion) coming from reduced payments to hospitals. Two important mechanisms to achieve this anticipated cost savings were through reduced payments for avoidable re-admissions and for hospital-acquired conditions.

Avoidable re-admissions

Avoidable re-admission rates in the US received national attention during the debate preceding PPACA, helped by a published study analyzing 2004

Medicare claims data which showed that 20% of Medicare fee-for-service patients were re-admitted within 30 days of discharge, with an estimated cost of $17.4 billion for unplanned readmissions.[2] The PPACA allows Centers for Medicare and Medicare Services (CMS) to withhold from 1–3% of payments to hospitals with high readmission rates. Hospitalist programs should monitor and implement components of proven strategies, such as Care Transitions Program, Projects RED or BOOST[3–5] to reduce their readmission rates.

Hospital-acquired conditions

The PPACA also contains provisions to penalize hospitals with high rates of hospital-acquired conditions, which include, among others, advanced stage pressure ulcers, catheter-associated central line infections, and Foley-catheter related urinary tract infections. Other chapters in this textbook address these conditions and present strategies for prevention.

Clinical Documentation

The revenue cycle for hospitals starts with the admission and is entirely driven by the clinical documentation of the diagnoses and procedures treated and performed (Table 1). Specificity and comprehensiveness are critical for ensuring accurate coding, which then drives reimbursement and publicly-reported quality data (US News, HealthGrades, HospitalCompare). More so, CMS is mandating a transition to the International Classification of Diseases, 10th Revision, Clinical Modification (ICD-10-CM) in October 2014, which will require even greater diagnostic and procedural specificity to map to the appropriate ICD-10 code.

MS-DRG

In the United States, CMS adopted a new DRG system in 2007, MS-DRG (Medicare-Severity), which includes a triad for most DRGs based upon

Table 1. Clinical Documentation Pearls

Unable to Code	Acceptable to Code
LUL infiltrate	LUL pneumonia
Sputum culture positive for Klebsiella, will start antibiotics	Klebsiella pneumonia
Hgb 5.2; transfused	Acute or chronic blood loss anemia
Emaciated; total protein/albumin low; nutrition supplements started	Severe protein calorie malnutrition
ABG 7.22/68/44; will treat accordingly	Acute respiratory failure, acidosis
Will rehydrate patient	Dehydration
BP 70/40 on dopamine for support	Shock or septic shock
No overt CHF; will continue lasix and digoxin	Chronic systolic cHF
Unable to void; cathed for 600 mL	Acute urinary retention
↓K; give 3 runs of IV KCl	Hypokalemia

Table 2. Triad of Pneumonia Diagnosis Related Groups

MS-DRG	Description	Weight	*Payment
193	Pneumonia with MCC	1.4378	$7189
194	Pneumonia with CC	0.9976	$4988
195	Pneumonia w/o CC/MCC	0.7095	$3548

* Assumes a base rate equal to the national average of approximately $5000.

a list of important secondary diagnoses, termed complications/co-morbidities and major complications/co-morbidities (cc's and mcc's). A relative weight is assigned to each DRG and is directly proportional to the hospital's payment through Medicare Part A (see Table 2). A patient admitted for pneumonia complicated by hyponatremia as a secondary diagnosis, for example, would group to DRG 194, while a co-morbid stage 3 sacral pressure ulcer, present on admission, would group to DRG 193. Failing to correctly document the latter would result in a 50% lower payment to the hospital. In addition, the case mix index (CMI) would be 50% lower (CMI being the average of the relative weights of a sample of DRGs). Had the pressure ulcer developed during the admission, it would not have been eligible as an mcc. If there wasn't a 2nd mcc, then the DRG would group to the lower-weighted DRGs.

APR-DRG

In addition to sometimes serving as cc's and mcc's in the MS-DRG algorithm, secondary diagnoses are important to document because they are also used when data are "severity-adjusted." Using APR-DRG (All Patient Refined), patients are classified into one of four severity of illness (SOI) scores (1–4 corresponding to minor, moderate, major and extreme). This SOI score is then used to calculate an expected mortality for a group of hospital patients, which is used to calculate a mortality index (actual/expected mortality), which is preferably < 1. In most *US News* and *World Report* rankings of top US hospitals, for example, the mortality index accounts for 1/3 of the score.

Satisfaction Surveys

Increasing attention is also being paid to customer service and perceived quality. HCAHPS (Hospital Consumer Assessment of Healthcare Providers and Systems) is a national survey in the US that asks Medicare patients about their experiences during a recent hospital stay. The results are now publicly-reported on its website www.hospitalcompare.hhs.gov, including a question asking whether a patient's doctor "always" communicated well.

Medical Necessity

Recovery Audit Contractor (RAC)

Commercial payers and government regulators are focusing more attention than ever before on evaluating the medical necessity of delivered healthcare services, with the primary intent to avoid payments for medically unnecessary services. Hospitals face the brunt of this scrutiny, with the massive federal RAC (Recovery Audit Contractor) program incentivized to recoup overpayments through a contingency fee contract. This means that hospitalists must be careful to clearly document the clinical rationale for the reason for admission and continued hospitalization. Short stays are a major audit target, the argument being that the patient may have been able to be safely cared for at a lower acuity level setting. For example, a patient admitted for pneumonia who is treated with a dose of IV antibiotics and discharged the following day to complete a course of oral antibiotics may or may not have required hospitalization. Clinical documentation of the various patient-specific risk factors, such as hypoxemia, co-morbid chronic systolic heart failure, other chronic advanced stage medical conditions, and/or a high pneumonia severity index (PSI) score is essential in order to justify the appropriateness of the hospitalization.

Concurrent Review

Commercial insurance companies in the US typically require prompt notification of admission of their members and have a concurrent review process where case managers provide information (based on what clinicians write) about the patient's condition and need for hospitalization to obtain authorization (i.e. "if what you say turns out to be so, we will approve payment for the admission"). Sometimes, this requires the physician to participate in a telephonic peer-to-peer clinical review with the commercial insurance medical director.

Retrospective Denial

Programs such as the RAC, and other audits (Office of the Inspector General, Justice Department, and others) involve issuance of medical necessity denials after discharge, requiring hospitals to go back and review the medical record and determine whether or not to appeal the denial. If appealed, the physician is often asked to participate in the process.

Dashboards

Doctors understand data and appreciate a healthy dose of competition. The physician dashboard is a powerful tool that leverages these factors to manage the program, drive improvements, and demonstrate effectiveness.

Dashboard data can be tracked on a monthly basis, shared both individually and in aggregate, and may include:

- Productivity measures such as discharge volume and RVUs (relative value units) based on level of professional billing.
- Efficiency measures such as observed/expected LOS and discharge order time.
- Utilization measures such as medical necessity denial and one-day stay rates and direct hospital costs.
- Satisfaction measures such as patient and referring clinician satisfaction scores.
- Quality measures such as re-admission and mortality rates.

Hospitalists should work with hospital leadership to carefully select the most appropriate measures and determine how data are defined, collected and reported.[6]

Aligning Interests

In addition to assuming leadership roles in care quality, hospitalist programs are in a unique position to leverage their growth and diverse skill sets with hospital administration in a number of ways. For example, hospitalists can often best serve as the physician advisor in utilization management, a required role in Medicare's conditions of participation, ensuring the appropriate utilization of resources for Medicare patients.

A physician champion is also needed in hospitals' clinical documentation improvement programs to ensure accurate and comprehensive documentation and coding. A physician advisor with experience and credibility amongst the clinical staff is critical to the program's success, which is typically accompanied by a sizable return on investment for the hospital.

A third key role often best filled by a hospitalist is that of the physician champion for the Health Information Management (coding) department, where a physician with a deep familiarity with hospital care assists with insurance company and government DRG denials. Similar to medical necessity denials described above, these denials involve the allegation of a coding error, typically a diagnosis code that was included without supporting clinical documentation. By removing the code, the DRG is often changed to a lower-weighted one. The physician champion can assist in appealing these denials, educating coders about the clinical context of the charts they are abstracting, and educating physicians about the relationship between documentation, coding, billing, and publicly-reported quality data.

References

1. http://www.ama-assn.org/amednews/2009/09/07/bise0910.htm Hospital profit margins improving. A study shows that fewer institutions are in the red and that cash reserves are increasing. By Victoria Stagg Elliott. AMD news staff. *Posted Sept. 10, 2009.*
2. Jencks SF, Williams MV, Coleman EA. (2009). Rehospitalizations among Patients in the Medicare Fee-for-Service Program. *N Engl J Med* 360(14): 1418–1428.
3. Care Transitions Program http://www.caretransitions.org. Eric A. Coleman, MD, MPH. The Division of Health Care Policy and Research 13611 East Colfax Avenue, Suite 100 Aurora, CO 80045–5701.
4. Project RED (Re-Engineered Discharge) http://www.bu.edu/fammed/projectred/index.html. Brian Jack, MD Principal Investigator Brian.Jack@bmc.org
5. Project BOOST (Better Outcomes for Older adults through Safe Transitions) http://www.hospitalmedicine.org/ResourceRoomRedesign/RR_CareTransitions/CT_Home.cfm Mark V. Williams, MD, FHM Principal Investigator Advisory Board Co-Chair Professor & Chief, Division of Hospital Medicine Northwestern University Feinberg School of Medicine Chicago, IL BOOST@hospitalmedicine.org
6. Measuring Hospitalist Performance: Metrics, Reports, and Dashboards. Society of Hospital Medicine's Benchmarks Committee White Paper. http://www.hospitalmedicine.org

Chapter 14

Inpatient Documentation and Coding

Steve K. Sigworth, and Ira M. Helenius**

Key Pearls

- Medical necessity should always drive documentation and coding.
- Coding and documentation rules are interpreted differently at different institutions. When needed, an institution's compliance office can be contacted to determine institution-specific rules.
- A chief complaint is required at each coding level, and if it is missing; the note will not meet the requirements of any level.
- Initial visits level 2 and 3 must have a complete history component, which requires: 4+ HPI, 10+ ROS and 3 PFSH.
- No ROS is required for discharge day services or level 1 subsequent visit; all others require a ROS.

Introduction

One difficult aspect of inpatient medicine is the practice of coding and billing for the services provided. Unfortunately, the instructions for coding and billing set forth in the United States by the Center for Medicare and Medicaid Services (CMS) are vague and unintuitive, leading to significant complexity associated with these codes. Furthermore, coding is

*Mount Sinai School of Medicine, New York, NY.

generally NOT taught during residency and must be learned quickly in the first weeks of becoming an attending physician.

This brief chapter is designed to explain the basic concepts of documentation and coding utilizing regulations for coding promoted by CMS in their 1995 and 1997 guidelines. Importantly, variations of interpretation of these guidelines exist between hospitals, states and regions. It is important to become familiar with an organization's compliance department and review their interpretations of the guidelines. This will enable adherence to their interpretation of the CMS rules and allow for correct documentation and coding.

Hospitalist Coding

Reimbursements for hospital services are divided into two categories. The first is the "facility" fee. This is typically based on a Diagnosis-related Group (DRG) payment, which is determined upon a review of the medical record and procedural services after discharge. The second is the "professional" fee. This fee is for services rendered by the physician during hospitalization and is determined by reference to the physician's progress notes. These notes are assigned an Evaluation and Management (E&M) code depending on the complexity of the service rendered.

CMS requires that "medical necessity" drive each E&M code. This means that one should only perform and document in a note those services that are medically necessary for the patient. As the rules surrounding documentation become more familiar, medical complexity will indeed be the driver behind the determination of the correct code for professional services.

There are three basic categories of E&M codes used during a hospitalization: Initial Visit Codes (99221, 99222, 99223); Subsequent Visit Codes (99231, 99232, 99233); and Discharge Day Codes (99238, 99239). The exact code used for the former two are typically chosen based on the complexity of the patient's problem, while the discharge day code is time-based.

Documenting E&M Codes for Initial and Subsequent Visits

Medical documentation notes are made up of four components:

- Chief Complaint
- History
- Physical Exam
- Medical Decision Making

Chief Complaint

The Chief Complaint is typically the medical condition or symptoms that necessitated the admission. Importantly, the chief complaint is required on every note for which a bill is submitted.

History

The History component has three elements:

- History of Present Illness (HPI)
- Review of Systems (ROS)
- Past Family, Social History (PFSH)

The **HPI** contains the descriptors that pertain to the context of the Chief Complaint. Examples include timing, location, duration, quality, context, severity, modifying factors and associated signs and symptoms. To meet the requirement for any Initial Visit Code, at least four of these descriptors must be documented.

The **ROS** is a query of signs/symptoms of 14 recognized body systems. The highest level ROS requires documentation of at least 10 of these systems. The systems include:

- Constitution (fever/weight loss)
- Eyes
- Ears, Nose, Mouth, Throat

- Cardiovascular
- Respiratory
- Gastrointestinal
- Genitourinary
- Musculoskeletal
- Skin/Breast
- Neurological
- Psychiatric
- Endocrine
- Heme/Lymph
- Allergy/Immunology

The **PFSH** contains information pertaining to past medical, family and social history. To meet the higher level initial visit codes (99222 and 99223), all three must be documented.

Physical Exam

There are two options for documentation of the physical exam as set forth by CMS: the 1995 rules and the 1997 rules. In both sets of rules, the physical exam can be documented using 12 body systems. The 1995 rules are often more easily applicable to a general exam. Although there is much variation, most compliance departments agree that the highest level exam (comprehensive exam) includes at least eight body systems. The body systems are:

- Constitutional (Vital Signs, general)
- Eyes
- Ears, Nose, Mouth, Throat
- Cardiovascular
- Respiratory
- Gastrointestinal
- Genitourinary
- Musculoskeletal
- Skin

- Neurological
- Psychiatric
- Heme/Lymph/Immunology

Medical Decision Making

There are three elements of **Medical Decision Making**, but only two of the three need to be achieved to reach each Medical Decision Making level:

- Diagnoses: Number of diagnoses or treatment options
- Data: Amount/complexity of reviewed information
- Risk: Morbidity/mortality

The **diagnosis** element is the number of documented diagnoses**.** New and worsening problems are given two or more points, whereas existing or stable problems count as one point. A problem is considered new for billing purposes if it is new to the hospitalist's group, even if the diagnosis is not new to the patient. This is important when determining the code for admission notes. For example, when patient is admitted for cellulitis, stable congestive heart failure would be considered a new diagnosis and count as three points.

The **data** element pertains to the number of data points reviewed or ordered.

Data Points

- Laboratory (includes pathology)
- Radiology
- Cardiopulmonary diagnostics
- Independent interpretation of diagnostic/radiology test
- Communication with other MD regarding the patient
- Obtaining history from someone other than the patient
- Summarizing old records

The overall **risk** is determined by the highest level of risk in one of three categories (Table 1) and is assigned a level of Low, Moderate or High. CMS has published a comprehensive risk table.[1]

Table 1 Examples from CMS Risk Table

	Low Risk	Moderate Risk	High Risk
Presenting Problem	One stable chronic illness or an uncomplicated acute illness	One or more chronic illnesses with mild exacerbation or an undiagnosed new problem with uncertain prognosis	An acute or chronic illness with severe exacerbation or medical severity that may be life threatening
Diagnostic Procedure	Non-cardiac imaging with contrast	Cardiac stress testing	Diagnostic endoscopy with risk factors
Management Options	Over-the-counter drugs	Prescription drug managements	Parenteral controlled substances

One can argue that most hospitalizations are the result of a severe medical condition that may be a threat to life, therefore most initial inpatient visits should qualify as high risk.

Determining Which Code to Use

Once the note has been documented, the appropriate E&M code must be determined. For all notes, a chief complaint or reason for the visit must be documented. For initial visit notes, all three of the other components (History, Physical Exam, Medical Decision Making) of the note are required and therefore the component with the lowest level determines the code. For subsequent visit notes, only two of the three components are required and therefore the lowest level component can be dropped and the code is determined by the lower of the two remaining components.

Tables 2 and 3 summarize the elements required for initial and subsequent visit notes. The data in these tables are generalizations. An institution's compliance department may have more specific coding tools to help choose coding levels, in particular with respect to the physical exam.

Table 2 Inpatient Initial Visit

	99221	99222	99223
History			
CC	cc	cc	cc
HPI	4	4	4
ROS	Problem pertinent + 2	10	10
PFSH	1	3	3
Physical Exam	Detailed exam	Comprehensive exam	Comprehensive exam
Medical Decision Making (need 2 of 3)			
Diagnoses	1–2	3	4
Data Points	0–2	3	4
Overall Risk	low	mod	high

Documenting E&M Codes for Discharge Day Visits

The discharge day note requires four different components.

- Hospital Course
- Final Examination
- Discharge Medication Reconciliation
- Preparation of discharge records

All the components listed above must be described when documenting a discharge note. If the time required for the physician to complete these components was 30 minutes or less, then code 99238 should be used. If the time required was greater than 30 minutes, code 99239 should be used and the time spent documented in the note.

Documenting E&M Codes for Consultation Visits

Before 2010, an additional set of consult codes (99251–5) was used in the United States to document new consult visits. However, as of 2010, CMS

Table 3 Inpatient Established Visit

	99231	99232	99233
History			
CC	cc	cc	cc
HPI	1–3	1–3	4
ROS	0	1	2+
PFSH	0	0	0
Physical Exam	Problem focused exam	Expanded problem Focused exam	Detailed exam
Medical Decision Making			
(need 2 of 3)			
Diagnoses	1–2	3	4
Data Points	0–2	3	4
Overall Risk	low	mod	high

no longer recognizes these codes, though the codes are still recognized by some carriers. For Medicare, all initial hospital codes now require the accepting physician to attach modifier "AI" to their initial hospital code (99221–3), and consultant visits for these patients now require a new visit code without the AI modifier. The rules regarding consultative codes are detailed by CMS.[2]

Conclusion

Do not despair. The process of first determining the code, then documenting only the necessary components to meet the level of that code, becomes easier and more intuitive with practice and experience. It remains extremely important to understand the institutional interpretation of the CMS guidelines and be familiar with the institution's compliance office to better incorporate specific documentation requirements when needed.

For more information access the official CMS Medical Learning Network site: http://www.cms.hhs.gov/MLNEdWebGuide/25_EMDOC.asp

References

1. Center for Medicare and Medicaid Services. Evaluation and management services guide 2006 http://www.cms.hhs.gov/mlnproducts/downloads/eval_mgmt_serv_guide.pdf (see page 20) Accessed April 3, 2011.
2. Center for Medicare and Medicaid Manual System, Subject: Revisions to Consultation Services Payment Policy http://www.cms.gov/manuals/downloads/clm104c12.pdf (see section 30.6.10) Accessed April 3, 2011.

Chapter 15

Non-Physician Practitioners in the Hospital Setting

*Alan S. Briones**

Key Pearls

- Nurse Practitioners (NPs) and Physician Assistants (PAs) are autonomous Non Physician Providers (NPPs) that can deliver high quality patient care in collaboration with physicians.
- Utilization of NPPs is a strategic measure that can increase efficiency and decrease the escalating cost of healthcare.
- The most common barriers and impediments to a successful NPPs-Physician collaboration in clinical practice are a physician's lack of knowledge of NPPs role and scope of practice, poor physician attitude towards NPPs, and patient and family reluctance of receiving NPP care.
- There is a growing recognition of the importance of the role played by NPPs among patients and physicians.
- The three major types of NPPs-Hospitalist Practice model are academic center model, community hospital model and private physician model.

Definition of Non-Physician Practitioners (NPPs)

The term NPPs is loosely defined as practitioners who render care to patients but are not physicians, so consist of a broad category of healthcare practitioners, including Nurse Practitioners (NPs), Physician Assistants

*Mount Sinai School of Medicine, New York, NY, USA.

(PAs), Clinical Psychologists, Clinical Social Workers, Physical and Occupational Therapists, Nurse Midwives, and Speech Language Pathologists. The scope of practice, licensure and credentialing requirements for each NPPs are established by the state laws of the jurisdiction in which the NPPs practice.[1] In many settings, however, the term NPPs is generally used to refer to NPs and PAs, and the collaboration of hospitalists with these practitioners will be the focus of this chapter.

In the hospital setting, the NPs/PAs practices have expanded due to regional shortages of physicians, efforts to reduce the cost of healthcare, and decrease in graduate medical education funding. With the limitation of work hours of interns and house staff physicians, more NPs and PAs are expected to assume patient care responsibilities.

Quality and Cost-Effectiveness of NPs and PAs Care

NPs and PAs are autonomous high quality alternative healthcare providers who practice in all the specialties of Medicine and Surgery, and in the ambulatory care, acute and subspecialty care, emergency room and long-term care settings. For the hospitalist, the physician-NPP collaboration is a widely used model of care in the hospital setting and has the potential to enhance efficiency and reduce costs.

Research has shown that NPs and PAs practices have been shown to demonstrate patient outcomes that were similar compared to physicians.[2–5] In a study of five primary care clinics, Mundinger[2] and colleagues showed that in patients who were randomly assigned to either NPs or physicians, at the end of six months and one year, no significant differences were found in the patient health status, health service utilization, hemoglobin A1C for patients with diabetes, peak flow for patients with asthma, and patient satisfaction scores.

In a comparison of eight quality measures of HIV care provided by NPs and PAs versus physicians,[4] six of the eight quality measures did not statistically differ between NPs/ PAs and either infectious disease specialists or generalist HIV experts. Adjusted rates of purified protein derivative testing and Pap smears were statistically significantly higher for NPs and PAs than for physicians. Furthermore, NPs and PAs had statistically significantly higher performance scores than generalist non-HIV experts on six of the eight quality measures.

Roy[5] demonstrated that among hospitalized medical patients, the quality and efficiency of patient care on a PAs/Hospitalist service were comparable to those of the traditional house staff services. No differences were seen in inpatient mortality, ICU transfers, readmissions, patient satisfaction and length of stay.

In a recent study that compared patient satisfaction with care provided by NPs, PAs, and physicians in the Veteran's Health Systems, the satisfaction scores increased when more NPs provided care, but were slightly higher or remain the same when PAs were involved.[6]

The cost of healthcare in the United States of America is one of the highest in the world, surpassing $2.3 trillion in 2008.[7] The use of NPPs is a strategic cost cutting measure. Overall, the annual salary and cost of education of NPPs are lower as compared with those for physicians. In surveys carried out 2009, the estimated annual salary of hospitalists is $215,000[8]; $90,900 for physician assistants[9]; and $90,200 for nurse practitioners.[10]

In a 2004 study of 26 primary care practices with a volume of approximately two million visits annually by 206 providers, the total labor costs per visit were lower in practices where NPs and PAs were utilized.[11] In a three-year analysis of the healthcare costs associated with an on-site NP in a primary care practice, savings were estimated at $1,089,466 per year.[12] Furthermore, the NPs-Hospitalist team was associated with decreased length of stay and improved hospital profit as compared with the "usual care" by a hospitalist.[13]

NPPs Roles and Responsibilities

NPs and PAs have expanded their roles and responsibilities over time. PAs were historically utilized and trained in a military setting, assisting surgeons in the care of wounded and injured soldiers. NPs were born from highly skilled and clinically experienced nurses who have been mentored by physicians during the 1950s and early 1960s to augment the need for primary care services in medically underserved areas.[14]

The primary role of NPs and PAs within hospitals is to assist the hospitalist and other attending physicians in the management of hospitalized patients. During the first few years of employment, recent graduates traditionally work under the close direct supervision of a physician. Attending physicians should be readily available to answer questions and provide backup. The attending physicians should also be actively involved in the initial care, management and treatment decisions and plans for discharge of the patient, particularly early in hospitalization and while the patients are unstable. However, as the NPPs gain more clinical experience and acumen, they typically become more independent and autonomous.

NPPs may work independently and manage hospitalized patients on their own, with appropriate consultations with physicians about complex cases. Alternatively, NPPs may work closely with the physician and be primarily responsible for specific tasks assigned to them (e.g. follow-up of test results, consulting specialists, implementing discharge planning).

NPPs are also often utilized to help provide 24-hour coverage to the critical needs of hospitalized patients, particularly when fewer or no physicians are available in-house.

Autonomy and Scope of Practice

NPs are registered nurses with an advanced master's degree and clinical training to provide preventive and acute care in the hospital. NPs perform services as authorized by a state's nurse practice act which varies from state-to-state, with some states having independent practice for NPs (not requiring any physician involvement), and some requiring a collaborative practice agreement with a physician.

NPs Responsibilities Include[15]:

- Taking health histories and performing complete physical examinations
- Diagnosing and treating common acute and chronic diseases
- Interpreting laboratory results and diagnostic tests
- Prescribing medications

- Rendering patient education
- Preventive counseling on medical care and health maintenance
- Referring patients to subspecialty care when indicated.

Similarly, PAs have advanced education and clinical training and experience to diagnose and treat acute and chronic illnesses. They always work as members of a physician-directed team. Their scope of practice is determined by four parameters: education and experience; state law; facility policy; and the supervising physician's delegating decisions.[16] PAs roles are varied and depend on the institution's needs.

General Types of NPPs Models of Care[17]

NPPs in Academic Centers

The NPPs work in teams, with ratios varying from 2–3 NPPs to 1 physician. This practice model is similar to resident/attending model where an NPPs act as the primary provider, working very autonomously and independently in medical decision making. Besides admitting and following up on patients, writing notes and placing orders, interpreting lab tests, and communicating with other providers, consultants and families, they also perform simple bedside procedures such as thoracentesis, paracentesis and arterial blood gas, etc. The NPPs communicate frequently with the physician who is available constantly for consultation, whenever necessary. The NPPs may also be integrated in a team with house staff residents/physicians and performs the duties of an intern. Encounters are usually billed as shared visits.

NPPs in Small Community Hospital

The NPPs collaborate with the physician, and patient encounters are jointly done. The NPPs responsibilities depend on NPPs comfort and experience. The billing is done by the physicians under their provider numbers for 100% reimbursement. The average number of patient visits or census is low (less than 10 per day). NPPs are less autonomous in medical decision making.

NPPs in Private Physician Hospitalist Service

NPPs are usually employed by the hospital and are supervised by the "Hospitalist group," but they provide care for patients admitted to the "Private Attending Service." The private physicians are mainly responsible for their patients and NPPs services are strategically used by them when they are in their private offices during the day. The NPPs role is collaborative. Billing is done by the private physicians.

Potential Pitfalls of Collaboration

The most common barriers and impediments to a successful NPPs or PAs–Physician collaboration in clinical practice are:[18]

- Physician's lack of knowledge of NPs/PAs role and scope of practice
- Poor Physician attitudes towards NPs/PAs
- Poor communication and lack of respect
- Patient and family reluctance of NPs/PAs care

Continuing physician education and awareness through special sessions in scientific meetings, in hospital board meetings, and potentially requiring this for state board licensure or Hospital Medicine board certification are some means of overcoming these barriers. Moreover, resident house staff physicians are more exposed and educated early during residency training regarding the roles of NPs and PAs in patient care. To improve patient and family acceptance of NPPs, physicians can help by educating them on the NPPs role, responsibilities and scope of practice.

Reimbursement and Billing

As recognition of their autonomy, NPs and PAs services are reimbursed by Medicare in three ways:

1) NPPs may bill directly for their services under the physician fee schedule and their employers receive a percentage (typically 85%) of the fee schedule payment.

2) NPPs services may be billed incident to physician services, in which case the physicians bill for the services at 100 percent of the fee schedule payment, even though NPP provided the services.

NPPs services may be included in the payment bundle for services provided in hospitals or skilled nursing facilities.[19]

References

1. Benesch K, Morris D , Hyman D. (2010) Non-Physician Practitioners: A bridge to the future of healthcare. Health Lawyers Weekly. March 19, 2010 Vol. VIII Issue 11.
2. Mundinger MO, Kane RL, Lenz ER, *et al.* (2000) Primary outcomes in patients treated by nurse practitioners or physicians. *JAMA* **283**: 59–68.
3. Horrocks S, Anderson E, Salisbury C. (2002) Systematic review of whether nurse practitioners working in primary care can provide care equivalent to doctors. *BMJ* **324**: 819–823.
4. Wilson IB, Landon BE, Hirschhorn LR, *et al.* (2005) Quality of HIV care provided by nurse practitioner, physician assistants and physicians. *Ann Intern Med* **143**: 729–736.
5. Roy CL, Liang CL, Lund M, *et al.* (2008) Implementation of a physician assistant/hospitalist service in an academic medical center: Impact on efficiency and patient outcomes. *J Hosp Med* **3**: 361–368.
6. Budzi D, Lurie S, Singh K, Hooker R. (2010) Veterans' Perceptions of Care by Nurse Practitioners, Physician Assistants, and Physicians: A Comparison From Satisfaction Surveys. *J Am Acad Nurse Pract* **22**: 170–176.
7. Centers for Medicare and Medicaid Services, Office of the Actuary, National Health Statistics Group, National Health Care Expenditures Data, January 2010. Retrieved March 2010 at http://www.cms.gov/nationalhealthexpenddata/01_overview.asp?
8. 2010 SHM/MGMA salary compensation survey for adult hospitalist medicine (data based 2009). Retrieved March 2011 at http://thehappyhospitalist.blogspot.com/2010/09/hospitalist-salary-compensation-survey.html

9. Best Jobs in America-CNNmoney.com survey 2009. Retrieved March 2011 at http://money.cnn.com/magazines/moneymag/bestjobs/2009/snapshots/2.html
10. American Academy of Nurse Practitioners (2010). Documentation of quality nurse practitioner care. Retrieved March 2011 at www.anp.org.
11. Roblin OW, Howard DH, Becker ER, *et al.* (2004) Use of midlevel practitioners to achieve labor cost savings in the primary care practice of an MCO. *Health Services Research* **39**: 607–626.
12. Chenoweth D, Martin N, Pankowski J, *et al.* (2008) Nurse Practitioner Services: Three-Year Impact on Health Care Costs. *Journal of Occupational & Environmental Medicine* **50**: 1293–1298.
13. Cowan M, Shapiro M, Hays R, *et al.* (2006) The Effect of a Multidisciplinary Hospitalist/Physician and Advanced Practice Nurse Collaboration on Hospital Costs. *Journal of Nursing Administration* **36**: 79–85.
14. Baer ED. (1999) Philosophical and historical bases of advanced practice nursing roles. In: Mezey MD, McGivern DO, eds. Nurses, nurse practitioners: Evolution to advanced practice. 3rd ed. New York: Springer.
15. NP scope of Practice: American College of Nurse Practitioners. Retrieved March 2011 at http://www.acnpweb.org/i4a/pages/index.cfm?pageid=3465
16. PA Scope of Practice. American academy of Physician assistants. Retrieved March 2011 at http://www.aapa.org/advocacy-and-practice-resources/state-government-and-licensing/scope-of-practice.
17. NPP-Society of Hospital Medicine Practice Models. Retrieved June 23, 2011 at http://www.hospitalmedicine.org/AM/Template.cfm?Section=Non_Physician_Providers&Template=/CM/HTMLDisplay.cfm&ContentID=25093
18. Clarin OA. (2007) Strategies to Overcome Barriers to Effective Nurse Practitioner and Physician Collaboration. *Journal for Nurse Practitioners* **3**: 538–548.
19. Medicare payments to Nurse practitioners and Physician assistants. (2002) Retrieved March 2011 at http://www.medpac.gov/documents/jun02_NonPhysPay.pdf

Hospitalist as Educator

Chapter 16

Teaching Tips and Pearls

*Lisa Coplit**

Key Pearls

- Keep teaching relevant for learners and tap into their motivations.
- Teach often in small doses: Two minutes on the go, using the patient as the context, can be more useful than an hour in the classroom.
- When teaching different levels of learners at the same time, try a variety of techniques to make sure everyone is engaged.
- Utilize the five Microskills of Clinical Teaching to ensure an effective teaching encounter when time is limited: Get a Commitment, Probe for Supporting Evidence, Teach General Rules, Reinforce What Was Right, Correct Mistakes.
- When giving feedback, remind your learner that your intention is to help them succeed; keep your observations specific, and help create a plan for improvement.

Our role as teachers is a privilege and brings some of the greatest personal rewards to the practice of medicine, yet it can be easy to neglect on a busy inpatient service. This chapter is meant to serve as a primer on clinical teaching, provide straightforward recommendations to enhance effectiveness as a teacher, provide references for more in depth study of teaching, and help make teaching an integral part of daily life in the hospital for busy hospitalists.

*Quinnipiac University School of Medicine, Hamden, CT, USA.

Table 1. General Principles to Maximize Efficiency

Principle	Actions
Make your teaching relevant	1. Diagnose your learner before you teach 2. "Target then Teach" 3. Choose topics that are relevant to the learner's experience, interests, and knowledge gaps 4. Use cases and problems that help solve real clinical problems 5. Have learners identify their own learning needs (self-directed learning)
Use small "Teachable Moments" frequently	1. Discuss 1–2 key teaching points just before, during, or after seeing a patient 2. Model (demonstrate and explain) an exam technique in a patient with clinical findings 3. Use the Microskills of Clinical Teaching — see below 4. Give learners opportunities for skill practice in your presence and provide feedback 5. Ask learners to reflect on their own practice

There are two overarching concepts that can help teaching to be more efficient, deliberate, and effective (see Table 1). One simple key to teaching in any setting, and the backbone of adult learning theory, is to keep your teaching relevant for your learners.[1,2] Relevance can mean different things, such as needing information to take care of a patient, academic interest in the topic, and learning for the boards. Hospitalists are surrounded by what is most relevant — acutely ill patients with a variety of diseases; immediately necessary treatments; complex social issues that need your intervention in a matter of days; ethical dilemmas, medical systems issues and errors; etc. Osler knew this without the benefit of studying learning theory: "In what may be called the natural method of teaching, the student begins with the patient, continues with the patient, and ends his studies with the patient, using books and lectures as tools, as means to an end.[3]" However, teachers may be tempted to go to their comfort zone and teach what they know, rather than what the learner needs to know. This approach robs teachers of time because they may be teaching what learners feel is already obvious to them, or teaching so far above the learners' level that they cannot connect to the content.

To ensure that the time you spend teaching is efficient and relevant, take the time to find out what your learner wants and needs to learn. Irby and Wilkerson call this timesaving rule "Target then teach"[4] where the teacher uses questions and observations to direct his or her teaching. Begin by asking questions to help you determine what your learners already know: "Why do you think he has pneumonia?" "Have you ever seen the effects of hyperkalemia on an ECG?" "What is the most appropriate next test?" Next, conduct a 2-minute observation of your learner interacting with the patient. Inform the patient and the learner that you are briefly observing for teaching purposes and debrief afterwards. Lastly, direct your teaching based upon what you have learned. This intuitive 3-step process will help you "diagnose" your learner's needs, and give you the information you need to choose among the countless possible topics that arise each day with each learner.

Second, consider that good teaching can happen in small doses. The belief that teaching requires an hour in the classroom or at the bedside during a formal teaching session can inhibit us from grasping the *teachable moments*. Most clinicians remember being on-call as a medical student, busily moving through the hallways on the way to the emergency room to see a new patient with their resident, and reviewing the differential diagnosis of chest pain or the meaning of pre-test probability in a patient who may have had a pulmonary embolism. For many students and residents, these exciting but brief teaching moments are the most memorable and effective because they have immediate relevance to their patients and the learning is based on their direct experience.[5,6] Two minutes on the go may be more meaningful than an hour in the classroom because contextual learning deepens learning experiences.[7]

The clinical teacher's role is critical because experiential learning depends heavily on the facilitation of learning by the teacher and not simply the exposure to patients.[4,6–8] As an example, after evaluating a patient whose labs just returned and reveal evidence of a microangiopathic hemolytic anemia and thrombocytopenia, the teacher may ask the team, "Let's review the five criteria for TTP and decide whether she meets the criteria."

These two principles can help you translate learning theory into effective practical teaching. Keep your teaching relevant and take advantage of small "teachable moments" frequently.

Tips for Teaching that Won't Slow you Down (Too Much)

While every clinical setting could be described as busy, the inpatient setting usually adds acuity and increased severity of a patient's illness to the equation, making the time pressures uniquely challenging to the hospitalist physician.[9] Below are some teaching techniques that can help you maximize teaching for your learners despite the pressures of time, and take advantage of the teaching opportunities on the wards (see also Table 2).[7,9–13]

Teaching Different Levels of Learners

Teaching different levels of learners simultaneously is the classic model of inpatient teaching. It is also one that can prove to be the most daunting to faculty who are eagerly trying to ensure that all learners on the team are engaged and actively learning. Some of the methods that your best clinical teachers used are undoubtedly those recommended in the literature.[9,11,13,14] While considering the following options, try using more than one method. While it may be easier and more comfortable using one teaching method, changing teaching formats keeps you and your learners more engaged, and reaches different types of learners.

Suggestions:

1. Explain how you will be conducting rounds and your expectations. For example:
   - *Everyone will be involved so that we're all contributing and learning from each other.*
   - *I'll be asking lots of questions and it's ok to be wrong, but I expect you to try to reason through the questions or think about how to find the answer.*

Table 2. Tips for Teaching with Limited Time

Teaching Technique	Actions	Example
Orient your learners on Day 1 and establish goals (Saves time later)	1. Explain the daily schedule 2. Introduce team to each other, nurses, etc. 3. Clarify your expectations for rounds, presentations, write-ups 4. Ask learners for their goals ⟹ 5. Share your learning goals	• *Are there any particular topics that we should focus on this month?* • *What types of experiences have been most useful to you in attending rounds (bedside rounds, review of radiology studies, etc?*
Create a productive learning environment (i.e. A stimulating learning setting where learners feel comfortable to verbalize their ideas and knowledge gaps)	1. Introduce yourself and others 2. Use learners' names 3. Encourage participation (invite learner's opinions and questions, ask ⟹ questions, praise independent thinking, state your desire for participation) 4. Engage your learners/audience: Speak clearly, make eye contact, use an animated voice, avoid sitting/standing in one place 5. Acknowledge your own limitations ⟹	*Do you have any questions about our session yesterday?* *I also had trouble learning to diagnose acid-base problems. Let me show you what helped me.*
Create interest in the topic	1. Show enthusiasm for your topic and learners a. Why do you like it? b. Why did you choose to teach it? ⟹ c. How is it relevant to them?	*Acid-base problems are my favorite topic to teach — they affect almost every patient in the hospital and figuring out the problems is fun once you understand the basics.*
Center the teaching around the learner's needs	1. Take time to diagnose your learner before you teach 2. Choose topics that are relevant to the ⟹ learner's experience, interests and knowledge gaps	*Jen, since you're going into OB/Gyn, you will undoubtedly see patients with heart failure. Let's focus on the physical exam findings today.*

(*Continued*)

Table 2 (*Continued*)

Teaching Technique	Actions	Example
Let others help you teach	1. Use consultants' expertise (include teaching about how to ask a clinical question) 2. Ask all learners on the team to teach 3. Search the literature as a team during a teaching session	*Mike, why don't you look up the diagnostic criteria for SLE, and Maria, can you look up the recent article on early vs. late initiation of dialysis on patient survival to help us decide whether we should call renal before discharging your patient?*
Use modeling to demonstrate skills	1. Demonstrate a physical exam skills 2. Demonstrate communication skills, history taking, or patient counseling skills 3. Demonstrate procedural skills 4. Demonstrate written communication skills (note writing, consult writing)	*I want you to watch how I break bad news to this patient and let's talk afterwards about what you observed and how it went.*
Verbalize your thought process	1. Think out loud to explain your reasoning process for diagnostic or treatment decisions	*I'm debating whether this patient needs a cardiac catheterization or continued medical management.*
	2. Include the alternatives that you are considering and why you are excluding them	*His angina is stable and relatively well controlled on meds, but the stress test suggests the area of ischemia is larger. Let's call cardiology to evaluate him for a cath.*

(*Continued*)

Table 2. (*Continued*)

Teaching Technique	Actions	Example
Create Teaching Scripts	1. Mini-lectures (5–10 min) on the most common topics (Anemia, hyponatremia, acute renal failure, etc) 2. Focus on diagnosis or management 3. Use them as a teachable moment when it's relevant to a patient's case	
Extend the case	1. Ask "What if…" questions 2. Illustrate how the context changes the diagnostic possibilities and teaches clinical reasoning ⇨ 3. Helpful for sign out rounds with housestaff because it can help predict potential unrecognized outcomes	• *What if the patient's creatinine was 3 instead of 1?* • *What if the patient was 60 instead of 20?* • *What if you start treatment and the patient starts seizing?* • *What will you do if the patient spikes a fever tonight? Why?*
Ask higher level (reasoning) questions	1. Requires your learners to analyze data and apply information, unlike a recall (pimping/factual) question 2. Allows you to evaluate your learners clinical reasoning skills ⇨ 3. Demonstrates to learners the types of questions to be asking themselves	• *Why do you think this patient has jaundice?* • *Why did you rule out hepatitis?* • *How do you treat heart failure in a patient with aortic stenosis?*

(*Continued*)

Table 2. (*Continued*)

Teaching Technique	Actions	Example
Teach and role model other important topics that impact learners and patients	1. Address the hidden curriculum *The customs and unspoken actions that learners experience* 2. Functioning on the wards *Time management, use of technology, relationships with other healthcare providers* 3. Professionalism *Your responsibilities to patients and colleagues, and your attitudes and behaviors* 4. Empathy 5. Effective use of the literature 6. Communication skills, including *oral and written presentations*	

- *Explain how you will ask questions and who is responsible for answering the questions.*
- *Stop me if you have any questions.*

2. Ask level appropriate questions to all — Start with the most junior learners (differential diagnosis, pathophysiology) and increase the "clinical difficulty" of the questions with each level of learner (advanced differential diagnosis for interns and management, advanced management and recent literature for residents). If a senior learner is not able to answer a question, avoid allowing a more junior learner to attempt it because this may embarrass the resident and affect group dynamics.
3. Consider aiming high — Target your teaching to the intern and resident level which allows more junior learners to see what they will eventually be expected to know, but allow junior learners to ask clarifying questions.
4. Have them teach each other — Vary how often, how much, and who will teach.

5. Make the resident your "teaching assistant" — Many are very up to date on recent literature and subspecialty medicine.
6. Let the team work together to guide the discussion — Generate a list of problems/learning issues from a case presentation and allow the team to decide which you will discuss.
7. When the team is separated (such as post-call), take advantage of that time and dedicate some teaching to the level of learners left on the team.
8. Remember that everyone needs to learn and review the basics — The most common medical conditions, physical findings, diagnosis and treatment. The techniques above can help to ensure active learning for all, but don't hesitate to teach "bread and butter" medicine.

The Microskills of Clinical Teaching

The Microskills of Clinical Teaching is a practical, well studied, well known, learner-centered teaching model designed for time-limited clinical teaching settings.[15–17] It is also called the One Minute Preceptor referring to the ability of the attending to use five short steps to facilitate a quick, yet effective teaching encounter. It is most useful after a case presentation and allows the teacher to evaluate the learner's level and knowledge, teach important concepts, and provide meaningful feedback to learners.

Example of the Microskills in Action

A medicine resident covering medical consults presents a patient to the medicine consultation attending:

Mrs. M. is a 62-year-old woman with diabetes and hypertension who is post-op day #3 from a right fem-pop bypass. Her nurse called me at 7 am today because she was complaining of heartburn. She said that she felt burning and pressure in her lower chest for an hour and did have some nausea. She doesn't have any cardiac history, has a history of GERD, and had some relief with Maalox. Her BP was a little elevated at 145/90, HR

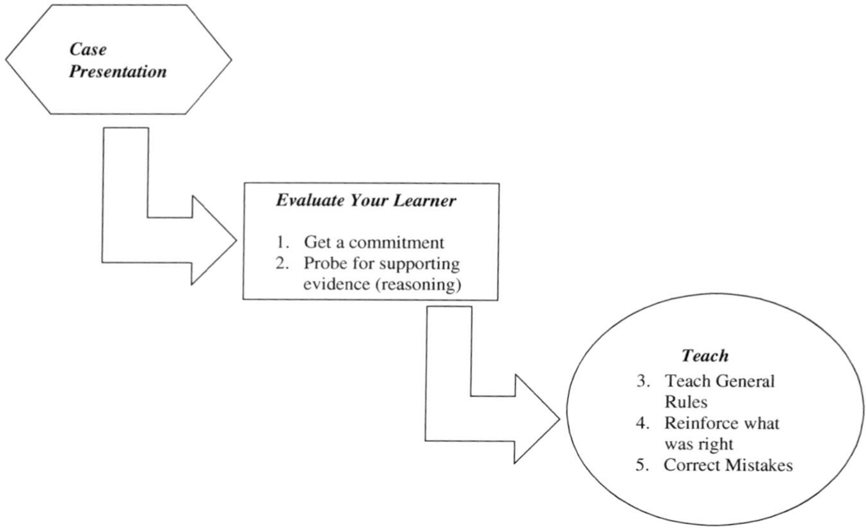

85, and the rest of her vitals were normal. Her exam was unremarkable and her ECG was unchanged. Her labs are pending.

1. *Get a Commitment*

Attending: *What do you think is going on?*
Resident: *I think it's probably GERD, but I'm not sure.*

2. *Probe for Supporting Evidence*

Attending: *What led you to that conclusion?*
Resident: *She said that this feels similar to her usual heartburn which is the most compelling piece of history to me and her ECG is unchanged.*

Attending: *Do you feel comfortable ruling out a cardiac cause of her pain?*

Resident: *That is next on my differential. As I said, her ECG is unchanged but she has LVH and some flipped t waves at baseline. Her pre-op stress test was unremarkable, but it wasn't diagnostic because she's on a beta blocker. She has a family history of CAD and she is diabetic, so I realize that she can have an atypical presentation, but I still think this is GERD.*

3. *Teach General Rules* (Focus on one to two general concepts that can be applied to other patients in the future)

Attending: *You're probably right, but I'm concerned about her risk factors. Each time I create a differential diagnosis, I try to include the most likely and the most concerning possibilities. The fact that she has known vascular disease means that we can assume she also has CAD, so she is at a fairly high risk of having perioperative ischemia after vascular surgery. I think our suspicion is high enough to at least warrant checking her cardiac enzymes and a follow-up ECG.*

4. *Reinforce What was Right*

Attending: *You did an excellent job of distilling a complicated case into a succinct and logical presentation, and you used all of the information to create a reasonable differential diagnosis.*

5. *Correct Mistakes*

Attending: *The next time you see a patient with postoperative chest pain, especially after vascular surgery, remember to have a low threshold for working up and treating ischemia.*

Pearls for Giving Meaningful Feedback with Less Stress

Regardless of whether evaluations of learners need to be formally documented, feedback is an essential part of teaching that cannot be separated from the learning process. Feedback provides learners with direction, helps them assess whether they are meeting their goals, and provides them with the benefit of your wealth of experience and knowledge to help them achieve their educational goals.[6,18,19] Faculty often forget or avoid giving necessary negative/corrective feedback because it can be time consuming and unpleasant, but there are several guidelines for giving feedback that can make the process more comfortable for the teacher, and more useful for the learner.

Guidelines for Effective Feedback:

1. Commit to a specific date and time to give global feedback with each team of housestaff/students (e.g. one attending rounds at the midpoint and the end).
2. Let your learners know what to expect at the beginning of the rotation:
   - Your goals — You will be basing your feedback upon these goals.
   - Relevance of feedback — Feedback will help them reach their goals and everyone has room for improvement.
   - Your role — To work with them and help them improve (you are their ally).
   - Their role — To assess their own performance, ask for help, discuss their assessment at your formal feedback sessions, and possibly give you feedback.
3. Be specific — Effective feedback explains to the learner what he/she is doing right and what needs improvement.

   Examples of Specific Feedback

   - *It seems that you're having difficulty with organization during the day which is keeping you here late each night.*
   - *Your write-ups are excellent because they are well organized, your HPI tells a logical story and your assessment explains your thought process.*
   - *I'm concerned about your attitude towards the nurses because you often make negative comments about them to your interns.*
   - *I've noticed that the chief complaints in your write-ups often don't address the actual symptoms of the patient at presentation, but rather focus on the first thing the patient says — for instance, for Mr. P who presented with complaints of dizziness and your chief complaint was "my cardiologist told me to come in." It may require using a bit of interpretation. We'll work on this for the next few patients you see until it makes sense.*

- Use the feedback sandwich if it makes you more comfortable (positive, negative positive OR positive negative, action plan), but make sure your message is not lost in the sandwich.
- Ally with your learners:
    - o *I want you to be successful and we'll work on this together.*
    - o *How can I best help you achieve this?*
- Have the learner create a plan for improvement — Ask the learners how you can help them improve but have a plan ready in case they need your help.
    - o *For the next week, lets go over your "To Do List" together right after rounds. The first two days I'll help you prioritize your list, then you will take over and we'll touch base at the end of each day.*

Making Time for Teaching

The most helpful approach is to remember that great teaching occurs in small moments and can be woven into the fabric of your clinical responsibilities. However, it can also be very helpful to plan out protected time for teaching.

Suggestions:

- Plan time for teaching that is sacred (Nothing but a patient emergency will cut it short or interrupt it). Examples:
    - o Attending rounds
    - o 5 minutes at the beginning of work rounds
    - o 5 minutes at the end of work rounds
    - o End of the day (around 4 pm)
    - o 20 minutes on "no admit" days for clinical skill teaching at the bedside
    - o Once a week at lunchtime for everyone on the team to present the topics they researched that week.

- Your big teaching commitments are attending/teaching rounds but consider making your own small commitments. Examples:
    - Teach about one patient per day
    - Ask one higher level (reasoning) question per patient
    - Give one teaching pearl per patient on rounds
    - Prepare 5–8 short teaching scripts (see above) and try to teach each one once per rotation
    - Teach one physical exam skill per day.
- Role model what you expect of your learners.

  Most teaching happens when the teacher is not trying because teachers are incredibly influential role models for their learners. Many clinicians easily recall their best professors as inspiring role models and exceptional caregivers. They often provided valuable insights into the care of patients just by observing them interacting with their patients. Learning in the inpatient setting is a powerful experience and the attitude with which the physician teacher approaches each day and each patient can set the standard for their team.

References

1. Knowles, MS, Holton EF III, an RA. Swanson. (1998) *The Adult Learner*. Gulf Publishing, Houston.
2. Kaufman DM. (2003) ABC of learning and teaching in medicine: Applying educational theory in practice. *BMJ* **326**: 213–216.
3. William O. (2003) The hospital as a college, in Aequanimitas, 315. In: Silverman M, (ed), *The Quotable Osler*. American College of Physicians Pr, Philadelphia.
4. Irby DM, Wilkerson L. (2008) Teaching when time is limited. *BMJ* **336**(7640): 384–7.
5. Kolb D, Fry R. (1975) Towards an applied theory of experiential learning. In: Cooper C, (ed), *Theories of Group Processes*. J Wiley; London, pp. 33–58.

6. Ende J, ed. (2010). *Theory and Practice of Teaching Medicine*. ACP Pr, Philadelphia.
7. Skeff KM, Stratos GA, eds. (2010) *Methods for Teaching Medicine*. ACP Pr, Philadelphia.
8. Wimmers P, Schmidt H and Splinter T. (2006) Influence of clerkship experiences on clinical competence. *Med Educ* **40**: 450–8.
9. Wiese, J, ed. (2010) *Teaching in the Hospital*. ACP Pr, Philadelphia.
10. The Stanford Faculty Development Program in Clinical Teaching Skills, Stanford University, Leland, 1998.
11. Kroenke K. (1992) Attending rounds. *J Gen Int Med* **7**: 68–75.
12. Bowen JL. (2006) Educational strategies to promote clinical diagnostic reasoning. *NEJM* **355**(21): 2217–2225.
13. Weinholtz, D and Edwards, J. (1992) *Teaching During Rounds: A Handbook for Attending Physicians and Residents*. The Johns Hopkins University Press; Baltimore.
14. Detsky AS. (2009) The art of pimping. *JAMA* **301**(13): 1379–1381.
15. Neher JO, Gordon CC, Meyer B and Stevens N. (1992) A five-step "microskills" model of clinical teaching. *J Am Board Family Pract* **5**(4): 419–424.
16. Aagaard E, Teherani A and Irby D. (2004) Effectiveness of the one-minute preceptor model for diagnosing the patient and the learner: Proof of concept. *Acad Med* **79**: 42–9.
17. Furney SL, Orsini AN, Orsetti KE, *et al*. (2001) Teaching the one-minute preceptor. A randomized controlled trial. *J Gen Intern Med* **16**(9): 620–4.
18. Ende J. (1983) Feedback in clinical medical education. *JAMA* **250**: 777–81.
19. Hewson M, Little M. (1998) Giving feedback in medical education: Verification of recommended techniques. *J Gen Intern Med* **13**: 111–6.

Chapter 17

Teaching at the Bedside

Somnath Mookherjee and Brad A. Sharpe*

Key Pearls

- Bedside teaching can be a highly valuable educational experience and is generally well received by patients, learners and teachers.
- Before the bedside teaching session, the teacher should determine the two to three specific teaching goals for the session.
- Before starting, the teacher should explain the goals and structure of the encounter to the learners and patient.
- To stay patient-centered and maximize efficiency, the teacher should ask the patient to try to maintain a list of questions, and if necessary, return after the teaching encounter to address all issues completely.
- After the session, the teacher should provide direct feedback by listing one behavior that the learner did well and should continue and one behavior that the learner should modify or not continue.

Introduction

Bedside teaching is one of the most challenging skills for the teaching hospitalist. Yet, teaching at the bedside is essential to transform learners into outstanding clinicians.[1] Moreover, as all bedside teaching occurs in a clinical context, it is uniquely suited for the teaching of several core competencies in hospital medicine. First, the learner can benefit from

*University of California, San Francisco, CA, USA.

real world demonstrations of professionalism, including optimal communication strategies with patients, family and nurses. Second, key aspects of the physical examination can be demonstrated and interpreted in the context of clinical decisions. Third, patient safety may be emphasized at the bedside. For example, teachers may point out the presence or absence of foley catheters or sequential compression devices.

Published literature suggests that bedside teaching is well received by all involved. Patients tend to value bedside oral case presentations, and there is no evidence that they object to having their care discussed in their presence.[2,3] Learners find the bedside useful in learning many competencies and their appreciation tends to be greater the more they are exposed to bedside teaching.[4,5] Finally, teachers who use this technique feel that it is effective and rewarding.[6]

Despite these benefits, bedside teaching is underutilized.[5] Barriers include the perception that bedside teaching is inefficient; fear that the patient will feel objectified in front of an audience of learners; and learner discomfort in "performing" in front of a group.[7] In this chapter, we present a simple framework to overcome these barriers and to optimize teaching at the bedside. This framework can be modified and applied to the multiple forms of bedside interactions, including bedside oral case presentations by students or housestaff, "on the fly" interactions with the patient and learner, and dedicated teaching visits to the bedside. In addition, we list common pitfalls in bedside teaching and offer strategies to overcome them (Table 1).

Framework

Set the Stage with Learners — What to Do Before Entering the Room

For bedside teaching to be successful, the teacher must be prepared and set the stage before entering the room. The teacher should have a general strategy ahead of time and fine-tune the specific plan in collaboration with the learners.

Table 1. Common Pitfalls in Bedside Teaching

Pitfall	Strategies to Avoid or Overcome
Patient is made to feel that their care is secondary to educational priorities.	Orient the patient and ask permission for bedside teaching. Clarify that while there is an educational component on a teaching service, the patient's care is paramount. Thank the patient for his or her contribution to medical education.
Patient asks you questions (instead of the learner).	Allow the learner to be at the forefront by taking a step back from the group. Look to the learner when questions are raised. Maintain patient centeredness by summarizing and agreeing or modifying the learner's responses.
Patient has multiple questions, encounter takes longer than planned.	Ask the session leader not to invite the patient to interrupt with questions or clarifications. Rather, encourage the patient to write down questions so they can all be addressed at the same time. Assure the patient that all questions will be addressed at the conclusion of the encounter.
You are uncertain if your physical examination finding is "correct."	Describe your findings as accurately as possible. If you are not sure how to interpret what you are seeing, share that with the team. By expressing a plan for how you intend to improve that particular skill, you will be demonstrating practice-based learning, a key competency for trainees.

1. *Establish your goals ahead of time*

Pre-determine the teaching goals for specific patients (e.g. demonstration of the physical examination for ascites in a patient with cirrhosis, modeling of patient-centered communication in a patient with end-stage metastatic cancer).

2. *State your established goals clearly to the group*

Entering a patients room without all providers having the same plan can be inefficient and confusing — it is useful to pre-label the bedside encounter as both a teaching and patient care-related activity. Pause outside the room and clearly state the goals: "I am going to demonstrate how to examine patients for the presence of ascites and I want everyone to practice the techniques as well."

3. *Define roles and responsibilities*

Identify who is to make introductions and lead the conversation with the patient. If the encounter is to be a bedside presentation, it may be appropriate to have the presenter practice what they will say to the patient to orient them to the plan (see ***Explain the goals and structure of the encounter*** below).

4. *Establish that there will be debriefing and feedback after the encounter*

Constructive feedback is best accepted if the process is normalized and expected. Clearly state you will be providing feedback when you come out of the room. For example, consider stating the following, "After you summarize the plan for the patient, we'll come out of the room and I'll give you feedback on how I think you did."

Orient the Patient — What to Do When you Enter the Room

1. *Introductions*

The designated team member taking the lead should introduce the patient to the group and then have each person introduce himself or herself; this should include names, level of training, and role in the patient's care.

2. *Explain the goals and structure of the encounter to the patient*

This is especially important if a bedside oral case presentation is planned. If unstructured, these encounters may take longer than planned and bias learners against future bedside presentations. For example, "I am going to formally present your case to my attending and the rest of the team. We will do a brief exam and then summarize our plan. It will be more efficient if you can write down your questions as they come up, so we can address everything when we wrap up. Is this plan OK with you?"

3. *Elicit any additional goals from the patient*

This is important to maintain the patient-centered tone of the interaction. All additional goals raised by the patient should be addressed. However, due to time constraints, sometimes it is more appropriate for the attending to take the responsibility of returning later.

Key Principles to Follow at the Bedside

1. *Follow your pre-arranged structure*

Allow the designated learner to lead the conversation. The conversation is unlikely to be exactly the same as you envision, but rather than interrupting and re-directing (unless absolutely necessary), formulate how to convey your observations as feedback to the learner after the encounter. If the goal of the encounter is a bedside presentation, avoid interruptions to ask questions by taking notes; many questions will be answered simply by waiting. Any additional questions can be asked at the conclusion of the presentation.

2. *Maintain patient respect*

Ask patient for permission before involving learners in interactions with the patient or in discussing the patient's case. For example, state to the patient, "Is it OK if I show the rest of the group some physical examination findings?" or "We like to think about medical problems by making a list of possible diagnoses — is it OK if we do that right now?" Avoid the use of medical jargon and be sure to define terms if necessary.

3. *Maintain learner respect*

Involve all learners and defer to the designated leader whenever possible.

Debrief — Outside the Room

1. *Provide learner-specific feedback*

Elicit the designated leader's self-evaluation of their performance by asking, "How did you think that went?" or "Which aspects of that interaction went well? What would you want to do differently in the future?" List one behavior that the learner did well and should continue, and one behavior that the learner should modify or not continue. Summarize two or three key teaching points from the encounter.

2. *Elicit feedback about the session*

Ask participants how they felt the session went. Make a specific plan to overcome any shortcomings in the next session.

Summary

Effective bedside teaching is a valuable tool for attending hospitalists in both community and academic practice. In the era of work hour restrictions for trainees in graduate medical education, teaching at the bedside can be an efficient way to teach key competencies. Community hospitalists can also use bedside teaching to improve the skills of nurses, physician's assistants, and other practitioners. By following a simple framework in which the hospitalist first sets the stage with learners, orients the patient, follows a pre-determined session structure, and debriefs afterwards, hospitalists can optimize teaching at the bedside.

References

1. Ramani S. (2003) Twelve tips to improve bedside teaching. *Med Teach* **25**(2): 112–5.
2. Simons RJ, Baily RG, Zelis R, Zwillich CW. (1989) The physiologic and psychological effects of the bedside presentation. *N Engl J Med* **321**(18): 1273–5.
3. Lehmann LS, Brancati FL, Chen MC, Roter D, Dobs AS. (1997) The effect of bedside case presentations on patients' perceptions of their medical care. *N Engl J Med* **336**(16): 1150–5.
4. Gonzalo JD, Masters PA, Simons RJ, Chuang CH. (2009) Attending rounds and bedside case presentations: medical student and medicine resident experiences and attitudes. *Teach Learn Med* **21**(2): 105–10.
5. Crumlish CM, Yialamas MA, McMahon GT. (2009) Quantification of bedside teaching by an academic hospitalist group. *J Hosp Med* **4**(5): 304–7.
6. Petersen K, Rosenbaum ME, Kreiter CD, Thomas A, Vogelgesang SA, Lawry GV. (2008) A randomized controlled study comparing educational outcomes of examination room versus conference room staffing. *Teach Learn Med* **20**(3): 218–24.
7. Williams KN, Ramani S, Fraser B, Orlander JD. (2008) Improving bedside teaching: findings from a focus group study of learners. *Acad Med* **83**(3): 257–64.

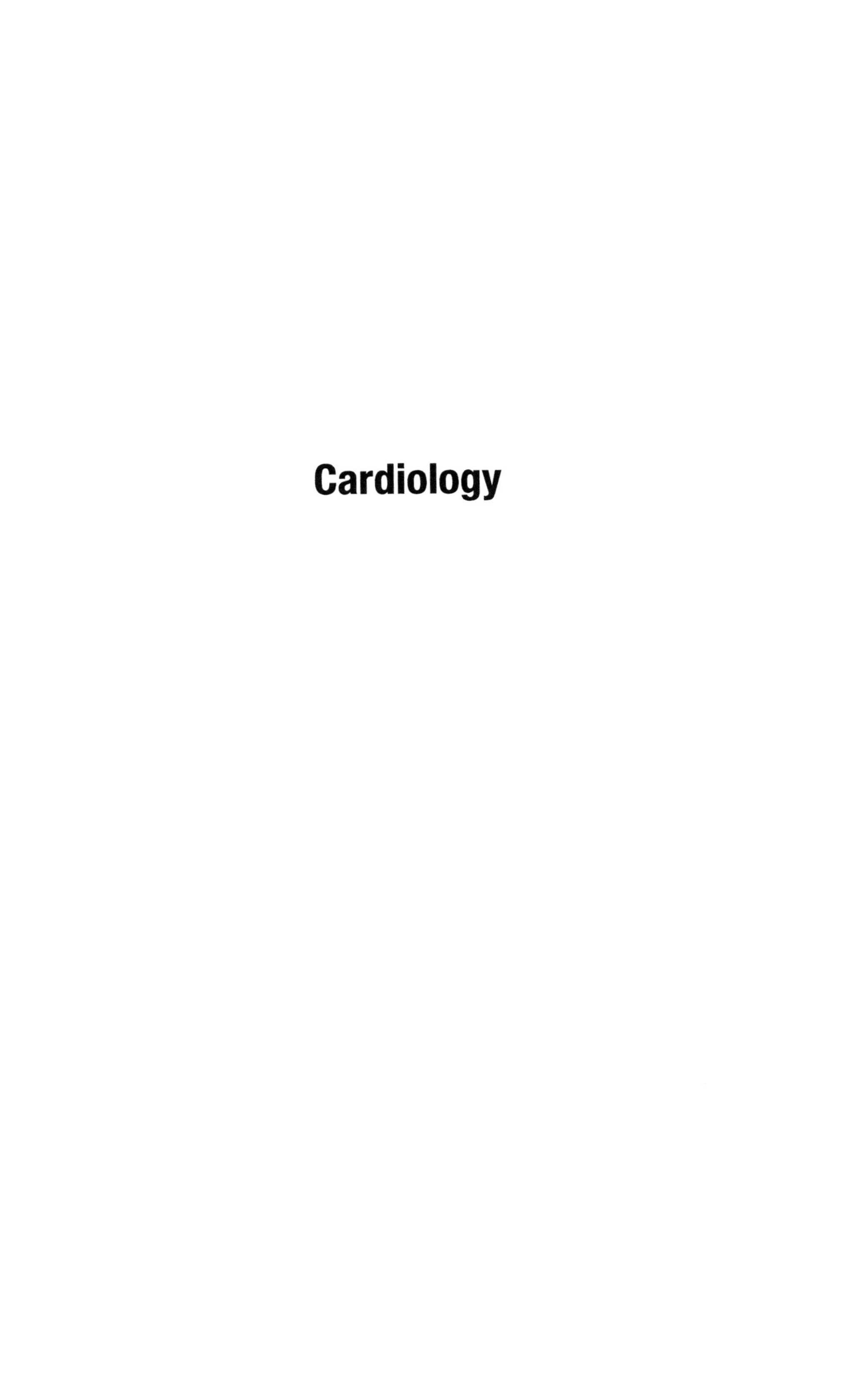

Cardiology

Chapter 18

Approach to Chest Pain

*Kevin G. Dunsky**

Key Pearls

- Cardiovascular causes of chest pain include myocardial ischemia, aortic dissection, myocarditis, pericarditis and coronary spasm.
- Myocardial perfusion imaging, which includes two common agents, thallium-201 and technetium-99 sestamibi, increases the diagnostic accuracy of stress testing.
- Stress echocardiography looks at stress-induced decreases in wall motion which may indicate underlying coronary ischemia. These results are similar to SPECT imaging.[6]
- Perhaps the greatest utility of cardiac computed tomography is its strong negative predictive value. Various studies have shown the negative predictive value to be 96–100%.
- Although there is no evidence that chest pain units decrease adverse outcomes, they may reduce length of stay and rate of hospital admissions.

Chest pain remains a diagnostic challenge to the physician in both the — inpatient and outpatient setting. It is a common complaint and the ramifications for the patient can range from a minimal issue to a life-threatening disorder.

*Mount Sinai School of Medicine, New York, NY, USA.

Key History Elements and Physical Exam Findings

As is true in all of medicine, the history and physical examination are critical in making the proper diagnosis. The duration, location and quality of the pain should always be determined. One should ask if the pain is related to food and whether or not it occurs during coughing or deep inspiration. It is important to know if anything exacerbates or relieves the pain. Associated symptoms such as dyspnea, nausea, vomiting and radiating pain should be included when talking to the patient.

Special attention to the physical exam needs to be performed. Just by looking at the patient, one can assess for diaphoresis or cyanosis. Taking blood pressures in both arms is important because this can provide clues to the presence of an aortic dissection. Simple inspection of the chest wall for lesions indicating the presence of herpes zoster is important. Crepitus indicating the presence of subcutaneous air may be seen in the presence of an esophageal rupture. Proper auscultation of the lungs can help diagnose congestive heart failure or the possible presence of a pneumothorax.

Friction rubs can help to diagnose pericarditis. The presence of an S3 can indicate the presence of congestive heart failure, whereas an S4 is present in myocardial ischemia and at times in diastolic dysfunction. Simple palpation of the abdomen can help identify potential problems such as masses or organomegaly. Right upper quadrant tenderness may increase the likelihood of cholecystitis.

Differential Diagnosis

Chest pain can be caused by a variety of disorders. Essentially, any input through the thoracic autonomic ganglia can cause chest pain. Esophageal rupture is a critical disorder and should be considered. Chest X-ray and esophagography can often aid in confirming this diagnosis. Peptic ulcer disease and gastroesophageal reflux may also masquerade as chest pain. Pancreatitis and biliary tract disease should also be considered. Pancreatitis is often associated with an elevated amylase or lipase. Patients with biliary disease often present with recurrent right upper quadrant pain or pain after eating. It is quite uncommon that exertion would elicit any of these findings.

Pulmonary etiologies, including pleuritis and pneumonia, may also present as chest pain. Pain during breathing or coughing may be seen in pleuritis. Fevers and productive sputum are often seen in patients with pneumonia. Life-threatening pulmonary disorders such as a pulmonary embolism is always of great concern. Various diagnostic tools are available to diagnose pulmonary embolism. Clinical risk predictors include signs and symptoms of deep venous thrombosis, tachycardia, immobilization for more than three days, hemoptysis, previous deep venous thrombosis or pulmonary embolus, or surgery within four weeks.[1] Diagnostic tools include a V/Q scan or CT angiogram. A tension pneumothorax can also be a life-threatening disorder and this is often diagnosed clinically as well as on a routine chest X-ray.

Musculoskeletal disorders such as costochondritis and trauma can cause chest pain and should be considered. Herpes zoster can clearly cause chest pain and in fact the chest pain, may precede the vesicular rash by several days.

Cardiovascular causes clearly need to be identified due to the possible fatal implications. Thus, myocardial ischemia and aortic dissection are two findings that can clearly cause chest pain. Myocarditis and pericarditis should also be included in this list. Intermittent or constant chest pain that is exacerbated by breathing is commonly described in patients with pericarditis. It is often worse in the supine position and is relieved by the patient leaning forward. A friction rub may be present on physical exam. Myocardits is often associated with fever and a recent infection. Coronary artery spasm may cause chest pain that may be indistinguishable from a person experiencing an acute coronary syndrome.

Since heart disease is a leading cause of mortality, it is essential to identify whether such a diagnosis can be confirmed. Identifying risk factors such as hypertension, hypercholesterolemia, tobacco use, diabetes and an early family history of coronary artery disease should always be carried out. A full physical, ECG and cardiac biomarkers such as troponins should be obtained. If the chest pain is not related to exertion whatsoever, it is less likely that the pain is due to an acute coronary syndrome. It should be noted, however, that critical disease can be caused from silent ischemia, and the patient may not exhibit any of the usual signs or symptoms of chest pain.

Cardiac Testing

Stress testing is a significant tool in diagnosing heart disease. An exercise stress test will attempt to reproduce the chest pain and assess for ECG changes which may be indicative of coronary ischemia. The American College of Cardiology and the American Heart Association performed a meta-analysis of the diagnostic accuracy of exercise stress testing involving 24,045 patients who underwent both coronary angiography and exercise stress testing. The results indicated a mean sensitivity of 68% and a mean specificity of 77%. If patients with previous MI's were excluded, the mean sensitivity was 67% and the mean specificity was 72% of exercise stress testing for diagnosing coronary artery disease.[2]

Myocardial perfusion imaging, which includes two common agents, thallium-201 and technetium-99 sestamibi, increases the diagnostic accuracy of stress testing. The ACC/AHA guidelines report that when both exercise and pharmacologic stress tests with SPECT imaging are compared with angiography, the test is 87–89% sensitive and 73–75% specific for significant stenosis (>50%).[3] Vanzetto performed a six year follow-up study which showed that in patients with a normal thallium-201 perfusion study, the rate of myocardial infarction or death was only 0.88%.[4] Iskander performed a meta-analysis which showed that a normal technetium-99 sestamibi imaging result was associated with a 0.6% cardiac event rate per year.[5]

Stress echocardiography looks at stress-induced decreases in wall motion which may indicate underlying coronary ischemia. A study by Fleischmann showed that stress echocardiography had a sensitivity of 85% and a specificity of 77% as compared with coronary angiography. Although this test is operator dependent, these results are similar to SPECT imaging.[6]

Cardiac computed tomography can measure calcification in the walls of the coronary arteries. The amount of calcium is expressed as an Agatston score. If any calcification is present, the test is considered positive. Calcium scores greater than 1000 are associated with increases in morbidity and mortality. In fact, such a score indicates a patient having a 20% chance of suffering a myocardial infarction or cardiac death within a year. However, it should be noted that a high score does not necessarily mean that there is an obstructive lesion. A positive scan indicates athero-sclerosis, but that does not mean significant obstruction is present.[7]

Perhaps the greatest utility of this test is its strong negative predictive value. A negative test has a 96–100% negative predictive value for obstructive lesions.[8] Thus, patients with a normal study are unlikely to have significant stenosis. This can be of great help to physicians evaluating chest pain patients in acute settings.

Chest Pain Units

Patients often present to the Emergency Department with complaints of chest pain. Chest pain units have been developed to help physicians choose which patients would benefit from further testing and inpatient admission. Protocols including a history and physical, observation period and serial measurements of serum biomarkers are used to help improve risk stratifying this patient population. Although there is no evidence that chest pain units decrease adverse outcomes, there are a number of trials which indicate that they may reduce length of stay and rate of hospital admissions. As a result, chest pain protocols for evaluating patients with suspected acute coronary syndromes (ACS) and chest pain in the Emergency Department received a Class I recommendation by the 2010 American Heart Association Guidelines for Cardiopulmonary Resuscitation and Emergency Cardiovascular Care.[9]

Conclusion

Chest pain is a common presentation that all physicians face. The differential diagnosis is wide and includes many different etiologies, including pulmonary, gastrointestinal, infectious as well as cardiac. A careful history and physical will help to narrow the diagnosis. Since cardiac disease is a leading cause of mortality, it is essential to make the proper diagnosis. The various imaging tests described above will greatly help the physician to make the proper diagnosis and as a result help to facilitate the proper care of the patient.

References

1. Wells PS, Anderson DR, Rodger M, *et al.* (2000) Derivation of a simple clinical model to categorize patients' probability of pulmonary embolism: Increasing the model utility with the SimpliRED*D*-dimer. *Thromb Haemost* **83**: 418.
2. Gianrossi R, Detrano R, Mulvihill D, *et al.* Exercise-induced ST depression in the diagnosis of coronary artery disease. A meta-analysis. *Circulation* **80**: 87–98.
3. Gibbons RJ, Balady GJ, Beasley JW, *et al.* (1997) ACC/AHA Guidelines for Exercise Testing. A report of the American College of Cardiology/American Heart Association Task Force on Practice Guidelines (Committee on Exercise Testing). *J Am Coll Cardiol* **30**(1): 260–311.
4. Vanzetto G, Ormezzano O, Fagret D, *et al.* (1999) Long-term additive prognostic value of thallium-201 myocardial perfusion imaging over clinical and exercise stress test in low to intermediate risk patients: Study in 1137 patients with 6-year follow-up. *Circulation* **100**(14): 1521–7.
5. Iskander S, Iskandrian AE. (1998) Risk assessment using single-photon emission computed tomographic technetium-99m sestamibi imaging. *J Am Coll Cardiol* **32**(1): 57–62.
6. Fleischmann KE, Hunink MG, Kuntz KM, *et al.* (1998) Exercise echocardiography or, exercise SPECT imaging? A meta-analysis of diagnostic test performance. *JAMA* **280**(10): 913–20.
7. Pletcher MJ, Tice JA, Pignone M, Browner WS. (2004) Using the coronary artery calcium score to predict coronary heart disease

events: A systematic review and meta-analysis. *Arch Intern Med* **164**: 1285–1292.

8. Budoff MJ, Achenbachs S, Roger S, *et al*. (2006) Assessment of coronary artery disease by cardiac computed tomography. A scientific statement from the American Heart Association Committee on Cardiovascular Imaging and Intervention, Council on Cardiovascular Radiology and Intervention, and Committee on Cardiac Imaging, Council on Clinical Cardiology. *Circulation* **114**: 1761–1791.
9. O'Connor, Robert E. *et al*. (2010) Part 10: Acute coronary syndromes: 2010 American Heart Association Guidelines for Cardiopulmonary Resuscitation and Emergency Cardiovascular Care. *Circulation* **122**: S787–S817.

Chapter 19

Acute Coronary Syndrome

Phillip A. Erwin, Rajeev L. Narayan* and Bruce J. Darrow**

Key Pearls

- Acute coronary syndromes include unstable angina, non-ST-elevation myocardial infarction, and ST-elevation myocardial infarction.
- Diagnosis of acute coronary syndrome is made on the basis of clinical evaluation and targeted testing, including electrocardiogram and Troponin.
- Transition from medical stabilization to early revascularization is indicated for ACS patients with higher clinical risk.
- Transition to outpatient recovery includes optimization of multiple medications and additional non-medical therapies.
- Appropriate management of MI patients forms the basis of assessment of hospital performance and quality of care.

Definitition and Pathophysiology

Myocardial infarction (MI) occurs when myocardial ischemia leads to cardiac myocyte death. MI is diagnosed when biomarkers of myocyte necrosis (primarily cardiac troponins) are detected in association with clinical symptoms of myocardial ischemia.[1] It is important to recognize that elevated Troponin levels alone are not sufficient for diagnosis of MI — clinical context is required. As shown in Table 1, MI is classified according to its presumed etiology. Type 1 MI is caused by an intracoronary event that leads to complete coronary obstruction, whereas Type 2

*Mount Sinai School of Medicine, New York, NY, USA.

Table 1. Types of Myocardial Infarction (MI)

1.	Coronary event leading to MI.
2.	Mismatch between myocardial oxygen demand and supply.
3.	Sudden death with evidence of myocardial ischemia that occurs before serum markers of myocardial necrosis can be drawn.
4a.	PCI-related elevation of biomarkers.
4b.	MI secondary to in-stent thrombosis.
5.	MI related to CABG surgey.

Thygesen K, Alpert JS, White HD; Joint ESC/ACCF/AHA/WHF Task Force for the Redefinition of Myocardial Infarction. (2007) Universal definition of myocardial infarction. *J Am Coll Cardiol* **50:** 2173–2195.

MI results when myocardial oxygen demand exceeds supply, such as in a patient with stable obstructive coronary disease and severe anemia.[1]

Acute coronary syndrome (ACS) describes a continuum of ischemia. Myocardial ischemia without myocardial necrosis — and therefore without biomarker elevations — is classified as unstable angina (UA). Once ischemia progresses to cell necrosis, biomarkers become elevated and non ST-elevation MI (NSTEMI) is diagnosed. ST-elevation MI (STEMI) is the result of complete coronary artery occlusion, with characteristic electrocardiogram (ECG) findings and positive biomarkers.[2]

Diagnosis

Evaluation of the patient with suspected ACS focuses on confirming or excluding the diagnosis, and instituting treatment according to the patient's risk of an adverse outcome.[2] Diagnosis, prognosis and management are driven by the ECG, history, exam, and cardiac biomarkers.

ECG Evaluation

The ECG should be the first parameter analyzed because characteristic ECG findings can direct history-taking and will determine acute management (e.g. expedited revascularization of a patient with STEMI). Comparison with old ECGs is helpful when evaluating T-wave changes or determining whether Q-waves or left bundle-branch block (LBBB) are new. The ECG in ACS can be dynamic, so even if the first ECG is non-diagnostic, serial ECGs can be useful in securing a diagnosis.[2] Regardless, a lack of ECG changes — even when taken during chest pain episodes — does not exclude myocardial infarction.[2,3] ECG changes characteristic of UA/NSTEMI include new ST-segment depressions ≥ 0.5 mm in multiple leads, T-wave flattening or T-wave inversion.[2] STEMI is defined as ST elevation of ≥ 1 mm in two or more contiguous precordial leads or adjacent limb leads, usually with reciprocal ST depressions.[4] New or presumed new LBBB should be managed in the same way as STEMI.[4]

History

Symptoms typical of ACS include retrosternal chest pain or pressure that may radiate to the arms (usually left) or jaw. Chest pain or pressure may be associated with dyspnea, diaphoresis, nausea, epigastric discomfort, or fatigue — although any of these symptoms may occur in isolation without chest pain.[2,5,6] The symptoms typically worsen with exertion and improve with rest or nitrates.[7] Less consistent with ACS is pain that is positional, pleuritic, described as sharp or stabbing, or is reproducible with palpation.[7] Nonetheless, these symptoms are not absolute and their presence or absence is not diagnostic in isolation. In particular, women and diabetics may present with atypical symptoms.[2] The history should elicit the duration of the symptoms, risk factors for coronary artery disease, and contraindications to treatments such as thrombolysis or nitrates.[2]

Physical Exam

At the time of presentation, findings consistent with ACS or a poor prognosis can guide management (e.g. S3, hypotension, pulmonary edema).[8] The exam may also reveal a non-coronary cause of symptoms such as uncontrolled hypertension, arrhythmia, pericarditis, or aortic dissection.

It is important to document not only abnormalities, but also the absence of signs of complications of MI that may appear later in the patient's hospital course (e.g. murmur of ventricular septal defect).

Cardiac Biomarkers

Evaluation of ACS symptoms should include serum Troponin measurement. Detection of Troponin has both diagnostic and prognostic value. Troponin may not be detectable for several hours from the start of MI, so it is not until three negative sets of Troponin levels have been drawn 6–8 hours apart that MI can be excluded.[2,7] Nonetheless, it is important to recall that troponin levels can be elevated from a non-ACS cause, such as myocarditis.[1]

Initial Treatment and Stabilization

Initial treatment should begin when the diagnosis of ACS is suspected and should be guided by the patient's risk of mortality from a cardiac event.[2,8] The TIMI Risk Score is a validated predictor of outcome in UA/NSTEMI (see Table 2). Aspirin (162–325 mg) should be given promptly to every patient undergoing evaluation for ACS unless there is a contraindication; clopidogrel may be substituted in case of aspirin allergy.[2] Control of pain with nitrates or opiates is standard treatment, but is not clearly associated with improved outcome.[2]

UA/NSTEMI

All patients with a high risk of UA/NSTEMI and without contraindications should be given clopidogrel 300–600 mg, unfractionated or low-molecular weight heparin, and a high-dose statin.[2,9] Beta-blockers may be given if not contraindicated by bradycardia or heart failure.[2] It is reasonable to consult a cardiologist before biomarker result if the patient is hemodynamically unstable or has refractory pain, or once ACS is diagnosed. Determination of whether the patient will undergo conservative versus early invasive management (cardiac catheterization with possible revascularization within 48 hours of presentation) should be guided by risk factors and

Table 2. TIMI Risk Score for UA/NSTEMI (1 Point Each)

Age ≥ 65
≥ 3 risk factors for CAD (HTN, HL, DM, smoking, family history)
Documented coronary stenoses ≥ 50%
Aspirin use in past 7 days
≥ 2 anginal episodes in past 24 hr
ST deviation greater than 0.5 mm
Elevated cardiac biomarkers

Antman EM, *et al.* (2000) The TIMI Risk Score for Unstable Angina/Non-ST Elevation MI. *JAMA* **284:** 835–842.

clinical circumstances. Patients with TIMI risk scores ≥ 3 (Table 2), hemodynamic instability, PCI within six months, prior coronary bypass surgery, ejection fraction <40%, sustained ventricular tachycardia, or recurrent angina should be considered for an early invasive strategy.[2,4,10] Patients managed conservatively can be medically optimized before further risk stratification and a follow-up appointment with a cardiologist.

Stress testing with adjunct imaging may be utilized safely in low TIMI risk patients (specifically those with negative serum biomarkers and without dynamic ST-T deviations) to help stratify patients and determine suitability for percutaneous intervention.[2] In patients with low clinical suspicion of disease, this can be performed on an inpatient or outpatient basis. In those patients suspected of having obstructive coronary disease, stress testing may be safely performed after the acute event has resolved and should be performed as an inpatient procedure to allow for rapid risk assessment and treatment planning. Use of stress testing in this sense should be thought of as assisting with risk stratification and allowing clinicians to decide if invasive therapy is warranted.[2]

STEMI

Patients with STEMI should have their management discussed immediately with a cardiologist to determine whether they are candidates for percutaneous intervention (PCI), thrombolysis, or conservative management. If PCI is available, or the patient can be rapidly transferred to a hospital performing

PCI, patient outcomes are better than with thrombolysis. Concurrent medical therapy is otherwise similar to treatment of NSTEMI.[4] Addition of a glycoprotein IIb/IIIa antagonist may be made at the discretion of the consulting cardiologist.[11]

Transition to Maintenance Therapy

Hospital discharge marks the transition from treatment for ACS to outpatient management of stable chronic ischemic coronary disease. In addition to medical therapy, lifestyle modifications, smoking cessation, and participation in cardiac rehabilitation are recommended.[2,12]

Medications for secondary coronary prevention include antiplatelet agents; aspirin (75–325 mg daily) forms the foundation.[2,12] In addition to aspirin, clopidogrel (75 mg daily) for up to one year after an acute coronary syndrome has been shown to be beneficial in secondary prevention.[2,4,12] Indefinite use of beta-blockers has been shown to reduce cardiac events and should be prescribed before discharge.[2,4] High-dose statin therapy with target low-density lipoprotein-cholesterol (LDL-C) below 70–100 mg/dl should also be instituted prior to discharge if not contraindicated.[2,9,12]

An echocardiogram is usually the test of choice to determine cardiac function and guide transitional therapy. For patients with left ventricular ejection fraction less than 40%, ACE-Inhibitors (ACE-I), have a mortality benefit[4] and are indicated. In those patients who are intolerant of ACE-I's, angiotensin receptor blockers (ARBs) may be substituted.[4] Finally, in STEMI patients with left ventricular dysfunction, eplerenone, an aldosterone antagonist, has been shown to reduce mortality.[2,12,13] The use of these medications should be offset by clinical parameters that may limit their use, including hypotension, bradycardia, or hyperkalemia. Additionally, these medications may require outpatient titration to achieve maximum benefit.

Quality Measures in Acute Coronary Syndromes

As the above treatments are recognized as standard of care for patients with ACS, regulatory groups have established core measures for hospital

Table 3. National Hospital Inpatient Quality Measures for Myocardial Infarction

1. Administration of aspirin at arrival and at discharge.
2. ACE-I or ARB prescribed at discharge for LVEF < 40%.
3. Smoking cessation counseling.
4. Beta-blocker prescribed at discharge to patients without contraindications.
5. Fibrinolysis administered within 30 min of hospital arrival for STEMI patients at institutions where PCI is unavailable and in whom delays in transfer are expected.
6. Primary PCI for patients presenting with STEMI to institutions capable of performing such procedures within 90 min of arrival.
7. LDL-Cholesterol assessment on admission.
8. Lipid-lowering therapy (e.g. statins) prescribed at discharge

Krumholz HM *et al.* (2008) ACC/AHA 2008 performance measures for adults with ST-elevation and non-ST-elevation myocardial infarction: A report of the American College of Cardiology/American Heart Association Task Force on Performance Measures (Writing Committee to Develop Performance Measures for ST-Elevation and Non-ST-Elevation Myocardial Infarction). *J Am Coll Cardiol* **52**: 2046–99.

performance in the care of patients with acute MI.[13] Table 3 summarizes the core measures established by the Center for Medicare and Medicaid Services and The Joint Commission. These guidelines are subject to regular review; Table 3 lists requirements as of January 2012.

References

1. Thygesen K, Alpert JS, White HD. (2007) Joint ESC/ACCF/AHA/WHF Task force for the redefinition of myocardial infarction. Universal definition of myocardial infarction. *J Am Coll Cardiol* **50**: 2173–2195.
2. Anderson JL, *et al.* (2007) ACC/AHA 2007 guidelines for the management of patients with unstable angina/non–ST-elevation myocardial infarction — executive summary: A report of the American College of Cardiology/American Heart Association Task Force on Practice Guidelines (Writing Committee to Revise the 2002 Guidelines for the Management of Patients With Unstable Angina/Non–ST-Elevation

Myocardial Infarction) developed in collaboration with the American College of Emergency Physicians, American College of Physicians, Society for Academic Emergency Medicine, Society for Cardiovascular Angiography and Interventions and Society of Thoracic Surgeons. *J Am Coll Cardiol* **50**: 652–726.

3. Turnipseed SD, *et al.* (2009) Frequency of Acute Coronary Syndrome in patients with normal electrocardiogram performed during presence or absence of chest pain. *Acad Emerg Med* **16**: 495–499.
4. Antman EM, *et al.* (2004) ACC/AHA Guidelines for the management of patients with ST-elevation myocardial infarction — Executive Summary. *Circulation* **110**: 588–636.
5. Panju AA, *et al.* (1998) Is this patient having a myocardial infarction? *JAMA* **280**: 1256–1263.
6. Swap, CJ, Nagurney, JT. (2005) Value and limitation of chest pain history in the evaluation of patients with suspected acute coronary syndromes. *JAMA* **294**: 2623–2629.
7. Cannon CP, and Lee TH. (2008) Approach to the patient with chest pain. In: Libby P, *et al.* (eds), *Braunwald's Heart Disease, 8th ed.* Saunders Elsevier, Philadelphia: pp. 1195–1206.
8. Antman EM, *et al.* (2000) The TIMI risk score for unstable angina/non-ST elevation MI. *JAMA* **284**: 835–842.
9. Cannon CP, *et al.* (2004) Intensive versus moderate lipid lowering with statins after acute coronary syndromes. *N Engl J Med* **350**: 1495–1504.
10. Cannon CP, *et al.* (2001) Comparison of early invasive and conservative strategies in patients with unstable coronary syndromes treated with the glycoprotein IIb/IIIa inhibitor tirofiban. *N Engl J Med* **344**: 1879–1887.
11. Keeley EC, Boura JA, Grines CL. (2003) Primary angioplasty versus intravenous thrombolytic therapy for acute myocardial infarction: A quantitative review of 23 randomised trials. *Lancet* **361**: 13–20.
12. Kushner FG, *et al.* (2009) Focused Updates: ACC/AHA guidelines for the management of patients with ST-elevation myocardial infarction (updating the 2004 guideline and 2007 focused update) and

ACC/AHA/SCAI guidelines on percutaneous coronary intervention (updating the 2005 guideline and 2007 focused update): A report of the American College of Cardiology Foundation/American Heart Association Task Force on Practice Guidelines. *J Am Coll Cardiol* **54**: 2205–2241.

13. Krumholz HM, *et al.* (2008) ACC/AHA 2008 performance measures for adults with ST-elevation and non–ST-elevation myocardial infarction: A report of the American College of Cardiology/American Heart Association Task Force on Performance Measures (Writing Committee to Develop Performance Measures for ST-Elevation and Non–ST-Elevation Myocardial Infarction). *J Am Coll Cardiol* **52**: 2046–99.

Chapter 20

Acute Decompensated Heart Failure

Gabriel Sayer and Sean P. Pinney*[†]

Key Pearls

- Acute decompensated heart failure can occur in patients with preserved or impaired left ventricular systolic function, and is associated with an increased risk of subsequent rehospitalization and mortality.
- The initial patient evaluation should include an assessment of volume status, adequacy of perfusion and triggers that led to decompensation.
- Management can be guided by physical examination and rarely requires pulmonary artery catheterization.
- Diuretics are the mainstay of therapy alleviating symptoms of congestion, and inotropes are reserved for the minority of patients who present with hypotension and low cardiac output.
- Prior to home discharge all patients should be educated about their medications, dietary restrictions, weight monitoring and followup appointments.

Introduction

Heart failure hospitalizations significantly burden the healthcare system. They account for more than one million admissions yearly in the United States, often with high levels of in-hospital morbidity and mortality, particularly among the elderly.[1] They signify a deleterious turn in an individual's

*Massachusetts General Hospital, Boston, MA, USA.
[†]Mount Sinai School of Medicine, New York, NY, USA.

natural history of chronic heart failure. Nearly half of all patients hospitalized with acute decompensated heart failure will be rehospitalized within six months of discharge. One quarter to one third of patients will die from heart failure within one year of discharge.[2,3] This chapter will outline the diagnostic and therapeutic approaches to managing hospitalized heart failure patients, and will discuss the important transition back to the outpatient setting.

Clinical Profiles

There are three general profiles that describe patients with decompensated heart failure (Fig. 1).[4] The first is characterized by volume overload with pulmonary and/or peripheral congestion usually associated with systemic hypertension, so-called "warm and wet." The second profile refers to patients who are "cold and wet." They show signs of hypoperfusion with diminished pulses, cool skin and congestion with a normal or reduced blood pressure. The third profile is that of a profoundly reduced cardiac output with renal failure, poor mentation, hypotension and other signs of cardiogenic shock. These patients are referred to as "cold and dry." These

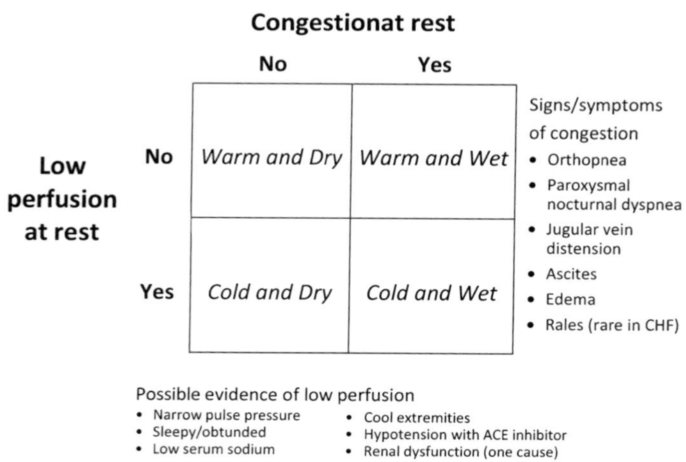

Fig. 1. Description of four possible hemodynamic profiles in congestive heart failure based on evidence of congestion and perfusion on physical examination. Adapted, with permission, from Stevenson.[4]

clinical profiles are present in all forms of heart failure and occur in patients regardless of their systolic function. However, cardiogenic shock is more commonly seen in patients with decreased systolic function.

The understanding of the demographic and clinical characteristics has been informed by two large clinical registries of patients hospitalized with heart failure (Table 1).[5] In general, these patients are of advanced age and suffer from other chronic medical conditions, such as hypertension, coronary artery disease, diabetes and chronic kidney disease. About half have a normal or near-normal ejection fraction. Men and women are affected in nearly equal numbers. The most common presenting complaint is dyspnea, and most patients have pulmonary vascular congestion or peripheral edema. Typically, the systolic blood pressure is elevated. Overt cardiogenic shock is rare.

Diagnostic Strategies

The initial approach when encountering a patient with acute heart failure is to quickly ascertain volume status, adequacy of perfusion, and triggers that led to decompensation.

Table 1. Clinical Characteristics of Patients Admitted with Acute Heart Failure, Based on Data from the ADHERE and OPTIMIZE-HF Registries

Mean Age	74 Years
Men	48%
Coronary artery disease	55%
Hypertension	72%
Diabetes	43%
Atrial fibrillation	31%
Renal insufficiency	30%
COPD	30%
Hyponatremia	25%
Mean systolic blood pressure	143 mmHg
Dyspnea at rest	40%
Rales	65%
Peripheral edema	66%

Heart failure is a condition typified by expansion of extracellular volume. Signs and symptoms of volume overload are present in most patients with acute heart failure. Typically, hospitalized patients will report recently experiencing exertional dyspnea, orthopnea, paroxysmal nocturnal dyspnea or lower extremity edema. Signs of congestion that may be present on exam include an elevation of the jugular venous waveform, inspiratory crackles, palpable hepatomegaly, ascites or peripheral edema. Occasionally, pulmonary edema may be present in a chest radiograph, but not appreciated when auscultating the lungs. The reason for this apparent paradox is a result of enhanced lymphatic drainage of the lung. The presence of Kerley B lines, the horizontal densities present at the periphery of the lung bases on a chest radiograph, is a reflection of increased fluid in the lymphatic system. Chest radiographs are also helpful in identifying cardiomegaly and pleural effusions, typically more common on the right side than the left. While not exclusively a sign of volume overload, a third heart sound (S3 gallop) is a specific finding for decompensated heart failure which often identifies those patients at higher risk of further hemodynamic compromise.

Of similar importance to assessing volume status is determining the adequacy of perfusion and, by extension, of cardiac output. Manifestations of a reduced cardiac output include low blood pressure, cool extremities with thready or absent pulses and diminished capillary refill. A cloudy sensorium or altered mental status may indicate a reduction in cerebral perfusion. Worsening renal function with elevations of BUN and creatinine is often a sign of reduced renal perfusion. Based on this assessment of fluid status and adequacy of perfusion, patients can be classified into the three profiles that will help guide the treatment decisions discussed below.[4]

In addition to assessing the severity and duration of symptoms, it is also important to identify potentital etiologies that triggered decompensation (Table 2). The most common precipitants of heart failure admissions are myocardial ischemia, pulmonary infections and failure to adhere to medical therapy or a low sodium diet. Myocardial ischemia is frequently present and occasionally underappreciated as a trigger of decompensation. Increased myocardial wall stress from elevations in ventricular filling

Table 2. Factors Precipitating Admission for Acute Heart Failure

Myocardial ischemia
Arrhythmias
Uncontrolled hypertension
Pneumonia or respiratory process
Worsening renal function
Nonadherence to medications
Nonadherence to diet
Pulmonary embolus
Nonsteroidal anti-inflammatory drugs
Excessive alcohol or illicit drug use
Endocrine abnormalities (diabetes, thyroid)
Other infections

pressures leads to increased myocardial oxygen demand. This demand may be great enough to produce ischemia even in the absence of epicardial coronary artery stenosis. Elevations in serum troponin have been associated with an increased risk of in-hospital mortality.[6] Not all triggers of decompensation are associated with the same risk of in-hospital mortality. For example, dietary indiscretions and medication noncompliance are associated with a much lower risk of in-hospital mortality than worsening renal function or pneumonia.[7]

Determining whether a patient is experiencing dyspnea as a result of heart failure or from another cause, such as pulmonary disease, can be challenging. Plasma levels of brain natriuretic peptide (BNP) are sometimes useful in these situations.[4] If a plasma BNP level is less than 50 pg/ml, the cause of dyspnea is unlikely to be related to heart failure. On the other hand, when serum levels of BNP are elevated above 100 pg/ml, heart failure is more likely, but other etiologies of dyspnea still need to be considered. Serum levels of BNP may be elevated above 100 pg/ml in the setting of advancing age, kidney disease, pulmonary embolism and pulmonary artery hypertension. For these reasons, one must rely on the history and physical examination, more than blood tests, to properly diagnose decompensated heart failure.

Outcomes of Acute Heart Failure

Patients hospitalized with heart failure receive treatment that improves symptoms, but whose effect on mortality is uncertain. On average, patients spend about four days in hospital and report feeling better by the end of their stay. Nonetheless, 40% have residual symptoms by the time of discharge and about 5% feel no better, or may even feel worse,[9] which may reflect an inability to completely decongest patients. Although 70% of hospitalized patients receive intravenous diuretics, only half will lose more than 2 kg of weight and as many as 20% will be sent home with a weight that is unchanged or higher than their admission weight.[9] Leaving the hospital congested and symptomatic sets the stage for future hospitalizations. Currently, one out of every four patients will be rehospitalized within one month of their discharge.

Admission for acute decompensated heart failure carries with it a significant risk of mortality. During hospitalization, approximately 4% of patients will die, and 10% will die within three months of discharge.[9] Patients with systolic dysfunction experience a slightly higher rate of hospital mortality compared to those with heart failure and preserved systolic function. Patients with systolic dysfunction are also more likely to require intensive care unit admission and spend more days in hospital.

Predictors of increased in-hospital mortality have been identified (Table 3).[10] They include signs of congestion, such as jugular venous distention or an elevated pulmonary capillary wedge pressure, and elevated levels of BNP. Hyponatremia, with serum sodium less than 135 meq/L, and a positive cardiac troponin assay are also poor prognostic signs.[6] Two of the strongest predictors of mortality in acute heart failure are impaired renal function and hypotension on admission. One simple clinical algorithm uses only three measurements at presentation (BUN above or below 43 mg/dL, systolic blood pressure above or below 115 mmHg and serum creatinine above or below 2.75) to discriminate patients into low, intermediate and high risk groups in terms of in-hospital mortality.[11] Identifying at-risk subgroups helps to inform treatment decisions and, when appropriate, facilitate discussions about advanced therapies such as mechanical support and transplantation.

Table 3. Predictors of Mortality for Patients Admitted with Acute Heart Failure*

Systolic blood pressure	Admission and early postdischarge SBP inversely correlates with postdischarge mortality. The higher the BP, the lower both in-hospital and postdischarge mortality.
Renal dysfunction	Associated with a two- to threefold increase in postdischarge mortality. Worsening renal function during hospitalization or soon after discharge is also associated with an increase in in-hospital and postdischarge mortality.
Coronary artery disease	Extent and severity of CAD appears to be a predictor of poor prognosis.
Elevated serum troponin level	Results in a threefold increase in in-hospital mortality, a twofold increase in postdischarge mortality, and a threefold increase in the rehospitalization rate.
Elevated plasma BNP	Elevated natriuretic peptides associated with increased resource utilization and mortality.
Prolonged QRS on electrocardiogram	Increase in QRS duration occurs in approximately 40% of patients with reduced systolic function and is a strong predictor of early and late postdischarge mortality and rehospitalization.
Hyponatremia	Defined as serum sodium <135 mmol/L, occurs in approximately 25% of patients, and is associated with a two- to threefold increase in postdischarge mortality.
Evidence of congestion at discharge	An important predictor of postdischarge mortality and morbidity.
Functional capacity at discharge	Predischarge functional capacity, defined by the 6 min walk test, is emerging as an important predictor of postdischarge outcomes.

*Adapted, with permission, from Ref. 10.

Management of Acute Heart Failure

The goals of therapy for decompensated heart failure are to:

- Alleviate symptoms;
- Improve volume status and hemodynamics;
- Optimize chronic therapy;
- Educate patients about their medicines and self-assessment;
- Initiate a disease management program when possible.

Treatment for acute heart failure should be initiated soon after arrival. Identification and treatment of coexisting conditions, such as infections, arrhythmias and myocardial ischemia, is essential. If an acute coronary syndrome is present, clinicians should consider early revascularization to prevent further deterioration of cardiac function. It is appropriate to consider reducing or temporarily discontinuing administration of ACE-I, ARBs and/or aldosterone antagonists in the setting of worsening renal function. This is particularly true for patients receiving intravenous diuretics, or combinations of diuretics, which may further worsen azotemia. In the absence of cardiogenic shock, beta-blockers should be maintained at the same outpatient dose whenever possible. Reducing the dose or eliminating beta-blockers during acute heart failure hospitalization may result in poorer outcomes.

A pulmonary artery catheter can provide information about volume status and response to therapy, but its routine use in clinical trials proved to be of no benefit.[12] Placement of these catheters should be reserved for patients with uncertain volume status and evidence of impaired perfusion or those who may require evaluation for cardiac transplantation or mechanical circulatory support.

Diuretics

Loop diuretics are the first agents used to treat acute heart failure. When administered intravenously, they rapidly alleviate dyspnea, often before producing an effective diuresis. These diuretics block the reabsorption of sodium in the thick, ascending loop of Henle. They have a relatively short half-life and once tubular concentration falls sodium reabsorption resumes. Patients should be treated promptly with doses sufficient to increase urine output to optimize volume status. It is important to regularly assess a patient's volume status and the adequacy of perfusion by recording daily urine output, body weight and orthostatic blood pressure. Patients should have regular blood sampling to monitor serum levels of electrolytes, particularly potassium and magnesium, which may become depleted.

Although loop diuretics improve symptoms of acute heart failure, their effect on mortality is uncertain and has never been studied in a large clinical trial. The potential to harm may be more than a theoretical side effect. There has been a reported direct association between the daily dose of a loop diuretic and the observed mortality. This relationship is a key input into the Seattle Heart Failure Model, used to assess mortality risk in heart failure patients.[12] Loop diuretics reduce plasma volume, which in turn lowers cardiac output. The kidney senses a reduction in perfusion, releasing renin, which subsequently increases angiotensin II. This increase in neurohormonal activation is potentially deleterious, but restoration of euvolemia quickly leads to sustained reductions in these counterregulatory neurohormones.

Clinicians frequently encounter patients who inadequately respond to diuretics. There are several potential explanations for this diuretic resistance. Nonsteroidal anti-inflammatory drugs (NSAIDs) reduce the efficacy of diuretics and when used concomitantly can precipitate acute renal failure. Excessive dietary sodium and water intake may occasionally explain the discrepancy between increases in urine output and lack of weight loss. Patients with chronic kidney disease have a blunted responsiveness to diuretics and require higher initial doses. Elevations in central venous pressure beyond 18 mmHg can lead to renal congestion and a reduction in GFR. This is one instance where the use of loop diuretics can improve GFR by reducing CVP to near-normal levels.

There are several strategies to overcome diuretic resistance. If urine output is inadequate with the initial loop diuretic dose, subsequent doses should be doubled until a diuresis occurs. Addition of a thiazide diuretic can be an effective way to block sodium reabsorption at other sites of the nephron. Delivering loop diuretics as a continuous intravenous infusion avoids rebound tubular sodium reabsorption and produces a steady diuresis. On occasion, it may be necessary to measure cardiac filling pressures and resting hemodynamics in those instances where doubt exists as to a patient's true volume status and cardiac output. Addition of a vasodilator or inotrope may be indicated in cases of a reduced cardiac output to increase both renal perfusion and GFR.

An alternative way to reduce congestion is to mechanically remove fluid. Ultrafiltration uses a pressure gradient across a semipermeable membrane to remove fluid. The composition of this fluid contains more sodium than that produced by loop diuretics. Although clinical experience with this device is limited, in one study ultrafiltrated patients spent fewer days in hospital and required repeat heart failure hospitalizations less often than patients receiving loop diuretics.[13] Current barriers to widespread use of ultrafiltration include its more invasive nature, need for vascular access, telemetry or intensive care unit monitoring and cost.

Vasodilators

Vasodilators are effective drugs for treating acute decompensated heart failure, because they quickly improve the loading conditions on the heart. They act by relaxing vascular smooth muscle cells and in so doing reduce systemic vascular resistance and increase venous capacitance. By lowering both afterload and preload, vasodilators reduce ventricular volumes, myocardial wall stress and oxygen demand. The efficiency of cardiac contraction improves and cardiac output increases. Vasodilators also decrease the severity of mitral regurgitation, when present, and further lower pulmonary capillary pressure. Unlike diuretics, vasodilators may decrease neurohormonal stimulation. They are usually reserved for patients who have more pronounced symptoms upon presentation or persistent symptoms in spite of treatment with intravenous diuretics. Vasodilators work particularly well in patients with significant hypertension. They should be used cautiously in patients with a reduced blood pressure and are contraindicated in cardiogenic shock.

Currently, three vasodilators are used for the treatment of acute heart failure: nitroglycerin, sodium nitroprusside and nesiritide. Nitroglycerin produces vascular relaxation by first being converted to nitric oxide, which in turn signals cyclic guanosine monophosphate (cGMP) production. It is primarily a venodilator, but is often used in patients with acute coronary syndromes because of its ability to dilate coronary arteries. Its use may be limited by headache, hypotension and tachyphylaxis. When it is employed to treat heart failure, much higher doses than those used in treating myocardial ischemia are required. Sodium nitroprusside works through a similar mechanism as nitroglycerin, but is a more potent arterial dilator. As a result, it is more likely to produce hypotension and it should be administered only in an intensive care unit with continuous arterial blood pressure monitoring. Nitroprusside may worsen myocardial ischemia by producing coronary steal and reflex tachycardia. Prolonged infusion may result in thiocyanate toxicity, particularly in patients with impaired renal function. Nesiritide is a recombinant form of B-type natriuretic peptide which lowers pulmonary capillary wedge pressure more quickly than nitroglycerin while alleviating dyspnea to a similar degree.[14] It has a longer half-life than nitroglycerin or nitroprusside and requires minimal, if any, dose titration. Its primary side effect is hypotension, which can be mitigated by omitting an initial bolus.

Inotropes

Inotropes enhance cardiac contractility by promoting actin–myosin bridging in myocardial cells. Dobutamine and dopamine work through beta-1 receptors, stimulating the production of cyclic adenosine monophosphate (cAMP) and increasing intracellular calcium. Milrinone is a phosphodiesterase-3 inhibitor that prevents breakdown of cAMP. In addition to its myocardial effects, milrinone produces vascular smooth muscle cell relaxation and vasodilation. As opposed to the catecholamines, milrinone leaves the beta-receptor unoccupied and allows for concomitant therapy with a beta-blocker. This approach may be particularly useful when transitioning hospitalized patients off inotropes to chronic medical therapy. Inotropes should be reserved for patients with poor peripheral perfusion where augmenting cardiac output is required to restore an adequate circulation and relieve symptoms.

All inotropes possess significant side effects. They elevate the heart rate, promote tachyarrhythmias and, in the case of milrinone, produce hypotension. Increases in the heart rate and contractility increase myocardial oxygen demand and may worsen ischemia. As in chronic heart failure, routine inotrope use increases mortality and is strongly discouraged.[15]

Transition Home

Hospitalization for acute heart failure offers a "teachable moment" for clinicians to instruct patients about living with heart failure. Spending adequate time teaching patients and their families about triggers of heart failure, prognosis, importance of compliance, and identifying signs and symptoms of clinical worsening can often reduce the need for subsequent hospitalization. Prior to going home, all patients should receive written discharge instructions that address:

- Dietary restrictions;
- Activity level;
- Discharge medications;
- Followup appointments;
- Daily weight monitoring;
- What to do if symptoms worsen.

Clinicians should ensure that patients have achieved euvolemia and are receiving optimal doses of ACE/ARB and beta-blockers. The ventricular rate of atrial fibrillation should be controlled. Whenever possible, hospitalized heart failure patients should be referred to an outpatient disease management team. Taking the time to complete these steps in accordance with clinical practice guidelines will ensure a safe, high-quality discharge.

Conclusion

Treating acute heart failure patients remains a clinical challenge. Current therapies effectively improve symptoms, but have uncertain effects on mortality. Applying the evidence-based approaches outlined above and summarized in Fig. 2 should help improve outcomes for these complex patients.

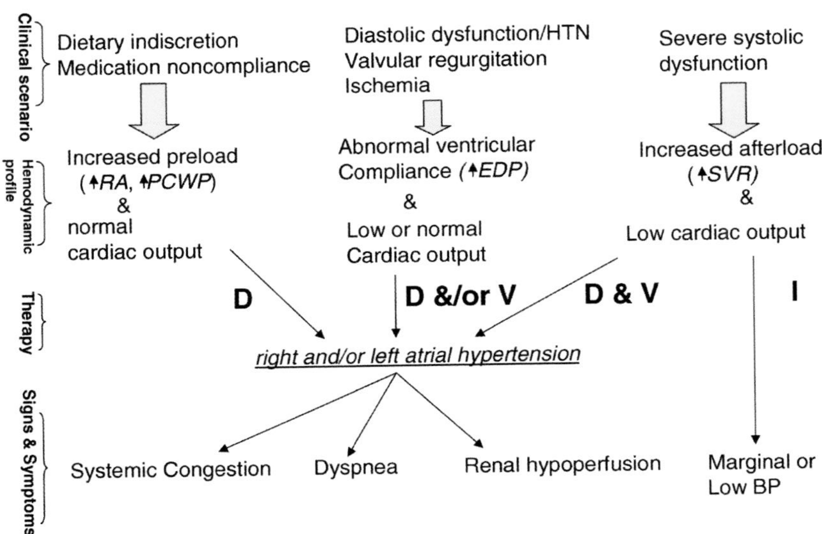

Fig. 2. Putting it all together: the pathophysiology and treatment of decompensated heart failure. **D** = diuretic therapy or mechanical volume removel; **V** = vasodilator therapy; **I** = inotropic therapy (Reprinted, with permission, from Ref. 17.)

References

1. Lloyd-Jones D, Adams R, Carnethon M, *et al.* (2009) Heart disease and stroke statistics — 2009 update: A report from the American Heart Association Statistics Committee and Stroke Statistics Subcommittee. *Circulation* **119**: 480–486.
2. Krumholz HM, Parent EM, Tu N, *et al.* (1997) Readmission after hospitalization for congestive heart failure among Medicare beneficiaries. *Arch Intern Med* **157**: 99–104.
3. Goldberg RJ, Ciampa J, Lessard D, *et al.* (2007) Long-term survival after heart failure: A contemporary population-based perspective. *Arch Intern Med* **167**: 490–496.
4. Stevenson LW. (1999) Tailored therapy to hemodynamic goals for advanced heart failure. *Eur J Heart Fail* **1**: 251–257.
5. Gheorghiade M, Zannad F, Sopko G, *et al.* (2005) Acute heart failure syndromes: Current state and framework for future research. *Circulation* **112**: 3958–3968.
6. Peacock WFt, De Marco T, Fonarow GC, *et al.* (2008) Cardiac troponin and outcome in acute heart failure. *N Engl J Med* **358**: 2117–2126.
7. Fonarow GC, Abraham WT, Albert NM, *et al.* (2008) Factors identified as precipitating hospital admissions for heart failure and clinical outcomes: Findings from OPTIMIZE-HF. *Arch Intern Med* **168**: 847–854.
8. Maisel AS, Krishnaswamy P, Nowak RM, *et al.* (2002) Rapid measurement of B-type natriuretic peptide in the emergency diagnosis of heart failure. *N Engl J Med* **347**: 161–167.
9. Fonarow GC, Abraham WT, Albert NM, *et al.* (2007) Influence of a performance-improvement initiative on quality of care for patients hospitalized with heart failure: Results of the Organized Program to Initiate Lifesaving Treatment in Hospitalized Patients with Heart Failure (OPTIMIZE-HF). *Arch Intern Med* **167**: 1493–1502.
10. Gheorghiade M, Pang PS. (2009) Acute heart failure syndromes. *J Am Coll Cardiol* **53**: 557–573.

11. Fonarow GC, Adams KF, Jr., Abraham WT, *et al.* (2005) Risk stratification for in-hospital mortality in acutely decompensated heart failure: Classification and regression tree analysis. *JAMA* **293**: 572–580.
12. Levy WC, Mozaffarian D, Linker DT, *et al.* (2006) The Seattle Heart Failure Model: Prediction of survival in heart failure. *Circulation* **113**: 1424–1433.
13. Costanzo MR, Guglin ME, Saltzberg MT, *et al.* (2007) Ultrafiltration versus intravenous diuretics for patients hospitalized for acute decompensated heart failure. *J Am Coll Cardiol* **49**: 675–683.
14. Publication Committee for the VMAC Investigators (Vasodilatation in the Management of Acute CHF). (2002) Intravenous nesiritide vs nitroglycerin for treatment of decompensated congestive heart failure: A randomized controlled trial. *JAMA* **287**: 1531–1540.
15. Cuffe MS, Califf RM, Adams KF, Jr., *et al.* (2002) Short-term intravenous milrinone for acute exacerbation of chronic heart failure: A randomized controlled trial. *JAMA* **287**: 1541–1547.
16. Konstam MA, Gheorghiade M, Burnett JC, Jr., *et al.* (2007) Effects of oral tolvaptan in patients hospitalized for worsening heart failure: The EVEREST Outcome Trial. *JAMA* **297**: 1319–1331.
17. Yancy CW. (2008) Vasodilator therapy for decompensated heart failure. *J Am Coll Cardiol* **52**: 208–210.

Chapter 21

Valvular Heart Disease

Mark Harrison[†] *and Lane Duvall*[*]

Key Pearls

- With the aging of the US population, the four major types of valvular heart disease (aortic stenosis, aortic regurgitation, mitral stenosis and mitral regurgitation) will continue to increase in prevalence. Transthoracic echocardiography plays a key role in making the diagnosis.
- In patients with severe symptomatic aortic stenosis, (as manifested by syncope, shortness of breath, or angina), surgical valve replacement is the best current treatment option.
- Mitral stenosis is usually caused by rheumatic heart disease and therapy is targeted towards reducing CHF symptoms and decreasing the risk of thromboembolism.
- Aortic regurgitation presents variably, depending on the underlying etiology and natural history.
- Mitral regurgitation is caused by a wide number of entities. Medical therapy is centered around relieving pulmonary congestion, but when patients become symptomatic, they may benefit from surgical repair or replacement of the valve.

*Mount Sinai Medical Center, New York, NY, USA.
[†]The Hudson Valley Heart Center, Poughkeepsie, NY, USA.

Introduction

Valvular heart disease includes a group of congenital or acquired conditions characterized by abnormal valvular function (stenosis, regurgitation, or both) which can cause significant morbidity and mortality.[1–2] While the exact prevalence is unknown, estimates have identified up to 5 million Americans affected, with the number expected to increase as the population ages.[3–4] Transthoracic echocardiography plays a key role in making the diagnosis.[5–6]

Aortic Stenosis (AS)

A normal trileaflet aortic valve allows for unobstructed flow between the left ventricle and the aorta. Under certain pathologic circumstances, aortic stenosis develops, in which the valve can narrow and prevent complete opening, impeding normal blood flow.

Etiology

In the United States, the most common cause of AS is progressive calcification and degeneration of the valve occurring with age. "Senile" AS usually presents in the seventh through ninth decade of life. Worldwide, rheumatic fever can be a cause of AS, presenting in the third through fifth decade of life, and usually accompanied by mitral valve disease. Due to recurrent inflammation, the valve progressively narrows through fibrous contracture and fusion of adjacent cusps. Finally, a congenital cause of AS occurs in patients with a bicuspid aortic valve, consisting of two cusps instead of three. Occurring in 1–2% of people, bicuspid aortic valves are especially prone to the formation of calcium deposits and bicuspid AS usually presents in the 40s and 50s.

History and Physical

Symptoms of aortic stenosis tend to develop gradually. Ultimately, patients with progressive disease experience the classic triad of chest pain, syncope, and congestive heart failure (CHF).

In patients with angina, the five-year mortality rate is 50%. Syncope can be attributed to poor cardiac output, decreased cerebral blood flow, or cardiac arrhythmias. After a syncopal event, the median survival is three years. Finally, for individuals with symptoms of CHF, the prognosis is extremely poor, with a two-year mortality of 50% if the valve is not replaced. Symptoms of heart failure may occur from a combination of systolic dysfunction, diastolic dysfunction, or both.

On examination, patients with aortic stenosis typically have a harsh systolic crescendo-decrescendo murmur heard at the right upper sternal border which radiates to both carotids. Advanced disease is suggested by a diminished S2, late peaking murmur, and weak and delayed carotid pulses.

Diagnosis and Testing

The standard evaluation for patients with suspected AS includes an ECG, chest X-ray (CXR) and an echocardiogram. In advanced aortic stenosis, the 12-lead ECG will often reveal left ventricular hypertrophy; however, it is not present in all patients. On CXR, cardiomegaly and calcification of the aorta and aortic valve support the diagnosis of AS.

Ultimately, echocardiography can confirm the clinical diagnosis of aortic stenosis. Beyond assessing the degree and severity of valve narrowing, echo provides additional information on ventricular size, systolic and diastolic function, valve leaflet number, valve morphology, and the degree of calcification. Cardiac catheterization can be used for hemodynamic confirmation of severity if needed.

Treatment

The initial management of patients with significant AS presenting with congestive heart failure includes monitoring, supportive oxygen, intravenous access, and diuretics. For patients with angina, measures should be taken to relieve the chest discomfort, which may include administration of oxygen, nitrates, and beta blockers. Importantly, blood pressure lowering agents should be used with caution as patients with significant AS do not have the ability to augment their cardiac output to compensate for a significant drop in blood pressure.

Ultimately, severe symptomatic AS is treated surgically through valve replacement. The operative mortality varies significantly depending on age and co-morbidities. For those patients deemed high risk, percutaneous valvuloplasty represents a less invasive approach to temporarily improve symptoms; however, no mortality benefit has been demonstrated with this technique.

Mitral Stenosis (MS)

Mitral stenosis is a narrowing of the mitral valve opening that impedes blood flow from the left atrium to the left ventricle during diastole.

Etiology

The most common cause of mitral stenosis is rheumatic heart disease. After the initial episode of rheumatic fever, a latency period of 20–40 years occurs until the onset of symptoms. Given the widespread use of antibiotics in the United States, the incidence has decreased significantly over time. However, it still poses a significant problem in developing countries.

Rarer causes of MS include malignant carcinoid, congenital MS, and collagen vascular diseases, such as systemic lupus erythematosis and rheumatoid arthritis.

History and Physical

Unless the degree of stenosis is severe, patients are asymptomatic at rest. Certain clinical situations which increase the heart rate such as pregnancy, exercise, hyperthyroidism, rapid atrial fibrillation, and fever can all lead to reduction in ventricular filling time during diastole. This leads to diminished cardiac output and causes a decline in functional capacity, dyspnea, orthopnea, and fatigue. Elevated left atrial pressure predisposes patients to the development of atrial fibrillation, and pulmonary edema.

Cardiac examination for MS is best conducted with the patient in the left lateral decubitus position with the stethoscope applied to the cardiac apex. An accentuated S1 and variable S2 is followed by an opening snap with an accompanying diastolic, low-pitched, rumbling murmur. Other physical findings are related to the degree of heart failure (i.e. elevated JVP, peripheral edema) and the presence of atrial fibrillation (irregular heart beat).

Diagnosis and Testing

Initially, echocardiography is the diagnostic study of choice to assess for the presence of mitral stenosis. Echocardiography can identify the severity and etiology of MS as well as morphologic features of the valve, subvalvular structures, and pulmonary hypertension. On occasion, cardiac catheterization is indicated to determine the severity of MS and pulmonary pressures, when clinical and echocardiographic assessments are discordant.

ECG is an insensitive method to detect MS, but may reveal atrial fibrillation, left atrial enlargement and/or right ventricular hypertrophy. On CXR, patients with advanced disease often demonstrate left atrial or pulmonary artery enlargement and pulmonary congestion.

Treatment

Medical therapy for MS is directed at decreasing the heart rate, reducing CHF symptoms (most frequently with diuretics), and decreasing the risk of thromboembolism. Rate control, especially in patients with atrial fibrillation often requires the use of beta blockers, calcium channel blockers, and/or digoxin. Systemic anticoagulation for patients with mitral stenosis and ongoing atrial fibrillation is indicated indefinitely. For patients in sinus rhythm, the severity of MS and the degree of left atrial enlargement is often considered in the decision to anticoagulate.

Aortic Regurgitation (AR)

Aortic regurgitation may result from intrinsic abnormalities of the aortic valve, the ascending aorta, or both. Typically, AR worsens over an extended period of time, but acute onset AR does occur and often in a dramatic fashion.

Etiology

Congenital bicuspid aortic valves, rheumatic heart disease, and collagen vascular diseases are predisposing valvular conditions that can lead to progressive AR. Senile valvular changes, which are almost always accompanied by AS, can also lead to regurgitation. One of the important causes of acute AR is infective endocarditis.

Entities that primarily affect the aortic root distal to the valve can cause dilation and produce regurgitation. These include aortic dissection, Marfans disease, thoracic aneurysms, and syphilis aortitis.

History and Physical

Aortic regurgitation presents variably depending on the underlying etiology and natural history. Acute AR typically presents with tachycardia and severe dyspnea from pulmonary edema. A brief diastolic murmur is sometimes auscultated. In acute AR, patients should be evaluated for acute aortic dissection and/or endocarditis.

In those with chronic disease, the degree of symptoms is dependent on the amount of left ventricular compensation. Those who have advanced disease describe shortness of breath with exertion and fatigue. On physical exam, classic features of chronic AR include a widened pulse pressure (often > 100 mmHg), diastolic decrescendo murmur at the upper sternal border, and an Austin-Flint murmur which is a low-pitched diastolic murmur at the apex. Water-hammer pulses, uvular bouncing, femoral bruits and pulsations in the nail beds (Quinckes pulse) can also be appreciated.

Diagnosis and Testing

Similar to other valvular lesions, the ECG and CXR are often nonspecific. A transthoracic echocardiogram (TTE) is indicated to assess the severity of AR, left ventricular size and function, dimension of aortic root, leaflet morphology and evidence of endocarditis. On the basis of TTE findings, transesophageal echocardiography can be used to clarify the presence of vegetation on the valve or aortic dissection. Depending on the clinical scenario and institution, MRI/CT can also be utilized to evaluate the aorta when dissection is suspected.

Treatment

Aortic valve surgery is indicated for patients with increased left ventricular size, reduced LV function, or symptomatic aortic regurgitation. Medical therapy plays a limited role. Vasodilators (i.e. ACE inhibitors, Hydralazine, peripherally acting calcium channel blockers) can be used to improve hemodynamics. Patients who present in decompensated heart failure require diuretics to relieve pulmonary congestion. Appropriate antibiotics are indicated when endocarditis is present.

Mitral Regurgitation (MR)

The mitral valve is a complex anatomic structure composed of an annulus, two leaflets and a subvalvular apparatus (chordate tendineae and papillary muscles). Disruption of any one of these components can lead to mitral regurgitation.

Etiology

Mitral regurgitation etiologies can be organized into six major categories: (a) *Degenerative*, which is a primary pathology of the valve itself (i.e. mitral valve prolapse); (b) *Dilated cardiomyopathy,* where regurgitation results from widening of the left ventricle and dilation of the mitral valve annulus; (c) *Ischemic*, syndromes in which ischemia or infarction of papillary muscles disrupt mitral valve functioning; (d) *Rheumatic*, which is often associated with concomitant MS; (e) *Infective endocarditis*, that destroys the leaflet tissue; and (e) *Other*, including congenital anomalies of the valve (i.e. cleft) and hypertrophic cardiomyopathy with obstruction.

History and Physical

Similar to other valvular disease, MR will present variably based on the natural history of the underlying pathology. Acute MR will present with significant shortness of breath from pulmonary edema. In the chronic setting, mitral regurgitation can be asymptomatic for years. As the disease progresses, patients report dyspnea with exertion, palpitations (often from atrial fibrillation) and other symptoms of heart failure.

On examination, a systolic murmur can be heard best at the apex with radiation to the axilla. The murmur is often but not always holosystolic. Crackles on lung exam, lower extremity edema, elevated JVP, and auscultation of an extra heart sound, can identify patients with concomitant heart failure.

Diagnosis and Testing

All patients with suspected significant MR should undergo an ECG (to assess for the presence of LVH, left atrial enlargement, and atrial fibrillation) and CXR (for inspection of cardiac size and degree of pulmonary edema). Confirmatory echocardiography evaluates the degree and etiology of regurgitation. On occasion a right and left heart catheterization is indicated to further elucidate the severity, and cause of MR as well as measure pulmonary artery pressures.

Treatment

Severe acute mitral regurgitation often requires stabilization in an intensive care setting with aggressive afterload reduction through IV nitroprusside and on occasion, an intraortic balloon pump. Diuretics are usually needed to relieve pulmonary congestion. In stable patients, oral vasodilators such as ACE inhibitors, angiotension receptor blockers, or hydralazine can achieve the desired effect. Depending on the natural history and etiology of MR, patients may benefit from surgical repair or replacement of the valve. Indications for surgery include the presence of symptoms, a reduced ejection fraction, LV dilatation, pulmonary hypertension, or atrial fibrillation. When technically feasible, mitral valve repair is preferred.

References

1. Bonow RO, Carabello BA, Kanu C, *et al.* (2006) ACC/AHA 2006 guidelines for the management of patients with valvular heart disease: A report of the American College of Cardiology/American Heart Association Task Force on Practice Guidelines (writing committee to revise the 1998 Guidelines for the Management of Patients With Valvular Heart Disease): developed in collaboration with the Society of Cardiovascular Anesthesiologists: endorsed by the Society for Cardiovascular Angiography and Interventions and the Society of Thoracic Surgeons. *Circulation* **114**: e84–e231.
2. Maganti K, Rigolin VH, Sarano ME, *et al.* (2010) Valvular heart disease: Diagnosis and management. *Mayo Clin Proc* **85**: 483–500.
3. Braunwald E, Bonow RO. (2012) *Braunwald's Heart Disease: A Textbook of Cardiovascular Medicine*. Saunders; Philadelphia, pp. xxiv, 1961. p.
4. Hurst JW, Fuster V, Walsh RA, *et al.* (2011) *Hurst's the Heart*. McGraw-Hill Medical; New York, p. 2 v. (xxix, 2444, I–2480 p.).
5. Otto CM, Schwaegler RG, Freeman RV. (2011) *Echocardiography Review Guide: Companion to the Textbook of Clinical Echocardiography*. Saunders, Philadelphia, PA, p. p.
6. Otto CM, Pearlman AS. (1995) *Textbook of Clinical Echocardiography*. W.B. Saunders, Philadelphia: p. xiv, 404 p.

Chapter 22

Atrial Fibrillation and Flutter

Kabir Bhasin and Jonathan L. Halperin**

Key Pearls

- Atrial fibrillation (AF) is the most common sustained arrhythmia and is associated with considerable morbidity and increased mortality. Atrial flutter is less common.
- Immediate cardioversion is indicated when AF causes hemodynamic instability manifested as angina, acute heart failure or shock.
- Rate control can usually be achieved by administering beta-blockers or nondihydropyridine calcium channel blockers (diltiazem or verapamil) to slow conduction across the AV node. Digitalis or amiodarone may used for this purpose in patients with heart failure.
- Anticoagulant therapy is the most effective stroke prevention strategy and should be employed whenever the risk of thromboembolism exceeds the risk of bleeding.
- Catheter ablation is the most effective way to achieve sustained maintenance of sinus rhythm, but as an invasive procedure it carries risks that must be considered in case selection.

*Mount Sinai Medical Center, New York, NY, USA.

Introduction

Atrial fibrillation (AF) is a sustained supraventricular arrhythmia in which normal atrial electrical activity is replaced by multiple, rapid, irregular areas of depolarization throughout the atria. Atrial flutter is a more organized form of rapid atrial depolarization. Both result in loss of organized atrial contraction and variable, often rapid, ventricular depolarization. Clinical manifestations result from impaired hemodynamics secondary to loss of atrioventricular synchrony, progressive ventricular dysfunction due to tachycardia, and increased risk for ischemic events due to embolism of a thrombus arising from stasis in the left atrium.

Epidemiology

AF is the most common sustained arrhythmia, affecting over 2 million individuals in the United States. The overall prevalence is 1%, higher in men and increasing with age from 0.1% among adults under 55 years old to 9% of those over 80.[1] The incidence of AF also increases with age, accruing to an estimated lifetime risk of approximately one in four.[2] Atrial flutter is less common and usually more transient.

AF and atrial flutter may cause symptoms of palpitation, fatigue, and impaired exercise tolerance and are associated with higher rates of mortality. The risk of stroke is approximately fivefold greater than that for otherwise comparable patients in sinus rhythm, and is most pronounced in those over age 75 and in those with certain comorbid conditions. Several observational studies have demonstrated that AF nearly doubles the risk of premature death.[3]

Etiologies and Associated Conditions

Although there are several competing theories on the mechanism of AF, its initiation and maintenance depend on two conditions: (1) an electrical trigger (a manifestation of increased excitability) necessary for initiating the arrhythmia and (2) an abnormal myocardial substrate, typically involving atrial fibrosis and electrical remodeling with or without dilation, allowing for re-entrant circuits.[3] Many, if not all, of the etiologic and predisposing factors contribute to one or both of these conditions. AF typically originates in the left atrium near the ostia of the four pulmonary veins. Typical atrial flutter involves a large re-entrant circuit in the right atrium, usually in the region of the tricuspid isthmus.

Clinical Findings

History and Physical Examination

In the evaluation of patients with AF or atrial flutter, the clinical history should:

- Characterize the pattern of arrhythmia as paroxysmal or persistent;
- Define the impact of associated symptoms;
- Identify possible etiologies and predisposing factors;
- Estimate the risk of thromboembolism and response to previous treatment.

Symptoms may include palpitation, fatigue, dyspnea, or reduced exercise capacity. Many patients are asymptomatic, with the arrhythmia identified incidentally.

Physical examination may confirm the diagnosis and identify contributory causes (e.g. hyperthyroidism) or consequences (e.g. heart failure or shock). A pulse deficit (the difference between the apical heart rate and the peripheral pulse rate) provides information about the adequacy of rate control and ventricular function. Auscultation may demonstrate associated valvular disease, heart failure, or pulmonary disease.

Electrocardiogram

Diagnosis is based on the ECG demonstrating disorganized atrial electrical activity in the form of fibrillatory waves or the more organized rapid pattern of atrial flutter and the absence of P waves. The ventricular response to AF is typically irregular, whereas the response to atrial flutter may be regular. The electrocardiogram is also used to identify comorbid cardiovascular conditions, such as chamber hypertrophy, myocardial ischemia or infarction, pre-excitation and conduction defects.

Echocardiography

Transthoracic echocardiography (TTE) is useful mainly for evaluating chamber dimensions and function, excluding valvular disease, and detecting pulmonary hypertension. It is less sensitive than transesophageal echocardiography (TEE) for detecting thrombi in the left atrium and left atrial appendage. Hence, TTE cannot substitute for TEE to expedite cardioversion.

Additional Laboratory Evaluation

Serum electrolytes, renal, thyroid and liver function, and the hemogram should be measured in all patients with AF or atrial flutter to identify potential provocative factors and comorbid illness and to aid pharmacological management. Exercise testing, ambulatory rhythm (e.g. Holter) monitoring, and electrophysiological testing may be useful in selected cases for guiding therapy.

Management

Optimum management of patients with AF or atrial flutter involves, in order of priority, adequate control of the ventricular response, selection of appropriate antithrombotic therapy, and judicious decisions about the value and approach to rhythm control. Immediate cardioversion to restore sinus rhythm is indicated only when acute hemodynamic instability (angina, heart failure, or shock) develops as a consequence of the arrhythmia or in patients with pre-excitation due to an accessory conduction pathway resulting in extremely rapid ventricular response that threatens to degenerate into ventricular tachycardia or fibrillation.

It was long presumed that restoration and maintenance of sinus rhythm (rhythm control strategy) would be superior to rate control for prevention of stroke and mortality in patients with AF. However, several randomized trials have failed to validate this hypothesis, largely because of the inherent toxicity of most antiarrhythmic drugs, the risk associated with invasive approaches like catheter-based ablation, and the risk of thromboembolism associated with asymptomatic recurrence of AF after withdrawal of anticoagulation.[4,5]

Rate Control

The goals of rate control therapy are to alleviate symptoms associated with AF and prevent the development of tachycardia-mediated cardiomyopathy. In one study, the composite rate of death from cardiovascular causes and hospitalization for heart failure was not reduced with more aggressive efforts to control the heart rate compared with more lenient control.[6] Optimally, however, in managing patients with AF, AV-nodal blocking medication should be administered as needed to slow the heart rate to 60–80 beats per minute (bpm) at rest and less than 120 bpm with moderate exertion.[3]

Beta-blockers and the nondihydropyridine calcium channel blockers diltiazem or verapamil are typically chosen for this purpose. Beta-blockers may aggravate bronchospasm, however, and, like calcium channel blockers, may aggravate hypotension associated with AF. Calcium channel blockers should be avoided in patients with impaired LV systolic function, whereas bisoprolol, extended-release metoprolol, and carvedilol have each been shown to reduce mortality in patients with LV dysfunction.[3,7] Digoxin is less effective for control of the ventricular response during exercise, but is indicated in patients with heart failure due to impaired systolic LV function. The antiarrhythmic agent amiodarone, and, to a lesser extent dronedarone, also slow the ventricular response to AF, but the latter is contraindicated in patients with decompensated heart failure.[8,9] In general, AV-nodal blocking drugs should be avoided in patients with preexcitation due to the Wolff–Parkinson–White syndrome, because of the risk that facilitating rapid conduction along an accessory pathway could lead to ventricular fibrillation.

Stroke Risk Assessment

Certain clinical risk factors are more pertinent than the pattern of AF (paroxysmal, persistent, or permanent) in stratifying stroke risk. All patients with AF should be evaluated for risk factors associated with thromboembolism and candidacy for long-term anticoagulant therapy. Among several models developed to estimate the risk of thromboembolism in patients with AF or atrial flutter, the most widely used is the $CHADS_2$ score, which assigns points as follows:

- History of heart failure or reduced LVEF: 1 point
- Hypertension: 1 point
- Age >75 years: 1 point
- Diabetes: 1 point
- History of stroke, TIA, or systemic embolism 2 points

The $CHADS_2$ scoring system and other risk prediction tools were developed at a time when warfarin was the sole oral anticoagulant available. The approximate prevalence and stroke rates without anticoagulation associated with various $CHADS_2$ risk categories are shown in Table 1; current recommendations for antithrombotic therapy issued by several North American professional societies are presented in Table 2. As new oral anticoagulants are introduced that carry a lower risk of intracerebral hemorrhage, the balance of risk and benefit may shift, such that many patients who in the past might be treated with aspirin, including those in the moderate-risk strata, may benefit from anticoagulant therapy. This is an area of future research, and new risk stratification models are likely to arise.

There is less consensus about risk factors for bleeding during anticoagulation than about stroke risk stratification, but several schemes have

Table 1. The CHADS2 Stroke Risk Score for Patients with Nonvalvular Atrial Fibrillation

	Score	Prevalence [%]
Congestive Heart Failure	1	32
Hypertension	1	65
Age greater than 75 years	1	23
Diabetes	1	18
Stroke	2	10
Moderate to High Risk	≥2	50–60
Low Risk	0–1	40–50

[Adapted from: VanWalraven C *et al.* (2003) *Arch Intern Med* 163: 936.]
*Nieuwlaat R *et al.* (2006) EuroHeart survey, *Eur Heart J* (e-published).

Table 2. Summary of Recommendations for Antithrombotic Therapy for Prevention of Stroke and Systemic Embolism in the Guidelines Published by the American College of Cardiology, American Heart Association and European Society of Cardiology

Risk Category	Recommended Therapy
No risk factors CHADS$_2$ = 0	Aspirin, 81–325 mg qd
One moderate risk factor CHADS$_2$ = 1	Aspirin, 81–325 mg/d or Warfarin (INR 2.0–3.0, target 2.5)
Any high risk factor or >1 moderate risk factor CHADS$_2$ ≥2 or Mitral stenosis	Warfarin (INR 2.0–3.0, target 2.5)
Prosthetic valve	Warfarin (INR 2.5–3.5, target 3.0)

[Fuster V *et al.* (2006) *J Am Coll Cardiol* 48: 854–906.] The European guidelines were modified in 2010.

been developed. For patients at high risk of thromboembolism who are unable to sustain chronic anticoagulation, left atrial appendage occlusion devices are under investigation, but the safety, efficacy, and indications for these devices have not been clearly established.[16]

Antithrombotic Therapy

Although anticoagulation is more effective than antiplatelet therapy with aspirin across all risk strata, patients at very low risk of stroke may not gain sufficient benefit to warrant the inconvenience and risk of bleeding associated with warfarin. The combination of aspirin and clopidogrel is less effective than warfarin and is associated with greater risk of bleeding than aspirin, but was more effective than aspirin alone in a study of patients who were unwilling or considered ineligible to take a vitamin K antagonist.[15] The selection of antithrombotic therapy to employ is individualized based on age and other risk factors.

The most extensively studied anticoagulant is the vitamin K antagonist warfarin, which in clinical trials yielded, on average, a 68% reduction in the risk of stroke compared to a placebo or no treatment.[10] Unfortunately, despite this dramatic benefit, approximately 36%–47% of candidates for anticoagulation do not receive warfarin therapy.[11–13] The relatively low rate of use is likely multifactorial. Beyond concerns over hemorrhage, warfarin interacts with multiple foods and drugs, requires frequent coagulation monitoring, and often results in anticoagulation outside the target range of intensity.

The need for a safe, effective, and convenient oral anticoagulant has long been recognized and the key targets identified for study have been coagulation factors IIa (thrombin) and Xa. The first of the novel oral anticoagulants to receive FDA approval was dabigatran etexilate, a prodrug that is activated after ingestion to directly inhibit thrombin. In the open label RE-LY trial of patients with nonvalvular AF, dabigatran etexilate, 150 mg twice daily, appeared superior and a lower dose of 110 mg twice daily was noninferior to warfarin for prevention of stroke and systemic embolism. The higher dose of dabigatran was not inferior to warfarin in terms of major bleeding, and the most-feared complication of anticoagulant therapy, intracerebral hemorrhage, occurred less often with dabigatran than with warfarin.[14] The FDA approved dabigatran etexilate, 150 mg twice daily, for patients with AF who have one or more stroke risk factors and adequate renal function (creatinine clearance >30 ml/min); a lower dose of 75 mg twice daily was approved for patients with impaired renal function (15–30 ml/min) based on pharmacokinetic models, but this dose regimen has not been clinically evaluated; the dose of 110 mg twice daily has not been approved for use in the U.S. Approximately 10% of patients receiving dabigatran experienced dyspepsia, and rates of colonic bleeding were higher with dabigatran than with warfarin in the RE-LY trial. Rivaroxaban was the first oral direct factor Xa inhibitor to garner FDA approval for clinical use. In the ROCKET AF trial, rivaroxaban was non-inferior to warfarin for prevention of stroke or systemic embolism in patients with non-valvular atrial fibrilllation. While there was no significant difference in overall rates of major bleeding with rivaroxaban as compared with warfarin, the factor Xa inhibitor was associated with less intracranial and fatal hemorrhage.[17] The FDA approved rivaroxaben in a dose of 20 mg once daily for patients with creatinine clearance greater than 50 mL/min. For those with moderately impaired renal function (creatinine clearance between 15 and 49 mL/min), a lower dose of 15 mg once daily is available. A subsequent trial evaluating the factor Xa inhibitor, apixaban, also demonstrated benefit as compared with warfarin and another involving edoxaban is in progress. These agents may also become available as therapeutic alternatives to warfarin.

Rhythm Control

Given the potential toxicity of antiarrhythmic drugs, efforts to restore and maintain sinus rhythm are typically reserved for patients with AF of recent onset (< 1 year), hemodynamic instability, or persistent symptoms despite adequate rate control. There are two components to the strategy of rhythm control: cardioversion and maintenance of sinus rhythm.

Cardioversion

Restoration of sinus rhythm can be accomplished by either direct current cardioversion (DCCV) or administration of pharmacological agents. The former involves delivery of an R-wave-synchronous biphasic electrical shock (usually 100–200 J) while the patient is sedated. DCCV is relatively safe and initial success exceeds 90%; sustained sinus arrest or sinus bradycardia follows < 1% of procedures.[18]

The Vaughan–Williams class IC drugs (flecainide and propafenone) block sodium channels and are effective in restoring sinus rhythm, increasing the success of DCCV, and preventing early recurrence of AF. These agents carry potential proarrhythmic toxicity, leading to *torsades de pointes* ventricular tachycardia and ventricular fibrillation in patients with ischemic heart disease, left ventricular hypertrophy, or heart failure. In addition, an initial vagolytic effect may accelerate the ventricular response to AF, requiring concurrent treatment with AV-nodal blocking agents. The class III antiarrhythmic drugs ibutilide and dofetilide, which inhibit potassium channels, can be used in patients with ischemic heart disease or heart failure, but also possess proarrhythmic potential requiring in-hospital initiation and close monitoring of the QTc interval.[18] Amiodarone is effective and relatively free of proarrhythmic toxicity, but initiation of treatment is time-consuming and myriad extracardiac side effects limit its long-term use.

Regardless of the method of cardioversion, antithrombotic therapy is necessary for reducing the risk of stroke and systemic embolism associated with restoration of organized atrial mechanical activity. When possible, patients with AF for longer than 48 hr should be anticoagulated (INR >2) for at least 3 weeks prior to cardioversion. When earlier cardioversion is indicated, TEE should be performed to exclude a thrombus in the LAA. Since termination of AF may be followed by an uncertain period of "stunning" (atrial mechanical arrest), anticoagulation should be in effect at the time of cardioversion and continued for at least 3–4 weeks afterward and longer for patients with risk factors for thromboembolism because of the possibility of recurrent AF with or without symptoms.[19]

Maintenance of sinus rhythm

Long-term antiarrhythmic drug therapy is not indicated after cardioversion for most patients with a first-detected episode of AF. For those

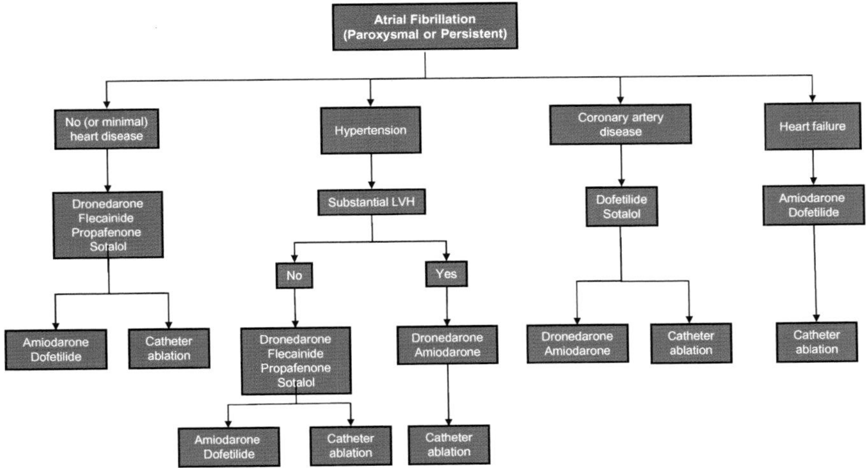

Fig. 1. Antiarrhythmic therapy for maintenance of sinus rhythm in patients with paroxysmal or persistent atrial fibrillation.

[Adapted from: Fuster V *et al.* (2006) *J Am Coll Cardiol* 48: 854–906.]

Note: Drugs are listed alphabetically rather than in order of preference or efficacy; catheter ablation may be an appropriate initial choice for carefully selected, very symptomatic patients.

with symptomatic recurrent AF, however, selection of antiarrhythmic medication is based on the pattern of AF and comorbid conditions, as summarized in Fig. 1. The role of catheter ablation, in which the ostia of the pulmonary veins are electrically isolated from the left atrium, has not been fully established. The method appears generally more effective than antiarrhythmic drug therapy, but is associated with a risk of major complications, including thromboembolism, perforation leading to hemopericardium or tamponade, and esophageal injury. It is usually reserved for otherwise healthy patients with little associated structural heart disease in whom disabling symptoms of AF have not responded sufficiently to one or more antiarrhythmic drugs, but may be an appropriate initial strategy in carefully selected patients who are very symptomatic of the arrhythmia when drug therapy is considered a less desirable option (Table 3).[3,20] Ablation of typical atrial flutter is more

Table 3. Patient Selection for Catheter-based Ablation of Atrial Fibrillation (Courtesy of Dr. Hugh Calkins.)

Variable	Better Candidate	Less Optimal Candidate
Symptoms	Highly symptomatic	Minimally symptomatic
Class I and III drugs failed	≥1	0
AF type	Paroxysmal	Long-standing persistant
Age	Younger (<70 years)	Older (≥70 years)
LA size	Smaller (<5.0cm)	Larger (≥5.0 cm)
Ejection fraction	Normal	Reduced
Congestive heart failure	No	Yes
Other cardiac disease	No	Yes
Pulmonary disease	No	Yes
Sleep apnea	No	Yes
Obesity	No	Yes
Prior stroke/TIA	No	Yes

straightforward and is associated with less risk, in part because transseptal catheterization is not required.

Future Trends

The population with AF is expanding rapidly as patients live longer with more advanced heart disease and this will continue unless more effective prophylactic measures are developed. Stroke is the most pressing concern but new drugs and devices promise to expand treatment more broadly across the population at risk. More effective drugs, procedures, and devices are available but their relative safety and efficacy may differ for defined patient subgroups and comparative cost-effectiveness analyses are in an early stage of development.

References

1. Go AS, Heyleck EM, Phillips KA, *et al.* (2001) Prevalence of diagnosed atrial fibrillation in adults: National implications for

rhythm management and stroke prevention: The Anticoagulation and Risk Factors in Atrial Fibrillation (ATRIA) Study. *JAMA* **285**: 2370.

2. Miyasaka Y, Barnes ME, Gersh BJ, *et al.* (2006) Secular trends in incidence of atrial fibrillation in Olmsted County, Minnesota, 1980 to 2000, and implications on the projections for future prevalence. *Circulation* **114**: 119.
3. Fuster V, Ryden LE, Cannom DS, *et al.* (2006) ACC/AHA/ESC 2006 guidelines for the management of patients with atrial fibrillation: A report of the American College of Cardiology/American Heart Association Task Force on Practice Guidelines and the European Society of Cardiology Committee for Practice Guidelines (Writing Committee to Revise the 2001 Guidelines for the Management of Patients with Atrial Fibrillation): Developed in collaboration with the European Heart Rhythm Association and the Heart Rhythm Society. *Circulation* **114**: 257.
4. De Denus S, Sanoski CA, Carlsson J, *et al.* (2005) Rate versus rhythm control in patients with atrial fibrillation: A meta-analysis. *Arch Intern Med* **165**: 258.
5. Calkins H, Brugada J, Packer DL, *et al.* (2007) HRS/EHRA/ECAS expert consensus statement on catheter and surgical ablation of atrial fibrillation: Recommendations for personnel, policy, procedure and follow-up. A report of the Heart Rhythm Society (HRS) Task Force on catheter and surgical ablation of atrial fibrillation. *Heart Rhythm* **4**: 816.
6. Van Gelder IC, Hessel F, Groenveld MD, *et al.* (2010) Lenient versus strict rate control in patients with atrial fibrillation. *N Engl J Med* **362**: 1363.
7. Torp-Pederson C, Poole-Wilson PA, Swedberg K, *et al.* (2005) Effects of metoprolol and carvedilol on cause-specific mortality and morbidity in patients with chronic heart failure: COMET. *Am Heart J* **149**: 371.
8. Kober L, Torp-Pederson C, McMurray JJV, *et al.* (2008) Increased mortality after dronedarone therapy for severe heart failure. *N Engl J Med* **358**: 2678.

9. Hohnloser SH, Crijns HJGM, van Eickels M, *et al.*, on behalf of the ATHENA investigators. (2009) Effect of dronedarone on cardiovascular events in atrial fibrillation. *N Engl J Med* **360**: 668.
10. Hart RG, Pearce LA, Aguilar MI. (2007) Meta-analysis: Antithrombotic therapy to prevent stroke in patients who have nonvalvular atrial fibrillation. *Ann Intern Med* **146**: 857.
11. Birman-Deych E, Radford MJ, Nilasena DS, Gage BF. (2006) Use and effectiveness of warfarin in Medicare beneficiaries with atrial fibrillation. *Stroke* **37**: 1070.
12. McCormick D, Gurwitz JH, Goldberg RJ, *et al.* (2001) Prevalence and quality of warfarin use for patients with atrial fibrillation in the long-term care setting. *Arch Intern Med* **161**: 2458.
13. Goto S, Bhatt DL, Röther J, *et al.*; REACH Registry Investigators. (2008) Prevalence, clinical profile, and cardiovascular outcomes of atrial fibrillation patients with atherothrombosis. *Am Heart J* **156**: 855.
14. Wallentin L, Yusuf S, Ezekowitz MD, *et al.*, on behalf of the RE-LY investigators. (2010) Efficacy and safety of dabigatran compared with warfarin at different levels of international normalised ratio control for stroke prevention in atrial fibrillation: An analysis of the RE-LY trial. *Lancet* **376**: 975.
15. Connolly S, Pogue J, Hart R, *et al.* (2006) Clopidogrel plus aspirin versus oral anticoagulation for atrial fibrillation in the atrial fibrillation clopidogrel trail with ibersartan for prevention of vascular events: ACTIVE-W. *Lancet* **367**(9526): 1903.
16. Holmes DR, Reddy VY, Turi ZG, *et al.*, on behalf of the PROTECT-AF investigators. (2009) Percutaneous closure of the left atrial appendage versus warfarin therapy for prevention of stroke in patients with atrial fibrillation: A randomised non-inferiority trial. *Lancet* **374**: 534.
17. Patel MR, Mahaffey KW, Garg J, *et al.* (2011) Rivaroxaban versus warfarin in nonvalvular artial fibrillation. *N Engl J Med* **365**: 883.
18. McNammara RL, Tamariz LJ, Segal JB, *et al.* (2003) Management of atrial fibrillation: Review of the evidence for the role of pharmacologic

therapy, electrical cardioversion, and echocardiography. *Ann Inter Med* **139**: 1018.

19. Gallagher MM, Hennessy BJ, Edvardsson N, *et al.* (2002) Embolic complications of direct current cardioversion of atrial arrhythmias: Association with low intensity of anticoagulation at the time of cardioversion. *J Am Coll Card* **40**: 926.
20. Camm AJ, Kirchhof P, Lip GYH, *et al.*; The Task Force for the Management of Atrial Fibrillation of the European Society of Cardiology (ESC). (2010) Guidelines for the management of atrial fibrillation. *Eur Heart J* [doi:10.1093/eurheartj/ehq278].

Chapter 23

Arrhythmias: Supraventricular Tachycardias, Ventricular Tachycardias and Bradyarrhythmias

*Avi Fischer**

Key Pearls

- Even nonlethal arrhythmias, such as atrial fibrillation, should be treated by direct current (DC) cardioversion if thought to be responsible for a patient's unstable condition.
- An electrophysiology (EP) study provides information about the presence of arrhythmias and the effectiveness of pharmacologic therapy, and for the prediction of the future risk of sudden cardiac death.
- When deciding to implant a permanent pacemaker (PPM), it is important to ascertain that symptoms are due to the rhythm disturbance.
- During a supraventricular tachycardia (SVT), it is important to decide whether the rhythm is regular or irregular and to attempt to identify the presence of a P-wave as this often provides clues about the diagnosis.
- It is important to identify whether structural heart disease is present in the patient with ventricular tachycardia (VT), as the treatment offered is often dictated by the presence of structural abnormalities.

*Mount Sinai School of Medicine, New York, NY, USA.

Introduction

There are numerous mechanisms important in the genesis of atrial and ventricular arrhythmias. It is critical for all healthcare providers to appreciate that any rhythm that is responsible for hemodynamic instability should be treated using advanced cardiac life-support algorithms. Even nonlethal arrhythmias, such as atrial fibrillation, should be treated by synchronized direct current (DC) cardioversion if thought to be responsible for a patient's unstable condition. This chapter will focus on arrhythmias commonly encountered in inpatients, concentrating on treatment strategies.

Role of the Electrophysiology Study

Electrophysiology (EP) testing is performed to establish a mechanism for a particular arrhythmia — either tachycardia or bradycardia. Additionally, EP testing is often utilized to guide the treatment strategy, whether antiarrhythmic drug therapy, cardiac rhythm device implantation or ablation. It may be performed to characterize the function of the sinus node, the atrioventricular (AV) node and the His–Purkinje or specialized conduction system in the heart to guide treatment for bradyarrhythmias. Furthermore, it is used to induce tachyarrhythmias and allow for characterization, differentiation of the mechanism of the arrhythmia, and to facilitate ablation of the substrate of the arrhythmia. With the advent of cardiac rhythm device and catheter ablation technologies, these treatments have become the mainstay of arrhythmia management. The procedure is performed via a transvenous approach using venous access obtained most often via the femoral veins. Multiple flexible, multipolar electrode catheters are positioned in specific sites within the heart, and recording and stimulation performed. The study can provide important information about the presence of arrhythmias, evaluate the effectiveness of pharmacologic therapy of an arrhythmia, predict the future risk of sudden cardiac death and assess the need for an implantable cardiac rhythm device such as a pacemaker or defibrillator.

Bradyarrhythmias

There are a variety of conditions causing bradyarrhythmias that are transient and reversible. Reversible causes of bradycardia include the use of drugs such as beta-blockers, calcium channel blockers and other antiarrhythmic agents, electrolyte disturbances or myocardial infarction. It is always important to exclude any metabolic or pharmacologic contributors prior to making the decision to implant a permanent device.

Specific clinical settings may warrant the placement of a temporary transvenous pacemaker. Temporary pacing may be required in the setting of acute myocardial infarction, prophylactically in the patient at risk for developing progressive conduction disturbances, and for symptomatic bradycardia in the patient without a reversible cause who is awaiting placement of a permanent device. A summary of the general indications for temporary pacing can be seen in Table 1. Once reversible causes have been excluded, even a single episode of symptomatic bradycardia may be enough to indicate a permanent pacemaker implant, but symptoms must be clearly due to the rhythm disturbance.

Tachyarrhythmias

Supraventricular Arrhythmias

One of the most important methods for evaluating the mechanism of any arrhythmia is analysis of atrial activity on the surface electrocardiogram (ECG) and identification of the morphology of the P wave and QRS

Table 1. Pacing Common Diagnoses of Regular Narrow Complex Tachycardias

In acute myocardial infarction:

- Medically refractory sinus node or A node or AV node dysfunction causing symptomatic bradycardia
- Mobitz II second-degree AV block with anterior infarction
- Third-degree AV block with anterior infarction
- New bifascicular block
- Alternating bundle branch block

complex. Often the inferior limb leads II, III, aVF as well as precordial lead V1 are best for identifying P waves. Narrow complex tachycardias are characterized by having a QRS duration of 100 ms or less. When evaluating a supraventricular tachycardia, it is also useful to identify whether the rhythm is regular or irregular, as this often offers clues about the diagnosis. An irregularly irregular rhythm is most often indicative of atrial fibrillation, but may also represent a multifocal atrial tachycardia.

Further dividing regular narrow complex tachycardias into those with a short RP interval and those with a long RP interval may help in generating a differential diagnosis and treatment plan (Table 2). The RP interval is assessed by identifying the position of the P wave on the surface ECG and its position relative to the QRS (R wave). Short RP tachycardias have the P wave either "buried" in the QRS or present after the QRS in the T wave such that the RP interval is shorter than the PR interval (Fig 1).

Regular Narrow Complex Tachycardia with a Short RP Interval

There are three main tachycardia types that manifest as regular, narrow and with a short RP interval (RP < PR interval). These tachycardias include

Table 2. Indications for Temporary Pacing

In the absence of myocardial infarction:

- Medically refractory symptomatic bradycardia, sinus node dysfunction, second- or third-degree AV block
- Third-degree AV block with wide QRS escape rhythm, ventricular rate < 50 bpm or signs of hypoperfusion

Prophylactic

- New AV block or bundle branch block with acute endocarditis (especially aortic valve)
- Perioperatively in patient with history of syncope and with bifascicular block
- To allow treatment with drugs that worsen bradycardias

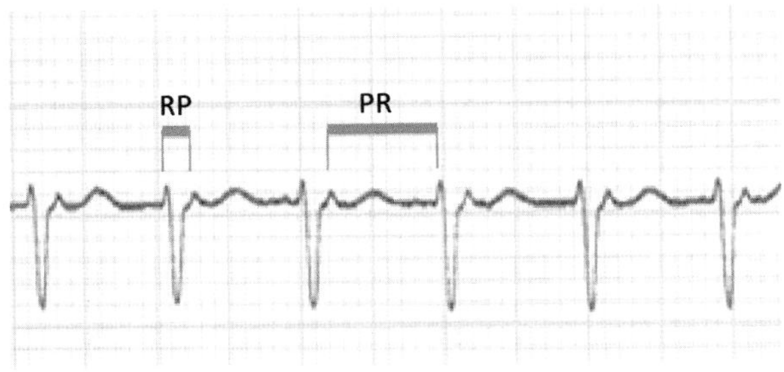

Fig. 1. Measurement of the RP and PR intervals on the surface electrocardiogram. Black lines indicate the P wave and the R wave used to measure these intervals.

typical AV-nodal re-entrant tachycardia, AV re-entrant tachycardia and an atrial tachycardia with a first degree AV block where the P wave occurs late in the QRS complex or within the T wave.

AV-nodal re-entrant tachycardia

AV-nodal re-entrant tachycardia (AVNRT) is a common arrhythmia occurring in young, healthy individuals with no structural heart disease. It is more common in females, and patients often describe abrupt onset and offset of palpitations and tachycardia. Mechanistically, there are two pathways of AV nodal conduction present (slow and fast), and the typical form consists of anterograde conduction over the slow pathway and retrograde conduction over the fast pathway. As retrograde conduction of the impulse back to the atria is rapid, the P wave either is not visible because it occurs simultaneously with the QRS or is seen in the terminal portion of the QRS (Fig. 2). Acutely, vagal maneuvers, adenosine or AV-nodal blockers such as calcium channel or beta-blockers are effective therapies for termination of the arrhythmia. For long-term management, AV-nodal blockers are most effective and can be used either on a daily or "as needed" basis when tachycardia occurs. Other antiarrhythmics can be used either alone or in conjunction with AV-nodal blocking agents. Catheter ablation of the slow AV-nodal pathway is curative in 95% of patients, but a complete AV block can complicate slow pathway ablation in 0.5%–1% of patients.[1]

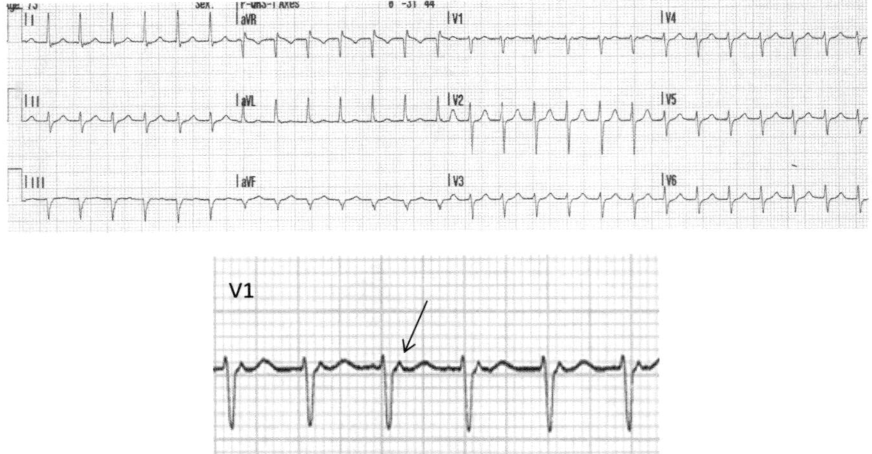

Fig. 2. Twelve-lead electrocardiogram of a narrow complex tachycardia with P waves seen in the terminal portion of the QRS complex. The arrow in the magnified trace of lead V1 identifies a clearer image of the P wave.

AV re-entrant tachycardia

AV re-entrant tachycardia (AVRT) involves an accessory atrioventricular connection or pathway such as that seen in the Wolff–Parkinson–White (WPW) syndrome. Patients with WPW have the characteristic "delta wave" seen on the surface ECG, associated with a short PR interval of less than 120 ms, a slurred upstroke of the QRS indicating pre-excitation (delta wave), a broad QRS and secondary ST and T wave changes (Fig. 3). In patients with WPW, the most common arrhythmia is AVRT that utilizes the AV node for antegrade conduction and the accessory pathway for retrograde conduction. As with AVNRT, this tachycardia often has abrupt onset and offset and is characterized by a short RP interval. The presence of alternation in the amplitude of the QRS complexes (QRS alternans) on the surface ECG during tachycardia points to AVRT as the mechanism, but this finding is not limited to AVRT. The location of the accessory pathway is along the lateral mitral valve annulus in approximately 50% of cases, in the posteroseptum in 25%, along the lateral tricuspid valve annulus in 25% and in the anteroseptum in 2%.[2] Acutely, vagal maneuvers,

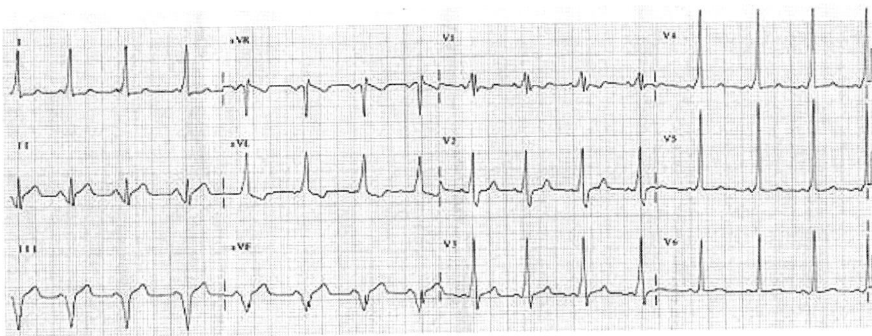

Fig. 3. Twelve-lead electrocardiogram from a patient with Wolff–Parkinson–White. Note the short PR interval, the slurred upstroke of the initial portion of the QRS complex and the nonspecific T wave changes.

adenosine or AV-nodal blockers such as calcium channel or beta-blockers are effective therapies for termination. Chronically, AV-nodal blockers are most effective and can be used either on a daily or "as needed" basis when tachycardia occurs. Catheter ablation of the accessory pathway is curative in 95% of patients and an AV block is uncommon except when ablating anteroseptal pathways as these are located close to the AV node.[2]

Atrial tachycardia

In contrast to AVNRT and AVRT, the mechanism of atrial tachycardia (AT) is most often not re-entrant and patients are often older and may have structural heart disease. As a result of increased automaticity, an impulse arises from an ectopic focus in either the right or left atrium. Often the tachycardia is incessant in nature and, depending on the rate of the AT, can occur with 1:1 AV conduction. Bursts of nonsustained tachycardia can often occur and P wave morphology can often be seen most clearly in the initiating beat (Fig. 4).

The morphology of the P wave on the surface ECG is often helpful in predicting the location of the ectopic focus. In particular, inverted P waves in limb leads I and aVL suggest the presence of a left atrial focus. Acutely, adenosine will terminate 10%–15% of ATs and AV-nodal blockers are

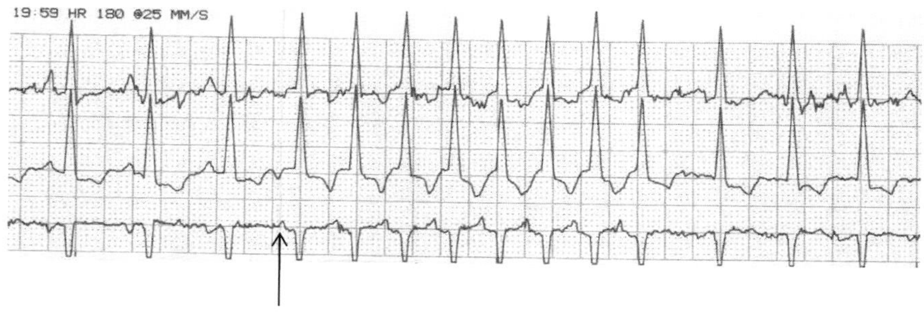

Fig. 4. Telemetry recording of a run of atrial ectopic beats. The arrow indicates the first atrial ectopic beat with a P wave morphology different from that present in sinus rhythm.

effective therapies for controlling the ventricular rate. However, chronic therapy of an ectopic AT often involves the use of an antiarrhythmic agent and/or catheter ablation. The choice of antiarrhythmic varies with the clinical characteristics of the patient and may include amiodarone, sotalol or agents such as flecainide or propafenone. Depending on the location of the ectopic focus and the experience of the operator, the success rates for ablation approach 80%–85%.[3]

Ventricular Arrhythmias

The definition of sustained ventricular tachycardia (VT) is a ventricular rhythm at a rate of ≥100 bpm lasting at least 30 s in duration. VTs are categorized as occurring in the setting of structural heart disease and in the "normal heart." It is important to identify whether structural heart disease is present in the patient with VT, as the treatments offered may be very different. Structural heart disease is most commonly the result of coronary artery disease and prior myocardial infarction; however, VT may also occur in the setting of a nonischemic cardiomyopathy. In addition, it is critical to differentiate between the occurrence of monomorphic VT and of polymorphic VT or ventricular fibrillation. Over the last several years, there have been a number of genetic conditions, such as the long QT syndromes (LQTSs), Brugada syndrome and catecholaminergic polymorphic

VT (CPVT), that occur in younger patients with a structurally normal heart. The VT seen in these patients is polymorphic rather than monomorphic and these patients constitute a unique population of patients, each with a specific treatment approach beyond the scope of this chapter.

Ventricular Tachycardia in the Absence of Structural Heart Disease (Idiopathic VT)

It is important to understand that monomorphic VT which occurs in the setting of a structurally normal heart carries a good prognosis. The VTs occurring in these patients can be subdivided into those with a left bundle branch block (LBBB) morphology and those with a right bundle branch (RBBB) morphology. In general, VTs with an LBBB morphology arise from the right ventricle (RV) and those with an RBBB, from the left ventricle (LV).

Left bundle branch block VT

The most common anatomic location of an LBBB morphology VT is the right-ventricular outflow tract (RVOT). The typical ECG of this VT has an LBBB morphology with an inferior axis and characteristic upright QRS complexes in the inferior limb leads (Fig. 5). This VT often occurs in young patients, is often provoked by exercise and frequently is repetitive. As mentioned previously, this form of VT is not associated with increased mortality or risk of sudden death. Patients can be treated pharmacologically, as this arrhythmia is often responsive to beta-blockers, calcium channel blockers, adenosine and vagal maneuvers. Induction of this VT by programmed electrical stimulation may be difficult and specific maneuvers in the EP laboratory are often required for provocation. Radio frequency ablation of the VT focus can be performed as a curative therapy, with the success rates of ablation being 90%–95%.[4]

Right bundle branch block VT

A less common form of idiopathic VT, also associated with an excellent long-term and low risk of sudden death, involves the Purkinje tissue in the

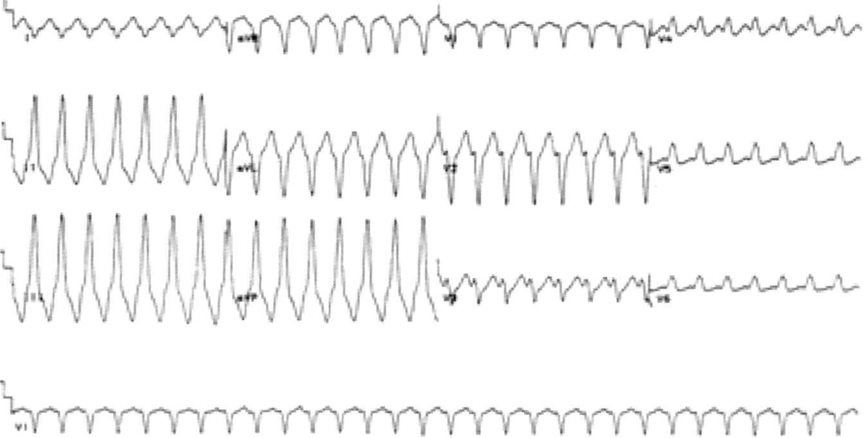

Fig. 5. Twelve-lead electrocardiogram of right-ventricular outflow tract (RVOT) VT. The QRS morphology in lead V1 has a left bundle branch (LBBB) morphology and the QRS is upright in leads II, III, aVF is inferior.

LV. This form of VT is often paroxysmal and is less likely to be induced by exercise. Induction of this arrhythmia in the EP laboratory occurs in almost 90% of cases (as opposed to LBBB VT). Classically, this form of VT is responsive to verapamil but other antiarrhythmic agents, specifically class III antiarrhythmics, are often used. Catheter ablation for this form of VT is highly successful.

Ventricular Tachycardia in the Presence of Structural Heart Disease

Ischemic cardiomyopathy

The most common setting for VT in patients with coronary artery disease (CAD) is postmyocardial infarction. Patients who present with VT in the setting of CAD and myocardial infarction (MI) often have a significant reduction in left-ventricular function, which is a significant predictor of long-term mortality in these patients. The presence of myocardial scarring and fibrosis as a result of MI acts as the substrate for re-entrant ventricular arrhythmias. There have been numerous large multicenter trials that have positioned the implantable cardioverter defibrillator (ICD) as the first-line therapy for patients with CAD and a reduced ejection fraction of ≤35%, even in the absence of VT.[5] Based on the results of these trials and the overwhelming evidence that these devices significantly reduce the incidence of sudden death, these devices are implanted for primary prevention in select patients.

In addition to the use of ICDs, antiarrhythmic drugs can be employed in the patient with VT in the setting of ischemic heart disease to suppress recurrent VT. Often antiarrhythmics are initiated in response to ICD shocks, but radio frequency ablation of the VT substrate is being performed more commonly as a means of reducing ICD therapies in patients with recurrent VT. Re-entrant VT in the setting of an ischemic cardiomyopathy is often easily and reproducibly induced in the EP laboratory, allowing for mapping of the precise location of the substrate of the VT. The success rates for ablation of VT show that it is often a more definitive therapy that reduces the need for long-term antiarrhythmic medications.

Nonischemic cardiomyopathy

Left-ventricular function is an important determinant of mortality in patients with a nonischemic cause of cardiomyopathy. The presence of asymptomatic nonsustained VT is almost universal in patients with nonischemic cardiomyopathy, with the incidence increasing as the New York Heart Association (NYHA) functional class worsens. As is the case with ischemic cardiomyopathy, ICD therapy is the first-line treatment for patients with nonischemic cardiomyopathy and an LV ejection fraction of ≤ 35%, even in the absence of VT.[5] Data from large randomized trials have demonstrated the mortality benefit of primary prevention ICD implantation in this patient population. It is important to rule out reversible causes of cardiomyopathy in the nonischemic patient prior to implanting a permanent device. The approach to treating recurrent VT in the nonischemic patient is similar to that in the patient with ischemic cardiomyopathy. Often antiarrhythmics are used as first-line therapy, but ablation is becoming a more widely accepted approach to treating VT in these patients.

References

1. Clague JR, *et al.* (2001) Targeting the slow pathway for atrioventricular nodal re*entrant tachycardia: Initial results and long-term follow-up in 379 consecutive patients. *Eur Heart J* **22**: 82–88.
2. Lee PC, *et al.* (2006) Electrophysiologic characteristics and radiofrequency catheter ablation in children with Wolff–Parkinson–White syndrome. *Pacing Clin Electrophysiol* **29**: 490–495.
3. Hsieh MH, Chen SA. Catheter ablation of focal atrial tachycardia. In: Zipes DP, Haissaguerre M, (eds). *Catheter Ablation of Arrhythmias* 2nd ed. Futura, Armonk, New York, pp. 185–203.
4. Joshi S, Wilber DJ. (2005) Ablation of idiopathic right ventricular outflow tract tachycardia: Current perspectives. *J Cardiovasc Electrophysiol* **16**(Suppl 1): S52–S58.
5. Bardy GH, *et al.* (2005) Amiodarone or an implantable cardioverter-defibrillator for congestive heart failure. *N Engl J Med* **352**: 225–237.

Chapter 24

Malignant Hypertension

Adam Harris and Michael C. Kim*[†]

Key Pearls

- Severely elevated blood pressure with evidence of end organ damage is a hypertensive emergency; medications should be administered parenterally and pressures should be reduced by 25% within the first 4 hours.
- Symptoms occur acutely, as the result of several positive feedback mechanisms that contribute to a rapid rise in blood pressures.
- A wide variety of clinical presentations are possible based on underlying disease states, including hypertensive encephalopathy, MI, aortic dissection, renal failure, vision disruptions and salt imbalances.
- Hypertensive encephalopathy is very common in patients with malignant hypertension but is a rapidly reversible condition if treated in a timely fashion; neurological symptoms include headache, nausea, vision loss, projectile vomiting, restlessness, confusion, drowsiness and seizures.
- Treatment options differ based on underlying organ damage and thus it is critical to discern these conditions rapidly through physical exam, radiology and laboratory testing.

*Stony Brook School of Medicine, Stony Brook, NY, USA.
[†]Mount Sinai Medical Center, New York, NY, USA.

Introduction

Malignant hypertension (also known as accelerated hypertension) is defined as severely elevated blood pressure (BP) (>180/120 mmHg) associated with papilledema. In situations where there is evidence of organ failure, it is considered a hypertensive emergency and a rapid reduction in BP is required to minimize damage. However, if the patient presents with severely elevated BP, but no acute end organ damage, it is considered a hypertensive urgency and BP can be reduced more slowly.[2,7]

Incidence and Etiology

Malignant hypertension occurs in approximately 1% of the hypertensive population. It could develop *de novo* but this is unlikely.[9,11] Although patients with secondary hypertension account for only 5% of the hypertensive population, they represent up to 40% of patients who present with malignant hypertension.[8] Furthermore, patients with secondary hypertension, and others who were previously normotensive, develop organ damage at lower BPs and earlier in the course of their hypertensive conditions when compared to patients with underlying chronic hypertension who have developed adaptations to withstand higher pressures.[3] Thus, the onset of malignant hypertension is more correlated with the rate at which BP changes than any absolute BP.[1–3] (Table 1)

Pathophysiology

Hypertensive emergencies are the result of rapid intense systemic vasoconstriction with profound volume depletion.[1,10] Severely elevated BP exceeds the vascular autoregulatory ability to protect microvasculature. When this occurs, several positive feedback mechanisms are set off exacerbating already high pressures, thus symptoms manifest very rapidly (Fig. 1).

Under conditions of extreme hypertension, autoregulation, which normally protects vascular endothelium from elevations in BP through vasoconstriction, is no longer able to compensate. High pressures are

Table. 1.[1,7] Causes of Hypertensive Emergencies

- Essential hypertension (most common)
- Renal disease
  Chronic pyelonephritis
  Primary glomerulonephritis
  Vasculitis
  Microscopic polyarteritis nodosa
  Wegner's granulomatosis
  Hemolytic uremic syndrome
  Thrombotic thrombocytopenic purpura
  Systemic sclerosis
  Systemic lupus erythematosus
- Renovascular disease
  Renal artery stenosis (atheromatous or fibromuscular dysplasia)
  Polyarteritis nodosa
- Pregnancy
  Severe pre-eclampsia/eclampsia
- Endocrine
  Pheochromocytoma
  Cushing's syndrome
  Renin-secreting tumors
  Primary hyperaldosteronism
- Drugs
  Cocaine or other sympathomimetics
  Erythropoietin
  Cyclosporin
  Abrupt withdrawal of centrally acting α2-adrenergic agonist
  Interactions with nonselective monoamine-oxidase inhibitors
- Central-nervous-system disorders
  Head injury
  Cerebral infarction/hemorrhage
  Brain tumors

transmitted to microvasculature, leading to endothelial damage and fibrinoid necrosis with intimal proliferation. These changes lead to luminal narrowing, increasing peripheral resistance.[9] In the kidney the transmission of such pressure to capillary beds results in pressure natriuresis and

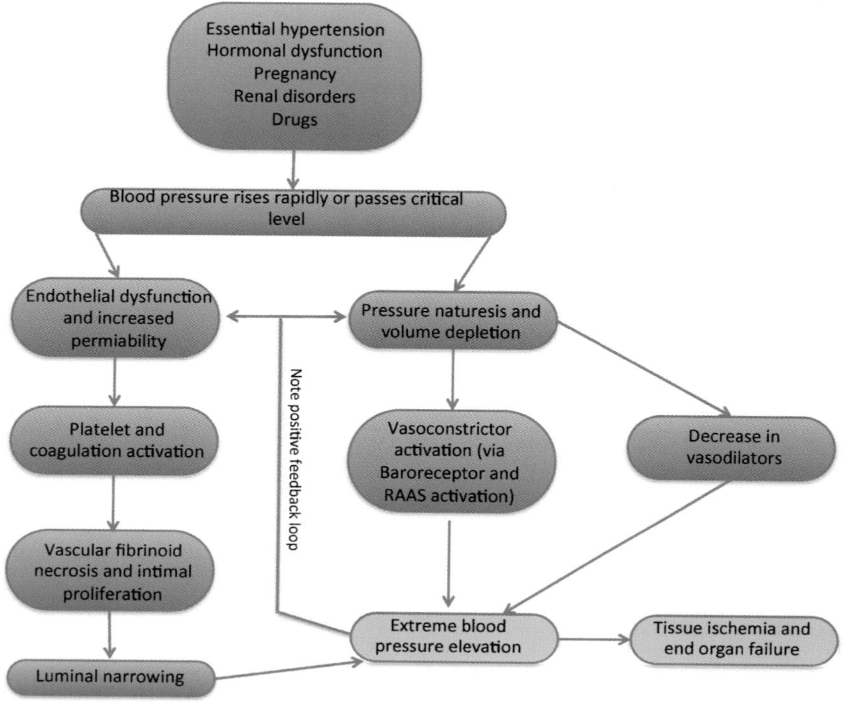

Fig. 1.[7] Pathophysiology of malignant hypertension.

subsequent volume depletion. The resulting hypovolemia further induces systemic vasoconstriction as well as activates the rennin–angiotensin–aldosterone system (RAAS). Angiotensin activation causes vasoconstriction and stimulates aldosterone secretion, leading to salt retention, elevating BPs and possibly resulting in cardiac complications.[3] Lastly, for reasons which are not entirely clear, under conditions of extreme pressure, endothelial vasodilitory function is lost.[1]

Clinical Presentation

Patients presenting with malignant hypertension can have diastolic pressures that range from 100 to 180 mmHg and systolic pressures from 150 to 290 mmHg. Other clinical manifestations of malignant hypertension are highly variable depending on underlying hypertensive conditions and its effects on particular organ systems. Generalized presentation includes weakness and malaise. Weight loss and salt imbalances are often the result of volume depletion.[2]

Ophthalmic Manifestations

35%–60% of patients presenting with malignant hypertension complain of vision loss, likely the result of papilledema — optic disk swelling resulting from high intracranial pressure.[2,10] Other ophthalmic changes include cotton-wool spots, flame hemorrhages and the presence of a macula star.

Neurological Changes (Hypertensive Encephalopathy)

Acute hypertensive encephalopathy is common in patients presenting with malignant hypertension. More than 60% present with headaches and 30% complain of dizziness.[2] Other neurological symptoms include nausea, projectile vomiting, restlessness, confusion, drowsiness and seizure. Hypertensive encephalopathy is believed to be the result of a "breakthrough" of cerebral autoregulation. This results in an interruption of the blood–brain barrier and consequently cerebral edema along with local changes in ionic and neurotransmitter concentrations, which leads to neurological impairments.[10]

Cardiovascular Complications

Heart failure leading to pulmonary edema is present in about 11% of patients. The abrupt rise in BP dramatically increases cardiac wall stress, which results in elevated oxygen demand, leading to myocardial ischemia and possible infarct, particularly in patients with underlying coronary artery disease. In addition, secondary hyperaldosteronism may result in hypokalemia and associated cardiac abnormalities. Finally, although uncommon, aortic dissection is also a possibility and represents the most rapidly fatal complication.[1,2]

The Kidney

As noted earlier in our discussion of the rennin–angiotensin system, renal involvement is common in malignant hypertension, but can be highly variable in presentation. Proteinuria and elevated creatinine are common, but often in the nonnephrotic ranges[2]; however, malignant nephroclerosis is possible. Furthermore, renal artery stenosis may be the precipitating factor in the oversecretion of renin and subsequently the onset of malignant hypertension.[10]

Hematological Changes

As erythrocytes travel through the damaged vasculature, they tend to lyse, resulting in microangiopathic hemolytic anemia. Hypokalemia is possible due to aldosterone oversecretion and while renin levels can be reduced fairly quickly, aldosterone levels may remain elevated for some time, presenting in subsequent weeks as what appears to be primary hyperaldosteronism.[2]

Clinical Evaluation (Table 2)

Treatment

When treating severely elevated BP, the distinction between a hypertensive emergency and a hypertensive urgency becomes very important.

Hypertensive Urgency (Table 3)

If no end organ damage can be detected, the patient is considered to have presented with a hypertensive urgency. Antihypertensive medication should be administered orally, initially at very low doses with incremental increases to avoid excessive BP reduction. The goal of treatment is to lower the BP by 25% to around 160/100 mmHg within 24 hr. After the initial administration, the patient should be monitored for several hours and discharged. A followup examination should be done within the next 1–2 days.[2,7]

Table 2.[2,7] Focused Physican Exam Elements and Laboratory Tests in the Evaluation of Malignant Hypertension

History	Physical	Laboratory Testing
• Current hypertensive condition.	• BP should be measured in both arms (a large difference is suggestive of aortic dissection) and in the supine and standing positions (orthostatic hypotension is indicative of volume depletion).	• ***Renal function***: serum electrolyte, blood urea nitrogen and creatinine levels should be assessed, as well as performing a urinalysis and urine sediment examination.
• Cardiovascular history. • Baseline BP and previous organ damage • Medications, particularly antihypertensive prescription and compliance — cessation of β-blockers or central sympatholytic agents may have resulted in rebound hypertension.	• Fundoscopic examination should be performed to identify retinopathy characteristic of malignant hypertension. • Cardiovascular examination should aim to identify new murmurs which may indicate recent myocardial ischemia. • Pulmonary rales suggest heart failure. • Abdominal bruits, particularly in patients with a history of atherosclerotic plaque in any vasculature, can indicate renal artery stenosis, a possible underlying cause of their hypertensive emergency. • A careful neurological examination is of paramount importance. Hypertensive encephalopathy presents with flapping tremor, delirium, nausea and headache, and must be ruled out.	• ***Hematological condition***: a complete blood count and smear to identify potential microangiopathic hemolytic anemia. • ***Cardiovascular condition:*** an electrocar diogram should be obtained for all patients presenting with severe hypertension to reveal possible myocardial ischemia/infarct and possible left-ventricular hypertrophy resulting from underlying chronic hypertension. Also, a chest X-ray to evaluate pulmonary congestion and mediastinum widening suggestive of aortic dissection. • ***Neurologic condition***: a CT scan of the head without contrast (to avoid precipitating acute renal failure) should be performed in any patient with neurological symptoms.

Table 3.[7] Specific Drugs for Hypertensive Urgencies

Drug	Mechanism of Action	Onset/Peak Effect	Dosage (until desired BP is achieved)	Adverse Effects
Captopril	Angiotensin-converting enzyme (ACE) inhibitor	15–30 min/ 30–90 min	25 mg initial oral dose, incremental doses of 50–100 mg every 90–120 min	Cough, hypotension, hyperkalemia, angioedema, contraindicated in bilateral renal artery stenosis
Nicardipine	Calcium channel blocker	½–2 hr	30 mg oral dose, every 8 hr	Palpitations, flushing, dizziness, constipation
Labetalol	α1- and β-adrenergic antagonists	1–2 hr	200 mg oral dose, every 3–4 hr	Nausea dizziness
Clonidine	α2-adrenergic receptor agonist	15–30 min/ 2–4 hr	0.1–0.2 mg initial oral dose, 0.05–0.1 mg every hour, maximum dose of 0.7 mg	Sedation, orthostatic hypotension

Hypertensive Emergency (Table 4)

If end organ damage is detected, it is a hypertensive emergency. The patient should be admitted to intensive care and have an arterial line placed for accurate BP reading.[1] Parenteral drug administration should begin immediately, with the goal of reducing the mean arterial pressure by 10% during the first hour and an additional 15% within the next 2–3 hr to a diastolic pressure of approximately 100mmHg. The initial fall in the BP should not exceed 25%.[7] Because many patients presenting with malignant hypertension have profound volume depletion, vasodilatation can result in a very rapid reduction in the BP, leading to cardiac and cerebrovascular hypotension. Thus, patients with volume depletion should be placed on an intravenous saline regimen to restore blood volume and decrease RAAS

Table 4.7 Specific Drugs for Hypertensive Emergencies

Drug	Mechanism	Onset/Duration	Dosage (until desired BP is achieved)	Side Effects	Notes
Sodium nitroprusside	Nitric oxide compound	Immediate/2–3 min	0.25–5 µg/kg/min IV	Nausea, vomiting, *cyanide intoxication*, increased intracranial pressure, methemoglobinemia	Due to rapidity of onset and direct dilation of both arteries and veins, nitroprusside is considered to be the first-line drug for most hypertensive emergencies.[4]
Fenoldopam mesylate	Dopamine-1 receptor agonist	<5 min/30 min	Initial dose 0.1 mcg/kg per min; titrate at 15 min intervals depending upon the blood pressure response	Headache, flushing, tachycardia, ST-T wave abnormalities (Primarily T-wave inversion) hypokalemia	Unique in its ability to increase renal perfusion, and thus is recommended in patients with renal failure. Contraindicated in patients with glaucoma.[5]
Nitroglycerin	Nitric oxide compound	2–5 min/5–10 min	5–100 µg/min IV (requires special delivery system due	Headache, tachycardia, flushing, tachyphylaxis, methemoglobinemia	Used primarily in patients with acute coronary syndrome or

(*Continued*)

Table 4.[7] *(Continued)*

Drug	Mechanism	Onset/Duration	Dosage (until desired BP is achieved)	Side Effects	Notes
			to drug binding to tubing)		pulmonary edema, otherwise not considered to be first-line therapy.[12]
Enalaprilat	ACE inhibitor	<30 min/12–24 hr	0625–2.5 mg every 6 hr IV	Cough, hypotension, angioedema, taste changes, hyperkalemia	Active form of enalapril, therefore contraindicated in pregnancy and bilateral renal artery stenosis. Due to variability in patient volume status and renin activity, may be response unpredictable.[6]
Hydralazine	Direct vasodilator, arterial only	10 min/1–4 hr	5–20 mg IV bolus every 4–6 hr	Tachycardia, flushing, headache, sodium and water retention, increased intracranial pressure, aggravation	Use is *limited primarily* to pregnancy (pre-eclampsia) due to unpredictability of response. Administer

(Continued)

Table 4.[7] *(Continued)*

Drug	Mechanism	Onset/Duration	Dosage (until desired BP is achieved)	Side Effects	Notes
				of angina	with β -blocker to prevent reflex sympathetic discharge.[12]
Nicardipine	Calcium channel blocker	5–15min/4–6 hr	5 mg/hr, increasing by 2.5 mg/hr every 5 min to a maximum of 15 mg/hr	Tachycardia, headache, flushing, local phlebitis	Has been shown to increase myocardial perfusion and stroke volume. Also recommended treatment for ischemic stroke in patients with BP>220 mmHg systolic or 120 mmHg diastolic.[12]
Esmolol	β-adrenergic blocker	1–2 min/10–30 min	500 μ g/kg bolus injection IV; 50–100 μ g/kg/min by infusion. May repeat bolus after 5 min or increase infusion rate;	Hypotension, nausea, bronchoconstriction, first-degree atrioventricular block	Ultrashort-acting, but metabolized by RBCs and therefore anemic pts will have longer half-life. Particularly useful in postoperative patients to prevent hemodynamic instability.[12]

(Continued)

Table 4.[7] *(Continued)*

Drug	Mechanism	Onset/Duration	Dosage (until desired BP is achieved)	Side Effects	Notes
Labetalol	α-, β-adrenergic blocker	5–10 min/3—6 hr	20–80 mg IV bolus every 10 min; 0.5–2.0 mg/min IV infusion	Bronchoconstriction, heart block, vomiting, exacerbation of heart failure	
Phentolamine	α-adrenergic receptor blocker	1–2 min/10–30 min	5–15 mg IV bolus	Tachycardia, flushing, headache	
Clevidipine	Arterial calcium channel blocker	2–4 min/5–15 min	Initial dose IV infusion of 1–2 mg/hr maintenance dose 4–6 mg/hr	Dizziness, drowsiness, headache; nausea, vomiting, severe allergic reactions	Does not reduce cardiac filling pressures or reflex tachychardia.[12]

ECG = electrocardiogram; IM - intramuscular; IV = intravenous; RBCs = red blood cells; BP = blood pressure.

activation. Drug choice and subsequent therapy for patients presenting with malignant hypertension are dependent on specific end organ damage. Traditionally, in the absence of specific comorbidities, the most commonly used drugs for hypertensive emergencies are IV labetolol and nicardipine. However, recently, clevidipine, a fast acting calcium channel blocker, has become the drug of choice for most practitioners. Clevidipine is metabolized by esterases in blood and extravascular tissue. Its clearance will therefore be unaffected by renal or hepatic failure, which may be present during hypertensive emergencies. Furthermore, because it is selective for arterial calcium channels, it preserves cardiac function while reducing cardiac afterload and maintaining preload. When the BP is under control, the patient should be switched to oral therapy and treated on an outpatient basis with the goal of reducing the diastolic pressure gradually to approximately 90 mmHg over 1–3 months. Finally, secondary causes should be investigated, particularly in young patients.[2]

Specific Situations (Table 5)

Acute kidney failure. This may be the cause or effect of malignant hypertension. Given that there is potential for renal recovery, immediate antihypertensive therapy is of paramount importance in patients presenting with acute renal failure. While lowering BP is paramount, one must be careful to maintain euvolemia so as to avoid ischemic damage. In order to provide the best chance for renal recovery, patients should be placed on dialysis and have their BP kept under control. Fenoldopam is generally used in acute kidney failure because it has been shown to maintain or increase renal perfusion while lowering BP.[7]

Hypertensive encephalopathy. Patients presenting with hypertensive encephalopathy require rapid reduction in BP. Therefore, the mean BP should be lowered by 20% or to 100–110 mmHg diastolic pressure within the first hour.[1] Special care must be taken in elderly patients and patients with essential hypertension, as they are more prone to hypoperfusion at lower pressures.[2] In the case of patients who present with seizures, the use

Table 5.[7,12] Drug of Choice for Specific Hypertensive Complications

Type of Emergency	First-Line Drug	Second-Line Drug
Subarachnoid hemorrhage	Nimodipine	Labetalol
Cerebral vascular event	Nicardipine	Nitroprusside, enalaprilat
Acute renal failure	Fenoldopam	Nicardipine
Aortic dissection	α-blocker + nitroprusside	Labetalol, trimethaphan
Pulmonary edema	Nitroglycerin (β blockers and other drugs that decrease cardiac output should be avoided)	Nitroprusside ± ACE inhibitor
Cardiac ischemia	Nitroglycerin ± β-blocker	Nitroprusside, labetalol
Pre-eclampsia	Methyldopa magnesium sulfate (do not use with calcium channel blocker)	Hydralazine ± β-blocker
Pheochromocytoma	Phentolamine	Nitroprusside + β-blocker

of anticonvulsants is reasonable and will itself help to lower the BP.[7] Hypertensive encephalopathy is a rapidly reversible condition if treated in a timely fashion. If symptoms do not abate within 6–12 hr of normalization of the BP, other causes for the encephalopathy should be investigated.

Aortic dissection. This is the most rapidly fatal complication of malignant hypertension. BP should be reduced rapidly and aggressively, to a systolic pressure of 100–110 mmHg. The therapeutic goal is to reduce shear stress on the aortic wall by lowering both the BP and the heart rate.[1] This can be accomplished by using a combination of β-blockers and vasodilators like sodium nitroprusside. β-blockers should be administered first.[2]

References

1. Vaughan CJ, Delanty N. (2000) Seminar: hypertensive emergencies. *The Lancet* **356**: 411–17.
2. Kitiyakara C, Guzman NJ. (1998) Malignant hypertension and hypertensive emergencies. *J. Am. Soc. Nephrol.* **9**: 133–142.

3. Flemin S. (2000) Malignant hypertension — the role of paracrine rennin — angiotensin system. **192**: 135–139.
4. Archer SL, Huang JM, Hampl V, *et al.* (1994) Nitric oxide and cGMP cause vasorelaxation by activation of a charybdotoxin-sensitive K channel by cGMP-dependent protein kinase. *Proc. Nat. Acad. Sci.*; **91**(16): 7583.
5. Murphy MB, Murray C, Shorten GD. (2001) Fenoldopam: a selective peripheral dopamine-receptor agonist for the treatment of severe hypertension. *N Engl J Med* **345**(21): 1548.
6. Hirschl MM, Binder M, Bur A, *et al.* (1995) Clinical evaluation of different doses of intravenous enalaprilat in patients with hypertensive crises. *Arch Intern Med* **155**(20): 2217.
7. Vaidya CK, Ouelette JR. (2007) Hypertensive urgency and emergency. *Hospital Physician, Resident Grand Rounds* **43**: 43–50.
8. Edmunds E, Beevers DG. (2000) What has happened to malignant hypertension? A disease no longer vanishing. *J. Hum. Hypertens.* **14**: 159–161.
9. Kumar V, Abbas AK, Fausto N, Aster J. (2009) *Robbins and Cotran Pathologic Basis of Disease*, 8th ed. WB Saunders, Philadelphia, PA.
10. Izzo JL Jr, Sica DA, Black HR. (2008) in the essentials of high blood pressure. *Hypertensive Primer 4th ed.* Lippincott Williams and Wilkins, Philadelphia, PA.
11. Bennett NM, Shea S. (1988) Hypertensive emergency: Case criteria, sociodemographic profile, and previous care of 100 cases. *Am J Public Health* **78**: 636–40.
12. Varon J (2008) Treatment of acute severe hypertension: current and newer agents. *Drugs* **68**(3): 283.

Chapter 25

Syncope

Prashant Vaishnava and Marc Miller**

Key Pearls

- The most common cause of syncope is neurocardiogenic (i.e. vasovagal), and the primary purpose of the evaluation of the patient presenting with syncope is to exclude the presence of underlying structural heart disease.
- A meticulous history and directed physical examination are paramount in identifying the cause of syncope.
- The presence of prodrome or postepisode fatigue are the hallmarks of neurocardiogenic syncope.
- The diagnosis of an arrhythmic cause of syncope hinges upon the ECG documentation of a rhythm disturbance at the time of symptoms, and the frequency of symptoms dictates the type and duration of ambulatory monitoring.
- The clinical utility and diagnostic yield of tilt table testing and electrophysiologic testing is low, particularly in patients with no underlying structural heart disease.

Introduction

Failure of the systemic circulation to generate adequate cerebral hypoperfusion may result in syncope, a transient and brief loss of consciousness associated with a loss of postural tone and followed by spontaneous recovery. While syncope is a common symptom, accounting for up to 6% of

*Mount Sinai School of Medicine, New York, NY, USA.

hospitalizations, an underlying cause is not identified in up to one-third of patients. Meticulous history and directed physical examination are paramount in the evaluation and should center upon establishing the presence of arrhythmia or structural heart disease, which have emerged as the most important predictors of death among patients presenting with syncope.[1–4]

In the general population, the most common cause of syncope is vasovagal or neurocardiogenic, a phenomenon associated with hypotension and/or bradycardia.[5–7] The gold standard for diagnosing an arrhythmic cause of syncope is electrocardiographic (ECG) demonstration of the rhythm disturbance at the time of symptoms. The type and duration of ambulatory ECG monitoring — Holter, event, or implantable loop monitoring — is dictated by the frequency of symptoms. Tilt table testing and electrophysiologic studies, while limited by variable sensitivity, specificity and diagnostic yield, may be useful aids in the evaluation of syncope for select patients.

Patient History

Meticulous history taking begins with establishing that syncope is actually the presenting complaint by excluding dizziness, presyncope and vertigo, which do not result in a loss of consciousness or postural tone. Emphasis should be given to the circumstances immediately preceding the syncopal episode and may suggest a particular etiology. A sequential record of the details of the event, including eyewitness descriptions, is often useful. A loss of consciousness that is precipitated by pain, exercise, micturition, defecation, deglutition, or stress is often neurocardiogenic in origin.

Neurocardiogenic, or vasovagal, syncope is triggered by a reflex increase in vagal efferent activity and sympathetic withdrawal. Often the first sign of impending vasovagal syncope, facial pallor, results from reduced skin blood flow occurring secondary to vasoconstriction mediated by the sympathetic nervous system. This is followed by other premonitory signs and symptoms, which include diaphoresis, restlessness, and difficulty with concentration.

A prolonged period of unconsciousness (often exceeding five minutes), observed rhythmic or clonic movements, and disorientation after the event may indicate seizure as the diagnosis. Tonic-clonic movements may also be seen in non-neurological causes of syncope. Transient ischemic attacks rarely result in syncope, though in the presence of occlusive carotid artery disease, hypotensive transient ischemic attacks have been reported. Posture-related syncope is often ascribed to orthostatic hypotension. Volume depletion, medications that alter vascular tone and heart rate, neurodegenerative diseases (e.g. Parkinson's disease), or secondary autonomic dysfunction (as seen in diabetes mellitus) may result in orthostatic hypotension. Carotid sinus hypersensitivity is a consideration, particularly with an aging population, and should be suspected with syncope provoked by head rotation or pressure on the carotid sinus (as with tumors, shaving, or tight collars).[8] A careful medication history may reveal the addition of new drugs, particularly antiarrhythmic or antihypertensive agents, which may provoke proarrhythmia or orthostasis, respectively.

Physical Examination

Physical examination may also provide important clues that point toward a particular cause for the syncope. Blood pressure and heart rate in the supine, sitting, and standing positions, initially and after three minutes with attention to reproduction of symptoms, may suggest orthostatic hypotension. Evaluation of the carotid impulse may suggest aortic stenosis if it is parvus or tardus, and the presence of a carotid bruit may signify obstructive carotid arterial disease. Carotid sinus massage in the supine and/or upright positions leading to an exaggerated drop in heart rate may suggest carotid sinus hypersensitivity, but should not be attempted in the patient with a suspected ipsilateral carotid artery stenosis or recent cerebrovascular accident. Cardiovascular examination may reveal a harsh crescendo-decrescendo systolic murmur with softening of the second heart sound that is consistent with aortic stenosis. Alternatively, a systolic murmur that intensifies with the Valsalva maneuver is associated with

Table 1. Clinical Features Suggestive of Specific Causes of Syncope

Historical Features	
Loss of consciousness precipitated or following pain, exercise, micturition, defecation, deglutition, or stress	Neurocardiogenic
Facial pallor	Neurocardiogenic
Premonitory signs, including diaphoresis, restlessness, nausea, or difficulty with concentration	Neurocardiogenic
Prolonged period of unconsciousness (often exceeding 5 min)	Seizure
Observed rhythmic or clonic movements	Seizure
Antecedent history of volume depletion	Orthostatic hypotension
Known history of neurodegenerative disease	Orthostatic hypotension/autonomic insufficiency
Loss of consciousness provoked by head rotation or with massage on the carotid sinus (as with shaving or tight collars)	Carotid sinus hypersensitivity
Objective Features	
Relative hypotension in the standing position, when compared to supine and sitting positions	Orthostatic hypotension
Parvus and/or tardus carotid arterial pulse	Aortic stenosis
Carotid bruit	Obstructive carotid arterial disease
Exaggerated decrement in heart rate with carotid sinus massage (if not contraindicated)	Carotid sinus hypersensitivity
Systolic murmur with softening of the second heart sound	Aortic stenosis
Focal, localizing, and/or dynamic signs	Cerebrovascular accident

hypertrophic cardiomyopathy, from which a dynamic left ventricular outflow tract obstruction may result in syncope. Neurological assessment may suggest focal, localizing, or dynamic signs or symptoms that suggest a cerebrovascular accident; alternatively, neurodegenerative diseases like Parkinson's disease may result in autonomic insufficiency and are associated with particularly abnormal cognition and speech, motor strength, tremor and gait.

Table 1 contains a summary of the clinical features that are suggestive of specific causes of syncope.[6]

Cardiac Syncope: Arrhythmia and Structural Heart Disease

Abnormalities in cardiac rhythm or structural heart disease with obstruction of cardiac output may lead to syncope. In contrast to the prodromal symptoms that generally characterize vasovagal syncope, suddenness of onset without premonitory signs may be suggestive of syncope provoked by arrhythmias. Certain obstructive lesions (e.g. aortic stenosis or hypertrophic cardiomyopathy) may be associated with exertional syncope. Obstruction of cardiac output and arrhythmias frequently co-exist.

Among the pathologic entities that may lead to obstruction of cardiac output, aortic stenosis and hypertrophic cardiomyopathy warrant particular consideration, as follows:

1) **Aortic stenosis:** Angina pectoris, syncope, and heart failure are the classic symptoms of aortic stenosis. Once these symptoms develop, survival is limited; the median survival is only three years after syncope develops.
2) **Hypertrophic cardiomyopathy (HCM):** An important cause of sudden cardiac death among younger patients, HCM is a genetically determined myocardial disease. Syncope is a particularly ominous occurrence among patients with HCM and may result from supraventricular or ventricular arrhythmias, bradyarrhythmias, outflow tract obstruction, or an abnormal hemodynamic response to exertion.

Arrhythmic causes of syncope need to be considered. Bradyarrhythmias may occur as a consequence of either sinus node dysfunction or disorders of atrioventricular (AV) conduction. Regarding the former, sick sinus syndrome may manifest as sinus bradycardia or sinoatrial exit block. Bradycardia-tachycardia syndrome, in which there are features of sinus node disease and atrial arrhythmia, may frequently lead to syncope at the termination of the tachyarrythmia when there is overdrive suppression of the sinoatrial node. There are varying degrees of atrioventricular block, with different pathophysiologic mechanisms, electrocardiographic manifestations, and clinical consequences. First-degree atrioventricular block,

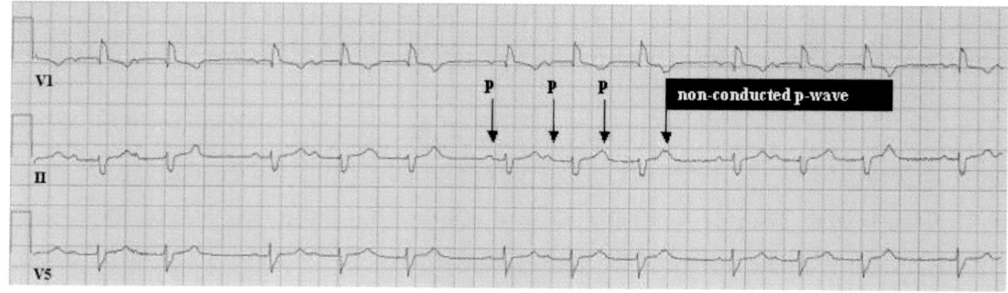

Fig. 1. Mobitz Type 1 AV block.

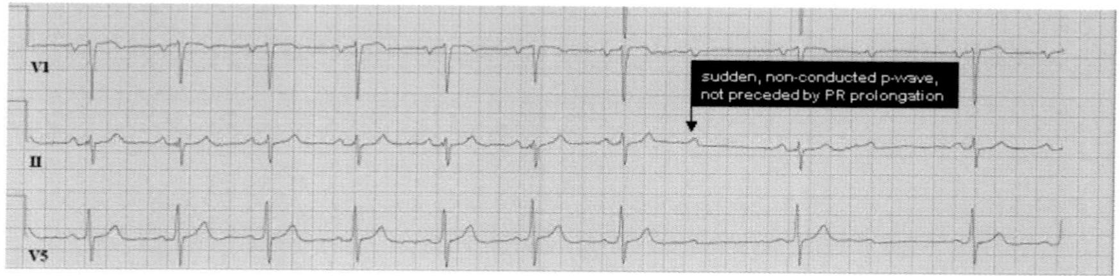

Fig. 2. Mobitz Type 2 second degree AV Block.

generally the result of delayed conduction within the AV node, appears as prolongation of the PR interval > 200 millseconds and carries an excellent prognosis.

Second-degree AV block of the Wenckebach type (i.e. Mobitz type 1) carries a similarly good prognosis, owing to an infra-nodal site of disease. Its electrocardiographic hallmark is progressive prolongation of the P–R interval prior to a nonconducted P wave (Fig. 1). The electrocardiographic hallmark of Mobitz type 2 second-degree AV block is a constant PR interval prior to a nonconducted P wave, and is generally caused by a block in the His-Purkinje system (Fig. 2). This form of atrioventricular block may often result in syncope and generally warrants permanent pacing, unless a reversible cause is apparent. Similarly, third-degree heart block is characterized by failure of all atrial activity to conduct to the ventricles, and it is manifested by atrioventricular dissociation (Fig. 3).

Just as bradyarrhythmias may reduce cardiac output and lead to cerebral hypoperfusion, ventricular tachycardia may lead to arrhythmic syncope. This malignant arrhythmia generally occurs in patients with

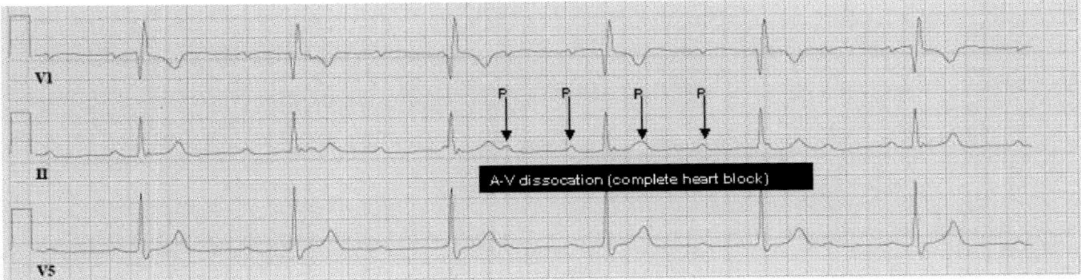

Fig. 3. Complete heart block.

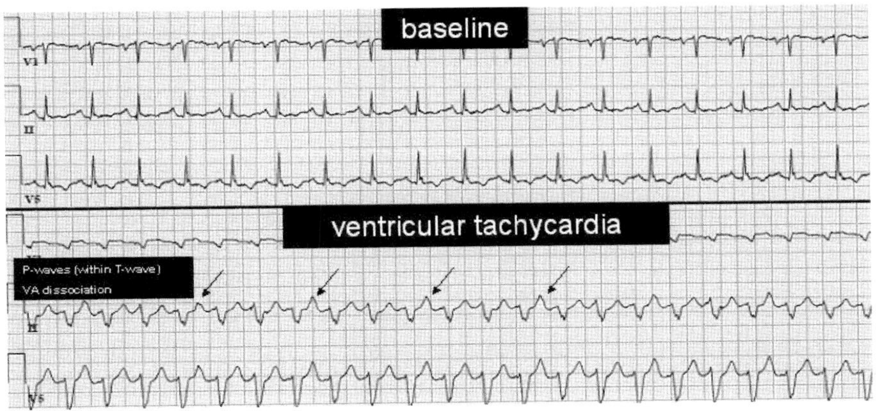

Fig. 4. Ventricular tachycardia.

underlying structural or ischemic heart disease (Fig. 4). On surface electrocardiography, the hallmarks of ventricular tachycardia include atrioventricular dissociation, easily discernible widening of the QRS complex, and concordance of QRS deflection. And while ventricular arrhythmias generally occur among those with diseased hearts, they may also be provoked by inherited channelopathies, in the absence of structural heart disease, and lead to syncope and sudden death.

The Long QT-syndrome (LQTS) and Brugada syndrome are two such channelopathies. LQTS, characterized by a prolongation of the corrected QT interval, QTc, to greater than 450 milliseconds may lead to syncope, presumably secondary to an episode of torsades de pointes, a polymorphic ventricular tachycardia (Fig. 5). Brugada syndrome, a heritable disorder of

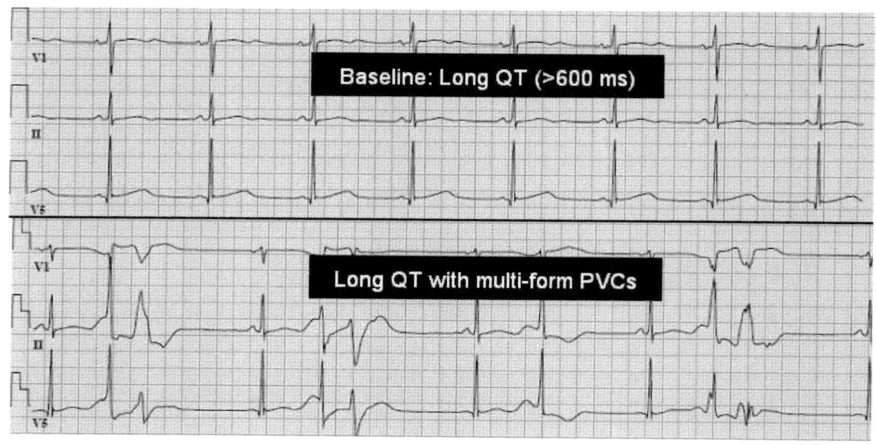

Fig. 5. Long QT.

the cardiac sodium channel, may also lead to syncope and is associated with characteristic electrocardiographic changes of ST elevation in the anterior precordial leads with an incomplete right bundle branch block. The distinctive ECG changes may be dynamic and/or provoked by certain factors (e.g., cocaine). Supraventricular tachyarrhythmias rarely cause syncope, unless there is concomitant cardiovascular disease, such as an obstruction to cardiac output.

Select Options for Monitoring and Diagnostic Evaluation

- **Routine laboratory testing:** Blood tests may reveal anemia or electrolyte derangements. Electrolyte deficits may cause or aggravate arrhythmias.
- **Noninvasive electrocardiographic monitoring:** A single resting ECG infrequently reveals the cause of a particular syncopal episode. Inpatient telemetry monitoring may reveal culprit arrhythmias more frequently. Often, noninvasive ambulatory ECG monitoring is necessary. Continuous Holter monitoring (for up to 72 hours) may reveal an

arrhythmic cause of syncope in up to 5% of patients. Long-term monitoring (lasting weeks or months) is often necessary, as rhythm disturbances may be transient.

- **Echocardiography:** When the presence or absence of an underlying structural heart disease cannot be determined by history and physical examination, transthoracic echocardiography may be indicated and offers valuable insight into biventricular and valvular function.
- **Electrophysiologic testing:** Such testing may allow for evaluation of sinus and AV node conduction, along with susceptibility to ventricular tachyarrhythmias, in patients thought to be at particularly high risk for recurrence of arrhythmic syncope. Candidates for electrophysiologic testing must be thoughtfully selected, as the yield of such invasive testing is particularly low among patients with no structural heart disease.
- **Tilt table testing:** Limited by its sensitivity, head-up tilt table testing may be a means to diagnose neurocardiogenic syncope in the setting of unexplained recurrent syncope. Tilt table testing is of limited value among individuals in whom the diagnosis of neurocardiogenic syncope is already strongly suggested on the basis of history-taking and physical examination.
- **Neurologic testing:** Computed tomography or magnetic resonance imaging of the brain may be indicated when a neurological basis of syncope is suspected and when focal neurologic findings are present. An electroencephalogram leads to a diagnosis in less than 2% of cases of syncope and is of limited utility.
- **Implantable device interrogation:** Patients with implanted devices (i.e. permanent pacemakers or cardioverter-defibrillators) presenting with syncope may benefit from bedside interrogation of their device when an arrhythmic cause of syncope is suspected. Bedside interrogation may also yield valuable information about the device's battery life and ability to sense intrinsic activity and capture appropriately. Manufacturer-specific device programmers are available.

References

1. Kapoor WN. (2000) Syncope. *N Engl J Med* **343**: 1856–62.
2. Kapoor WN. (2002) Current evaluation and management of syncope. *Circulation* **106**: 1606–09.
3. Kenny RA. (2003) Syncope in the elderly: Diagnosis, evaluation and treatment. *J Cardiovasc Electrophysiol* **14**: S74–77.
4. Mendu ML, McAvay G, Lampert R, *et al.* (2009) Yield of diagnostics tests by evaluating syncopal episodes in older patients. *Arch Inter Med* **169**: 1299–1305.
5. Strickberger SA, Benson W, Biaggioni I, *et al.* (2006) AHA/ACCF scientific statement on the evaluation of syncope. *Circulation* **113**: 316–27.
6. Soteriades ES, Evans JC, Larson MG, *et al.* (2002) Incidence and prognosis of syncope. *N Engl J Med* **347**: 878–85.
7. Sule S, Palaniswamy C, Aronow WS, *et al.* (2011) Etiology of syncope in patients hospitalized with syncope and predictors of mortality and rehospitalization for syncope at 27-month follow-up. *Clin Cardiol* **34**(1): 35–38.
8. Wieling W, Thijs RD, van Dijk N, *et al.* (2009) Symptoms and signs of syncope: A review of the link between physiology and clinical clues. *Brain* **132**: 2360–2642.

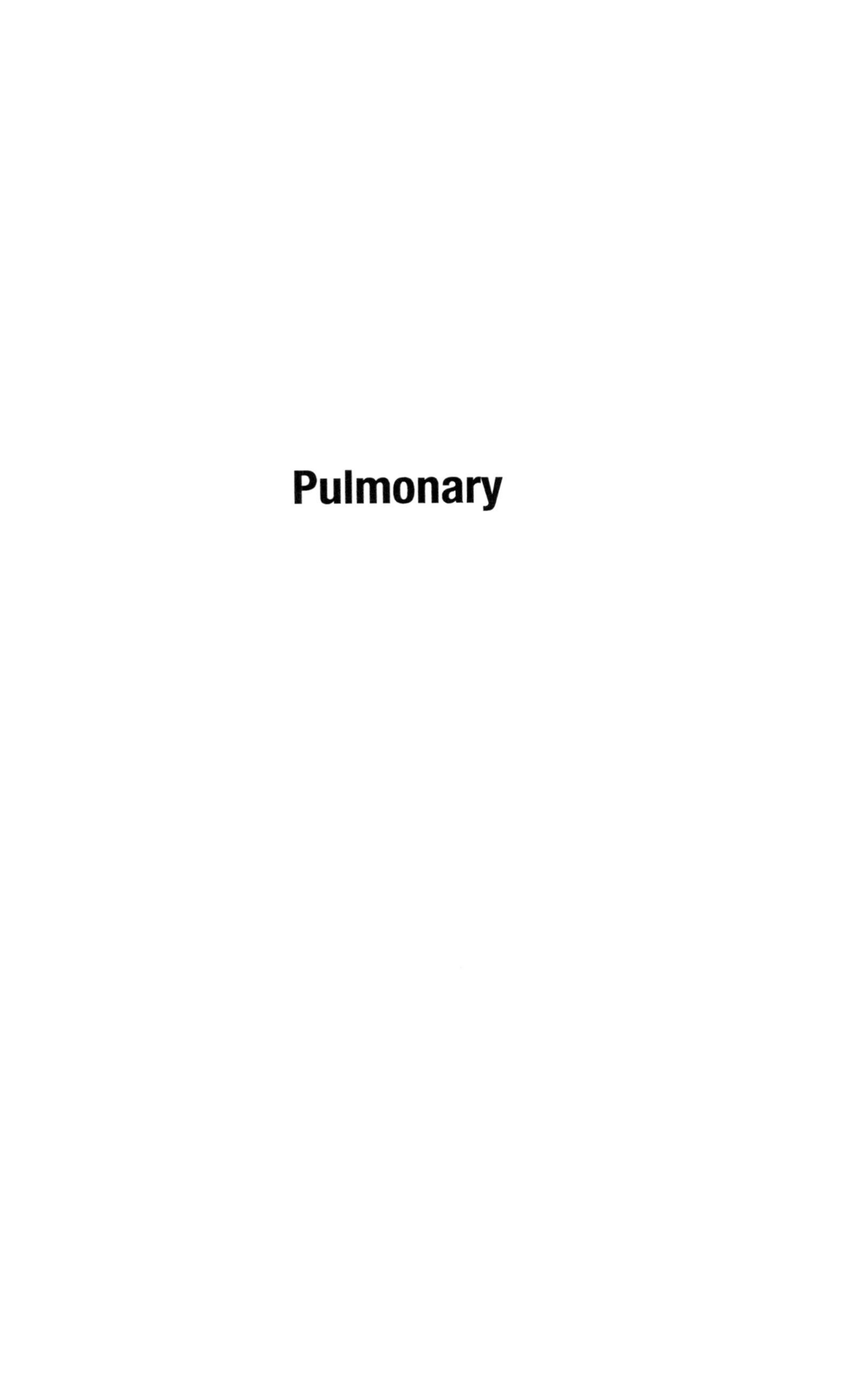

Pulmonary

Chapter 26

Approach to the Patient with Dyspnea

*Eric Barna**

Key Pearls

- In the majority of patients with dyspnea, the root pathophysiology is usually cardiac or pulmonary in nature.
- Dyspnea requires a thorough history and physical examination to guide the diagnostic approach and intervention.
- A chest X-ray should be routinely performed. The use of advanced diagnostic testing should be directed towards specific system involvement.
- The differential diagnosis for dyspnea is broad, but can be divided into more common systemic categories of disease processes.
- The hospitalist's initial approach to the severely dyspneic patient should involve recognition of the need for advanced airway management, potential triage to higher level of monitoring, and early goal-directed therapy for life-threatening etiologies.

DEFINITION: Dyspnea is multifactorial and complex, and can be defined as "a subjective experience of breathing discomfort that comprises qualitatively distinct sensations that vary in intensity."[1]

The spectrum of disease that can be embedded into the clinical presentation of dyspnea is extensive. These disease processes include

*Mount Sinai School of Medicine, New York, NY, USA.

asthma, COPD, interstitial-lung disease and cardiac dysfunction, as well as conditions beyond the cardiopulmonary system, and represent a large percentage of patients being admitted to medical services across the United States.

Pathophysiology

The mechanics of dyspnea rely on a complex set of interactions between the cerebral cortex and brain stem respiratory center and chemoreceptors. In order to better understand the physiologic mechanism as it relates to the clinical perception, it helps to view the respiratory system in three major functional roles[2–6]:

1) Efferent signaling: Signals that transmit to the muscles of respiration. This will determine the rate and depth of each breath. These efferent signals maintain sensitivity to any trigger that stimulates the respiratory centers, e.g. diabetic ketoacidocis, aspirin toxicity.
2) Ventilatory pump: These are the core anatomic components that allow for movement of pulmonary gasses; included herein are the muscles, bones, and luminal components of the airway. Pump failure may be a result of any disease process, external trigger or environmental factors that disrupt pump function. Examples include neuromuscular disorders such as Guillain-Barre syndrome, and myasthenia gravis.
3) Gas exchanger: Created by the anatomic surfaces that allow for exchange of oxygen and carbon dioxide, namely, pulmonary capillaries, and alveoli. It is at this level where localized impairment of gas exchanges through surface destruction, inflammation, or barrier formation lead to a sensation classically termed air gulping or air hunger. Examples include emphysema, pulmonary fibrosis, and congestive heart failure.

Table 1. The Qualitative Descriptor, and Associated Pathophysiologic Mechanism

Descriptor	Pathophysiology	Disease Process
Chest tightness, or constriction	Broncho constriction, interstitial edema	Asthma, myocardial ischemia
Increased work or effort of breathing	Obstructive airway disease, neuromuscular disease, reduced chest wall or pulmonary compliance	COPD, moderate to severe asthma, myopathy, pulmonary fibrosis
Air hunger, need to breathe, urge to breathe	Increased respiratory drive.	Heart failure, pulmonary embolism, moderate to severe asthma, COPD
Rapid shallow breathing	Decreased chest wall or pulmonary compliance	Interstitial fibrosis
Suffocating, smothering	Alveolar edema	Pulmonary edema

Diagnosis

Clinical History

The historical data gathered during the evaluation for dyspnea serves a key role in allowing the hospitalist to distinguish between pulmonary, cardiac, neuromuscular, or other root causes. The evaluation of the qualitative descriptors of dyspnea will aid in identifying plausible pathophysiologic etiologies (Table 1). The general history should be further tailored for the dyspneic patient to further elucidate the cause. Table 2 describes the key features of the medical history that should be emphasized for the dyspneic patient.

Physical Examination

The physical examination contains many features that can aid the diagnosis as well as assess the severity of dyspnea. Key features include the following:

Table 2. General History for the Dyspneic Patient

Components of General History	Targeting the Dyspneic Patient
General questions	Medication compliance, common triggers of comorbid conditions.
Past medical history	Cardiopulmonary comorbid conditions, prior intubation.
Time course	Sudden, gradual
Chest pain	Exertional or at rest, substernal or other location.
Cough and sputum production	Purulent, frothy, bloody, non productive vs. productive.
Medications	Medication changes, dosing adjustments, recent antibiotics.
Social history	Tobacco products may point towards a more chronic process. A clear drug history is also critical to evaluate for pulmonary effects of specific inhaled agents.

General Appearance:

- Ability to communicate in full sentences
- Anxious
- Use of accessory muscles
- Cyanotic appearance

Vital Signs:

- Hypotension
- Tachycardia
- Tachypnea
- Oxygen saturation

Chest:

- Air entry
- Paradoxical motion of chest wall

- Audible wheeze
- Stridor
- Crackles

Cardiac Exam:

- Jugular venous distention
- Audible murmur
- Audible S3
- Gallop
- Precordial impulse

Extremities:

- Peripheral edema
- Cyanosis
- Cool and clammy
- Clubbing

Neurologic:

- Altered mental status
- Focal neurologic deficit

Basic Diagnostic Testing

- Chest X-ray
- Electrocardiogram
- Cardiac enzymes (primary cardiac etiology is suspected)
- Brain natriuretic peptide (primary low cardiac output state suspected)
- Arterial blood gas (not routinely required), but useful when assessing need for intubation and mechanical ventilation, evaluating complex metabolic disturbances.

Advanced Diagnostic Testing

- Chest CT with IV contrast: If clinical suspicion of underlying pulmonary embolism is high and there is no existing contraindication to IV contrast exposure with respect to renal function, and or allergy.
- High resolution CT scan: For further evaluation of suspected underlying chronic interstitial lung disease.
- Ventilation perfusion scan: To be considered for evaluation of underlying pulmonary embolism, when patient cannot tolerate IV contrast.
- Pulmonary function testing: To better elucidate underlying restrictive vs. obstructive pulmonary disease.
- 2 Dimensional echocardiography: For further evaluation of suspected heart failure as root etiology of dyspnea.
- Cardiac catheterization: Left-sided for evaluation of underlying ischemic disease should primary root pathophysiology point to heart failure. Right-sided cardiac catheterization for further evaluation if suspicion of pulmonary hypertension exists.

Differential Diagnosis

The differential diagnosis for the patient presenting with dyspnea is broad. There are a few core diagnostic groupings that should serve as an initial template for the approach to the dyspneic patient (Table 3).

Early Management of the Acutely Dyspneic Patient

The cornerstone of initial management of the severely dyspneic patient relies on identifying and correcting the underlying disease process. The role of the hospitalist in evaluating the dyspneic patient especially in the acute setting is to improve the patients overall oxygenation, recognize the need for further advanced management of the airway, and initiate the appropriate treatment course early on. It is also essential to recognize the imminent and life-threatening etiologies of dyspnea and address these concerns rapidly.

Table 3. Differential Diagnosis of Dyspnea

Cardiac

- Ischemic heart disease (acute coronary syndrome)
- Congestive heart failure
- Decompensated heart failure with pulmonary edema
- Valvular disease
- Intracardiac shunting
- Arrhythmias
- Cardiac tamponade

Pulmonary

- Asthma (acute exacerbation)
- COPD
- Pulmonary embolism
- Interstitial lung disease
- Pulmonary hypertension
- Pulmonary infection
- Pulmonary hemorrhage
- ARDS
- Pulmonary oncologic process
- Pleural effusion
- Pneumothorax

Neuro/Psychiatric

- Neuromuscular disorders
- Stroke
- Anxiety with or without panic
- Hyperventilation
- Renal tubular acidosis

Key Management Strategies

- Initiate oxygen supplementation.
- Continue to monitor oxygenation closely.
- Recognize the need for advanced airway management, and possible need for Intensive Care Unit level of care.
- Patients with high clinical suspicion for pulmonary embolism and without contraindication to systemic anticoagulation should be started on heparin, while further imaging modalities are secured.

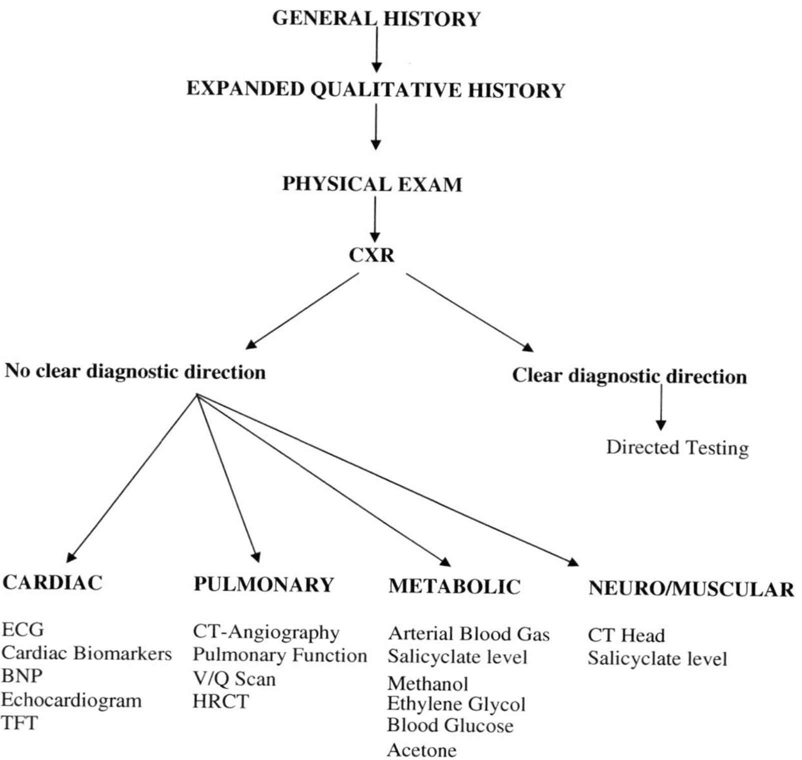

Fig. 1. Diagnostic approach to dyspnea.

References

1. Dyspnea. Mechanisms, assessment, and management: A consensus statement. American Thoracic Society. *Am J Respir Crit Care Med* 1999; **159**: 321.
2. Simon PM, Schwartzstein RM, Weiss JW, *et al.* (1989) Distinguishable sensations of breathlessness induced in normal volunteers. *Am Rev Respir Dis* **140**(4): 1021.
3. Banzett RB, Lansing RW, Reid MB, *et al.* (1989) Air hunger' arising from increased PCO2 in mechanically ventilated quadriplegics. *Respir Physiol* **76**(1): 53–67.

4. Banzett RB, Lansing RW, Brown R, *et al.* (1990) Air hunger' from increased PCO2 persists after complete neuromuscular block in humans. *Respir Physiol* **81**(1): 1–17.
5. Scano G. Stendardi L, Grazzini M, *et al.* (2005) Understanding dyspnea by its language. *Eur Respir J* **25**(2): 380–5.

Chapter 27

Asthma

*Gwen S. Skloot**

Key Pearls

- Prior severe exacerbations, multiple annual hospitalizations or Emergency Department visits, overuse of beta-agonist, poor perception of respiratory symptoms, other underlying cardiopulmonary or psychiatric illness, lack of a written action plan, mold sensitivity, low socioeconomic status and illicit drug use are all factors that increase mortality risk of an asthma exacerbation.
- Oxygen saturation and lung function (in all but the most severely ill patients) are key objective tests, while most other studies are not routinely required.
- The mainstay of inpatient asthma management includes systemic steroids, short-acting beta agonists, and supplemental oxygen.
- Consultation with an asthma specialist should be considered early in high-risk patients or those who do not respond to therapy as expected.
- Readiness for discharge hinges on return toward normal subjective and objective function (i.e. Peak Expiratory Flow Rate returns to 70% of predicted or personal best).

Introduction

Asthma is a chronic inflammatory disorder of the airways characterized by airway obstruction that is generally reversible, and by hyperresponsiveness

*Mount Sinai School of Medicine, New York, NY, USA.

to a variety of stimuli.[1] More than 22 million Americans are believed to have the disease.[2] Although it is encouraging that for the first time in decades, asthma death rates are decreasing,[3] morbidity remains quite high. Healthcare costs due to treatment of asthma in the acute care setting total a staggering $18 billion dollars per year.[3]

Definition, Precipitating Factors and Mortality Risk

Asthma exacerbations are defined by progressive worsening of respiratory symptoms such as shortness of breath, wheezing, cough and chest tightness, accompanied by decreases in lung function.[1] All patients with asthma are at risk for developing an acute exacerbation regardless of the underlying severity of their disease.[4] Respiratory viruses are recognized as the most important precipitating factor for acute exacerbations.

It is important to be familiar with patient characteristics predictive of increased mortality risk related to exacerbations.[1] Prior severe exacerbations with Intensive Care Unit (ICU) admission, multiple Emergency Department (ED) visits or hospitalizations within the year, using more than two canisters of short acting beta-agonist per month, poor perception of respiratory symptoms, lack of a written action plan, and mold sensitivity are historical factors associated with increased risk of death. Social factors such as low socioeconomic status or inner city residence, illicit drug use and major psychosocial problems are also important. Finally, other chronic cardiopulmonary disease or psychiatric illness can identify patients at high risk.

Evaluation of Patients Hospitalized with an Asthma Exacerbation

History

The clinician should take a focused history to determine the rate of progression of the exacerbation, the factors that may have precipitated the attack, the therapy that has been used and the time of the last dose.[1]

Attention should be paid to risk factors predictive of poor outcome. Comorbidities that can contribute to asthma such as allergic rhinitis, sinusitis, Gastroesophageal Reflux Disease (GERD), obesity, sleep disordered breathing and depression should be noted. The differential diagnosis of severe asthma[1,5] includes chronic obstructive pulmonary disease (chronic bronchitis or emphysema), cystic fibrosis, congestive heart failure (CHF), pulmonary embolism, vocal cord dysfunction, bronchiectasis, sarcoidosis, hypersensitivity pneumonitis and bronchiolitis obliterans.

Physical Examination

Examination should be targeted to confirm that the process is indeed an asthma exacerbation and to identify the severity of the attack. Physical findings typical of a severe asthma exacerbation are shown in Table 1.[1,4,6] Focus should be on the patient's level of alertness, hemodynamics, fluid status, and the presence of cyanosis, respiratory distress and wheezing. Some typical warning signs (tachypnea and tachycardia) may actually wane as a patient begins to fatigue. Patients may appear anxious and scared. Accessory muscle use is an indication of increased work of breathing. Although wheezing is generally thought of as a typical marker of an asthma attack, a quiet chest is more ominous.[7] and louder wheezing may actually be a sign of improvement.

Table 1. Physical Findings During a Severe Asthma Exacerbation

Difficulty talking in full sentences
Patient seated upright and unable to lie flat
Cyanosis and diaphoresis
Decreased level of consciousness
Confusion
Use of accessory muscles (sternocleidomastoid retraction)
Respiratory rate >30 breaths/min
Heart rate >120 beats/min or <60 beats/min with hypotension
Pulsus paradoxus (>15 mm Hg decrease with inspiration)
Quiet chest

Table 2. Indications for Specific Objective Testing in Inpatient Asthma Evaluation

Test	Patient Candidate
Lung Function:	
FEV_1 or PEF	All patients if possible
Pulse Oximetry	All patients
Chest Radiography	Suspect alternative diagnosis or complication (e.g. pneumonia, atelectasis, pneumothorax, etc.)
Laboratory Studies:	
ABG	Severe distress, suspected hypoventilation, $SpO_2 < 90\%$, FEV_1 or PEF $\leq 25\%$ predicted
CBC	Suspect infection
Serum electrolytes	Concurrent cardiovascular disease, on diuretic
Therapeutic Drug Monitoring	On methyxanthine formulation

FEV_1 = forced expiratory volume in 1 second; PEF = peak expiratory flow; ABG = arterial blood gas; SpO_2 = oxygen saturation by pulse oximetry; CBC = complete blood count.

Objective Testing

Very few tests are routinely recommended in the assessment of patients hospitalized for an asthma exacerbation. Table 2 summarizes the indications for lung function, chest radiography, and laboratory testing. Some measurement of lung function is helpful to stratify the severity of an attack and to assess response to therapy.[1] Spirometry (i.e., FEV_1) is preferable to peak expiratory flow (PEF) since the latter test cannot distinguish as well between obstructive disease and impairment due to other conditions (i.e., pneumonia or neuromuscular disease) or simply to reduced effort. FEV_1 or PEF should be measured upon admission and at least daily thereafter until discharge. In particular, measurement 15–20 minutes following bronchodilator is recommended with comparison to baseline. Large swings in lung function during a 24-hour period (i.e., morning and evening) are thought to portend a poorer prognosis. Patients with such fluctuations or those with baseline values <25% predicted and <10% increase after bronchodilator should be triaged for possible ICU transfer. Oxygen saturation should be monitored by pulse oximetry (SpO_2) in all patients. The goal should be to maintain SpO_2 >90% in all patients and >95% in pregnant women and in patients with cardiovascular disease.

In situations in which other respiratory conditions or complications are suspected (i.e., pneumonia, atelectasis, pneumothorax or pneumomediastinum), chest radiography can play a helpful role but otherwise should not be routinely ordered. Patients with severe respiratory distress, with hypoxia or persistently low lung function after treatment or, with suspected hypoventilation are candidates for arterial blood gas (ABG) monitoring. The most common finding is respiratory alkalosis.[4] A normal or elevated arterial carbon dioxide tension is an alarming finding that may signal respiratory muscle fatigue with impending respiratory failure. When the exacerbation is of longer duration, a compensatory nonanion-gap metabolic acidosis may be present.

Management of Patients Hospitalized with an Asthma Exacerbation

Medications

The mainstay of pharmacologic inpatient asthma management includes short-acting beta-agonists (SABA) and systemic corticosteroids. The frequency of administration of SABA depends upon improvement in airflow obstruction and associated symptoms. The onset of action is generally within five minutes and the duration, while uncertain in severe exacerbations, likely ranges between 3–6 hours.[4] Adverse effects include tremors and tachycardia or tachyarrthymias; therefore, more selective agents (i.e. levalbuterol) are preferred when high doses are required. SABA may be administered *via* metered dose inhaler (MDI) with a valved holding chamber (VHC) when the patient is cooperative and the exacerbation not severe. An MDI with a VHC is as effective as a nebulizer for treatment of acute asthma.[6] Four to eight puffs of an MDI are approximately equivalent to one nebulizer treatment. For severe asthma exacerbations or when the patient cannot cooperative effectively, nebulizer therapy is appropriate.

All hospitalized patients should receive systemic corticosteroids since these medications reverse airway inflammation and thus hasten recovery. High dose steroids are no longer considered advantageous and oral therapy is preferred, provided that gastrointestinal transit time or absorption is not compromised.[1] The total course of therapy may range from 3–10 days depending upon the severity of the exacerbation and the patient's response. There is no need to taper systemic steroids in patients who are treated for less than one week. The recommended dose of prednisone or the equivalent is 40–80 mg/day given in 1–2 divided doses until a PEF of 70% of predicted or personal best is achieved. Patients should continue on their inhaled corticosteroids while in the hospital.

Additional pharmacologic therapies have been studied as a possible way to avoid intubation though intubation should not be delayed once it is judged necessary. Such therapies include intravenous magnesium sulfate, heliox-driven albuterol nebulization, intravenous beta-2-agonists, intravenous leukotriene receptor antagonists and noninvasive ventilation. Only intravenous magnesium sulfate and heliox merit consideration at this time based on available data. These therapies should be reserved for patients with severe exacerbations who are not responding to traditional treatment.

Medications not recommended include methylxanthines and antibiotics (unless there are symptoms or signs of infection including purulent sputum, fever, or evidence of pneumonia). Although inhaled ipratropium bromide is recommended in the ED setting, it is not thought to be of additive benefit once a patient is hospitalized with an exacerbation.

Adjunct Therapy

Oxygen therapy is generally given until there is a demonstrable response to beta-agonist with improvement in symptoms, physical findings and lung function. Low-flow oxygen is usually sufficient and in fact, high-dose oxygen may precipitate hypercapnia in some patients.[8] Other adjunct therapies commonly employed in the past are no longer recommended. These include aggressive hydration, chest physiotherapy, mucolytics such as acetylcysteine since they may actually worsen cough or airflow obstruction, and sedation due to the risk of respiratory depression.

Monitoring Parameters

Patients hospitalized with an asthma exacerbation should be assessed frequently since acute deteriorations can occur. Evaluation should include monitoring of symptoms, vital signs, lung exam, pulmonary function and SpO_2 or ABG measurements as necessary.[1] Patients who are awake and alert, able to talk in full sentences without respiratory distress or accessory muscle use and who are able to lie down comfortably are manifesting improvement. Dyspnea may still be present but should occur only on exertion. Heart rate and respiratory rate should decrease to normal. Blood pressure should be normal without signs of pulsus paradoxus. While wheezing may persist in some patients, it is more important to note good air entry on examination. The goal for peak flow parameters is a return to ≥70% of predicted or personal best. Spirometry may still show obstruction but should be less severe. SpO_2 should exceed 95% on room air. In such a case, ABGs are not necessary. Indicators of improvement should be sustained for 60 minutes after the last SABA treatment.

Treatment of Comorbid Conditions

Certain comorbid conditions may complicate care of the hospitalized asthmatic. COPD or cardiovascular disease can lead to more severe illness or in the case of CHF, potential difficulty in identifying the patient's primary problem. Obese patients may be more at risk for worse outcomes related either to disease severity [9] or concurrent conditions such as GERD, obesity hypoventilation syndrome or obstructive sleep apnea syndrome (OSAS).[1] Such patients may have a blunted response to corticosteroids [10] and may be more likely to receive higher doses of therapy. Acute bacterial sinus infections can contribute to asthma exacerbations and should be treated with antibiotics. Although it is debatable whether GERD can worsen asthma, certainly patients with severe reflux symptoms should be treated with proton pump inhibitors.[1] Severe allergic rhinitis should be addressed with intranasal steroids. Patients with known OSAS should have continuous positive airway pressure (CPAP) continued in the hospital. In some cases, this may lessen nocturnal symptoms.

When to Consult a Specialist

Patients deemed to be at increased risk for mortality or those having a severe exacerbation should be evaluated by an asthma specialist early in the hospital course. In addition, patients who do not respond to initial therapy or those who clinically worsen at any time, merit evaluation by an asthma specialist. It is always better to err on the side of conservative management when considering a consultation.

Goals for Discharge

The primary goals in inpatient asthma management are to minimize symptoms, improve lung function and in general, return patients toward their baseline level of functioning. Optimally, asthma symptoms should have resolved at the time of discharge although in some patients, this will not be possible. PEF should have returned to ≥70% predicted or personal best prior to considering discharge. To reduce the likelihood of relapse and readmission, there should be a clearly outlined plan of care, including pharmacologic management at home and emphasis on the need for regular outpatient follow up with an appropriate physician (i.e. either primary care provider or an asthma specialist).

Prior to discharge, the patient's medicines should be converted to an outpatient regimen. Close observation for 24-hr is recommended after this adjustment. Discharge therapy should include continuation of oral systemic steroids to complete the prescribed course, initiation of inhaled corticosteroids in those patients naïve to this therapy prior to admission (this should be started while the patient is still in the hospital to facilitate appropriate inhaler use) and continuation of SABA for rescue.

Summary

The clinician should recognize risk factors that increase asthma mortality and should conduct a focused history and physical examination to quickly determine the severity of the exacerbation to triage care. Oxygen saturation and lung function are key objective tests to be done in almost all patients. The mainstay of therapy includes systemic steroids, SABA and supplemental oxygen. High-risk patients or those who do not respond to therapy as expected warrant early consultation with an asthma specialist. Readiness for discharge hinges on return toward normal subjective and objective function. Discharge planning should focus on both pharmacologic therapy and patient education. Proper evaluation and management of the patient hospitalized with an asthma exacerbation should improve outcomes and limit costs.

References

1. National Heart, Lung and Blood Institute. (2007) Expert panel report 3: Guidelines for the diagnosis and management of asthma: Full report NIH publication 08-4051.
2. Ginde AA, Espinola JA and Camargo CA. (2008) Improved overall trends but persistent racial disparities in emergency department visits for acute asthma, 1993–2005. *J Allergy Clin Immunol* **122**: 313–318.
3. Center for Disease Control and Prevention. (2009) Asthma prevalence and control characteristics by race/ethnicity — United States, 2002. *Morb Mortal Wkly Rep* **53**(7): 145–148.
4. Hallstrand TS, Fahy JV. (2002) Practical Management of acute asthma in adults. *Respir Care* **47**(2): 171–182.
5. Peters SP. (2010) Special considerations in adults for diagnoses that may coexist with or masquerade as asthma. *Ann Allergy Asthma Immunol* **104**: 455–460.

6. Lugogo NL, MacIntyre NR. (2008) Life-threatening asthma: Pathophysiology and management. *Resp Care* **53**(6): 726–735.
7. Shim CS, Williams MH Jr. (1983) Relationship of wheezing to the severity of obstruction in asthma. *Arch Intern Med* **143**(5): 890–892.
8. Chien JW, Ciufo R, Novak R, *et al.* (2000) Uncontrolled oxygen administration and respiratory failure in acute asthma. *Chest* **117**(3): 728–733.
9. Pakhale S, Doucette S, Vandemheen K, *et al.* (2010) A comparison of obese and nonobese people with asthma: Exploring an asthma-obesity interaction. *Chest* **137**: 1316–1323.
10. Sutherland ER, Goleva E, Strand M, *et al.* (2008) Body mass and glucocorticoid response in asthma. *Am J Respir Crit Care Med* **178**: 682–687.

Chapter 28

Hospital Management of COPD Exacerbations

*Neil Schachter**

Key Pearls

- COPD exacerbations requiring hospitalization account for about 6% of all episodes but nearly 50% of the costs.
- Five-year survival for patients requiring more than three hospitalizations is less than 40%.
- Comorbidities, particularly cardiovascular events and thromboembolic disease, are frequent reasons for admission of COPD patients and should be assessed for all patients hospitalized with a COPD exacerbation.
- Respiratory infection is the most common precipitating event of acute exacerbations and should be routinely treated.
- Comprehensive discharge planning is required to prevent early rehospitalization.

Introduction

Prior to the concerted effort on the part of many organizations to recognize important statistics that characterize this syndrome, there was a notable lack of concern about the incidence or severity of COPD. The numbers tell us that this is an important disease. Notably, there are an estimated 12 million Americans with diagnosed COPD, but an equal number are felt to have early with or undiagnosed disease. COPD is

*Mount Sinai Medicial Center, New York, NY, USA.

currently the third leading cause of death in the US, with over 120,000 deaths/year, 8 years earlier than anticipated. (*Centers for Disease Control (CDC) and Prevention's National Center for Health Statistics (NCHS)*, Deaths: Preliminary Data for 2010. http://www.cdc.gov/nchs/data/nvsr/nvsr60/nvsr60_04.pdf.) By the late 1990s, the mortality rate of COPD had risen by nearly 200% (compared to statistics from the 1960s), whereas that of all other major causes of death, including cardiovascular disease, and cancer, had significantly declined. The mortality rate of COPD 10 years after diagnosis remains greater than 50%. Finally, COPD is the primary cause for about 715,000 hospitalizations/year; it accounts for 16 million office visits annually and is responsible for direct medical costs of over US$20 billion half annually, about half of which are for hospitalizations.[1–4]

The Global Initiative for Chronic Obstructive Lung Disease (GOLD) was launched in 1998 as a collaboration between government agencies, scientific societies and industry, with a principal goal of producing recommendations for the management of COPD and has established itself as an authoritative source. Its iteration[3] defined COPD, as follows: "Chronic obstructive pulmonary disease (COPD), a common, preventable, and treatable disease, is characterized by persistent airflow limitation that is usually progressive and associated with enhanced chronic inflammatory response in the airways and the lungs to noxious particles and gases. Exacerbations and comorbidities contribute to the overall severity in individual patients." This concise definition de-emphasizes the prior (but still useful) concept of COPD as an umbrella term covering a number of clinical and pathologic syndromes, including emphysema (destruction of alveolar tissue), chronic bronchitis (chronic airway inflammation with symptoms of cough and phlegm), as well as some forms of asthma (particularly "adult" asthma with an irreversible obstructive component).

Clinical course. COPD is usually a disease of middle age, with the onset of symptoms in the patient's 50s or early 60s. In its classic presentation, it occurs 20 or 30 years after the patient has become addicted to cigarette smoking. Other irritants may be associated with the disease, such as occupational and environmental pollutants. Current smoking is not necessary for the onset of the disease but there is usually a history of at least 20–30 pack years of smoking. A small but significant subgroup have a hereditary condition (alpha-1 antitrypsin deficiency) which is associated with an earlier onset of the disease.

Because of the association with cigarette smoking and other pollutants with the development of COPD, comorbidities such as heart disease, diabetes, osteoporosis and lung cancer occur in a greater-than-expected number of these patients and frequently result in complications which contribute to the morbidity and mortality of this disease. An as-yet-poorly-defined predisposition may exist in patients who develop COPD; it is known as "systemic inflammation" and may contribute to the progression of the comorbidities as well as COPD itself.

Patients with COPD experience on average an accelerated loss of lung function which frequently parallels and may in part explain the progression of symptoms. In addition to this relatively continual progression of the disease, patients with COPD experience acute exacerbations which can accelerate the progression of the disease, leading to early disability and death.

Staging of the disease. Staging of the disease is important for several aspects of management. Based on spirometry, GOLD guidelines classify the disease into four stages of severity. Because all stages of the disease are defined by an obstructive component, the ratio of FEV1/FVC is required to be less than 0.7. Healthy individuals are able to exhale forcefully more than 70% of their forced vital capacity (FVC: the total amount of air that a person can forcefully exhale over a period of at least 6 s) in the first second (FEV1).

- Stage I (mild disease): FEV1 ≥ 80% of predicted
- Stage II (moderate disease): 50% ≤ FEV1 < 80% of predicted
- Stage III (severe disease): 30% ≤ FEV1 < 50% of predicted
- Stage IV (very severe disease): FEV1 < 30% of predicted, or less than 50% of predicted and the patient is suffering form respiratory failure.

Acute Exacerbations

Definition. COPD is characterized by intermittent episodes of deterioration known as acute exacerbations. These are heralded by a worsening of symptoms beyond the usual day-to-day variation characterized by:

- Increase in dyspnea;
- Increase in cough severity or frequency;
- Increase in sputum volume and/or character.

The typical exacerbation may be accompanied by constitutional symptoms (e.g. fever) and worsening of spirometric values (FVC and FEV1). The chest x-ray is usually unchanged unless pneumonia is the precipitating event.

Causes and risk factors. A majority of these episodes, particularly in patients with mild-to-moderate disease, can be handled in the outpatient setting. For patients with marginal respiratory reserve, respiratory failure can complicate the picture and requires hospital management. About 6% of patients with acute exacerbations will require hospitalization.[5,6] Hospitalization for COPD exacerbation is associated with a poor prognosis. Patients hospitalized on 1–2 occasions have a five-year survival rate of less than 60% and those with >3 hospitalizations have less than a 40% survival rate.

Specific indications for hospitalization have been proposed[7] by a joint position paper of the American Thoracic Society/European Respiratory Society (see Table 1).

Morbidity/mortality. The decision to hospitalize will depend on a number of considerations, including:

- *The baseline lung function of the patient.* Patients with severe or very severe disease will often be hypoxemic (requiring supplemental oxygen) in their baseline state as a result of reduced mechanical efficiency (obstruction, hyperinflation) and/or gas transport problems

Table 1. Specific Recommendations for Hospitalization and ICU Admission of the COPD Patient with Exacerbation[1]

Hospitalization

- The presence of high risk comorbid conditions, including pneumonia, cardiac arrhythmia, congestive heart failure, diabetes mellitus, renal or liver disease
- Inadequate response of symptoms to outpatient management
- Marked increase in dyspnea
- Inability to sleep due to symptoms
- Worsening hypoxemia
- Worsening hypercapnia
- Change in mental status
- Inability of the patient to care for himself or herself (lack of home support)
- Uncertain diagnosis
- Inadequate home care

ICU Admission

- Impending or actual respiratory failure
- Presence of other end organ dysfunctions (e.g. shock and renal, liver or neurological disturbances)
- Hemodynamic instability

(reduced diffusion and/or V/Q mismatch). Acute exacerbations can lead to abrupt decompensation resulting in the patient's usual supplemental oxygen being unable to keep their saturation at >90%. An abrupt change in saturation below the critical level can lead to pulmonary hypertension and cor pulmonale.

- *The nature of the precipitating event.* As many as two-thirds of acute exacerbations are attributable to respiratory infections (both bacterial and viral). Other precipitating factors include airway irritants such as smoking, pollutants, allergens (in patients with mixed disease asthma/COPD), as well as aspiration.
- *The presence of comorbidities.* Patients with COPD are prone to have comorbidities in a greater proportion than individuals of similar age and risk factors. In particular, cardiovascular disease, diabetes, lung cancer and thromboembolic disease (up to 30% of hospitalized patients) are frequent in this population and may be the precipitating events in acute exacerbations of COPD.

The role of exacerbations in the progression of COPD is clearly documented. Exacerbations in general and those associated with hospitalizations in particular lead to accelerated loss of lung function, re-exacerbation with frequent readmissions to hospital and, ultimately, increased mortality.[5–7]

Treatment of Acute Exacerbations

The treatment of the hospitalized patient with acute exacerbation involves identification and treatment of underlying causes of deterioration, reversing bronchoconstriction and inflammation by pharmacologic means, treating impending or actual respiratory failure with oxygen and/or assisted ventilation, preventing complications and assuring a smooth transition to posthospital management.

Antibiotics. A majority of COPD exacerbations are felt to be due to respiratory infection. Viruses, including rhinovirus, influenza, parainfluenza, coronavirus and adenovirus, are the most common isolates. With the exception of influenza, the isolation of a virus may not imply infection.

Bacterial infections account for up to half of the infections triggering acute exacerbations. Nontypeable *Haemophilus influenzae, Moraxella catarhallis* and *Streptococcus pneumoniae* are the most commonly isolated organisms associated with exacerbation. These are frequently difficult to isolate from sputum, and routine culture and examination of sputum smear and culture are not recommended. An exception is made for patients with suspected *Pseudomonas* infection. *Pseudomonas* as the cause of a COPD exacerbation is rare but tends to occur in the most severely compromised COPD patients, including patients with a prior history of *Pseudomonas* infection, receiving multiple courses of antibiotics, or with recent hospitalization for exacerbation. Patients hospitalized for COPD exacerbation should receive antibiotic therapy. Double blind studies with placebo control indicate that, overall, patients with exacerbations treated with antibiotics resolve more frequently compared to those receiving placebos. Patients with the most severe exacerbations were the most likely to experience the beneficial response to a course of antibiotic.[8,9] The choice of antibiotic depends on the level of suspicion for *Pseudomonas*. Patients without risk factors for *Pseudomonas* should receive a fluoroquinolone (e.g. levofloxacin, moxifloxacin) or a third generation cephalosporin (e.g. ceftriaxone, cefotaxime). Patients with risk factors for *Pseudomonas* should receive either a fluoroquinolone active against *Pseudomonas* (e.g. levofloxacin, ciprofloxacin), a fourth generation cephalosporin (e.g. ceftazidime, cefepime) or an antipseudomonal penicillin (e.g. piperacillin-tazobactam).

Isolation of the influenza virus should be treated with antiviral agents for which the current strain is susceptible. The antiviral agent zanamivir is contraindicated in patients with COPD.

Bronchodilators and inhaled corticosteroids. Inhaled beta-2 adrenergic bronchodilators with or without anticholinergic agents and inhaled corticosteroids are effective treatments for exacerbation of COPD. Short-acting bronchodilating agents (albuterol and/or ipratropium) are frequently the preferred agents used in the setting of hospitalized patients with COPD. They are usually administered by nebulizer either separately or in a combination solution. The latter has an additive effect, due to the separate mechanisms of action by which the agents promote smooth muscle relaxation. Their effective duration of action is about 4 hr and therefore need to be administered at regular intervals in order to have sustained bronchodilation. Use by other routes is usually avoided in the hospital setting. MDIs are difficult to employ in the sick COPD patient, and oral or parenteral administration of these agents has significant cardiovascular toxicity in this setting.

Many patients with severe or very severe COPD are maintained as outpatients on long-acting bronchodilator agents. Salmeterol and formoterol are two long-acting beta-2 adrenergic agents (LABAs) widely used in the treatment of COPD. Both drugs have a duration of action of approximately 12 hr. They are generally considered safe and effective for the treatment of COPD. Formoterol is also available for use as a nebulized solution. Furthermore, these agents are available in combination with an inhaled corticosteroid — fluticasone in the case of salmeterol, and budesonide or mometasone in the case of formoterol. Tiotropium is a long acting anticholinergic agent that is also often used in the outpatient treatment of COPD and may be used with LABAs to good effect. Maintenance of hospitalized patients on these longer-acting bronchodilating preparations with the use of short-acting bronchodilating agents (SABAs) every 4 hr on an as-needed basis may offer an alternative strategy to nebulized short-acting bronchodilators every 4 hr.

Methylxanthines (theophylline and aminophylline) can be administered orally or intravenously. They provide dose-dependent bronchodilation and can be titrated using serum levels. They may also have anti-inflammatory properties. Methylxanthines have lost favor in the treatment of airway obstruction because of their narrow window of the toxic-to-therapeutic ratio. They may nevertheless play a role in the refractory patient, as they may offer an alternative means of achieving airway relaxation independently of the beta and cholinergic receptors.

Oral and parenteral glucocorticoids. Concurrent use of glucocorticoid therapy by the intravenous or oral route is recommended for the initial treatment of severe exacerbations of COPD requiring hospitalization.[10,11] The exact mechanism of action is unclear; anti-inflammatory effects as well as resensitization of beta-adrenergic receptors may be involved. A list of commonly used steroid preparations administered for obstructive disease is shown in Table 2. High doses of steroids as well as prolonged use have recently been suggested to be no more effective than short term use with low doses. By contrast, the high dose intravenous route has been associated with higher rates of complications as well as increased hospital costs. In a retrospective study by Lindenauer,[12] oral doses of prednisone 20–60 mg once daily were as effective as an intravenous regimen.

Oxygen and assisted ventilation. Oxygen therapy is a fundamental part of the therapy for COPD exacerbations in the hospital. Adequate supplemental oxygen should be titrated to keep the patient's oxygenation at adequate levels ($SaO_2 > 90\%$; $PaO_2 > 60$ mmHg). A number of oxygen delivery systems allow for the accurate titration of oxygen so as not to cause suppression of

Table 2. Properties of Corticosteroids Commonly Administered to Treat COPD

Steroid	Relative Anti-Inflammatory Strength	Relative Mineralocorticoid Strength	Routes of Administration	Duration of Action (Systemic)
Hydrocortisone	1.0	1.0	IV, IM, oral	Short
Cortisone	0.8	0.8	IV, IM, oral	Short
Prednisone	2.5–3.5	0.8	Oral	Intermediate
Methylprednisolone	4.0–5.0	Less than 0.8	IV, IM, oral	Intermediate
Triamcinolone	4.0–5.0	0	IV, IM, oral	Intermediate
Dexamethasone	20–40	0	IV, IM, oral	Long

* Adapted from: Witek TJ, Schachter EN. (1994) *Pharmacology and Therapeutics in Respiratory Care*. WB Saunders, Philadelphia, PA.

the respiratory drive. These systems (preferably high flow Venturi masks) allow for reliable delivery of oxygen at F_IO_2 between 24 and 55%.[13] Because of the possible insidious development of hypercapnea, an arterial blood gas should be performed after the initiation of oxygen therapy in this setting (usually within an hour of establishing satisfactory oxygenation).

Noninvasive ventilation (NIV) in the setting of impending respiratory failure can stabilize patients with severe exacerbations and prevent the need for intubation with mechanical ventilation (Table 3). Initiation of this therapy requires skilled adjustment of noninvasive equipment and titration of pressures for patient comfort and is usually best accomplished in conjunction with a respiratory therapist.

Preventing complications. Patients with COPD have an excess of comorbidities, based on their frequent history of smoking and the possible effects of an as-yet-poorly-characterized chronic inflammatory state.[14] Cardiovascular disease is particularly common and may be the cause of morbidity and death in a large fraction of COPD patients admitted for acute exacerbation. Thromboembolic disease is a frequent complication of COPD exacerbation.[15,16] DVT has been documented in 11% of 196 patients admitted to a respiratory care unit, though most were

Table 3. Indications and Contraindications for NIV and Mechanical Ventilation[3]

Selection for NIV

- Moderate-to-severe dyspnea with use of accessory muscles and paradoxical abdominal motion
- Moderate-to-severe acidosis (pH < 7.35) and/or hypercapnia ($PaCO_2$ > 45 mmHg)
- Respiratory frequency > 25 breaths/min

Exclusion for NIV

- Respiratory arrest
- CV instability
- Change in mental status, uncooperative
- Aspiration risk
- Viscous or copious secretions
- Recent facial or gastroesophageal surgery
- Craniofacial trauma
- Nasopharyngeal abnormalities
- Burns
- Extreme obesity

Indications for Mechanical Ventilation with Intubation

- NIV failure
- Severe dyspnea, with use of accessory muscles and paradoxical respiration
- Respiratory rate > 35/min
- Life threatening hypoxemia
- Severe acidosis (pH < 7.25) and severe hypercapnia ($PaCO_2$ > 60 mmHg)
- Respiratory arrest
- Somnolence, impaired mental status
- CV instability
- Other complications (metabolic abnormalities, sepsis, pneumonia, PE, bacteremia, massive effusion)

asymptomatic. The frequency of PE during acute exacerbations of COPD has been estimated to be as high as 29% and PE accounts for up to 10% of deaths in COPD patients treated with long term oxygen. The high prevalence of this complication with acute exacerbations of COPD warrants the consideration of PE in exacerbations not responding to standard therapy, and that prophylaxis be routinely administered in these patients.

Assuring a smooth transition to posthospital management. Patients with COPD have a high incidence of rehospitalization.[5] The ideal length of hospitalization for acute exacerbation is not determined but patients should be stable both clinically and objectively (e.g. adequate gas exchange and decreased bronchodilator requirements) for at least 24 hr before discharge is considered. A written action plan with recommendations for the treatment of a repeat exacerbation is required. The care plan should be based on guidelines developed for the management of stable outpatient COPD, such as those described in the GOLD guidelines. Assessment of immunization status (influenza and *S. pneumonia*e) should be made before discharge and the patient immunized if indicated. Smoking cessation, if the patient is a current smoker, needs to be addressed. The patient should be evaluated for possible pulmonary rehabilitation at the time of discharge. Patients should be taught how to recognize acute exacerbation and given specific instructions on how to manage exacerbations. The patient's home situation should be fully addressed by home care and respiratory services. Home oxygen and visiting nurse services when needed should be in place, so that upon arrival at home the patient will not be without adequate resources. Medical followup should occur within 4–6 weeks.

Phophodiesterase IV inhibitors.

This newly developed class of agents has now been introduced for the management of COPD patients. Its role is not as yet totally defined but it is recommended by the GOLD Guidelines for patients with severe or very severe airway obstruction (GOLD 3 & 4). The expected outcome is to reduce the frequency and severity of exacerbations, and when taken in conjuction with long-acting bronchodilators, to modestly improve FEV1. GI side-effects and sleep disturbance are the most commonly reported side effects. The available product in the United States, roflumilast, is given orally 500 mcg once daily.[3,17]

Conclusions

Acute exacerbations of COPD, particularly those requiring hospitalization, are critical mileposts in the course of this disease. Early and appropriate management of these events — including treating their underlying cause, reversing the physiologic consequences (which include bronchospasm, respiratory failure and cor pulmonale) and limiting the consequences of comorbidities — is the challenge for the hospital-based physician. No less important is ensuring that the COPD patient has received all the preventive strategies prior to discharge and that a smooth transition back to the outpatient environment has been arranged.

References

1. Brown DW, Croft JB, Greenlund KJ, Giles WH. (2010) Trends in hospitalization with chronic obstructive pulmonary disease — United States, 1990–2005. *COPD* **7**(1): 59–62.
2. Centers for Disease Control and Prevention. (2008) Deaths from chronic obstructive pulmonary disease — United States, 2000–2005. *Morbidity and Mortality Weekly Report* **57**(45): 1229–1232.
3. Global Strategy for Diagnosis, Management and Prevention of COPD Updated 2011; http://www.goldcopd.com
4. Lenfant C. (2003) Shattuck lecture: clinical research to clinical practice — lost in translation? *N Engl J Med* **349**(9): 868–874.
5. Chenna PR, Mannino DM. (2010) Outcomes of severe COPD exacerbations requiring hospitalization. *Semin Respir Crit Care Med* **31**(3): 286–294. [Epub 2010, May 21].
6. Soler-Cataluña JJ, Martínez-García MA, Román Sánchez P, *et al.* (2005) Severe acute exacerbations and mortality in patients with chronic obstructive pulmonary disease. *Thorax* **60**(11): 925–931.
7. Celli BR, MacNee W; ATS/ERS Task Force. (2004) Standards for the diagnosis and treatment of patients with COPD: A summary of the ATS/ERS position paper. *Eur Respir J* **23**(6): 932–946.

8. Anthonisen NR, Manfreda J, Warren CP, *et al.* (1987) Antibiotic therapy in exacerbations of chronic obstructive pulmonary disease. *Ann Intern Med* **106**: 196–204.
9. Rothberg MB, Pekow PS, Lahti M, *et al.* (2010) Antibiotic therapy and treatment failure in patients hospitalized for acute exacerbations of chronic obstructive pulmonary disease. *JAMA* **303**: 2035
10. Davies L, Angus RM, Calverley PM. (1999) Oral corticosteroids in patients admitted to hospital with exacerbations of chronic obstructive pulmonary disease: A prospective randomised controlled trial. *Lancet* **354**(9177): 456–460.
11. Niewoehner DE, Erbland ML, Deupree RH, *et al.* (1999) Effect of systemic glucocorticoids on exacerbations of chronic obstructive pulmonary disease. Department of Veterans Affairs Cooperative Study Group. *N Engl J Med* **340**(25): 1941–1947.
12. Lindenauer PK, Pekow PS, Lahti MC, *et al.* (2010) Association of corticosteroid dose and route of administration with risk of treatment failure in acute exacerbation of chronic obstructive pulmonary disease. *JAMA* **303**(23): 2359–2367.
13. Schachter EN, Littner M, Luddy P, Beck GJ. (1980) Oxygen delivery systems in clinical practice. *Criti Care Med* **8**: 405–409.
14. Hurst JR, Perera WR, Wilkinson TM, *et al.* (2006) Systemic and upper and lower airway inflammation at exacerbation of chronic obstructive pulmonary disease. *Am J Respir Crit Care Med* **173**(1): 71–78.
15. Ambrosetti M, Ageno W, Spanevello A, *et al.* (2003) Prevalence and prevention of venous thromboembolism in patients with acute exacerbations of COPD. *Thromb Res* **112**(4): 203–207.
16. Rizkallah J, Man SF, Sin DD. (2009) Prevalence of pulmonary embolism in acute exacerbations of COPD: A systematic review and meta-analysis. *Chest* **135**(3): 786–793.
17. Calverley PM, Rabe KF, Goehring UM *et al.* (2009) Roflumilast in symptomatic chronic obstructive pulmonary disease: two randomised clinical trials. *Lancet* 29;374(9691): 685–94.

Chapter 29

Evaluation and Treatment of Diffuse Parenchymal Lung Disease

*June Kim and Timothy J. Harkin**

Key Pearls

- The American Thoracic Society (ATS) and the European Respiratory Society (ERS) have revised the classification of interstitial lung diseases (ILDs) and introduced the term "diffuse parenchymal lung disease" (DLPD).
- Special testing may be warranted to confirm occupational exposure (such as demonstration of ferruginous bodies in asbestosis from lung biopsies or a hypersensitivity panel for serologic evidence of immune reaction to organic antigens).
- Many patients who are referred to advanced lung disease programs for idiopathic lung disease are found to have an underlying systemic rheumatologic disease, such as rheumatoid arthritis, scleroderma, systemic lupus erythematosis, dermatomyositis, polymyositis, Sjogren's disease, or sarcoidosis.
- For patients with DPLDs who present with decompensated pulmonary symptoms, a chest CT angiogram can help rule out pulmonary embolism and identify infection, heart failure, or worsening of underlying lung disease. Early bronchoscopy should be considered for the prompt diagnosis and treatment of atypical lung infections.

*Mount Sinai School of Medicine, NY, New York, USA.

- Idiopathic pulmonary fibrosis (IPF) patients must be considered for early referral for lung transplantation, because there is no effective treatment and there is a very high risk of death from respiratory failure. Mean survival is approximately three years.

Introduction

Interstitial lung diseases (ILDs) are a heterogeneous group of disorders characterized by inflammation and/or fibrosis of the pulmonary interstitium, the microscopic space between alveolar epithelium and capillary endothelium. In 2002, the American Thoracic Society (ATS) and the European Respiratory Society (ERS) revised the classification of ILDs and introduced the term "diffuse parenchymal lung disease" (DLPD), and separated DLPD into four major categories (Fig. 1).

Each category has distinct clinical, radiographic, and pathologic characteristics, often presenting significant diagnostic challenges. An evaluation of a patient with DPLD therefore begins with early consultations with expert clinicians, radiologists, and pathologists who are well versed in these entities to determine the most likely diagnosis.[1,2]

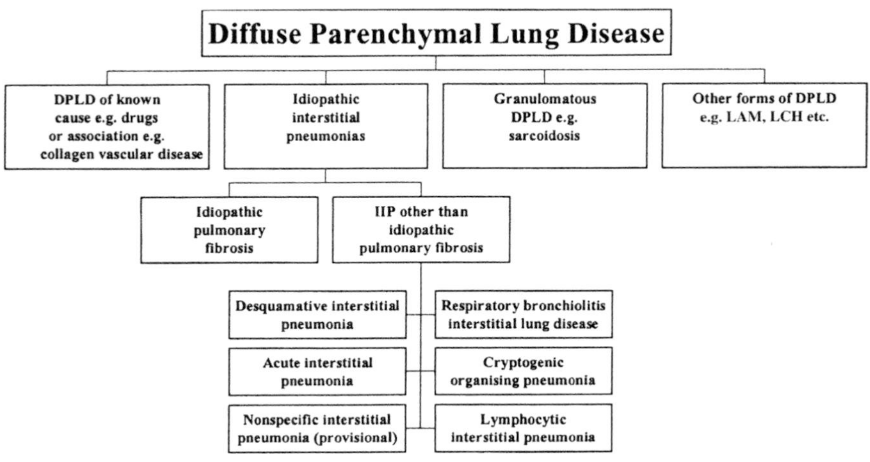

Fig 1. ATS/ER classification of diffuse parenchymal lung disease.[1]

The following is a brief summary of the clinical evaluation of patients with suspected DPLD and considerations for the diagnosis and management issues for the hospitalist.

Clinical Evaluation

History

An accurate diagnosis is essential to the appropriate management and prognostication of a DPLD patient. A comprehensive history is a critical component of this assessment, because at the most advanced stages of disease, many entities can be radiographically and pathologically indistinguishable from each other.

There are many medical agents that can cause DPLD (see Table 1).[3] Temporally linking exposure to the drug to the development of respiratory symptoms and radiographic findings is helpful in the diagnosis of drug-related DPLD. The inciting agent should be promptly discontinued if this is suspected. A complete updated list of medications that have been implicated in pulmonary disease is available at http://pneumotox.com.

Table 1. Drugs that Can Cause DPLD

Antibiotics	Cephalosporins, minocycline, nitrofurantoin, quinine
Rheumatologic treatments	Gold, leflunomide, methotrexate, NSAIDS, penicillamine, sulfasalazine, infliximab, etanercept
Cardiology	Amiodarone, angiotensin-converting enzyme inhibitors, aspirin, atenolol, statins
Oncology	Bleomycin, busulfan, chlorambucil, dasatnib, melphalan, imatinib, methotrexate, mitomycin C
Immunomodulators	Azathioprine, cyclophosphamide, erlotinib, gefitinib, interferons, rituxumab, sirolimus
Illicit drugs	Cocaine, heroin, intravenous talc, methadone
Miscellaneous	High concentrations of oxygen, inhaled or aspirated fat-containing substances (e.g. mineral oil), paraquat, radiotherapy

Adapted from Ref. 3.

History of exposure to asbestos at shipyards, while working with car brakes and installing insulation, to silica at construction sites or as a sandblaster, to coal dust among miners, to heavy metals in metal workers, and to organic/inorganic substances in farmers are just some examples of work-related exposures that can cause significant lung disease. It should be noted here that a typical history of hypersensitivity pneumonitis (immune reaction to organic dust) includes worsening of symptoms while at work or when repetitively exposed to a certain hobbies or locations. Similar symptoms are seen in occupational asthma, and this diagnosis should be considered as part of the differential diagnosis.

Patients can have indirect exposures as well, as exemplified by a landmark paper in 1979 by Selikoff's group, who found that 35% of household contacts of asbestos workers had radiographic evidence of asbestos exposure despite there being no direct exposure to the substance.[4] It was theorized that home contamination from shoes and work clothes was the source of asbestos exposure. Also, physicians must be wary that patients may not acknowledge their exposures or be unaware of inciting agents. For example, bird fanciers may not offer exposure history due to fear of being separated from their pets.

Special testing may ultimately be warranted to confirm occupational exposure (such as demonstration of ferruginous bodies in lung biopsis of asbestosis or lung biopsies or a hypersensitivity panel for serologic evidence of immune reaction to organic antigens).[5,6]

Particular attention to extrapulmonary signs and symptoms is also important to the diagnosis of patients with occult rheumatologic disease as a cause of ILD. Many patients who are referred to advanced lung disease programs for idiopathic lung disease are found to have an underlying systemic rheumatologic disease (see Fig. 2).[7] Clinicians should elicit signs and symptoms suggestive of rheumatoid arthritis, scleroderma, systemic lupus erythematosis, dermatomyositis, polymyositis, Sjogren's disease, sarcoidosis, or "overlapping" rheumatologic syndromes and pursue confirmatory testing with the guidance of rheumatology specialists (see Table 2).[8–17]

In addition, up to 10% of ILD patients meet criteria for "undifferentiated connective disease" (UCTD) but do not meet classically defined

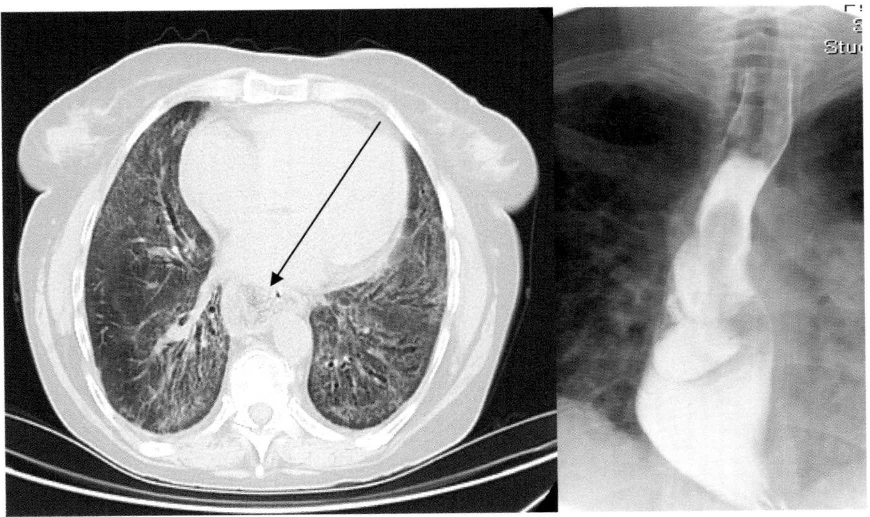

Fig. 2. Scleroderma-related DPLD: A woman with a history of Raynaud's phenomenon, dysphagia, and skin features suggestive of scleroderma. Chest CT demonstrated parenchymal disease typical of NSIP, an enlarged pulmonary artery (pulmonary hypertension), and an enlarged, dilated food-filled esophagus (arrow) that was later studied by esophagram.

criteria for a known rheumatologic illness. Recent data suggest that many patients with nonspecific interstitial pneumonia (NSIP) also meet criteria for UCTD.[22,23]

Similarly, patients with sarcoidosis, lymphangioleiomyomatosis, or pulmonary Langerhans cell histiocytosis (LCH) have unique clinical and radiographic features (see Table 2 and Figs. 3–5).

Idiopathic interstitial pneumonias are a distinct group of DPLDs of unknown etiology that requires a considerable amount of expertise to define and diagnose. However, it is critical to recognize the presentation of idiopathic pulmonary fibrosis (IPF), because it is the most common and most serious idiopathic interstitial pneumonia. IPF is found most commonly in males 40–70 years of age who have a previous smoking history and may have a familial clustering of pulmonary fibrosis. There is an important protypical clinical–radiographic presentation of this entity that allows the confirmation of this diagnosis without the need for a surgical

Table 2. Clinical Features and Tests that Aid in Differentiation of DPLD from Systemic Diseases[9–20]

Potential Etiology	Disease Specific Clinical Features and Summary of Diagnostic Criteria	Radiographic Spectrum in the Lung	Potential Clinical Testing	Potential Laboratory Data
Rheumatoid arthritis ACR (1987) criteria vs. CCP-7-replace rheumatoid nodules for early RF	***4 of 7 criteria*** Morning stiffness >1 hr Arthritis >3 joints Hand arthritis Symmetric arthritis Rheumatoid nodules (vs. Positive CCP) RF+ Radiographic changes	Pleural involvement Pericardial involvement Bronchiectasis and airways disease Interstitial lung disease UIP or NSIP pattern Small nodules Necrobiotic lung nodules	Hand x-ray (erosions)	Antinuclear antibody Rheumatoid factor Anti-CCP
Scleroderma 3 major categories **Limited SS sine scleroderma** **Limited cutaneous SS (CREST)** **Diffuse cutaneous** (LeRoy, 1988)	**Limited SS sine scleroderma** Raynaud's phenomena (RP) objective documentation or RP by history + nailfold capillaroscopy (dilation, avascular areas) and positive serology **Limited cutaneous SS** Above plus skin tautness of fingers, hands, forearms, legs, feet, toes, neck, and face	Interstitial lung disease, UIP or NSIP pattern Pulmonary artery enlargement (Pulm HTN with mosaicism and centrilobular nodules) Dilated esophagus	Nailfold capillaroscopy Swallowing studies Echocardiogram	Antinuclear antibodies with a nucleolar staining pattern (90% of SSc patients) Anticentromere (ACA), antitopoiso merase-I (Scl-70), anti-RNA poly merase, U3-RNP antibodies

(Continued)

Table 2. (*Continued*)

Potential Etiology	Disease Specific Clinical Features and Summary of Diagnostic Criteria	Radiographic Spectrum in the Lung	Potential Clinical Testing	Potential Laboratory Data
	CREST calcinosis, Raynaud's phenomenon, esophageal hypomotility, sclerodactyly, telangectasia			
	Diffuse cutaneous SS			
	RP within 1 year of onset of skin changes (puffy or hidebound)			
	Truncal and acral skin involvement			
	Presence of tendon friction rubs			
	Interstitial lung disease, oliguric renal failure, diffuse gastrointestinal disease, and myocardial involvement			
	Absence of ACA			
	Nailfold capillary dilatation and capillary destruction			
	Antitopoisomerase antibodies (30% of patients)			
Sjogren's disease	**Primary SS:** 4 of the 6 items below (I–IV) if at least IV	Lung cysts (LIP) Interstitial fibrosis,	"Keratoconjunctivitis sicca tests"	Antinuclear antibody

(*Continued*)

Table 2. *(Continued)*

Potential Etiology	Disease Specific Clinical Features and Summary of Diagnostic Criteria	Radiographic Spectrum in the Lung	Potential Clinical Testing	Potential Laboratory Data
	(histopathology) or VI (serology) is positive Or 3 of the 4 objective criteria items (items III–VI) **Subjective** I. Ocular symptoms (dry eyes >3 months; recurrent sensation of sand or gravel in the eyes, tear substitutes more than 3 times a day)	honeycombing and pulmonary fibrosis Small airways disease Risk of pseudolymphoma and lymphoma	Schirmer's I test, performed without anesthesia (<5 mm in 5 min) Rose bengal score or other ocular dye score (>4 according to van Bijsterveld's scoring system)	Antibodies to Ro(SSA) or La(SSB) antigens, or both Cryoglobulinemia Hypocomplementemia IgG4-positive lymphoproliferative syndrome
	II. Oral symptoms: dry mouth >3 months, persistently swollen salivary glands; frequently drink liquids to aid in swallowing dry food		Unstimulated whole salivary flow (<1.5 ml in 15 min)	
	Objective III. Ocular signs — positive result for at least one of the following two tests: 1. Schirmer's I test 2. Rose bengal score		Parotid sialography showing the presence of diffuse sialectasias (punctate, cavitary or	

(Continued)

Table 2. *(Continued)*

Potential Etiology	Disease Specific Clinical Features and Summary of Diagnostic Criteria	Radiographic Spectrum in the Lung	Potential Clinical Testing	Potential Laboratory Data
	IV. Histopathology: in minor salivary glands V. Salivary gland involvement: positive result for at least one of the following diagnostic tests: 1. Unstimulated whole salivary flow 2. Parotid sialography 3. Salivary scintigraphy VI. Antibodies to Ro(SSA) or La(SSB) antigens, or both		destructive pattern), without evidence of obstruction in the major ducts Salivary scintigraphy showing delayed uptake, reduced concentration and/or delayed excretion of tracer Possible gland biopsy	
Mixed Connective Tissue Disease	**Mixed connective tissue (overlap syndrome):** Combination of SLE, scleroderma or PSS, and polymyositis–dermatomyositis	Interstitial lung disease Pulmonary artery enlargement (Pulm HTN) with mosaicism and centrilobular nodules	Echocardiogram	Antinuclear antibody Anti-RNP antibodies titer (an RNAse-sensitive extractable >1:1600) Positive ANA (commonly >1:1000 and often greater than 1:10,000) speckled

(Continued)

Table 2. *(Continued)*

Potential Etiology	Disease Specific Clinical Features and Summary of Diagnostic Criteria	Radiographic Spectrum in the Lung	Potential Clinical Testing	Potential Laboratory Data
Systemic Lupus Erythematosis Diagnostic and Therapeutic Criteria Committee of the ACR, 1997	**4 or more of 11 criteria** 1. Malar rash 2. Discoid rash 3. Photosensitivity 4. Oral or nasopharyngeal ulceration 5. Arthritis (nonerosive arthritis 2 peripheral joints — tenderness, swelling, or effusion) 6. Serositis (pleuritis, pericarditis) 7. Renal disorder (persistent proteinuria or cellular casts) 8. Neurologic disorder (seizure psychosis) 9. Hematologic disorder anemia, leukopenia, (hemolytic lymphopenia, thrombocytopenia with absence of offending drug) 10. Immunologic disorder (anti-DNA ab, anti-Sm ab, antiphospholipid antibodies)	Pleural disease Pericardial disease Inflammatory pneumonitis (diffuse infiltrates/ consolidation/effusions with DAD on path) Diffuse alveolar hemorrhage (DAH) neutrophilic capillaritis; rapid resolution of findings Interstitial pulmonary fibrosis (not common) Pulmonary hypertension Diaphragmatic dysfunction (shrinking lung syndrome; high diaphragms); Pulmonary emboli with infarction	Plain radiographs of involved joints Renal ultrasonography to assess kidney disease Urine protein Urine sediment Echocardiography (pericardial disease and evidence of PE) Computed tomography (CT) (e.g. for abdominal pain, suspected pancreatitis)	Antinuclear antibodies (ANA), ANA is positive in significant titer (usually 1:160 or higher) in virtually all patients with SLE Antinuclear Ab Antiphospholipid antibodies Antibodies to double-stranded DNA Anti-Smith (Sm) antibodies Measurement of serum complement levels C3 and C4

(Continued)

Table 2. *(Continued)*

Potential Etiology	Disease Specific Clinical Features and Summary of Diagnostic Criteria	Radiographic Spectrum in the Lung	Potential Clinical Testing	Potential Laboratory Data
	11. Antinuclear antibody in the absence of drugs known to be associated with "drug-induced lupus" syndrome		Magnetic resonance imaging (neurologic involvement) Contrast angiography for vasculitis, medium-sized arteries	
Dermatomyositis/ PM	Symmetric proximal muscle weakness Typical rash of DM (only distinguishing clinical feature between DM and PM) ex. heliotrope rash Elevated serum muscle enzymes Myopathic changes on electromyography Characteristic muscle biopsy abnormalities	Aspiration PNA Interstitial lung disease UIP or NSIP pattern Consolidations (COP)	EMG Muscle biopsy	CPK Aldolase "Myositis panel": auto-Abs to synthetases encompassed anti-Jo-1, OJ, EJ, KS, PL7, and PL12 specificities Systemic sclerosis-specific

(Continued)

Table 2. *(Continued)*

Potential Etiology	Disease Specific Clinical Features and Summary of Diagnostic Criteria	Radiographic Spectrum in the Lung	Potential Clinical Testing	Potential Laboratory Data
	and absence of histopathologic signs of other myopathies			aAbs (aAbs to centromeres, topo I,Th, and RNA polymerases I/III) for overlap syndromes
Sarcoidosis	Diagnosis: Noncaseating granuloma in biopsy of two different organs (with all other causes of granulomas excluded) excluded or a positive Kveim test or Lofgren's syndrome (no biopsy needed) **Other signs and symptoms (organs affected)** Constitutional symptoms Lacrimal gland enlargement Skin findings: erythemanodosum, lupus pernio	Pulmonary Sarcoidosis Chest x-ray pattern 1. Stage 1: hilar adenopathy 2. Stage 2: hilar adenopathy with reticulonodular infiltrates 3. Stage 3: reticulonodular infiltrates 4. Fibrocystic lung disease	Kveim–Siltzbach test intradermally biopsy 4 wk FDG-PET or cardiac MRI for sarcoidosis of the heart MRI of the brain/ spine if concerned for neurosarcoidosis	ACE level is an insensitive and nonspecific test

(Continued)

Table 2. *(Continued)*

Potential Etiology	Disease Specific Clinical Features and Summary of Diagnostic Criteria	Radiographic Spectrum in the Lung	Potential Clinical Testing	Potential Laboratory Data
	Lymph node enlargement Cardiac symptoms including palpitations Neurologic symptoms, including uveitis and facial palsies Hepatosplenomegaly Liver disease Renal stones /renal disease Symptoms of hypercalcemia			
Lymphangioleio-myomatosis (LAM) (Johnson McCormack)	**Definite LAM** 1. Characteristic or compatible lung HRCT, and lung biopsy fitting the pathologic criteria for LAM 2. Characteristic lung HRCT and any of the following: a. Renal angiomyolipoma (kidney biopsy), thoracic or abdominal chylous effusion,	Multiple thin-walled round well-defined air-filled cysts	Abdominal CT vs. MRI for detection of angiomyolipomas, lymphangioleiomyomas, or lymphadenopathy Renal mass biopsy Lung biopsy LAM cells (smooth muscle cells) expressing markers of smooth muscle	

(Continued)

Table 2. *(Continued)*

Potential Etiology	Disease Specific Clinical Features and Summary of Diagnostic Criteria	Radiographic Spectrum in the Lung	Potential Clinical Testing	Potential Laboratory Data
	lymphangioleiomyoma, or lymphnode involved by LAM, and definite or probable tuberous sclerosis complex		and melanocytic differentiation, which are useful diagnosically	
	Heightened suspicion			
	Young female with recurrent pneumothorax or chylous effusion		Thoracocentesis of pleural effusion with triglyceride levels	
Pulmonary langerhans cell histiocytosis (LCH)	Young smoker	Reticular changes, micronodules measuring 2–5 mm, and diffuse cysts measuring up to 1 cm	Lung biopsy: stellate nodules with Langerhans cells and cysts Langerhans cells staining immunopositive for CD1a, Langerin, E-cadherin, and S100 Birbeck granules by electromicroscopy	

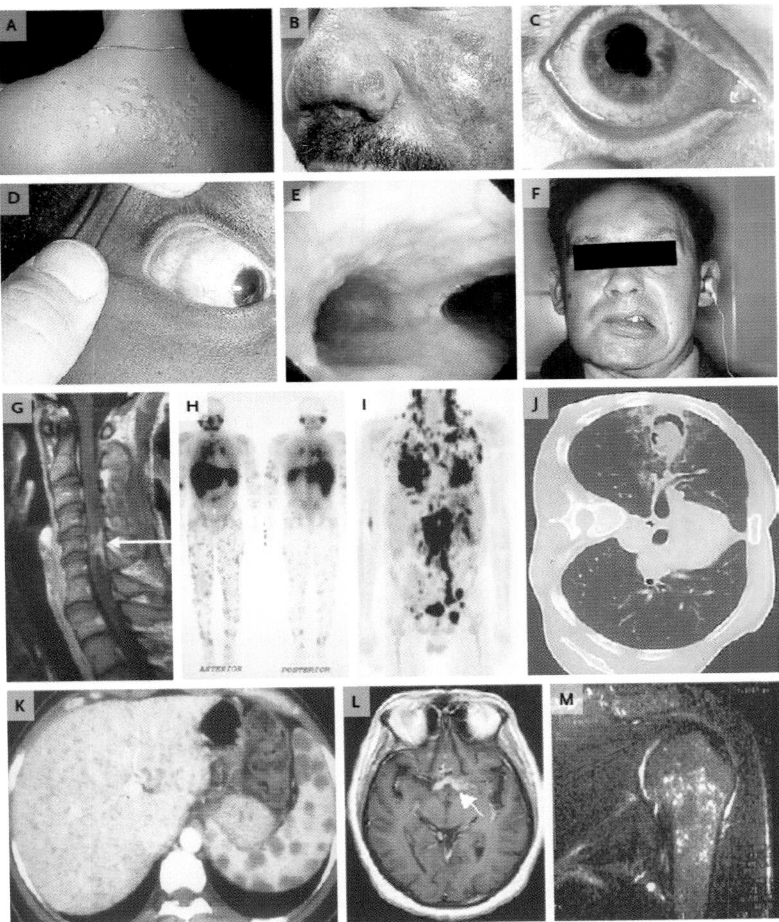

Fig. 3. Radiographic features and extra-pulmonary signs of possible sarcoidosis: (A) Waxy interscapular skin plaques; (B) lupus pernio; (C) anterior uveitis with synechiae; (D) enlarged, nodular lacrimal gland; (E) endobronchial cobblestoning; (F) ipsilateral peripheral facial-nerve and cranial-nerve involvement with hearing loss; (G) spinal cord mass on a T1-weighted MRI scan (arrow); (H) gallium scan demonstrating nasal, parotid, lung, liver, spleen, subcutaneous-nodule, and mediastinal and epitrochlear lymph-node involvement; (I) PET scan demonstrating hypermetabolism in the liver, spleen, and lymph nodes; (J) a right upper lobe cavity with a gravity-dependent aspergilloma; (K) abdominal CT scan demonstrating hypodense splenic nodules; (L) involvement of the optic chiasm seen on a gadolinium-enhanced MRI scan (arrow); (M) T1-weighted MRI scan demonstrating granulomatous involvement of the humerus. (From Reg. 18.)

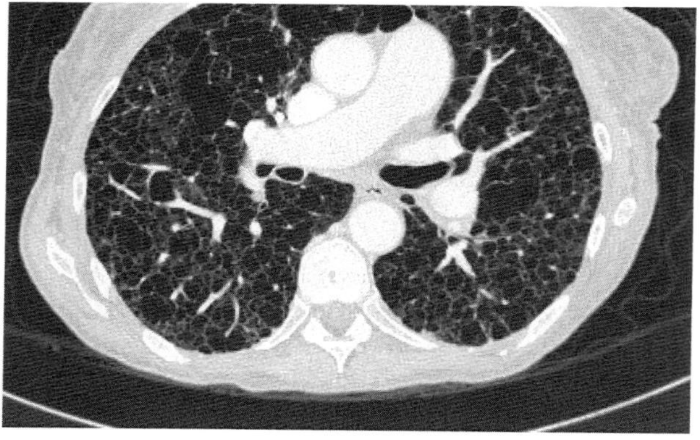

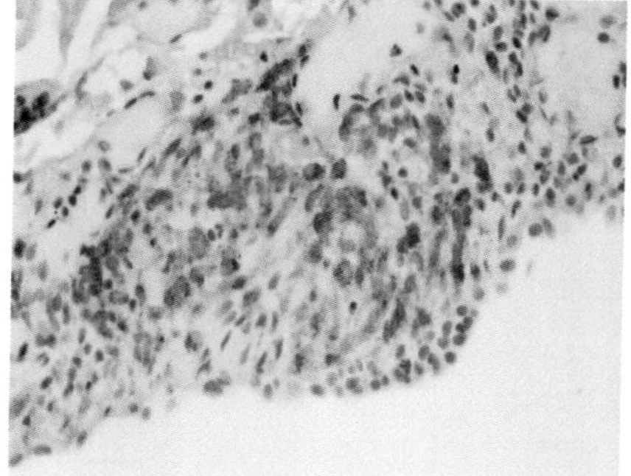

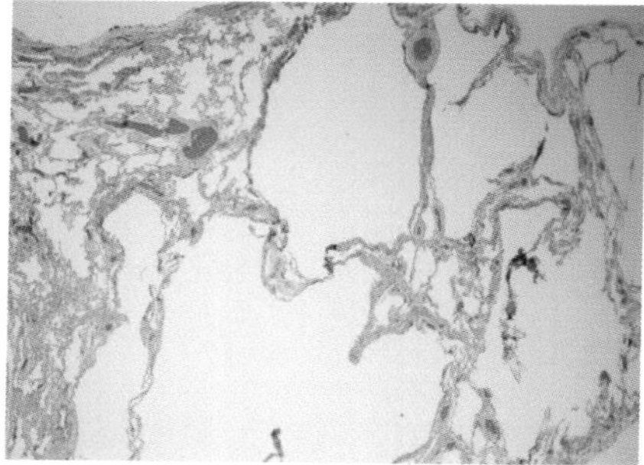

Fig. 4. Lymphangioleiomyomatosis (LAM): **A** young woman with recurrent pneumothorax, initially diagnosed with emphysema. Chest CT revealed diffuse thin-walled cysts. She was diagnosed with LAM via surgical lung biopsy. Histopathology: thin-walled cysts and nodules of LAM cells which stain for melanocyte marker HMB-45.

lung biopsy[24] (see Table 3 and Fig. 6). IPF patients must be considered for early referral for lung transplantation, because there is no effective treatment and there is a very high risk of death from respiratory failure (mean survival of about three years).[1,2,26] In addition, they are at risk of presenting with acute exacerbations of IPF, defined as acute, clinically significant respiratory deteriorations of unidentifiable cause that are associated with very high inpatient mortality.[25,27]

Some DPLDs are also associated with smoking (e.g. IPF, RBILD, DIP, LCH) or have familial clustering (e.g. IPF, sarcoidosis, Hermansky–Pudlak syndrome), which should be addressed in the history.

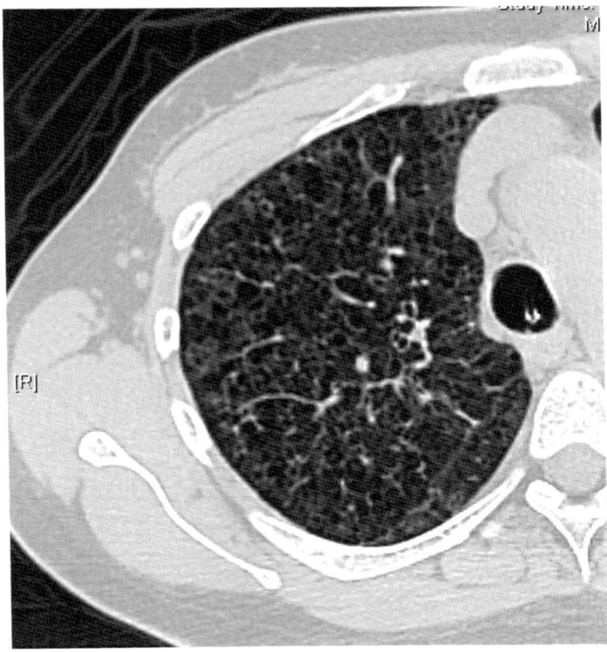

Fig. 5. Pulmonary Langerhans cell histiocytosis (LCH): A 39-year-old female referred for lung transplantation for progressive DPLD. Chest CT showed innumerable small cystic structures, reticular lines, coarsened interstitial markings, and diffusely scattered micronodules typical of LCH. Stellate lung nodules with Langerhans cells were found in her explanted lungs.

Lastly, it is important to note that other respiratory illnesses may share radiographic and pathologic features of DPLDs and should be excluded by history at the outset. Most DPLDs have a chronic course, with the exception of patients with acute interstitial pneumonia (AIP) who progress rapidly to respiratory failure in a matter of weeks or patients with IPF presenting with acute IPF exacerbation. Acute and subacute respiratory symptoms with diffuse chest radiographic findings can be caused by viral pneumonia, opportunistic infections (e.g. pneumocystis or CMV in an immunocompromised host), adult respiratory distress syndrome (ARDS), heart failure, transfusion-related acute lung injury, or diffuse alveolar hemorrhage. These should be expeditiously worked up and eliminated prior to considering a DPLD.

Table 3. ATS/ER Criteria for the Diagnosis of Idiopathic Pulmonary Fibrosis in the Absence of Surgical Lung Biopsy: the "Radiologic Diagnosis" of IPF

Major Criteria (all four need to be present)	Exclusion of other known causes of ILD, such as drug toxicities, environmental exposures, and connective tissue diseases Abnormal pulmonary function studies that include evidence of restriction (reduced VC, often with an increased FEV1/FVC ratio) and impaired gas exchange (decreased PaO_2, increased A-a gradient with rest or exercise, or decreased DLCO) Bibasilar reticular abnormalities with minimal ground glass opacities on HRCT scan Transbronchial lung biopsy or BAL showing no features to support an alternative diagnosis
Minor Criteria (at least 3 of 4 are needed)	Age >50 years Insidious onset of otherwise unexplained dyspnea on exertion Duration of illness >3 mth Bibasiliar, inspiratory crackles (dry or Velcro type)

Clinical Exam

A complete physical exam should be performed to seek classic findings for ILD, including dry crackles, evidence of pulmonary hypertension and cor pulmonale, and digital clubbing, but also to obtain subtle findings that may suggest associated systemic diseases (see Fig. 7).

Radiologic Evaluation

High-resolution chest CT (HRCT) with thin sections of 0.5–2.0 mm thickness with edge enhancement is the radiologic modality of choice for the evaluation of the pulmonary interstitium. It is frequently useful to also obtain images at end expiration and with prone positioning. Various terms are used by radiologists to describe radiographic findings on HRCTs (see Table 4).[28] The predominant pattern and distribution of these findings, and the presence of esophageal disease, lymphadenopathy, pleural/pericardial

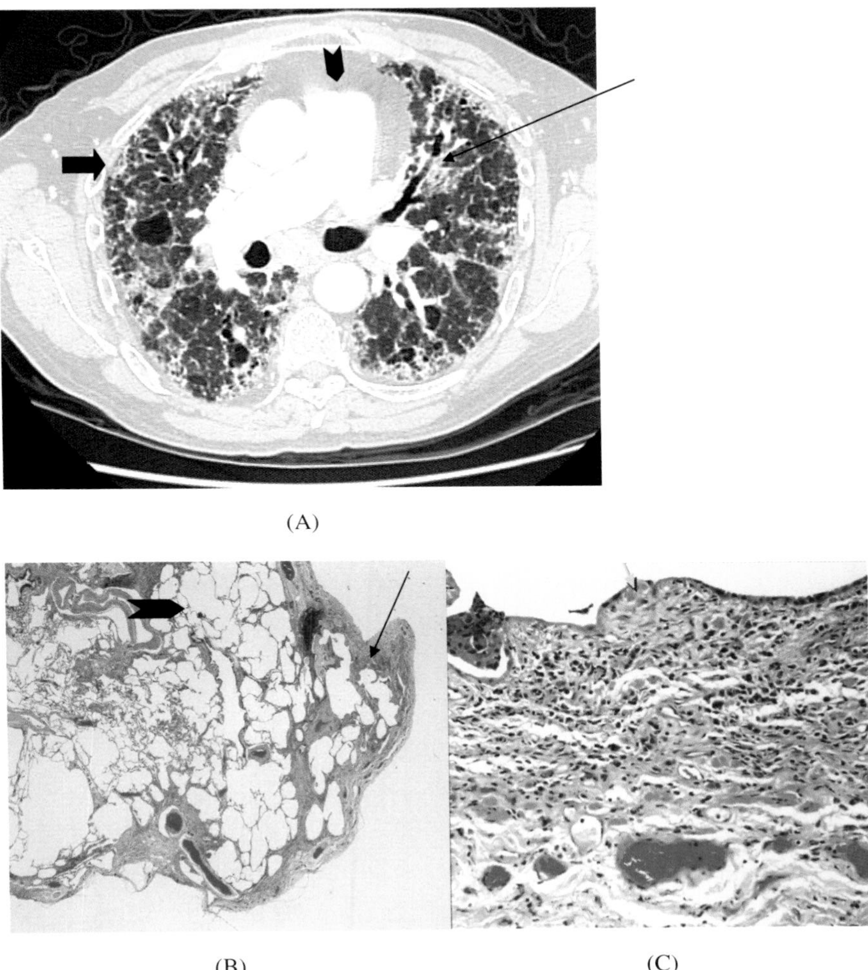

Fig. 6. Idiopathic Pulmonary Fibrosis (IPF). A 67-year-old male ex-smoker with IPF. Chest CT typical for advanced IPF/UIP: traction bronchiectasis (thin arrow), peripheral honeycombing (thick arrow), and subreticular lines, enlarged pulmonary artery suggestive of pulmonary hypertension (arrowhead). (B, C): Typical histopathology changes in IPF/UIP include heterogeneous appearance of lung tissue with alternating areas of normal lung (arrow head), honeycombing (black arrow) interstitial inflammation, and fibroblast foci (yellow arrow). (Pathology courtesy of Kevin Leslie, MD.)

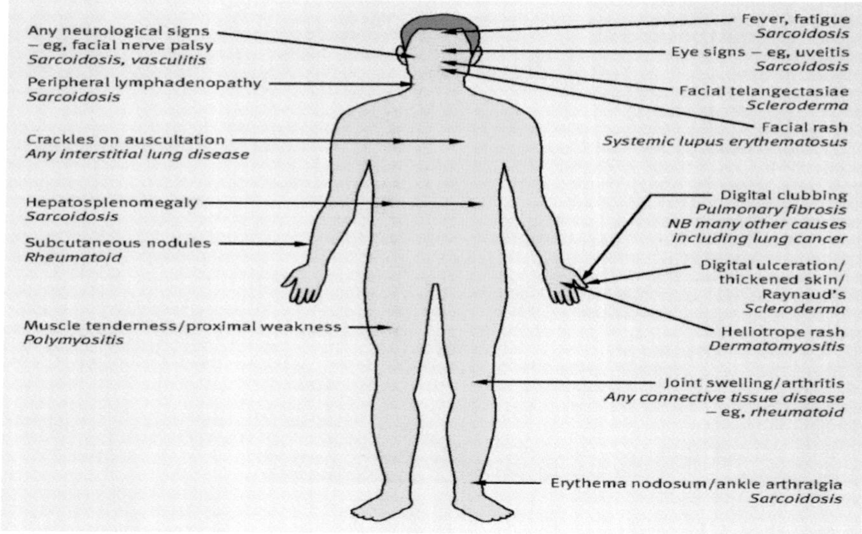

Fig. 7. Possible clinical manifestations of interstitial lung disease (borrowed from Dempsey *et al.*).

disease, or pulmonary artery enlargement can be helpful in the radiographic identification of different DPLDs.

HRCT also helps determine the need for a surgical lung biopsy (see Fig. 8). After known causes of DPLDs are ruled out, an HRCT that strongly suggests IPF does not necessarily require a lung biopsy in the right clinical context.

Pulmonary Function Testing, Echocardiography, Laboratory Data and Ancillary Testing

Baseline pulmonary function tests must be performed in DPLD to evaluate the presence of obstructive and restrictive dysfunction, and repeated to follow effects of therapeutic interventions. Spirometry with pre- and post-bronchodilator testing, lung volumes, and diffusion capacity (DLCO) should be specifically requested. A very low DLCO is generally a sign

Table 4. Terminology Frequently Used in Chest CT Radiology[28]

Consolidation	An increase in lung density that obscures underlying vessels. This indicates alveolar collapse or replacement of alveolar air with fluid or cells. Air bronchograms can be seen amidst the consolidated lung.
Ground glass	A hazy increase in lung density that does not obscure underlying vessels and is nonspecific. This can represent partial collapse or partial filling of alveoli, interstitial inflammation, increased capillary blood volume, or a combination of these. It can be nodular, focal/patchy, or diffuse.
Mosaic perfusion	Geographic differences in lung attenuation associated with air trapping or oligemia. This is not to be confused with ground glass opacity.
Traction bronchiectasis	Bronchial dilatation and bronchial irregularity in patients with pulmonary fibrosis. The traction of fibrotic lung tissue pulls on the bronchial walls.
Bronchiectasis	Bronchial dilatation. This is defined as a bronchial diameter greater than the diameter of the neighboring pulmonary arterial branch.
Interlobular septal thickening	Abnormal thickening of interlobular septae, surrounding the secondary pulmonary lobule with fibrosis, edema, or cell infiltration.
Intralobular septal thickening or intralobular lines	Fine, meshlike reticulation within the secondary pulmonary lobule. This can be an early sign of fibrosis or lung infiltration.
Macrocysts	Cysts greater than 1 cm.
Microcysts	Cysts less than 1 cm.
Honeycombing (Fig. 6A)	Cystic airspaces with clearly defined fibrous walls. This results from, or is associated with, pulmonary fibrosis and loss of lung architecture.
Subpleural lines / reticulation	Thin opacity close to the pleural surface, usually paralleling the pleurae. This can represent atelectasis or fibrosis in the nondependent lung.

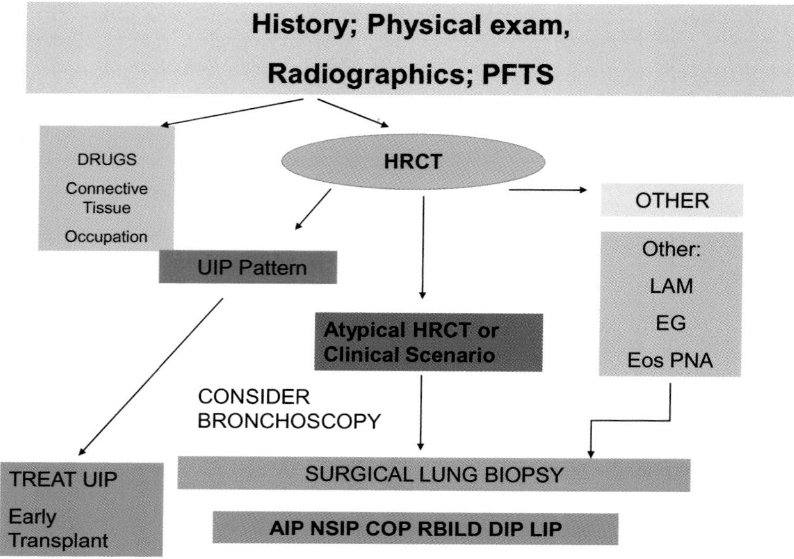

Fig. 8. Role of HRCT in the diagnostic process.

that the patient should be evaluated for oxygen supplementation therapy both at rest and on exertion. The 6 min walk test (6MWT) is helpful in assessing function and need for supplemental oxygen. Changes in the distance walked in 6 min and the degree of oxygen desaturation during 6MWT add prognostic information.[29]

An echocardiogram can help determine the presence of pulmonary hypertension and other concomitant cardiac factors that can contribute to respiratory symptoms. Right heart catheterization may be required, because echocardiography is not a sensitive or specific modality for detecting pulmonary hypertension.[30] This information is also important for aiding in a clinician's decision to refer a patient with DPLD for lung transplantation.[25]

Laboratory data and other ancillary testing should be obtained based on clinical and radiographic suspicion of disease (see Table 2).

Surgical Lung Biopsy

Transbronchial biopsies by bronchoscopy have a limited role in the histologic diagnosis of patients with DPLDs with the exception of sarcoidosis, hypersensitivity pneumonitis, LCH, and lymphangitic carcinomatosis. This is because the small amount of tissue obtained is generally insufficient for detecting the architecturally distinct histologic patterns of DPLDs. For example, transbronchial biopsies were able to detect UIP changes in only 9.3% of patients who went on to have confirmatory surgical lung biopsy (SLB).[31]

Although it is generally recommended that all patients with diffuse lung diseases of unknown cause that do not meet criteria for IPF be referred for SLBs, these are not uniformly performed due to fear of postoperative worsening of respiratory disease, and complications such as bronchopleural fistulas, hemothorax, infection, cardiovascular events, and even death (30-day risk 5%–7%).[32,33] Preoperative risk factors for postoperative death and complications include a diagnosis of UIP, mechanical ventilation prior to the operation, and the presence of an immunocompromised state. Preoperative lung physiology, unfortunately, does not help predict which patients are at higher risk for postoperative complications.[32,33] These risks have to be weighed against the benefits of SLB. After SLB, 40%–73% of cases result in a change in the clinical diagnosis.[32,33]

It is recommended that at least two areas in separate lobes of one lung with varying amounts of damage (area of unaffected and affected lung tissue) be sampled during SLB.

Management of DPLD

Management of DPLDs is disease-specific and generally requires the consultation of specialists familiar with these entities.

For the hospitalist, it is important to note that the mainstay of medical treatment for DPLDs is immunomodulatory agents that have significant side effects (e.g. leukopenia, hematuria, hyperglycemia, liver dysfunction, accelerated atherosclerosis/CAD, and increased risk of certain cancers) and can predispose the patient to atypical infections. Rheumatologic flares in CTD–ILD and sarcoidosis are also fairly common and should be treated appropriately.

Patients with DPLDs commonly present with decompensated cardiopulmonary symptoms. A CT angiogram of the chest may be helpful in ruling out pulmonary embolism in immobile patients and in determining if changes in the lung parenchyma represent infection, heart failure, or worsening of underlying lung disease. An infectious workup often requires early bronchoscopy for prompt diagnosis and treatment of atypical lung infections due to poor functional reserve in this population. Appropriate noninvasive testing for typical viral diseases and bacterial pneumonias (viral washings, sputum cultures, legionella urine antigen, mycoplasma studies, and blood cultures) should always be pursued prior to bronchoscopy. It should also be recognized that any extrapulmonary stressor can increase cardiopulmonary demands and be mistaken as a primary cardiopulmonary insult (e.g. urosepsis, pancreatitis).

IPF patients can present with an "acute IPF exacerbation." Proposed diagnostic criteria for acute exacerbation include subjective worsening of breathing over 30 days or less, new bilateral radiographic opacities, and the absence of infection or another identifiable etiology for respiratory decline.[24,26] This is a diagnosis of exclusion which may require extensive testing to rule out other etiologies.[24] Acute IPF exacerbations are associated with increased inpatient mortality, which can possibly be reduced with the use of early anticoagulation and possibly increased immunosuppression.[26] Similar exacerbations are described less commonly but can also be seen in other DPLDs. IPF patients should be promptly referred for lung transplantation due the high mortality associated with this disease.[25]

References

1. American Thoracic Society / European Respiratory Society International Multidisciplinary Consensus Classification of the Idiopathic Interstitial Pneumonias. (2002) *Am J Respir Crit Care Med* **165**(2): 277–304.

2. American Thoracic Society. (2000) Idiopathic pulmonary fibrosis: Diagnosis and treatment. International consensus statement. American Thoracic Society (ATS) and European Respiratory Society (ERS). *Am J Respir Crit Care Med* **161**(2 Pt 1): 646–664.
3. Dempsey OJ, Kerr KM, Remmen H, Denison AR. (2010) How to investigate a patient with suspected interstitial lung disease. *Br Med J* **340**: c2843.
4. Anderson HA, Lilis R, Daum SM, Selikoff IJ. (1979) Asbestosis among household contacts of asbestos factory workers. *Ann NY Acad Sci* **330**: 387–399.
5. Girard M, Cormier Y. (2010) Hypersensitivity pneumonitis. *Curr Opin Allergy Clin Immunol* **10**(2): 99–103.
6. Schwarz M, King, T. (2003) *Interstitial Lung Disease* 4th ed. BC Decker, London.
7. Castelino FV, Goldberg H, Dellaripa PF. (2010) The impact of rheumatological evaluation in the management of patients with interstitial lung disease. *Rheumatology* (Oxford) (Aug 4).
8. Franquet T. (2001) High-resolution CT of lung disease related to collagen vascular disease. *Radiol Clin North Am* **39**(6): 1171–1187.
9. Devaraj A, Wells AU, Hansell DM. (2007) Computed tomographic imaging in connective tissue diseases. *Semin Respir Crit Care Med* **28**(4): 389–397.
10. Liao KP, Batra KL, Chibnik L, *et al.* (2008) Anti-cyclic citrullinated peptide revised criteria for the classification of rheumatoid arthritis. *Ann Rheum Dis* **67**(11): 1557–1561.
11. LeRoy EC, Medsger TA Jr. (2001) Criteria for the classification of early systemic sclerosis. *J Rheumatol* **28**(7): 1573–1576.
12. Hachulla E, Launay D. (2010) Diagnosis and classification of systemic sclerosis. *Clin Rev Allergy Immunol* (Feb. 10).
13. Vitali C, Bombardieri S, Jonsson R, *et al.* European Study Group on Classification Criteria for Sjögren's Syndrome. (2002) Classification criteria for Sjögren's syndrome: A revised version of the European criteria proposed by the American–European Consensus Group. *Ann Rheum Dis* **61**(6): 554–558.

14. Petri M. (2005) Review of classification criteria for systemic lupus erythematosus. *Rheum Dis Clin North Am* **31**(2): 245–254, vi.
15. D'Cruz DP, Khamashta MA, Hughes GR. (2007) Systemic lupus erythematosus. *Lancet* **369**(9561): 587–596.
16. Dalakas MC. (1991) Polymyositis, dermatomyositis and inclusion-body myositis. *N Engl J Med* **325**(21): 1487–1498.
17. Mastaglia FL, Phillips BA. (2007) Idiopathic inflammatory myopathies: epidemiology, classification, and diagnostic criteria. *Rheum Dis Clin North Am* **28**(4): 723–741.
18. Iannuzzi MC, Rybicki BA, Teirstein AS. (2007) Sarcoidosis. *N Engl J Med* **357**(21): 2153–2165.
19. McCormack FX. (2008) Lymphangioleiomyomatosis: A clinical update. *Chest* **133**(2): 507–516.
20. Johnson SR. (2006) Lymphangioleiomyomatosis. *Eur Respir J* **27**(5): 1056–1065.
21. Allen TC. (2008) Pulmonary Langerhans cell histiocytosis and other pulmonary histiocytic diseases: A review. *Arch Pathol Lab Med* **132**(7): 1171–1181.
22. Kinder BW, Shariat C, Collard HR, *et al.* (2010) Undifferentiated connective tissue disease–associated interstitial lung disease: Changes in lung function. *Lung* **188**(2): 143–149.
23. Kinder BW, Collard HR, Koth L, *et al.* (2007) Idiopathic nonspecific interstitial pneumonia: Lung manifestation of undifferentiated connective tissue disease? *Am J Respir Crit Care Med* **176**(7): 691–697.
24. Hunninghake GW, Zimmerman MB, Schwartz DA, *et al.* (2001) Utility of a lung biopsy for the diagnosis of idiopathic pulmonary fibrosis. *Am J Respir Crit Care Med* **164**(2): 193–196.
25. Collard HR, Moore BB, Flaherty KR, *et al.* Idiopathic Pulmonary Fibrosis Clinical Research Network Investigators. (2007) Acute exacerbations of idiopathic pulmonary fibrosis. *Am J Respir Crit Care Med* **176**(7): 636–643.
26. Orens JB, Estenne M, Arcasoy S, *et al.* Pulmonary Scientific Council of the International Society for Heart and Lung Transplantation. (2006) International guidelines for the selection of lung transplant

candidates: 2006 update — a consensus report from the Pulmonary Scientific Council of the International Society for Heart and Lung Transplantation. *J Heart Lung Transplant.* **25**(7): 745–755.

27. Kubo H, Nakayama K, Yanai M, *et al.* (2005) Anticoagulant therapy for idiopathic pulmonary fibrosis. *Chest* **128**(3): 1475–1482
28. Argiriadi PA, Mendelson DS. (2009) High resolution computed tomography in idiopathic interstitial pneumonias. *Mt Sinai J Med* **76**(1): 37–52.
29. Flaherty KR, Andrei AC, Murray S, *et al.* (2006) Idiopathic pulmonary fibrosis: Prognostic value of changes in physiology and six-minute-walk test. *Am J Respir Crit Care Med* **174**(7): 803–809.
30. Fisher MR, Forfia PR, Chamera E, *et al.* (2009) Accuracy of Doppler echocardiography in the hemodynamic assessment of pulmonary hypertension. *Am J Respir Crit Care Med* **179**(7): 615–621.
31. Shim HS, Park MS, Park IK. (2010) Histopathologic findings of transbronchial biopsy in usual interstitial pneumonia. *Pathol Int* **60**(5): 373–377.
32. Lettieri CJ, Veerappan GR, Helman DL, *et al.* (2005) Outcomes and safety of surgical lung biopsy for interstitial lung disease. *Chest* **127**(5): 1600–1605.
33. Sigurdsson MI, Isaksson HJ, Gudmundsson G, Gudbjartsson T. (2009) Diagnostic surgical lung biopsies for suspected interstitial lung diseases: A retrospective study. *Ann Thorac Surg* **88**(1): 227–232.

Chapter 30

Pulmonary Hypertension

*Ajith P. Nair**

Key Pearls

- Pulmonary hypertension (PH) is defined by a mean pulmonary artery (mPA) pressure greater than 25 mmHg. Pulmonary arterial hypertension (PAH) is specified by a mPA >25 mmHg, pulmonary capillary wedge pressure <15 mmHg and pulmonary vascular resistance greater than 3 Woods Units.
- PH can be divided into five categories.
- Echocardiography and right heart catheterization with vasoreactivity testing are mandatory for the evaluation of PAH.
- PAH requires further investigation and specific therapy. PH from left-sided heart disease or lung disease requires treatment of the underlying disorder.
- Standard therapy for PAH includes diuretics, digoxin, anticoagulation, and supplemental oxygen. Calcium channel blockers are appropriate for patients who demonstrate vasoreactivity. Targeted therapy includes endothelin receptor antagonists, prostacyclin analogues and phosphodiesterase inhibitors.

Introduction

Pulmonary hypertension is characterized by increased resistance across the pulmonary circulation, which can lead to right ventricular (RV) failure

*Mount Sinai School of Medicine, New York, NY, USA.

through increased afterload. The pulmonary vascular abnormalities can result from a number of disorders, including cardiac, pulmonary or collagen vascular disease. Most hospitalized patients will have pulmonary hypertension secondary to left-sided heart disease (heart failure with preserved or abnormal systolic function). Further investigation is warranted for pulmonary hypertension that is due to pulmonary vascular disease or pulmonary arterial hypertension.

Definition

Pulmonary hypertension (PH) can be generally defined as an elevation in systolic pulmonary pressures greater than 35 mmHg or mean pulmonary artery pressures greater than 25 mmHg.[1] The disease can be pre-capillary, post-capillary or due to high cardiac output. Post-capillary pulmonary hypertension results from pulmonary venous congestion, which may result from left ventricular dysfunction or mitral valve disease. *Pulmonary arterial hypertension* (PAH) results from pre-capillary disease and is defined by a pulmonary arterial pressure >25 mmHg, a pulmonary capillary wedge pressure of <15 mmHg and pulmonary vascular resistance (PVR) of greater than 3 Woods Units.

The term *cor pulmonale* is used when pulmonary hypertension and cardiac dysfunction result from lung disease (e.g. chronic obstructive lung disease, connective tissues disease, and interstitial lung disease). *Eisenmenger's syndrome* occurs when right to left shunts associated with congenital heart disease reverse due to increasing pulmonary pressures.

Classification

Pulmonary hypertension can be acute or chronic, and the acute form usually results from pulmonary thromboembolic disease. The chronic forms of pulmonary hypertension can divided into five major categories (see Table. 1).[2]

Group I pulmonary arterial hypertension is characterized by disease of the small pulmonary arteries. Included are idiopathic pulmonary arterial hypertension (IPAH), which was formerly termed primary pulmonary

Table 1. Classification of Pulmonary Hypertension (Dana Point Clinical Classification of PH, 2008)

Group 1	Pulmonary Arterial Hypertension • Idiopathic PAH ("primary pulmonary hypertension") • Heritable pulmonary arterial hypertension (HPAH): BMPR2, ALK1, endoglin • Drug- and toxin-induced • Associated pulmonary arterial hypertension (APAH): Connective tissue diseases, HIV infection, Portal hypertension • Congenital heart disease • Schistosomiasis • Chronic hemolytic anemia • Persistent pulmonary hypertension of the newborn
Group 2	Left-sided Heart Disease • Systolic dysfunction • Diastolic dysfunction • Valvular disease
Group 3	Lung Disease or Hypoxemia • Chronic obstructive pulmonary disease • Interstitial lung disease • Other pulmonary diseases with mixed restrictive and obstructive pattern • Sleep-disordered breathing • Alveolar hypoventilation disorders • Chronic exposure to high altitude • Developmental abnormalities
Group 4	Chronic thrombotic and/or embolic disease
Group 5	Miscellaneous • Hematologic disorders: myeloproliferative disorders, splenectomy • Systemic disorders: sarcoidosis, pulmonary Langerhans cell • Metabolic disorders: glycogen storage disease, Gaucher disease, thyroid disorders • Others: tumoral obstruction, fibrosing mediastinitis, chronic renal failure on dialysis

hypertension; associated pulmonary arterial hypertension (APAH) from collagen vascular diseases; HIV; and portopulmonary hypertension; and heritable pulmonary arterial hypertension (HPAH). Mutations in bone morphogenetic protein receptor type 2 (BMPR2) have been identified as the primary cause of heritable PAH (HPAH). Drugs, including appetite suppressants containing aminorex, dexfenfluramine and fenfluramine, have been associated with an increased risk of PAH.

Secondary pulmonary hypertension usually results from cardiac or respiratory diseases. Increases in pulmonary blood flow through shunts or high output (e.g. dialysis fistulas or hepatic failure) or through venous congestion can lead to elevated pulmonary pressures. Lung disease can result in hypoxic vasoconstriction and the loss of pulmonary vasculature due to fibrosis. Pulmonary pressures can increase "out of proportion" to the degree of left-heart failure or lung disease, which may be due to intimal proliferation and increases in PVR.

Chronic thromboembolic pulmonary hypertension (CTEPH) is important to exclude as a cause of pulmonary hypertension as it can be potentially cured via thromboendarterectomy. Ventilation-perfusion scan has been shown to be a more sensitive test for detection of CTEPH than CT angiography. Embolic occlusion of the pulmonary vascular bed may also result from tumor metastases, schistosomiasis, filariasis, or talc or fiber embolism from intravenous drug use.

Clinical Presentation

The presentation of pulmonary hypertension is similar despite the multiple different etiologies of the disease. Dyspnea, fatigue, edema and exertional syncope are classic symptoms. RV ischemia may lead to angina. Patients with collagen vascular disease commonly have concomitant Raynaud's disease.

Physical examination findings include an increased intensity of the P2 component of the second heart sound, a right ventricular heave, a right-sided fourth sound, and murmurs of tricuspid and pulmonic valve regurgitation.

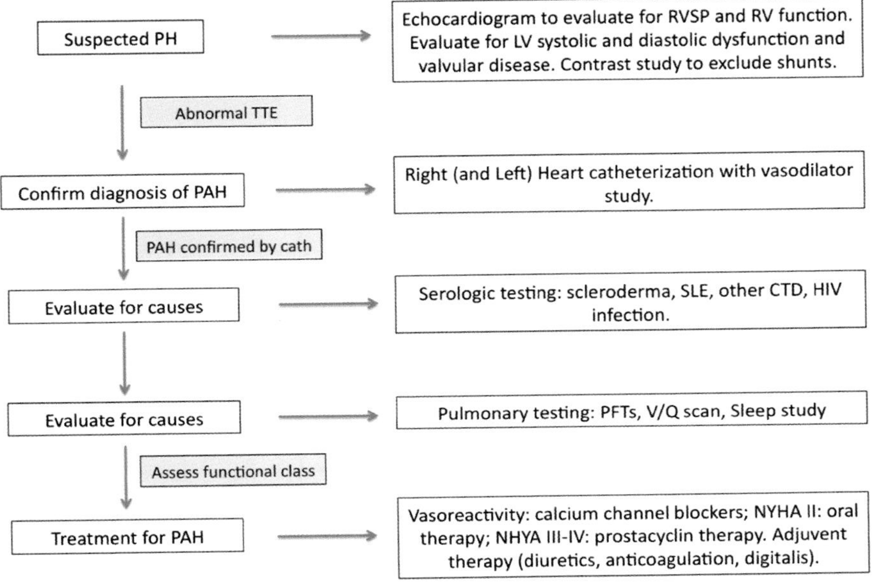

Fig. 1. Evaluation of suspected PH.

Distension of the jugular veins, a pulsatile liver, ascites, and peripheral edema usually indicate advanced right-sided failure.

Findings on chest radiograph are enlargement of the pulmonary trunk and hilar vessels and right-heart enlargement. The electrocardiogram may demonstrate right axis deviation, T wave inversions in the anterior precordial leads, right atrial enlargement, and RV hypertrophy.

Evaluation (see Fig. 1)

Echocardiography is essential to the diagnosis of pulmonary hypertension. The RV systolic pressure can be estimated via Doppler. It is important, however, to distinguish between PAH and PH from left-sided disease. Isolated RV enlargement and dysfunction and right atrial enlargement with normal LV function can be key indicators of PAH. Diastolic and systolic bowing of the septum are significant for RV volume and pressure overload, respectively.

The right-heart catheterization is the gold standard for the diagnosis of pulmonary hypertension. Catheterization is necessary to accurately measure the right atrial, right ventricular, and pulmonary arterial pressures, PVR and cardiac output. Diastolic dysfunction can be excluded through a normal wedge pressure or a left ventricular end diastolic pressure.

Once the diagnosis of pulmonary hypertension has been established, it is important to identify secondary causes of pulmonary hypertension that may be treatable. Ventilation-perfusion scanning is useful in excluding chronic thromboembolic disease. Pulmonary function testing with diffusion capacity can exclude restrictive or obstructive lung disease. Decreased diffusion capacity is an early marker of PAH and declines with worsening disease. Polysomnography is frequently performed as an outpatient to exclude obstructive sleep apnea. Laboratory testing includes work-up for scleroderma (anti-Scl-70, anti-centromere), systemic lupus erythematosus (ANA), rheumatoid arthritis (RF, anti-CCP), HIV infection and hepatitis. If indicated, further evaluation for hypercoaguable states or interstitial lung disease should be performed. Brain natriueretic peptide can be elevated with RV dysfunction and may be used to monitor disease progression.

Medical Treatment

General therapy to be considered for the pulmonary hypertension includes diuretics, cardiac glycosides, supplemental oxygen and anticoagulation.

Oral anticoagulation has been shown in a retrospective study by Fuster and colleagues to improve mortality in patients with idiopathic pulmonary arterial hypertension.[4] The target INR in these patients is 1.5 to 2.5 although patients with hypercoaguable states and chronic thromboembolic disease should be maintained at higher INRs (2.5 to 3.5).

Digitalis is commonly administered to patients who have evidence of RV dysfunction. Diuretics should be used in patients who exhibit clinical signs of right-heart failure. Excessive diuresis should be avoided as it can diminish cardiac output due to reduced preload. Patients who are grossly volume overloaded and have renal dysfunction should be considered for short-term ionotropic therapy (dobutamine, dopamine or milrinone). Supplemental oxygen is appropriate for patients with resting or exertional hypoxemia.

Calcium channel blockers (CCBs) are indicated for patients who demonstrate acute vasoreactivity. Less than 10% of patients with IPAH will be acute responders, however. Nifedipine, amlodipine and diltiazem are the preferred calcium channel blockers and should be titrated to the maximum tolerated doses. Calcium channel blockers should not be used empirically and only 50% of patients who are vasoreactive will be long-term responders to CCBs.

Targeted therapy for pulmonary hypertension includes prostacylcins, endothelin receptor antagonists and phosphodiesterase inhibitors.[5] These agents should be used after consultation with a pulmonary hypertension specialist. Prostacyclins used for PH include epoprostenol, treprostinil, and iloprost. Patients who have NYHA Class III to IV symptoms and significant right ventricular dysfunction with compromised cardiac outputs should be considered for epoprostenol. Epoprostenol (Flolan) is administered as a continuous infusion and acts as a pulmonary vasodilator. Additionally, it inhibits platelet aggregation, is an antiproliferative and acts as a cardiac iontrope.[6] It has a short half-life (6 minutes) and abrupt discontinuation may lead to rebound pulmonary hypertension and acute right ventricular failure. Treprostinil, which is a prostacyclin analogue with a longer half-life (240 minutes), may be administered as a continuous intravenous or subcutaneous infusion or as an inhaled therapy. Iloprost is an aerosolized prostacyclin that is administered six to nine times a day.

Endothelin promotes vasoconstriction and abnormal proliferation in pulmonary hypertension. The endothelin antagonists include bosentan, ambrisentan and sitaxsentan. The first two medications are approved for use in the US and differ in their specificity for endothelin receptors ETa and ETb. Bosentan, a non-selective agent, is administered twice daily and has been shown to reduced mortality and morbidity.[7] It has up to a 10% risk of hepatic dysfunction and monthly liver function tests are required. Ambrisentan, which has increased specificity for ETa, produces less hepatotoxicity although it can cause peripheral edema.[8]

Phosphodiesterase-5 (PDE-5) inhibitors enhance nitric oxide activity. Nitric oxide produces pulmonary vasodilatation, and PDE-5 inhibitors can produce selective pulmonary vasodilatation without significant systemic effects. Sildenafil (three times daily) and tadalafil (once daily) are approved for use in pulmonary hypertension.[9,10]

Combination therapies have been studied and should be considered for patients with severe pulmonary hypertension and right ventricular dysfunction who do not respond to monotherapy.

Surgical Treatment

For patients who are refractory to medical therapy, atrial septostomy and heart-lung or lung transplant should be considered. Atrial septostomy allows for decompression of the right ventricle and should be considered as a palliative measure or as a bridge to transplant. Ultimately, patients failing medical therapy should be referred for single- or double-lung transplant.

Prognosis

Left untreated, the median survival for pulmonary arterial hypertension is 2.8 years. Therapy for pulmonary hypertension can significantly alter the overall mortality and morbidity. Lung transplantation offers a five-year survival of 45–55%, and the rates of transplantation for PH have declined since the advent of PH-specific therapy.[11]

References

1. McLaughlin VV, Archer SL, Badesch DB, *et al.* (2009) ACCF/AHA 2009 expert consensus document on pulmonary hypertension a report of the American College of Cardiology Foundation Task Force on Expert Consensus Documents and the American Heart Association developed in collaboration with the American College of Chest Physicians; American Thoracic Society, Inc.; and the Pulmonary Hypertension Association. *J Am Coll Cardiol* **53**(17): 1573–619.

2. Simonneau G, Robbins IM, Beghetti M, *et al.* (2009) Updated clinical classification of pulmonary hypertension. *J Am Coll Cardiol* **54**(1 Suppl): S43–54.
3. Rich S, Brundage BH and Levy PS. (1985) The effect of vasodilator therapy on the clinical outcome of patients with primary pulmonary hypertension. *Circulation* **71**(6): 1191–6.
4. Fuster V, Steele PM, Edwards WD, *et al.* (1984) Primary pulmonary hypertension: Natural history and the importance of thrombosis. *Circulation* **70**(4): 580–7.
5. Barst RJ, Gibbs JS, Ghofrani HA, *et al.* (2009) Updated evidence-based treatment algorithm in pulmonary arterial hypertension. *J Am Coll Cardiol* **54**(1 Suppl): S78–84.
6. Barst RJ, Rubin LJ, Long WA, *et al.* (1996) A comparison of continuous intravenous epoprostenol (prostacyclin) with conventional therapy for primary pulmonary hypertension. The Primary Pulmonary Hypertension Study Group. *New Engl J Med* **334**(5): 296–302.
7. Rubin LJ, Badesch DB, Barst RJ, *et al.* (2002) Bosentan therapy for pulmonary arterial hypertension. *New Engl J Med* **346**(12): 896–903.
8. Galie N, Olschewski H, Oudiz RJ, *et al.* (2008) Ambrisentan for the treatment of pulmonary arterial hypertension: Results of the ambrisentan in pulmonary arterial hypertension, randomized, double-blind, placebo-controlled, multicenter, efficacy (ARIES) study 1 and 2. *Circulation* **117**(23): 3010–9.
9. Galie N, Ghofrani HA, Torbicki A, *et al.* (2005) Sildenafil citrate therapy for pulmonary arterial hypertension. *New Engl J Med* **353**(20): 2148–57.
10. Galie N, Brundage BH, Ghofrani HA, *et al.* (2009) Tadalafil therapy for pulmonary arterial hypertension. *Circulation* **119**(22): 2894–903.
11. Benza RL, Miller DP, Gomberg-Maitland M, *et al.* (xxxx) Predicting survival in pulmonary arterial hypertension: Insights from the Registry to Evaluate Early and Long-Term Pulmonary Arterial Hypertension Disease Management (REVEAL). *Circulation* **122**(2): 164–72.

Critical Care

Chapter 31

Sepsis: Manifestations and Management of the Host/ Pathogen Response

*Thomas H. Kalb**

Key Pearls

- Effective intervention in sepsis requires an integrated effort that includes early recognition, immediate fluids, appropriate antibiotics, source control, adequate monitoring of resuscitation end points, and supportive measures for multiple organ dysfunction.
- The adoption of a bundled management plan is associated with significantly improved survival.
- Every hour of delay in administration of appropriate antibiotics is associated with increased mortality in severe sepsis. Never withhold antibiotics in sepsis if signs of hypoperfusion are present.
- Source control is a time-sensitive, important component of early intervention.
- Shock in sepsis is multifactorial, and requires addressing preload deficits, evaluation of cardiac function with support of forward flow, and addressing defects in vasomotor tone.

* Feinstein Institute, Hofstra School of Medicine, NY, USA.

Introduction

Sepsis is the systemic response to infection. Severe sepsis and sepsis with shock reflect progressively life-threatening conditions that result from pathogen–host interaction. The incidence of sepsis is rising, with over 200,000 attributable deaths each year in North America. Early recognition and early initiation of therapeutic measures are key to successful management. This chapter outlines the basics of understanding what sepsis is and provides a brief evidence-based outline for initiating treatment and management skills including outcome analysis. Clinical controversies and opportunities for novel therapy are addressed.

Definitions, Pathophysiology, and Epidemiology

What Is SIRS/Sepsis/Severe Sepsis/ Sepsis with Shock

Sepsis is clinically defined as SIRS with a suspected or documented infection. SIRS (systemic inflammatory response syndrome) is a set of clinical features associated with systemic inflammation and innate immune activation.[1] Many patients who manifest SIRS criteria do not have an infectious etiology. For example, SIRS criteria are often met by patients with trauma or noninfectious inflammation such as pancreatitis.

The accepted consensus definitions for SIRS, sepsis, severe sepsis, and sepsis with shock (Table 1A) stem from consensus conference criteria.[1] More than 30% of patients meeting all four SIRS criteria at presentation progress to sepsis with shock. Signs of hypoperfusion and tissue dysoxia are the critical defining features of severe sepsis and sepsis with shock. Such clinical diagnostic schemes are required because there are no clinically validated biomarkers that substitute for or perform better than clinical markers of sepsis.

Mortality rises precipitously to the 30%–50% range in patients with suspected infection who manifest signs of severe sepsis and sepsis with shock.

Sepsis detection incidence is roughly equally divided between ED and hospitalized patients. Pneumonia is the most prevalent site of infection

Table 1A. SIRS and Sepsis Consensus Criteria[1]

SIRS:
Temperature (core temperature) >38.3°C or <36°C
Heart rate >90 beats/min
Respiratory rate >30 breaths/min
White cell count >12,000 cells/mm^3 or <4000 cells/mm^3
Sepsis = SIRS with suspected or documented infection
Severe sepsis = sepsis-associated organ dysfunction*
u/o <20 mL/hr;
Lactate >2.5,
SOFA score >4,
or hypotension
Septic shock = hypotension despite adequate fluid resuscitation (at least 20 mL/kg)
MAP<60
SBP <90 mmHg
SBP drop >40 mmHg from baseline

identified, followed by UTI, abdominal source, catheter related and others. Hundreds of mediators are known to be involved with the sepsis cascade.

Outcome is linked not only to the severity of sepsis, but also to the burden of comorbidities, and the timely introduction of effective therapy. Ultimately, outcome in sepsis is closely correlated with multiorgan failure. Multiple organ dysfunction syndrome (MODS) accounts for the diffuse organ involvement in sepsis. Cardiovascular dysfunction is most prominent at presentation, followed by pulmonary, renal, hematologic and hepatic, as well as metabolic and hypothalamic/pituitary derangements (see Table 1B for organ dysfunction consensus criteria).

What Causes Sepsis

Sepsis has been shown to result from pathogen associated molecular patterns (PAMPs) which bind and signal through pathogen response receptors.[2] For example, gram-negative bacterial lipopolysaccharide is recognized by TLR-4, which is expressed widely on innate immune effectors as well as many nonimmune cell types, such as endothelial

Table 1B. Diagnostic Criteria for Sepsis-Associated Organ Dysfunction Criteria Excerpted from 2001 International Sepsis Definitions Conference[1]

General parameters:
Altered mental status
Significant edema or positive fluid balance (>20 mL/kg over 24 hr)
Hyperglycemia (plasma glucose >110 mg/dL) in the absence of diabetes

Inflammatory parameters:
Normal white blood cell count with >10% immature forms
Plasma C-reactive protein >2 SD above the normal value

Hemodynamic parameters:
Arterial hypotension (systolic blood pressure <90 mmHg, mean arterial pressure <70, or a systolic blood pressure decrease >40 mmHg)
Mixed venous oxygen saturation >70%
Cardiac index >3.5l $min^{-1}m^2$

Organ dysfunction parameters:
Arterial hypoxemia (PaO_2/FIO_2 <300)
Acute oliguria (urine output <0.5 mL kg^{-1} h^{-1})
Creatinine increase >0.5 mg/dl
Coagulation abnormalities (INR > 1.5 or APTT >60 s)
Ileus (absent bowel sounds)
Thrombocytopenia (platelet count <100,000 uL)
Hyperbilirubinemia (plasma total bilirubin >4 mg/dL)

Tissue perfusion parameters:
Hyperlactatemia (>3 mmol/L)
Decreased capillary refill or mottling

cells. Cellular necrosis and damage associated molecular patterns (DAMPs) may also be recognized and result in amplification or may substitute for PAMP response, in part explaining the similar mediator profile in noninfectious etiologies of SIRS.

TLR-4 signaling results in a rapid transcriptional response through NF-κB and other transcription factors. NF-κ B activation triggers a cascade of mediators, including TNF-alpha. Experimentally, TNF-alpha infusion recapitulates all the lethal features of sepsis. Downstream from TNF-alpha, endotoxin related signaling involves hundreds of interrelated mediators.

The signaling through TLRs is rapid, complex, and involves multiple interwoven pathways for inflammation, metabolic pathways, and prothrombotic pathways. The clinical observation that inflammation triggers thrombogenicity has been understood within the context of an evolutionary connection between trauma and infection, wherein survival depends upon simultaneous hemostasis, restoration of immune barriers, and pathogen elimination.[3]

Adequate host defense against bacterial and nonbacterial pathogens is necessary for survival, and yet excess, systemic, dysregulated, or prolonged stimulation may result in the organ dysfunction that is seen in sepsis. Endotoxin induces its own counterregulation. Reflecting the complex nature of cellular response to pathogen, patients with sepsis manifest aspects of both proinflammatory and counterregulatory or compensatory anti-inflammatory responses.

One way to think about cellular response to pathogens in sepsis is to consider the endothelium a global "organ of injury," in that vessel injury and dysfunction contribute to gas exchange disturbance, hypotension, microcirculatory disturbance, mitochondrial decoupling, and diffuse organ damage. Thus, endothelial injury results in a disturbance in the pathway for oxygen uptake, delivery, and consumption.

What Causes Shock in Sepsis

Shock is clinically defined as acute hypoperfusion that results in organ dysfunction.

Several peptide and nonpeptide mediators of shock in sepsis have been identified, and early mediators such as TNF-alpha and excess iNOS may be amplified or substituted in their activity by late mediators such as adrenomedullin and HMGB1.

Patients with severe sepsis and shock often have multiple disturbances in perfusion that contribute to overall presentation and impact upon therapeutic decisions. In essence, three physiologic forms of shock comingle in patients with sepsis with shock.

Preload deficit is often the most prominent feature at initial presentation of shock in patients with severe sepsis or sepsis with shock. Venous return is a complex function of circulating blood volume, vasomotor tone, and blood flow distribution.[4] Thus, preload deficiency is not equivalent to hypovolemia, and all patients with signs of hypoperfusion require volume resuscitation irrespective of total body volume status.

Cardiac dysfunction in severe sepsis is estimated to occur early in as many as 25% of patients with severe sepsis and shock manifesting a low cardiac index despite fluid resuscitation. However, even in the absence of low output, many patients with sepsis will have myocyte dysfunction detected by troponin leak and poor contractility often with tachycardia.[5]

Vasodilatory shock with dysfunctional vasorelaxation and maldistribution of blood flow is accompanied by endothelial injury and capillary leak that results in extravascular fluid redistribution, V/Q mismatch, and ultimately in tissue dysoxia and mitochondrial dysfunction.[6] Table 2 outlines the three forms of shock in sepsis, pointing out the monitoring and management principles for intervention based on this physiological underpinning.

What Is the Cause of Microcirculatory Disturbance in Sepsis

Restoration of target levels of perfusion does not necessarily restore microcirculatory disturbance in severe sepsis. Survival is associated with restored microcirculatory flow, and the absence of restored capillary flow is an independent marker of mortality in sepsis.[7] Several pathological processes contribute to capillary dysfunction in sepsis, including increased thrombogenicity, disturbances in adhesiveness, rheology, autonomic tone, and mitochondrial dysfunction.

Sepsis Recognition and Intervention: Principles and Action Plan

Key Recognition Principles and Guidelines

Effective therapy is time-sensitive and requires accurate and early recognition of severe sepsis. The overall concept of early goal-directed

Table 2. Three Physiologic Forms of Shock with Sepsis

Form of Shock	Defining Physiology (gold standard measurement)	Surrogate Clinical Markers (*best clinical utility)	Primary Clinical Treatment	Clinical Comments
Preload shock	Low LVEDV <70 cm^3/m^2 (left ventricular end diastolic volume) determined by biplane contrast echocardiography	CVP <8 Wedge pressure <12 Stroke volume variation (SVV) >13% *IVC inspiratory collapsibility index >18% Passive leg raise Augmented stroke volume >12.5%	Isotonic crystalloid 20—30 mL/kg bolus (over 20 min optimally)	• Preload deficit most prominent form of shock at presentation. • Preload shock does not equal hypovolemia. • Static meausurement of LVEDV >70 does not preclude IVF response. • Wedge no better than CVP and CVP performs poorly to predict fluid responsiveness in sepsis.
Cardiac shock	Low contractility index (sBP/LVESVI) (by Doppler echocardiograpy)	*Low stroke volume <35 mL after volume resuscitation Low cardiac output <2.5 Low ejection fraction <45	Consider additional fluid challenge Consider inotropic support (dobutamine) Consider vasodilator (rarely employed)	• High cardiac output common after volume resuscitation though contractility defect, and troponin leak in up to 25%. • Chronotropy may offset benefit of dobutamine.

(*Continued*)

Table 2. (*Continued*)

Form of Shock	Defining Physiology (gold standard measurement)	Surrogate Clinical Markers (*best clinical utility)	Primary Clinical Treatment	Clinical Comments
Vasodilatory shock	Low peripheral (systemic) vascular resistance (by pulmonary artery catheter)	*MAP <65 mmHg after fluid bolus SBP <90 or 40 decreased from baseline after fluid bolus Poor capillary refill >2 s Mottled appearance	*Norepinephrine: begin at 2.5 mcg/min, increase by 2.5 every 5 min to therapeutic plateau/ maximal 20 mcg/min Dopamine: alternative primary agent Vasopressin: norepinephrine-sparing effect Corticosteroids: (hydrocortisone <300 mg/day) for pressor-dependent sepsis with shock	• Dopamine hampered by excess chronotropy. Vasopressin particularly useful if excess adrenergic chronotropy develops. • Avoid pure alpha adrenergic agents associated with drop in cardiac performance. • Corticosteroid provides pressor-sparing effect. Benefit debated.

therapy (EGDT), defined as a bundled care plan for the initial management of sepsis, has been widely adopted after a seminal publication by Rivers *et al.* from a single center showing impressive mortality benefit, though not all elements of the original description are universally adopted.

Over the ensuing decade, it has become generally agreed that the major advantage of bundled therapy is that a coordinated approach to sepsis improves implementation of therapy and provides a checklist to reduce omissions.[8] The major caveat to universal acceptance of bundled therapy is that the demonstrated benefit cannot be easily distinguished among constituent interventions, leaving open the possibility that some aspects are counterproductive or ineffective.

The core elements of EGDT, accepted by most, is the implementation of a system for early recognition and initiation of fluid resuscitation, antibiotics, and source control. Far more contentious are the debates that remain concerning resuscitation targets, monitoring tools, and adjunctive therapies such as blood product and inotropic therapy.

In the setting of ongoing debate over the implementation of EGDT, consensus statements such as the "Surviving Sepsis Campaign" provide useful guidelines from expert panels that examine and grade evidence, helping to demonstrate the data that support or limit evidence-based practice including EGDT in sepsis (Tables 3 and 4). The reader should be cautiously aware of the substantial debate among critical care experts. The major caveat for expert panel recommendations is that investigator bias and sponsorship may influence the interpretation of weighted evidence.[9]

No therapy bundle can be initiated until the patient is accurately recognized, so that a great deal of attention has recently been placed on sepsis prediction models that may enhance the process by which the early signs are picked up early and improve the "time zero" for EGDT implementation. If validated and automated, such algorithmic approaches raise the prospect of "pre-emptively" intervening with EGDT and may enhance the opportunity for targeted therapy that is active against early mediators of sepsis.[9]

Table 3. Initial Resuscitation and Infection Issues

Strength of recommendation and quality of evidence have been assessed using the GRADE criteria, presented in parentheses after each guideline
• Indicates a strong recommendation, or "we recommend"
○ Indicates a weak recommendation, or "we suggest"

Initial resuscitation (first 6 hours)
- Begin resuscitation immediately in patients with hypotension or elevated serum lactate >4 mmot/L; do not delay pending ICU admission (1C)
- Resuscitation goals (1C) CVP 8–12 mm Hg[a]
  Mean arterial pressure ≥ 65 mm Hg
  Urine output ≥0.5 mL-kg^{-1} hr^{-1}
  Central venous (superior vena cava) oxygen saturation ≥70% or mixed venous ≥65%
  ○ If venous oxygen saturation target is not achieved (2C)
  Consider further fluid
  Transfuse packed red blood cells if required to hematocrit of ≥30% and/or
  Start dobutamine infusion, maximum 20 μg kg^{-1} min^{-1}

Diagnosis
- Obtain appropriate cultures before starting antibiotics provided this does not significantly delay antimicrobial administration (1C)
  Obtain two or more BCs
  One or more BCs should be percutaneous
  One BC from each vascular access device in place >48 hrs
  Culture other sites as clinically indicated
- Perform imaging studies promptly to confirm and sample any source of infection, if safe to do so (1C)

Antibiotic therapy
- Begin intravenous antibiotics as early as possible and always within the first hour of recognizing severe sepsis (1D) and septic shock (1B)
- Broad-spectrum: one or more agents active against likely bacterial/fungal pathogens and with good penetration into presumed source (1B)
- Reassess antimicrobial regimen daily to optimize efficacy, prevent resistance, avoid toxicity, and minimize costs (1C)
  ○ Consider combination therapy in *Pseudomonas* infections (2D)
  ○ Consider combination empiric therapy in neutropenic patients (2D)
  ○ Combination therapy ≤3–5 days and de-escalation following susceptibilities (2D)
- Duration of therapy typically limited to 7–10 days; longer if response is slow or there are undrainable foci of infection or immunologic deficiencies (1D)
- Stop antimicrobial therapy if cause is found to be noninfectious (1D)

(*Continued*)

Table 3. (*Continued*)

Source identification and control

- A specific anatomic site of infection should be established as rapidly as possible (1C) and within first 6 hrs of presentation (1D)
- Formally evaluate patient for a focus of infection amenable to source control measures (e.g. abscess drainage, tissue debridement) (1C)
- Implement source control measures as soon as possible following successful initial resuscitation (1C) (exception: infected pancreatic necrosis, where surgical intervention is best delayed) (2B)
- Choose source control measure with maximum efficacy and minimal physiologic upset (1D)
- Remove intravascular access devices if potentially infected (1C)

GRADE, Grades of Recommendation, Assessment, Development and Evaluation; ICU, intensive care unit; CVP, central venous pressure; BC, blood culture.

[a]A higher target CVP of 12–15 mm Hg is recommended in the presence of mechanical ventilation or pre-existing decreased ventricular compliance.

With permission from Dellinger *et al.* (2008) *Crit Care Med* **36**: 296–327.

Table 4. Hemodynamic Support and Adjunctive Therapy

Strength of recommendation and quality of evidence have been assessed using the GRADE criteria, presented in parentheses after each guideline

- Indicates a strong recommendation, or "we recommend"
- Indicates a weak recommendation, or "we suggest"

Fluid therapy

- Fluid-resuscitate using crystalloids or colloids (1B)
- Target a CVP of ≥8 mm Hg (≥12 mmHg if mechanically ventilated) (1C)
- Use a fluid challenge technique while associtated with a hemodynamic improvement (1D)
- Give fluid challenges of 1000 mL of crystalloids or 300–500 mL of colloids over 30 mins. More rapid and larger volumes may be required in sepsis-induced tissue hypoperfusion (1D)
- Rate of fluid administration should be reduced if cardiac filling pressures increase without concurrent hemodynamic improvement (1D)

(*Continued*)

Table 4. (*Continued*)

Vasopressors

- Maintain MAP ≥ 65 mmHg (1C)
- Norepinephrine and dopamine centrally administered are the initial vasopressors of choice (1C)
- Epinephrine, phenylephrine, or vasopressin should not be administered as the initial vasopressor in septic shock (2C), Vasopressin 0.03 units/min may be subsequently added to norepinephrine with anticipation of an effect equivalent to norepinephrine alone
- Use epinephrine as the first alternative agent in septic shock when blood pressure is poorly responsive to norepinephrine or dopamine (2B)
- Do not use low-dose dopamine for renal protection (1A)
- In patients requiring, vasopressors, insert an arterial catheter as soon as practical (1D)

Inotropic therapy

- Use dobutamine in patients with myocardial dysfunction as supported by elevated cardiac filling pressures and low cardiac output (1C)
- Do not increase cardiac index to predetermined supranormal levels (1B)

Steroids

- Consider intravenous hydrocortisone for adult septic shock when hypotension responds poorly to adequate fluid resuscitation and vasopressors (2C)
- ACTH stimulation test is not recommended to identify the subset of adults with septic shock who should receive hydrocortisone (2B)
- Hydrocortisone is preferred to dexamethasone (2B)
- Fludrocortisone (50 μg orally once a day) may be included if an alternative to hydrocortisone is being used that lacks significant mineralocorticoid activity Fludrocortisone if optional if hydrocortisone is used (2C)
- Steroid therapy may be weaned once vasopressors are no longer required (2D)
- Hydrocortisone dose should be ≤300 mg/day (1A)
- Do not use corticosteroids to treat sepsis in the absence of shock unless the patient's endocrine or corticosteroid history warrants it (1D)

Recombinant human activated protein C

- Withdrawn from the market as of October 2011, based on negative results of PROWESS-SHOCK study that showed no benefit in adult patients with sepsis-induced organ dysfunction with clinial assessment of high risk of death.

GRADE, Grades of Recommendation, Assessment, Development and Evaluation; CVP, central venous pressure; MAP, mean arterial pressure; ACTH, adrenocorticotropic hormone; rhAPC, recombinant human activated protein C; APACHE, Acute Physiology and Chronic Health Evaluation.

(With permission from Dellinger *et al.* (2008) *Crit Care Med* **36**: 296–327.)

Key Intervention Principles

Aggressive fluid resuscitation combined with monitoring of preload deficit resolution is a key component of EGDT. All patients with severe sepsis or sepsis with shock should receive at least 25 ml/kg isotonic crystalloid (e.g. plasmalyte) as a bolus over <1 hr. No convincing outcome advantage to colloid administration has been demonstrated. A history of CHF, renal insufficiency, or other condition that predisposes to accumulation of extravascular lung water should not preclude an adequate fluid challenge in order to address acute hypoperfusion, through careful monitoring of respiratory status, and support with assisted ventilation offered for ventilatory compromise. Likewise, static indirect measures of preload sufficiency such as CVP or LVEDV do not predict accurately the response to fluid, and no perceived threshold value should preclude fluid challenge in patients who manifest signs of hypoperfusion.

Early and effective antibiotic administration is a critical time-sensitive component of EGDT. Delay in effective antibiotics is associated with significant mortality.[10] (Fig. 1).

After initial fluid resuscitation, patients who remain hypotensive should have pressors initiated. Norepinephrine is presently recommended, though vasopressin and dopamine are acceptable alternatives. Purported benefits of primary therapy with vasopressin have not been validated, though the addition of vasopressin infusion may allow a rapid decrease in the required norepinephrine dose. Consensus guidelines recommend avoiding unopposed or maximal alpha adrenergic agonists such as phenylephrine and do not advocate the use of dopamine for renal "protection."[11]

The use of inotropes to support cardiac contractility defects or to target indirect signs of tissue dysoxia such as $ScvO_2$ is a poorly defined element of EGDT, with limited data and poor clinical fidelity despite attractive physiological rationale. A conservative recommendation is to reserve dobutamine for patients with a cardiac index <2.5 L/min/m^2 despite adequate volume and pressor support.

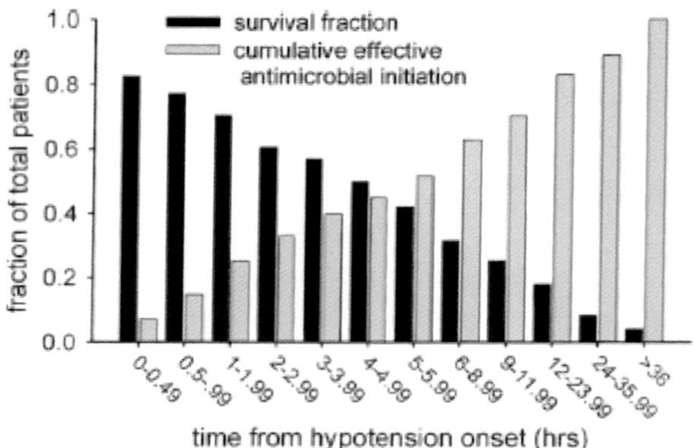

Fig. 1. Cumulative effective antimicrobial initiation following the onset of septic-shock-associated hypotension and associated survival. The x-axis represents time (hr) following the first documentation of septic-shock-associated hypotension. The black bars represent the fraction of patients surviving to hospital discharge for effective therapy initiated within the given time interval. The gray bray represent the cumulative fraction of patients having received effective antimicrobials at any given time point.

With permission from Kumar *et al.* (2006) *Crit Care Med* **34**: 1589–1596.

Role of Monitoring: What to Measure — When and How Reliable

Measurement of preload (LVEDV) by echocardiography is a relative measure of cardiac filling, though this is poorly predictive of volume responsiveness. Likewise, a static indirect measure of preload by CVP has poor discriminative capacity to identify patients who will respond to additional fluid administration with augmented stroke volume.[12] Respiratory cycle thoracic pressure variations influence volume and pressure estimates of preload, so that the greater the preload deficit, the greater the respiratory cycle variation. Several novel monitoring strategies have been offered that take advantage of dynamic respiratory cycle variation, and may provide a useful predictive index of preload deficit that is a better clinical determinant than CVP. Among dynamic indications of cardiac filling, the IVC collapsibility index has been shown to perform better than CVP in detecting preload deficit and predicting response to fluid bolus administration.[13]

Continuous measurement of $ScvO_2$, as a monitoring target of EGDT as described by Rivers *et al.* has not been widely adopted and requires specialized invasive monitoring. Moreover, among patients with septic shock who were treated to normalize central venous and mean arterial pressure, additional management to normalize lactate clearance, targeting at least 10% decreased lactate as a goal of an initial 6 hr of resuscitation, compared with management to normalize $ScvO_2$, did not result in significantly different in-hospital mortality.[14]

Other Therapeutic Considerations/Controversies

Transfusion of PRBCs is a controversial part of a bundled goal directed therapy that has not been independently validated. Although transfusion may increase oxygen content, it has limited or negative oxygen consumption benefit in the setting of microcirculatory disturbance in sepsis and critical illness.

Restrictive transfusion policy targeting Hgb >7.0 is recommended in sepsis and other critical illnesses that render patients at risk for ARDS and MODS, with associated augmented mortality risk.[15]

Guidelines such as the Surviving Sepsis Campaign currently maintain that hydrocortisone <300 mg/day should be administered for volume nonresponsive septic shock (Table 3). Nevertheless, no mortality benefit has been reproducibly demonstrated, perhaps owing to the inclusion of large numbers of patients who received etomidate which blocks steroid metabolism in the single trial that purported to show such a benefit. Cortrosyn stimulation testing is no longer recommended, based on the recognition that nonresponder information is obtained in retrospect and does not clearly predict a pressor-sparing effect.[16]

Initial enthusiasm for intensive insulin therapy to improve outcome in sepsis and septic shock has been tempered by poor reproducibility of benefit in multiple trials, largely attributed to the counterbalancing effect of excess hypoglycemia and an associated increased risk of death.[17] A prudent recommendation is to maintain BG <150 with careful attention to hypoglycemia by insuring adequate nutrition through the enteral or intravenous route.

For those patients who manifest oliguric renal failure, CVVH offers no benefit compared to intermittent hemodialysis in the absence of demonstrated hemodynamic intolerance to a trial of dialysis.[18]

The action of rAPC to improve outcome in severe sepsis is controversial, based on poor reproducibility of initial demonstration of benefit in a carefully selected cohort. Actions of APC in sepsis are thought to relate to anti-inflammatory properties as well as improvement in blood fluidity which may affect microcirculation. rAPC is considered possibly indicated in a carefully selected group of patients with a narrow timeline for initiation within the first 24 hr in patients with a compact clinical presentation, limited bleeding risk, and a high mortality estimate based on Apache II >25.[19]

Agents with vasodilatory properties have been purported to improve microcirculatory flow in sepsis, though the added clinical benefit of these interventions remains unclear. Such agents as dobutamine, cholinergic agonists, and therapy, which increase nitric oxide bioavailability (e.g. IV nitroglycerine), are undergoing investigation for this activity, though it has not-yet-demonstrated clinical value.

Targeted therapy aimed at interruption of individual inflammatory cascade elements (e.g. anti-TNF mAb) has been largely disappointing, with no mortality benefit in a wide variety of trials. Patients with severe sepsis invariably present after the initial innate response, which is short-lived and results in myriad downstream cascades including counterregulatory and potentially compensatory anti-inflammatory responses (CARS). The systems-based approach to cell signaling in sepsis has provided insight into the vast array of interwoven and time-sensitive signaling nodes and crosstalk which expose the complex task of clinically meaningful amelioration of sepsis by any strategy that targets early mediators of sepsis.[20]

Outcome Analysis and Prognosis

The prognostic assessment in sepsis is linked to the detection of multiorgan failure and is influenced by host factors related to comorbid illness and chronic illness. Genomic and epidemiologic characteristics contribute

Table 5. Sequential Organ Failure Assessment (SOFA) Score Schematic

SOFA Score	0	1	2	3	4
				With Respiratory Support	
Respiration, Pao_2/FIo_2 mm Hg	>400	≤400	≤300	≤200	≤100
Coagulation, platelets × $10^3/Vmm^3$	>150	≤150	≤100	≤50	≤20
Liver, bdlinibin, mg/dL (μmol/L)	<1.2 (<20)	1.2–1.9 (20–32)	2.0–5.9 (33–101)	6.0–11.9 (102–204)	>12.0 (>204)
Cardiovascular, hypotension	No hypotensdon	MAP <70 mm Hg	Dopamine ≤5 or dobutamine (any dose)[a]	Dopamine >5 or epinephrine ≤0.10 norepinephrine ≤0.1 [a]	Dopamine >l5 or epinephrire >0.1 or no repinephrine >0.1 [a]
Central nervous system, Glasgow Coma Scale score	15	13–14	10–12	6–9	<6
Renal, creatinine, mg/dL. (μmol/L)	<1.2 (<110)	1.2–1.9 (110–170)	2.0–3.4 (171–299)	3.5–1.9 (300–440)	>5.0 (>440)
Or urine output				or <500 mL/day	or <200 mL/day

MAP, mein arterial pressure.

[a]Adrenergic agents administered for ≥ 1 hr (doses given are in μg/kg/min).

With permission from: Dubois *et al.* (2006) *Crit Care Med* **34**(10): 2536–2540.

to host factor susceptibility to MODS and increased mortality in sepsis. For example, polymorphisms in TNF-alpha, a history of alcoholism, and African-American heritage have all been associated with worse outcome.

The action of rAPC in severe sepsis is controversial, based on poor reproducibility of initial demonstration of benefit in selected cohorts of septic patients. Actions of APC in sepsis are thought to relate to anti-inflammatory properties as well as blood fluidity properties that may affect microcirculatory disturbances in sepsis.[19] Until recently, rAPC was available as drotrecogin alpha [Xigris] for administration for carefully selected patients with severe sepsis with APACHE II >25. However, in a recently completed clinical trial, the PROWESS-SHOCK trial, drotecogin alpha [Xigris] failed to show a survival benefit. Results based on preliminary analyses done by Eli Lilly and Company, that were submitted to the FDA, showed a 28-day all cause mortality rate of 26.4% in Xirgis-treated patients as compared with 24.2% in placebo-treated patients, equivalent to a relative risk of 1.09; with a *p*-value of 0.31, which is not statistically significant. As a result, the FDA announced in October 2011 that Ely Lilly has voluntarily withdrawn drotrecogin alpha from the market and is no longer available for patient adminstration. Generating an APACHE II score had been utilized to assess the risk/benefit of rAPC administration, and may similarly be used to stratify patients for future novel therapeutics. Severity scoring systems have limited predictive power for individual patients at presentation, are limited to an ICU cohort, and may be logistically cumbersome to generate. Web-based severity score assistance is available from many sources (see www.medal.org). Simpler consolidated scoring modalities have been offered to improve routine incorporation into clinical activities.

Lastly, scoring schemes that also document the trajectory of response over time to therapy or accumulated organ dysfunction offer a better discriminator of outcome than initial admission screening modalities alone. The SOFA (Sequential Organ Failure Assessment) is presented in Table 5, and is more streamlined, with fewer physiologic variables than APACHE. SOFA assessment may inform decision making and adjust goals of care in patients who demonstrate progressive organ failure assessment despite resuscitative efforts.[21]

References

1. Levy MM, Fink MP, Marshall JC, *et al.* (2003) 2001 SCCM/ESICM/ACCP/ATS/SIS International Sepsis Definitions Conference. *Intensive Care Med* **29**: 530–538.
2. Kawai T, Akira S. (2007) TLR signaling. *Sem Immunol* **19**: 24–32.
3. Esmon CT. (2006) Inflammation and the activated protein C anticoagulant pathway. *Sem Thomb Hemost* **32**(Suppl 1): 49–60.
4. Jansen JRC, Maas JJ, Pinsky MR. (2010) Bedside assessment of mean systemic filling pressure. *Curr Opin Crit Care* **16**: 231–236.
5. Hunter JD, Doddi M. (2010) Sepsis and the heart. *Br J Anaesth* **104**(1): 3–11.
6. Landry DW, Oliver JA. (2001) The pathogenesis of vasodilatory shock. *New Engl J Med* **34**(8): 588–593.
7. Sakr Y, Dubois MJ, De BD, *et al.* (2004) Persistent microcirculatory alterations are associated with organ failure and death in patients with septic shock. *Crit Care Med* **32**: 1825–1831.
8. Jones AE, Brown MD, Trzeciak S, *et al.* (2008) The effect of a quantitative resuscitation strategy on mortality inpatients with sepsis: A meta-analysis. *Crit Care Med* **36**: 2734–2739.
9. Levy MM, Dellinger RP, Townsend SR, *et al.* (2010) The surviving sepsis campaign: Results of an international guideline-based performance improvement program targeting severe sepsis. *Crit Care Med* **38**: 367–374.
10. Gaieski DF, Mikkelsen ME, Band RA, *et al.* (2010) Impact of time to antibiotics on survival in patients with severe sepsis or septic shock in whom early goal-directed therapy was initiated in the emergency department. *Crit Care Med* **38**: 1045–1053.
11. Beale SJ, Hollenberg SM, Vincent JL, Parillo JE. (2004) Vasopressor and inotropic support in septic shock: An evidence-based review. *Crit Care Med* **32**(Suppl): S455–465.
12. Marik PE, Baram M, Vahid B. (2008) Does central venous pressure predict fluid responsiveness? A systematic review of the literature and the tale of seven mares. *Chest* **134**: 172–178.

13. Nagved AD, Merchant RC, Tirado-Gonzalez A, *et al.* (2010) Emergency department bedside ultrasonographic measurement of the caval index for noninvasive determination of low central venous pressure. *Ann Emerg Med* **55**: 290–295.
14. Jones AE, Shapiro NI, Trzeciak S, *et al.* (2010) Lactate clearance vs central venous oxygen saturation as goals of early sepsis therapy: A randomized clinical trial. *JAMA* **303**(8): 739–746.
15. Marik PE, Corwin HL. (2008) Efficacy of red blood cell transfusion in the critically ill: A systematic review of the literature. *Crit Care Med* **36**: 2667–2674.
16. Marik PE. (2009) Critical illness–related corticosteroid insufficiency. *Chest* **135**: 181–193.
17. Marik PE, Preiser J-C. (2009) Toward understanding tight glycemic control in the ICU. A systematic review and metaanalysis. *Chest* **137**: 544–551.
18. Cariou A, Vinsonneau C, Dhainaut J-F. (2004) Adjunctive therapies in sepsis: An evidence-based review. *Crit Care Med* **32**(Suppl): S562–S570.
19. Barie PS. (2008) Current role of activated protein C therapy for severe sepsis and septic shock. *Curr Infect Dis Rep* **10**: 368–376.
20. Gilchrist M, Thorsson V, Li B, *et al.* (2006) Systems biology approaches identify ATF3 as a negative regulator of Toll-like receptor 4. *Nature* **441**: 173–178.
21. Minne L, Abu-Hanna A, de Jonge E. (2008) Evaluation of SOFA-based models for predicting mortality in the ICU: A systematic review. *Critical Care* **12**(6): R161.

Chapter 32

Management of the Mechanically Ventilated Patient

Uma S. Ayyala

Key Pearls

- Modes of mechanical ventilation differ in how a breath is delivered, sustained, and terminated, as well as the degree of ventilatory support provided to a patient. Patients with specific clinical conditions may benefit from one mode over another.
- Patients who are mechanically ventilated require continuous hemodynamic as well as laboratory data to provide information about gas exchange.
- Supportive care of the mechanically ventilated patient includes adequate sedation and analgesia that can relieve pain and help prevent patient–ventilator dyssynchrony.
- Respiratory distress on the mechanical ventilator can be life-threatening and requires immediate attention. In addition to physical exam, laboratory and imaging data, evaluation of respiratory parameters such as peak and plateau airway pressures can help identify the root of distress.
- Liberation from the ventilator requires a patient to be clinically ready prior to initiating a spontaneous breathing trial. Successful weaning requires daily interruption of sedatives and a multidisciplinary, protocolized approach.

*Mount Sinai School of Medicine, New York, NY, USA.

Introduction

Respiratory failure requiring mechanical ventilation can be caused by a variety of medical conditions. Most commonly, mechanical ventilation is initiated for hypoxemic respiratory failure, hypercapnic respiratory failure, altered mental status requiring a stable airway, respiratory muscle fatigue, and bronchospasm. A thorough understanding of the modes and parameters of ventilators, as well as the management of complications from mechanical ventilation, is important in order to safely provide this therapy to patients.

Initiation of Mechanical Ventilation

Modes and Settings

Volume, pressure, and flow are three interrelated variables in all forms of mechanical ventilation. Modes of ventilation are differentiated by how inspiration is initiated (trigger variable), maintained (limit variable), and terminated (cycle variable). A breath is triggered by a preset variable — most often either pressure or flow. Then an inspiration is maintained and cycles to expiration once a preset measure of volume, pressure, flow, or time is met.

The three most common modes of mechanical ventilation are assist control ventilation (ACV), spontaneous intermittent mechanical ventilation (SIMV), and pressure support ventilation (PSV), as outlined in Table 1. ACV imposes the least amount of work of breathing for a patient and therefore is the most widely used mode.[1] In this mode, the ventilator supports every breath. A baseline respiratory rate (RR) is set, though the patient may breathe over this rate. The ACV mode can be either volume- or pressure-cycled. In volume-cycled ACV, a baseline RR, inspiratory flow, and tidal volume (TV) are designated with the dependent variable being airway pressure. Conversely, with pressure-cycled ACV, a peak inspiratory pressure (PIP), inspiratory time (T_i), and RR are set with TV as the dependent variable. This mode provides the advantage of controlling airway pressures but with the drawback of not guaranteeing a specific

Table 1. Modes of Mechanical Ventilation

Mode	Ventilator Support	Cycle Variable	Description
AC	Full	Volume or pressure	Preset: RR, TV or Pi, PEEP, inspiratory flow, FiO_2. Patent can overbreathe set rate and will receive set TV. Adv: For critically ill patients who require full ventilatory support. Disadv: May be more uncomfortable than partial support modes and requires sedation.
SIMV	Partial	Volume or pressure	Preset: RR, TV or Pi, PEEP, inspiratory flow or inspiratory time, PS for spontaneous breaths, FiO_2. Pt can overbreathe set rate and will receive PS. Adv: Better patient–ventilator synchrony; auto-PEEP less likely.
PSV	Partial	Flow	Preset: Pressure support level, PEEP, FiO_2. There is no set RR — pt must initiate a breath which delivers an inspiratory pressure until the inspiratory flow decreases to a preset threshold. Adv: Mode of weaning, more comfortable for pt. Disadv: Pt needs to be awake to trigger vent, not suitable for full mechanical ventilatory support.
T-piece	Spontaneous	None	No ventilator support at all — oxygen level is the only setting. Pt must breathe through ETT. Adv: Ideal mode for weaning.

TV and therefore minute ventilation. The SIMV and PSV modes provide less ventilatory support for patients but offer some advantages regarding patient comfort and use as weaning modalities (Table 1).

Once a mode of ventilation is decided on, other settings, such as RR, delivered oxygen (F_iO_2), positive end expiratory pressure (PEEP), and inspiratory flow, can be chosen (Table 2). When volume-cycled ACV is used, PIP and plateau pressure (P_{plat}) can be measured. PIP is the highest

Table 2. Glossary of Respiratory Parameters

Respiratory Parameter	Description
Respiratory rate (RR)	Normally set at 12–16. I↑RR to ↑ventilation. ↓RR used in "permissive hypercapnia" strategy.
Fraction of inspired oxygen (FiO_2)	Range 21%–100%. Initial ventilator settings should begin with 100% and titrate down to maintain PaO_2 of >60, O_2sat >90%.
Positive end-expiratory pressure (PEEP)	Positive pressure during expiration. Normal ventilator settings — physiologic PEEP of 3–5 mmHg. PEEP→↑functional residual capacity (FRC) — prevents atelectasis and improves oxygenation. Side effects: ↑intrathoracic pressure ◊↓venous return →↓preload.
Inspiratory flow rate	Usually set at 60 L/min. ↑flow to ↑expiratory time. ↑flow will ↑P_{peak}.
Inspiratory time	Set in pressure-cycled ventilation. Can alter inspiratory time to change I:E ratio.
I:E ratio	Normally 1:2. Change to 1:3–1:5 for obstructive lung disease. May increase inspiratory time in ARDS.
Peak inspiratory pressure (PIP)	Highest pressure during respiratory cycle. Function of both airway resistance and lung/chest wall/abdominal muscle compliance↑. ↓PIP → air leak in system. ↑PIP → either ↑airway resistance (mucus plugging, bronchospasm, occluded ETT) or ↑ P_{plat} (ARDS, pneumonia, pulmonary edema, pneumothorax, atelectasis).
Plateau pressure (P_{plat})	Measured at end of inspiration when airway resistance = 0. ↑P_{plat}→↓compliance of lung or chest wall.

pressure during respiration, reflecting two components: airway resistance and intrinsic compliance of the lung, chest wall, and abdomen.[2] P_{plat} is measured at end inspiration, when airway resistance is absent (zero flow), and is therefore a static measurement of lung, chest wall, and abdominal compliance.[2] PIP and P_{plat} become important when one is evaluating distress on the mechanical ventilator.

Monitoring and Supportive Care

Monitoring

Patients who are mechanically ventilated require daily clinical, radiological, and laboratory monitoring. In addition to a complete physical examination, clinical evaluation of patients should include observation for ventilator synchrony by assessing chest and abdominal movements. Radiographic monitoring after intubation is important, especially for confirming placement of the endotracheal tube. However, the frequency with which subsequent chest radiographs should be obtained is not yet defined, with some evidence supporting on-demand radiographs instead of daily chest radiographs.[3] Continuous pulse oximetry should be part of hemodynamic monitoring but can be inaccurate in patients who are hypothermic or hypotensive,[4] and should not replace arterial blood gas determinations of arterial oxygen tension (PaO_2). Daily arterial blood gases should be obtained to measure not only adequacy of oxygenation but also ventilation.

Supportive Care

Supportive care of the mechanically ventilated patient should encompass that of the critically ill patient, including sedation, stress ulcer prophylaxis, deep venous thrombosis prophylaxis, enteral nutrition, and measures to prevent nosocomial infections.[5] Of critical importance for these patients is adequate pain control. Pain may be due to the primary process requiring intubation (i.e. the surgical procedure and underlying medical condition) or from routine management, including placement of invasive catheters, suctioning of secretions, and turning to prevent decubitus ulcers. Pain can lead to increase in catecholamines, increase in oxygen consumption, and myocardial ischemia, and can manifest as impairment of vital signs as well as patient–ventilator dyssynchrony. No one sedative or analgesic has been proven to be superior to another in the critically ill population, and selection should be tailored individually. Sedatives commonly used include opiates, benzodiazapenes, propofol, neuroleptics, and dexmedetomidine. In specific instances, patients with ventilator dyssynchrony may require neuromuscular blocking agents to safely oxygenate and ventilate them. These drugs should be used with caution and always in conjunction with adequate sedation. Daily interruption of sedative infusions in addition to a daily spontaneous breathing trial has been proven to be of benefit in reducing days on the ventilator, ICU length of stay, and one-year mortality.[7]

Disease-Specific Conditions and Ventilator Management

The overall management of mechanical ventilation regardless of disease state includes: (1) titration of FiO_2 to the minimum required, (2) maintenance of low pressures to reduce barotrauma, (3) utilization of appropriate tidal volumes to reduce volutrauma, and (4) use of adequate PEEP to facilitate oxygenation. Initial ventilator settings for the majority of patients requiring invasive mechanical ventilation involve the ACV volume-controlled mode with a target TV of 8 ml/kg ideal body weight. Initially FiO_2 is set to 100% and PEEP is preset to 3–5 cmH_2O.

Obstructive Lung Disease

Mechanical ventilation initiated for acute exacerbations of asthma or chronic obstructive lung disease (COPD) requires careful attention, due to the potential for complications. In particular, patients with obstructive lung disease are at risk for high peak pressures, mainly from increased airway resistance. These pressures can lead to barotrauma manifesting as pneumothorax or pneumomediastinum. In addition, patients with obstructive lung disease can develop dynamic hyperinflation, where exhalation is not completed before initiation of the next breath. This leads to auto-PEEP, which can result in barotrauma as well as hemodynamic compromise (hypotension). A ventilatory strategy of "permissive hypercapnia" can prevent dynamic hyperinflation.[8] It employs a lower RR(8–10) and a higher flow rate (80–100 L/min) to allow for increased time for exhalation (I:E ratio of 1:3–1:5). The consequence of this lower RR is decreased minute ventilation leading to hypercapnia. Any patient with evidence of auto-PEEP and hemodynamic instability should be disconnected from the ventilator and allowed to fully exhale before altering parameters and reconnecting.

Acute Respiratory Distress Syndrome/ Acute Lung Injury

In patients who meet criteria for acute respiratory distress syndrome (ARDS)/acute lung injury (ALI), a lung-protective strategy is utilized. In a landmark trial, this approach of using a low TV (6 ml/kg IBW or less) compared to traditional TVs of 12 ml/kg to minimize volumtrauma from overdistension of alveoli and to limit airway pressures (goal plateau pressure <30) conferred an absolute mortality benefit of 8.8%.[9] Increasing levels of PEEP are used to prevent atelectasis and improve oxygenation. This ventilatory strategy results in hypercapnia which can be managed by increasing the RR.

Evaluation of Respiratory Distress in the Mechanically Ventilated Patient

Respiratory distress that develops in the mechanically ventilated patient can be a life-threatening emergency and must be attended to immediately. Clinically, such patients often have abnormal vital signs with evidence of tachycardia, tachypnea, or desaturation. Patients may be agitated, "bucking" the ventilator with dyssynchronous movements of the chest wall and abdominal musculature. There is a broad differential for respiratory distress in these patients that includes endotracheal tube or ventilator malfunction, inappropriate ventilator settings, inadequate sedation, intrinsic pulmonary pathology (e.g. bronchospasm, secretions, pneumothorax), or extrapulmonary processes (e.g. arrhythmias, sepsis).

Evaluation of respiratory distress in these patients should begin with determination of hemodynamic stability. If the patient is hemodynamically unstable, then he or she should be disconnected from the ventilator and manually ventilated with 100% oxygen. Close attention should be given to the ease with which ventilation can be provided. If resistance is met with each breath, the endotracheal tube may be obstructed and suctioning or even replacement of the tube may improve the patient's condition. If air is audible with each manually delivered breath, an air leak may be present and the endotracheal cuff may need to be inflated or the tube replaced to correct this problem. Other life-threatening conditions that must be addressed in the deteriorating patient include evaluation for tension pneumothorax and auto-PEEP. If clinical suspicion exists for tension pneumothorax (unilateral breath sounds, tracheal deviation, hemodynamic instability), then needle decompression needs to be performed.

In the stabilized patient, a more complete assessment can be performed (Fig. 1). This includes focused physical examination, chest radiography to evaluate tube placement and lung parenchyma, arterial blood gas to determine gas exchange, and an electrocardiogram to look for arrhythmia. Examination of the ventilator circuit and any triggered alarms can be helpful in localizing a cause for respiratory distress. The most common ventilator alarm activated is PIP. As discussed earlier, PIP, $P_{plat,}$ and the difference (PIP-P_{plat}) are values that can help identify the underlying cause of respiratory distress (Fig. 1).

Liberation from the Mechanical Ventilator

Liberation from the mechanical ventilator is a process that gradually transitions a patient from full ventilator support to spontaneous breathing. A patient's readiness to maintain spontaneous breathing is the first step in liberation from the ventilator (Table 3). Once the conditions are met, a spontaneous breathing trial can be initiated. In randomized controlled trials, both PSV and T-tube trials have been shown to be superior to SIMV as weaning modalities.[10,11] Coordinated efforts with the nurses, respiratory therapist, and physicians are integral to successful extubations.

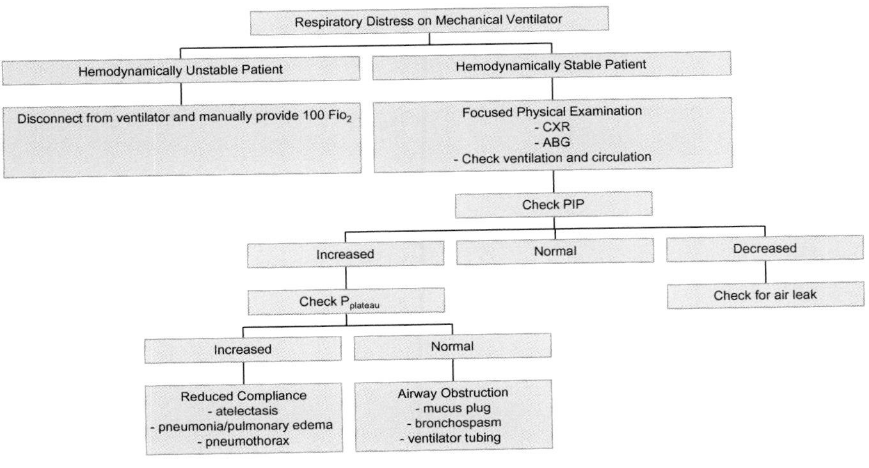

Fig. 1. Distress in the mechanically ventilated patient.

Table 3. Assessing Patient Readiness for a Spontaneous Breathing Trial

Clinical criteria:

- Underlying cause of respiratory failure has improved.
- Hemodynamic stability with HR 50–140, SBP 90–180 mmHg.
- SpO_2 >92% on FiO_2 < or = 40%.
- PEEP <5 cmH_2O.
- Patient can initiate his own breaths.
- Patient is alert and can follow simple commands.

Weaning parameter:

- Rapid shallow breathing index (RSBI): RR/TV (L)
  - To be performed while patient is spontaneously breathing. A value >105 breath/min/L predicts that a patient will fail a spontaneous breathing trial.[12]

References

1. Koh SO. (2007) Mode of mechanical ventilation: Volume controlled mode. *Crit Care Clin* **23**: 161–167.
2. Tobin, MJ. (1990) Respiratory monitoring. *JAMA* **264**: 244–251.
3. Hejblum G, Chalumeau-Lemoine L, Loos V, *et al*. (2009) Comparison of routine and on-demand prescription of chest radiographs in

mechanically ventilated adults: A multicentre, cluster-randomised, two-period crossover study. *Lancet* **374**(9702): 1687–1693.
4. Hinkelbein J, Genzwuerker HV, Fielder F. (2005) Detection of a systolic pressure threshold for reliable readings in pulse oximetry. *Resuscitation* **64**: 315–319.
5. Dellinger RP, Levy MM, Carlet JM, Bion J, Parker MM, Jaeschke R, Reinhart K, Angus DC, Brun-Buisson C, Beale R, Calandra T, Dhainaut JF, Gerlach H, Harvey M, Marini JJ, Marshall J, Ranieri M, Ramsay G, Sevransky J, Thompson BT, Townsend S, Vender JS, Zimmerman JL, Vincent JL. International Surviving Sepsis Campaign Guidelines Committee; American Association of Critical-Care Nurses; American College of Chest Physicians; American College of Emergency Physicians; Canadian Critical Care Society; European Society of Clinical Microbiology and Infectious Diseases; European Society of Intensive Care Medicine, *et al.* (2008) Surviving Sepsis Campaign: International guidelines for management of severe sepsis and septic shock. *Crit Care Med* **36**: 296–327.
6. Epstein J, Breslow MJ. (1999) The stress response of critical illness. *Crit Care Clin* **15**: 17–33.
7. Girard, TD, Kress JP, Fuchs BD, *et al.* (2008) Efficacy and safety of a paired sedation and ventilator weaning protocol for mechanically ventilated patients in intensive care (Awake and Breathing Controlled trial): A randomized controlled trial. *Lancet* **371**: 126.
8. Oddo M, Feihl F, Schaller MD, Perret C. (2006) Management of mechanical ventilation in acute severe asthma: Practical aspects. *Intensive Care Med* **32**(4): 501–510.
9. The Acute Respiratory Distress Syndrome Network. (2000) Ventilation with lower tidal volumes as compared with traditional tidal volumes for acute lung injury and the acute respiratory distress syndrome. *N Engl J Med* **342**(18): 1301–1308.
10. Esteban, A, Fructos F, Tobin MJ, *et al.* (1995) A comparison of four methods of weaning from mechanical ventilation. Spanish Lung Failure Collaborative Group. *N Engl J Med* **332**(6): 345–350.

11. Brochard L, Rauss A, Benito S, *et al.* (1994) Comparison of three methods of gradual withdrawal from ventilatory support during weaning from mechanical ventilation. *Am J Respir Crit Care Med* **150**(4): 896–903.
12. Meade M, Guyatt G, Cook D, *et al.* (2001) Predicting success in weaning from mechanical ventilation. *Chest* **120**(6S): 400S–424S.

Chapter 33

Glycemic Management in Critically Ill Patients

*Maria Skamagas**

Key Pearls

- Glucose goals in the critically ill patient: 140–180 mg/dL.
- A validated intravenous insulin protocol which incorporates current glucose, rate of glucose change, and current insulin infusion rate into adjustments of insulin infusion should be used. A hypoglycemia protocol should be incorporated.
- Glucose should be monitored every one hour after initiation of insulin infusion.
- HbA1c in the hyperglycemic critically ill patient should be measured to determine if there is pre-existing diabetes or whether elevated glucose is due to stress hyperglycemia.
- Intravenous insulin should be converted to subcutaneous insulin as the patient improves clinically. Patients with stress hyperglycemia on low dose insulin drip may only require correction insulin scale.

Critically ill patients are at risk for hyperglycemia, even if they do not carry a prior diagnosis of diabetes. Hyperglycemia is likely related to a host of factors, including counter-regulatory hormones such as cortisol and catecholamines; inflammatory cytokines; nutritional support (enteral and parenteral); and medications including glucocorticoids.[1]

*Mount Sinai School of Medicine, New York, NY, USA.

Hyperglycemia is associated with worse outcomes in the critically ill, and may be more deleterious in those without pre-existing diabetes.[2] There are some populations wherein intravenous (IV) insulin reduces blood glucose (BG) and appears to be beneficial in reducing mortality and/or infection: diabetics undergoing cardiothoracic surgery,[3,4] diabetics with myocardial infarction,[5] and non-diabetics undergoing cardiothoracic and general surgery.[6]

Based on large, randomized control trials, the optimal glucose range for improving outcomes in the critically ill is unknown and remains a moving target. In the NICE-SUGAR trial, surgical and medical critically ill patients suffered increased mortality and hypoglycemia when glucose targets of 80–110 mg/dL were applied.[7] Furthermore, the optimal glucose target may vary depending on the population type, i.e. medical versus surgical, diabetic versus non-diabetic. Current recommendations by the ADA/AACE are BG goal of 140–180 mg/dL in critically ill patients, using an IV insulin protocol with demonstrated efficacy and safety.[8] There are published insulin drip protocols using the lower glucose goal of 80–110 mg/dL,[9–11] and the newer goal of 140–180 mg/dL.[12]

Glucose Goals

- Glucose goals in the critically ill patient: 140–180 mg/dL.
- Consider initiating IV insulin infusion when glucose >180 mg/dL.

Insulin IV Infusion

A validated IV insulin drip protocol should be used, incorporating current glucose, rate of glucose change, and current insulin infusion rate into adjustments of the insulin infusion. A hypoglycemia protocol should be used.

- Insulin IV infusion: 100% bioavailable, immediate onset, duration of insulin action ~1 hour
- Insulin infusions come in different concentrations.

  Regular insulin 100 units mixed in 1000 mL of 0.9% NaCl (normal saline) → 1 unit insulin per 10 mL.

Regular insulin 100 units mixed in 100 mL of 0.9% NaCl (normal saline) → 1 unit insulin per 1 mL.
This concentration requires an infusion pump that can dispense ≤ 1mL/hour.

Glucose Monitoring

- Measure blood glucose (BG) every 1 hour.
- When BG is stable and no change in clinical status, nutrition, steroids, etc., consider reducing BG measurements to every 2 hours.
- Obtain blood from capillary/fingerstick and use bedside glucometer, OR obtain blood from venous/arterial source/catheter and measure BG on blood gas.
- Caveat: capillary BG measurements may be inaccurate in hypotensive/hypoperfused patients, severe edema, and patients receiving pressors.
- Check HbA1c to determine if patient has pre-existing diabetes or stress hyperglycemia.

Converting IV to Subcutaneous (SC) Insulin in Critically Ill[13]

- Convert to SC insulin when patient is clinically stable, off pressors, BG is stable, patient is ready to resume eating.
- Check BG before meals and at bedtime.
- If patient is not eating or is receiving tube feeds, check BG every 6 hours.
- Not to be used for diabetic emergencies (diabetic ketoacdosis and hyperglycemic hyperosmolar state).

Patients who do not have a prior diagnosis of insulin-requiring diabetes and who are receiving ≤1.5 units/hour of IV insulin, may not require transition to SC basal insulin. Consider starting correction insulin scale only, monitor BG, and initiate basal insulin if BG is not at goal.

These patients may require correction scale only, basal insulin only, or basal and mealtime insulin.

Calculation of SC Insulin Doses

1. **Total Daily Insulin Requirement**
   Determine the *average hourly rate* of IV insulin over last 6 hours and multiple rate × 20 hours
   Ex: 2 Units/hr × 20 hr = 40 Units = **Total Daily Insulin**
2. **Convert Total Daily Insulin to SC insulin**: 50% basal, 50% mealtime in divided doses.
   Ex: 40 units × 50% = 20 units

   BASAL: 20 Units glargine SC once daily
   Can also use detemir divided twice daily, or NPH divided twice daily (more hypoglycemia with the latter)

   MEALTIME: 20 ÷ 3 ≈ 6 Units rapid-acting insulin SC before meals
   Use only if patient is eating
   Use aspart, lispro, or glulisine
   If PO intake variable/poor, give less than this calculated dose
   Ex: Give 25–50% = 2–3 units after patient has eaten >25–50% meal

   CORRECTION INSULIN SCALE: Use before meals or every 6 hours
   Use aspart, lispro, or glulisine
   See Table 4 in Chapter 46 "Management of Diabetes and Hyperglycemia in Hospitalized Patients"

   ENTERAL NUTRITION (TUBE FEEDS): For patients on continuous tube feeds and insulin drip:
   Convert Total Daily Insulin to NPH insulin SC divided every 8 hours
   Ex: Total daily insulin of 40 units ÷ 3 ≈ NPH 13 units every 8 hours, give if tube feeds are infusing
   If tube feeds are inadvertently stopped, start IV Dextrose 10% and hold NPH.

3. **Discontinue IV insulin drip 2 hours after 1st dose of SC Basal Insulin**
4. **Hypoglycemia Orders** — See "Hypoglycemia" section in Chapter 46 "Management of Diabetes and Hyperglycemia in Hospitalized Patients."

References

1. Kavanagh BP, McCowen KC. (2010) Clinical practice. Glycemic control in the ICU. *N Engl J Med* **363**: 2540–6.
2. Egi M, Bellomo R, Stachowski E, *et al.* (2008) Blood glucose concentration and outcome of critical illness: The impact of diabetes. *Crit Care Med* **36**: 2249–55.
3. Furnary AP, Zerr KJ, Grunkemeier GL and Starr A. (1999) Continuous intravenous insulin infusion reduces the incidence of deep sternal wound infection in diabetic patients after cardiac surgical procedures. *Ann Thorac Surg* **67**: 352–60.
4. Furnary AP, Gao G, Grunkemeier GL, *et al.* (2003) Continuous insulin infusion reduces mortality in patients with diabetes undergoing coronary artery bypass grafting. *J Thorac Cardiovasc Surg* **125**: 1007–21.
5. Malmberg K. (1997) Prospective randomised study of intensive insulin treatment on long term survival after acute myocardial infarction in patients with diabetes mellitus. DIGAMI (Diabetes Mellitus, Insulin Glucose Infusion in Acute Myocardial Infarction) Study Group. *BMJ* **314**: 1512–5.
6. Van den Berghe G, Wouters P, Weekers F, *et al.* (2001) Intensive insulin therapy in the critically ill patients. *N Engl J Med* **345**: 1359–67.
7. The NICE-SUGAR Study Investigators. (2009) Intensive versus conventional glucose control in critically ill patients. *N Engl J Med* **360**: 1283–97.
8. Moghissi ES, Korytkowski MT, DiNardo M, *et al.* (2009) American Association of Clinical Endocrinologists and American Diabetes

Association consensus statement on inpatient glycemic control. *Endocr Pract* **15**: 353–69.

9. Goldberg PA, Siegel MD, Sherwin RS, *et al*. (2004) Implementation of a safe and effective insulin infusion protocol in a medical intensive care unit. *Diabetes Care* **27**: 461–7.
10. Wilson M, Weinreb J and Hoo GW. (2007) Intensive insulin therapy in critical care: A review of 12 protocols. *Diabetes Care* **30**: 1005–1011.
11. Portland: Portland Protocol. Providence Health Systems. Available from http://www.providence.org/oregon/programs_and_services/heart/portlandprotocol/e05protocol.htm
12. The NICE-SUGAR Study. Protocol available from https://studies.thegeorgeinstitute.org/nice/
13. Bode BW, Brathwaite SS, Steed RD, *et al*. (2004) ACE inpatient diabetes and metabolic control consensus conference. Intravenous insulin infusion therapy: Indications, methods, and transition to subcutaneous insulin therapy. *Endocr Pract* **10**: 71–80.

Renal

Chapter 34

Management of Hospitalized Patients with End-Stage Renal Disease

Anand C. Reddy, Sridhar R. Allam* and Brian D. Radbill**

Key Pearls

- Intradialytic hypotension is often secondary to excessive volume removal but may be a sign of an infected dialysis access, myocardial ischemia, or a significant pericardial effusion.
- Hemodialysis patients who present with a thrombosed AV access may be treated by an interventional radiologist or vascular surgeon in the outpatient setting and avoid hospital admission if they do not have an acute indication for dialysis.
- Hospitalized patients with advanced CKD should be educated about the risk of progression to ESRD and ideally seen by a nephrologist or CKD educator during their admission so that they may make early arrangements for future renal replacement therapy.
- Blood transfusions should be avoided in ESRD patients who are potential transplant candidates because of the risk of developing antibodies and rejecting a donor kidney in the future, but should be administered, if necessary, while the patient receives dialysis to avoid volume overload.
- Oral sodium phosphate solution bowel preps should never be used in patients with renal disease as these can cause acute phosphate nephropathy in patients with CKD, and severe hyperphosphatemia and hypocalcemia in patients with ESRD.

*Mount Sinai School of Medicine, New York NY, USA.

Introduction

Patients with end-stage renal disease (ESRD) are frequently hospitalized for conditions directly and indirectly related to their chronic kidney disease (CKD) or renal replacement therapy (i.e. hemodialysis, peritoneal dialysis, kidney transplantation). With an average of nearly two hospital admissions per patient-year, the adjusted ESRD hospitalization rate is four times higher than that of the general Medicare population.[1] As the number of patients with ESRD continues to grow in the United States, hospitalists can expect to see an increase in the number of ESRD-related admissions and must understand the specific care needs associated with this patient population.

Common Reasons for ESRD-related Hospitalization

Infections

ESRD patients are more susceptible to infections because of the adverse effects of uremia on the immune system; CKD/ESRD patients have a 3–4-fold higher risk of major infections and sepsis as compared to the general population.[2] In this section, we will limit our discussion to the management of dialysis access-associated infections. Other infections commonly seen in ESRD patients, such as pneumonia, are covered in other chapters.

Catheter-related Bacteremia

The overwhelming majority of vascular access-associated bloodstream infections in ESRD patients on hemodialysis (HD) are catheter-related bacteremias (CRBs). Patients typically present with fever and chills, often while receiving dialysis treatment through the infected catheres. Diagnosis of dialysis CRBs requires concurrent positive blood cultures from the dialysis catheter and a peripheral vein. In practice, obtaining blood cultures from the periphery is rarely done as ESRD patients have notoriously poor venous access. Empirical antibiotic therapy consists of vancomycin and an aminoglycoside or third-generation cephalosporin

Table 1. Commonly Used Empiric Antibiotic Regimens for Catheter-related Bacteremia in HD Patients* and Catheter-associated Peritonitis in PD Patients**

Mode of Dialysis	Gram Positive Coverage	Gram Negative Coverage
IHD (intermittent hemodialysis)	Vancomycin 20 mg/kg IV during last hr of dialysis followed by 10 mg/kg IV during last 30 min of each subsequent dialysis session. (Cefazolin 20 mg/kg IV after each dialysis can be used alternatively in units with low prevalence of MRSA)	Gentamicin or 1 tobramycin 1 mg/kg IV (not exceeding 100 mg), or ceftazidime 1 g IV after each dialysis session.
CAPD (continuous ambulatory peritoneal dialysis done manually)	Vancomycin 15–30 mg/kg IP every 5–7 days. (Cefazolin 15 mg/kg IP daily can be used alternatively in units with low prevalence of MRSA)	Gentamicin or tobramycin 0.6 mg/kg IP daily, or cefepime 1g IP daily
APD (automated peritoneal dialysis using cycler)	Vancomycin 30 mg/kg IP, followed by 15 mg/kg IP every 3–5 days. (Cefazolin 20 mg/kg IP daily can be used alternatively in units with low prevalence of MRSA)	Tobramycin 1.5 mg/kg IP once, then 0.5 mg/kg IP daily, or cefepime 1g IP daily

*Adapted from 2009 guidelines published by IDSA (Infectious Diseases Society of America).
**Adapted from 2010 guidelines published by ISPD (International Society of Peritoneal Dialysis); for patients with residual renal function (urine output >100 ml/day), dose should be increased by 25%. All antibiotics administered by intraperitoneal (IP) route should be used with long dwell of PD.

(see Table 1). In addition, management of a dialysis CRB typically involves catheter removal or catheter replacement via guidewire exchange because the risk of recurrence after antibiotic treatment alone is too high to attempt catheter salvage in most settings. If the patient is stable, most nephrologists prefer guidewire exchange over catheter removal because the results are similar and guidewire exchange preserves access sites which may otherwise be lost.[3]

Catheter-associated Peritonitis

Catheter-associated peritonitis (CAP) is seen in ESRD patients on peritoneal dialysis (PD) and often presents with fever, diffuse abdominal pain with peritoneal signs and cloudy dialysate effluent. Treatment consists of peritoneal lavage followed by the administration of intraperitoneal antibiotics (see Table 1). Patients with severe peritonitis or sepsis despite antibiotic treatment may require PD catheter removal and possibly conversion to HD until a new PD catheter can be placed. Of note, polymicrobial peritonitis is not typical and other diagnoses (e.g. bowel perforation, abscess) should be considered.

Volume Overload

Many ESRD patients are either anuric or have minimal residual renal function. Noncompliance with dietary salt and water restriction or the dialysis prescription may lead to life-threatening pulmonary edema, a common cause for hospital admission or presentation to the Emergency Department in ESRD. Pulmonary edema in ESRD is diagnosed clinically. An elevated brain naturetic peptide (BNP) level is of little use unless the "cut-off" value is adjusted upward to account for its decreased clearance in ESRD.[4] However, a normal BNP level has a high negative predictive value in virtually excluding heart failure in ESRD. Treatment typically involves emergent HD or ultrafiltration for volume removal.

Treatment of volume overload in ESRD patients on PD involves multiple short exchanges (1–2 hour dwells) with the dialysate containing a high dextrose concentration (4.5%) to maximize ultrafiltration and allow rapid volume removal.

Routine treatments for pulmonary edema, such as nitroglycerin and high-dose IV diuretics, in addition to oxygen therapy and/or BiPap, may be administered to ESRD patients — especially patients initiating dialysis who may still retain a significant degree of residual renal function — if hemodialysis therapy cannot be provided immediately.

Vascular Access Issues

An arteriovenous fistula (AVF) is formed by creating an anastomosis between an artery and a vein in a patient's arm. An arteriovenous graft (AVG) uses a synthetic graft to connect the artery and the vein in patients with suboptimal vasculature. Complications of AVFs and AVGs may occur immediately postoperatively due to the sudden alteration in peripheral blood flow or later due to the repeated cannulations involved with chronic use. These complications include steal syndrome, venous hypertension, high-output heart failure, pulmonary hypertension, access thrombosis, aneurysm or pseudoaneurysm formation, hemorrhage or access rupture, and infection.

Steal Syndrome

Placement of an AV access can result in distal hypoperfusion due to shunting ("steal") of arterial blood flow into the fistula. Acute ischemic symptoms characterized by an absent pulse or a cold extremity warrant immediate surgical correction to prevent the development of permanent injury. The treatment of choice is a distal revascularization with interval ligation (DRIL).[5] In this procedure, the artery is ligated distal to the arteriovenous anastomosis (thus preventing retrograde flow) and additional distal blood flow is provided by the bypass.

Aneurysms

Aneurysms and pseudoaneurysms develop in AVFs and AVGs, respectively. Multiple or large aneurysms or pseudoaneurysms may limit available cannulation sites and thereby risk functional access loss; however, the more serious concern is the risk of access rupture and subsequent catastrophic hemorrhage in the setting of a rapidly expanding or unstable lesion. Changes in the overlying skin (such as thinning, a shiny appearance, or eschar formation) signify an increased risk of access rupture and require immediate surgical evaluation.

Hyperkalemia

Potassium excretion is impaired in ESRD and hyperkalemia frequently develops. In addition to a low potassium diet, dialysis is considered the definitive treatment for hyperkalemia in patients with ESRD. However, because the initiation of acute hemodialysis may be delayed due to logistical reasons, a variety of temporizing measures must often be employed. These include:

- Cardiac membrane stabilization with intravenous calcium
- Potassium redistribution with insulin (with dextrose to prevent hypoglycemia)
- Potassium elimination with sodium polystyrene sulfonate (SPS; Kayexalate, Kionex).

SPS is a cation exchange resin that exchanges sodium for potassium in the large intestine and is excreted in the stool. Although SPS is frequently used to treat hyperkalemia in an inpatient setting, there are numerous reports of patients who have developed intestinal necrosis and bowel perforation after exposure to SPS in sorbitol as an enema and as an oral agent.[6] Therefore, this medication should be used judiciously, especially in patients with impaired bowel function (e.g. post-operatively).

Tips for Managing Hospitalized ESRD Patients

Orders

Daily Weights

The post-dialysis weight at which the patient is not volume overloaded (e.g. minimal or no edema) is termed the "dry weight." It is important to weigh ESRD patients daily so that the correct amount of ultrafiltrate may be removed when the patient is dialyzed.

Renal Diet

Despite the significant amount of solute removal achieved with chronic dialysis therapy, most ESRD patients must adhere to a strict diet and limited free water intake in order to prevent electrolyte imbalances such as hyperkalemia, hyperphosphatemia and hyponatremia. In addition, phosphorus binders are often required in order to reduce ingested phosphorus absorption. Lastly, when ESRD patients are NPO, maintenance IV fluids should not be routinely ordered as they can result in volume overload.

Labs

Because most dialysis patients have poor venous access and obtaining bloodwork is often challenging, physicians routinely ask that labs be drawn when the patient receives dialysis. However, while pre-dialysis chemistries may aid in prescribing the correct dialysis bath, drawing electrolytes post-dialysis can be misleading. Low potassium levels which may be observed immediately after dialysis increase over the next several hours, and immediate repletion may result in hyperkalemia.[7] This effect is more pronounced in patients with high pre-dialysis serum potassium concentration and in patients with massive intracellular release of potassium as seen in tumor lysis syndrome and rhabdomyolysis. In these instances, it is recommended to check serum potassium six hours after hemodialysis as these patients can develop rebound hyperkalemia and may require more frequent dialysis.

Medications

All medications that require renal excretion must be dosed properly in patients with ESRD in order to ensure efficacy and avoid toxicity. HD and PD offer variable drug clearance according to the size of the drug and degree of protein binding, and physicians should consult with a pharmacist before prescribing drugs which may require special dosing considerations. Commonly used outpatient medications in ESRD patients, such as phosphate binders, erythropoiesis stimulating agents, vitamin D derivatives and calcimimetics, should be continued during hospitalization if

Table 2. Reasons to Hold Commonly Used Outpatient Medications in ESRD Patients*

Medication	Indication for Use	When to Hold
Erythropoiesis-stimulating agents, (ESAs) (epoetin alfa, darbepoetin alfa etc.)	Anemia of chronic kidney disease	Hemoglobin >13 g/dL (consider when hemoglobin > 11 g/dL)
Phosphate binders (calcium carbonate, calcium acetate, sevelamer, lanthanum etc.)	Hyperphosphatemia	Serum phosphate <3.5 mg/dL or when patient is NPO as these agents only act by binding to phosphate present in food
Vitamin D derivatives (calcitriol, paricalcitol, doxercalciferol etc.)	Hyperparathyroidism	Intact PTH <150 or corrected total calcium >10.2 mg/dL or serum phosphate >6 mg/dL
Calcimimetics (cinacalcet)	Hyperparathyroidism	Corrected total calcium <8.4 mg/dL

*Adapted from the National Kidney Foundation Kidney Disease Outcomes Quality Initiative (NKF KDOQI).

they were adminstered prior to admission unless there are reasons to hold (see Table 2).

Some medications, such as low molecular weight heparin (LWMH), should be avoided altogether as serious bleeding complications have been reported. Certain opioids, including morphine, codeine and meperidine, should not be used because of the risk of accumulation of the parent drug or metabolites. Hydromorphone, fentanyl and methadone are better options for pain control in ESRD. Furthermore, because it is now recognized that preserving residual renal function in ESRD may be of significant benefit, nephrotoxic agents such as NSAIDs, aminoglycosides, and IV contrast dye should ideally be used sparingly or avoided when possible for patients who maintain any degree of urinary output.

Ancillary Studies

CT scans routinely require the use of hypersomolar intravenous contrast agents which may lead to volume overload in an under-dialyzed ESRD patient. Cardiac catheterizations, in particular, often use a large volume of contrast dye, especially when evaluating left ventricular function. Therefore, such procedures should be done in coordination with the nephrology team so that dialysis may be provided after the procedure in a timely fashion if necessary.

Gadolinium-containing contrast agents, used in magnetic resonance imaging, have been linked to a rare condition characterized by cutaneous and visceral fibrosis called nephrogenic systemic fibrosis (NSF) in patients with advanced kidney disease. There is currently no cure for NSF and use of gadolinium should be avoided in ESRD. If gadolinium is used, prompt dialysis post-procedure and then daily for the following 1–2 days should be considered, but whether aggressive hemodialysis prevents NSE is unknown.[8]

Opportunity for Renal Replacement Therapy Preparation and Re-Evaluation During Inpatient Hospitalization

Hospitalized patients with advanced CKD should be educated about the various types of chronic renal replacement therapy so that preparations may be made for future progression to ESRD. Arranging pre-emptive kidney transplantation may take several months or even years if a suitable donor cannot be identified. AVFs take several weeks to mature and the primary failure rate is significant. Furthermore, choosing between HD and PD is often a difficult decision for a patient. Initiating the conversation early, before an emergent situation develops, may help avoid significant morbidity later. In addition, establishing goals of care before an urgent indication for renal replacement therapy manifests is important so as to prevent initiating or continuing dialysis in a patient for whom there is no benefit.

References

1. Plantinga LC, Jaar BG. (2009) Preventing repeat hospitalizations in dialysis patients: A call for action. *Kidney Int* **76**(3): 249–251.

2. Naqvi SB, Collins AJ. (2006) Infectious complications in chronic kidney disease. *Adv Chronic Kidney Dis* **13**(3): 199–204.
3. Allon M. (2009) Treatment guidelines for dialysis catheter-related bacteremia: An update. *Am J Kidney Dis* **54**(1): 13–17.
4. Dhar S, Pressman GS, Subramanian S, *et al.* (2009) Natriuretic peptides and heart failure in the patient with chronic kidney disease: A review of current evidence. *Postgrad Med J* **85**(1004): 299–302.
5. Schanzer H, Eisenberg D. (2004) Management of steal syndrome resulting from dialysis access. *Semin Vasc Surg* **17**(1): 45–49.
6. Watson M, Abbott KC, Yuan CM. (2010) Damned If You Do, Damned If You Don't: Potassium Binding Resins in Hyperkalemia. *Clin J Am Soc Nephrol* **5**(10): 1723–1726.
7. Blumberg A, Roser HW, Zehnder C, Muller-Brand J. (1997) Plasma potassium in patients with terminal renal failure during and after haemodialysis; relationship with dialytic potassium removal and total body potassium. *Nephrol Dial Transplant* **12**(8): 1629–1634.
8. Leiner T, Kucharczyk W. (2009) NSF prevention in clinical practice: Summary of recommendations and guidelines in the United States, Canada, and Europe. *J Magn Reson Imaging* **30**(6): 1357–1363.

Chapter 35

Acute Kidney Injury

*Tonia K. Kim**

Key Pearls

- Specific laboratory tests, including the BUN/creatinine ratio, fractional excretion of sodium (FeNa), and the examination of the urinary sediment, can help distinguish between the different types of acute kidney injury (AKI) and determine the appropriate management.
- Recognizing risks of developing contrast-induced nephropathy (CIN) and employing strategies to help prevent CIN are important for minimizing renal damage.
- Anticipating some of the commonly seen electrolyte disturbances in AKI can help avert emergency situations.
- Certain medications and procedures should be avoided in AKI to prevent complications.
- Medications should be reviewed and adjusted throughout the course of AKI.

Introduction

Acute kidney injury (AKI) is defined as renal function deterioration over hours to days as measured by at least a 0.5 mg/dL creatinine increase over the baseline value or a >50% increase in creatinine over the baseline.

AKI represents a compelling spectrum of disease, owing to the frequency of its occurrence and the mortality with which it is associated.

*Mount Sinai School of Medicine, New York, NY, USA.

AKI is the current term for acute renal failure. AKI is very common in the hospital setting. One percent of patients have AKI at the time of hospital admission, 2%–5% develop AKI during hospital stay, and 4%–15% sustain AKI post-cardiopulmonary-bypass. The mortality rates for AKI can be staggering — as high as 80% in some postoperative patients. Prerenal AKI at hospital admission has been associated with approximately 7% mortality.[1]

All creatinine clearance calculations assume that the patient is in the steady state with regard to creatinine handling. In AKI, patients are not in the steady state. Therefore, the calculated creatinine clearance can be an overestimation of the patient's true glomerular filtration rate (GFR). If the patient's serum creatinine is rising every day, it is correct to assume that the patient's creatinine clearance is < 10 mL/min.

The relationship between the GFR and plasma creatinine is not linear.

- When the plasma creatinine is below 2 mg/dL, even a 0.5 mg/dL increase in creatinine represents a large decrease in the GFR.
- When the plasma creatinine is above 2 mg/dL, increases in it represent smaller decreases in the GFR.

Initial Workup of AKI

The primary tests to order upon recognition of AKI are:

- Chemistry panel including calcium, phosphorus, and liver function tests
- Urinalysis
- Random urine electrolytes, creatinine, osmolarity, and urea (if there is exposure to diuretics)
    - All from the same urine sample.
- Random urine protein/creatinine (urine P/C)
    - The urine P/C is an estimation of proteinuria and assumes there is a 1 g excretion of creatinine per day.
    - A random urine P/C of 1 is equivalent to 1 g of protein per day in a 24 hr urine collection.
    - Ensure that the units are identical in the numerator and denominator (either both are g/L or mg/dL). Otherwise, conversion is necessary for meaningful interpretation of the urine P/C.

  - The upper limit of normal is 0.2.
  - The nephrotic range is 3 or 3.5 or higher.
  - In AKI, the urine P/C can overestimate the true amount of proteinuria, because the amount of creatinine excreted can be significantly decreased.
  - The random urine microalbumin to creatinine ratio can also be used if the patient has relatively low levels of proteinuria. Microalbumin is measured in μg/dL and creatinine in mg/dL, resulting in the units of μg/mg.
- Renal and bladder ultrasound

The results of these initial tests will help guide the clinician in determining what further tests are needed. They will also lay the groundwork for discussion between the referring physician and the renal consultant in navigating the management of the patient.

Categories of AKI

- Prerenal AKI
- Intrarenal (intrinsic) AKI
- Postrenal AKI

Prerenal AKI

Definition

Prerenal AKI is AKI in which glomerular and tubular function remains intact but there is a problem in *renal perfusion*. The pathophysiology of prerenal AKI is reviewed in Fig. 1.

The clinical settings in which prerenal AKI is commonly seen are:

- Absolute decrease in effective arterial volume
  - GI or renal losses
  - Hemorrhage
- Relative decrease in effective arterial volume
  - Congestive heart failure
  - Cirrhosis (hepatorenal syndrome)

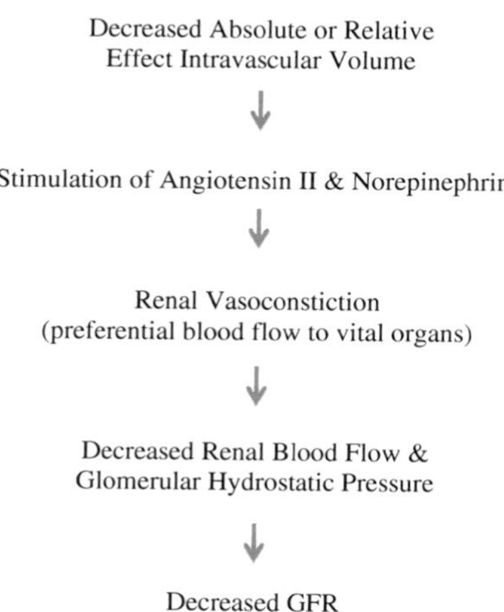

Fig. 1. Pathophysiology of prerenal AKI.

- Medications
  - Nonsteroidal anti-inflammatory drugs (NSAIDS) inhibit cyclo-oxygenase, thereby decreasing prostaglandin synthesis. The subsequent renal vasoconstriction decreases the GFR.
  - ACE inhibitors and angiotensin receptor blockers allow a greater magnitude of vasodilation in the efferent arteriole as compared with the afferent arteriole, leading to decreased GFR.
  - Tacrolimus and cyclosporine cause afferent arteriolar vasoconstriction.

Diagnosis

The diagnosis of prerenal AKI is best made by employing concepts in pathophysiology.[2] Table 1 lists laboratory tests that help delineate the diagnosis.

Treatment

- Fluid by mouth or intravenously. Isotonic solution is most effective in achieving intravascular repletion. Normal saline and intravenous fluid with sodium bicarbonate are appropriate choices. It is important to ensure that the fluid is isotonic (not hypertonic) (Table 2).

Table 1. Diagnosis of Prerenal AKI

Test	Prerenal AKI	Mechanism
Serum BUN: Cr	>20:1	Increase in proximal tubule sodium and water reabsorption. Water reabsorption increases the tubular fluid concentration of urea, leading to an increase in proximal tubular urea reabsorption down a favorable concentration gradient. Creatinine is not reabsorbed.
Urine sodium	<20 mEq/L	Decreased renal blood flow in the prerenal state is associated with an appropriate increase in proximal tubular sodium and water reabsorption. Since more sodium is reabsorbed, the urine sodium excreted is decreased.
Fractional excretion of sodium (FeNa) $\frac{U_{Na} \times P_{Cr}}{P_{Na} \times U_{Cr}} \times 100$	<1%	Since there is reabsorption of both sodium and water in prerenal states, sometimes the urine sodium will not be <20 mEq/L because the urine is so concentrated. Calculating the fractional excretion of sodium allows sodium handling to be assessed directly without the confounding effect of water reabsorption.
Urine osmolarity	>500 mOsm/kg or > serum Osm	Antidiuretic hormone (ADH) is stimulated by volume depletion, resulting in reabsorption of water (independent of sodium) at the collecting ducts.
Fractional excretion of urea (FeUrea) $\frac{U_{urea} \times P_{Cr}}{P_{urea} \times U_{Cr}} \times 100$	<35%	Loop diuretics (NaK2Cl transporter inhibitor at the loop of Henle) and thiazide diuretics (sodium chloride transporter inhibitor at the distal tubule) render the evaluation of urine sodium or FeNa less accurate. Urea is predominantly handled in the proximal nephron, thereby allowing the evaluation of the true volume status of the patient despite loop diuretics or thiazides.

Table 2. Isotonic Intravenous Fluids

IVF	Sodium Content	Important Elements to Monitor Before and During Infusion
Normal saline	154 mEq	• Excessive hydration with NS can be associated with a dilutional acidosis.
½ NS with 75 mEq sodium bicarbonate	152 mEq	• Avoid bicarbonate in lactic acidosis (unless pH < 7.1 or 7.2), because it can worsen lactic acidosis. • Alkalization can decrease ionized calcium. Ensure ionized calcium is normal or near-normal prior to infusion and monitor ionized calcium during infusion. • Alkalization can cause hypokalemia. Monitor potassium.
D5W with 150 mEq sodium bicarbonate	150 mEq	• Ensure lactic acidosis is not present. • Monitor ionized calcium as above. • Monitor glucose due to the D5W.
Plasmalyte or lactated ringers	140 mEq	• May want to avoid in AKI, given the potassium content (5 mEq/L).

- Reverse the underlying cause of hypoperfusion. Prerenal AKI with absolute decrease in effective arterial volume reverses relatively quickly with fluids. Optimizing cardiac output in CHF and hepatic function in cirrhosis can improve renal function. Prolonged prerenal AKI can lead to tubular damage, which can become irreversible.

Intrarenal (Intrinsic) AKI

Definition

Intrarenal AKI is AKI in which there is direct injury to kidney parenchyma.

There are certain aspects in the history or lab findings which will heighten suspicion that the AKI is intrarenal. The clinical settings in which intrarenal AKI is commonly seen are listed in Table 3.

Table 3. **Clinical Settings for Intrarenal (Intrinsic) AKI**

Part of Nephron Involved	Diseases	Features
Glomerular disease	Nephritic or nephrotic syndromes (nephritic diseases are more commonly associated with AKI than nephrotic)	• Proteinuria ≥3 or 3.5 g per day in nephrotic diseases; less in nephritic. • Presence of hematuria in nephritic diseases; not predominant feature in nephrotic. • Consider renal biopsy.
Interstitial disease	Acute interstitial nephritis (AIN)	• Associated with certain antibiotics (penicillins and cephalsporins).
Tubular disease	Acute tubular necrosis (ATN)	• Ischemic: hypotension • Toxic: IV contrast for CT scan and cardiac catheterization, aminoglycoside, other medications, myoglobin in rhabdomyolysis, hemoglobin in hemolysis.

Diagnosis

The urinalysis, urine electrolytes, and urinary sediment are key factors in making this distinction (Table 4).

Treatment

Removal of the inciting cause and supportive therapy are the core components of treatment of intrarenal AKI. Hyperkalemia is often encountered in AKI. The details of management of hyperkalemia are covered in a separate chapter. Obtaining an EKG is a critical step in the management. Hyperkalemic EKG changes warrant initiation of telemetry monitoring.

Table 4. Diagnosis of Intrarenal (Intrinsic) AKI vs. Prerenal AKI

Test	Prerenal AKI	Intrarenal AKI
Serum BUN: Cr	>20:1	< 20:1
Urine Na (mEq/L)	< 20	> 20
Fractional excretion of sodium (FeNa)	< 1%	> 1%
Urine osmolarity	>500 mOsm/kg or > serum Osm	~ 300 mOsm/Kg (very similar to plasma Osm)
Fractional excretion of urea (FeUrea)	<35%	>35%
Urine sediment	Normal	Glomerular: RBCs or RBC casts in nephritic diseases. Interstitial: WBCs or WBC casts in AIN. Tubular: muddy-brown granular casts in ATN.

Potassium should be frequently checked throughout the treatment, as repeat rounds of therapy to further decrease the potassium may be necessary. Hyperkalemia refractory to medical treatment is an important indication for dialysis.

Prevention of Contrast-Induced Nephropathy

The pathology of contrast-induced nephropathy (CIN) is ATN. The specific pathogenesis remains unclear. Toxic and ischemic injury mediated in part by reactive oxygen species is seen in animal and *in vitro* studies.[3]

The risk factors for developing CIN include:

- Chronic kidney disease (elevated baseline creatinine and/or proteinuria)
- Diabetes
- Age >75 years
- Volume depletion around the time of the contrast administration
- CHF

- Cirrhosis
- Hypertension
- NSAID use
- Hypotension
- Volume of contrast

Prognosis of CIN

Most cases of CIN occur within 24–72 hr of contrast administration. Creatinine can return to the baseline within 3–10 days. However, there are cases in which the creatinine remains above the baseline. Thirteen to 50% of patients with CIN who require dialysis after contrast exposure become dialysis-dependent.[4,5]

Prevention of CIN

- Low osmolar contrast medium at the lowest possible dose.
- Intravenous fluid with either normal saline or ½ NS. A dose commonly used is 1 mL/kg/hr 12 hr before contrast administration and 12 hr after administration.
- Intravenous fluid with bicarbonate
    - Some studies cite intravenous fluid with sodium bicarbonate (at 3 mL/kg/hr 1 hr bolus before contrast administration, then 1 mL/kg/hr for 6 hr after administration) as being superior to other forms of hydration.[6,7]
    - Can order ½ NS with 75 mEq of sodium bicarbonate. Can opt to lower the bolus dose, especially in elderly patients or any patient easily susceptible to volume overload.
- *N*-acetylcysteine — results of studies have been inconsistent, but report few adverse effects.[8] The most commonly used dose is 600 mg orally every 12 hr on the day before contrast, and every 12 hr on the day of contrast (for a total of four doses).

Postrenal AKI

Postrenal AKI is defined as AKI from the obstruction of urinary outflow tracts.

The clinical settings in which postrenal AKI is commonly seen are:

- Benign prostatic hypertrophy (BPH)
- Prostate cancer
- Cervical cancer
- Bladder or urological tumor
- Large bilateral kidney stones (rare) or obstructing kidney stones in the setting of a solitary kidney

The pathophysiology of postrenal AKI is based on Starling's forces. The driving force for the GFR depends on the glomerular hydrostatic pressure being greater than the capsular (Bowman's capsule) hydrostatic pressure. In postrenal AKI, the obstruction causes an increase in the capsular hydrostatic pressure, thereby decreasing the net outward pressure. This effect decreases the GFR.

Diagnosis

Placement of a Foley catheter or imaging with ultrasound can diagnose postrenal AKI.

Treatment

Foley catheter placement can treat postrenal AKI if the obstructing lesion is at or below the bladder neck. If the obstruction is above this level, percutaneous nephrostomies or surgical stent placement is required. Prompt relief of obstruction is critical, because the longer the obstruction is present, the lower the likelihood of returning to baseline creatinine will be.

Obstruction leads to tubular dysfunction and inability to reabsorb sodium and urea. After the obstruction is relieved, postobstructive diuresis (an osmotic diuresis) can occur from this additional solute. Therefore, it is very important to closely monitor urine output after relief of obstruction.

Intravenous Fluids for Postobstructive Diuresis

The kidney's ability to concentrate and dilute the urine is impaired in obstruction. In postobstructive diuresis, the most appropriate fluid is ½ NS. The rate of ½ NS can be 2/3 mL for every 1 mL of urine output. Frequent re-evaluation of urine output (at least every 8 hr) must be done to assess changes needed in the intravenous fluid rate. More frequent re-evaluation is required in large volumes of polyuria.

Parameters to Monitor in Postobstructive Diuresis

- Vitals: hypotension and tachycardia can result from falling behind in fluid repletion. Strict "ins and outs," daily weights, and lung exams are essential.
- Electrolyte and acid/base disturbances in postobstructive diuresis are outlined in Table 5.[9] Checking a chemistry panel at least every 8 hr is necessary. More frequent testing may be needed if the projected 24 hr urine output is excessive.

Medications and Procedures in AKI

It is prudent to avoid certain common medications and procedures in AKI (see Table 6). Since creatinine clearance is assumed to be < 10 mL/min in a patient whose creatinine is rising daily, medication dose adjustment is important in order to prevent possible untoward effects due to overdosage (such as antibiotics, digoxin, famotadine, allopurinol, or colchicine).

Renal Consult for AKI

Involving nephrologists earlier in the course of management may be beneficial if the initial tests show renal AKI, or if there are significant electrolyte or acid/base disturbances in any form of AKI. If there is significant proteinuria or hematuria in a patient with resolving or resolved prerenal AKI, a renal consult can determine if there is any underlying renal parenchymal disease. Nephrologists can also help determine if a renal

Table 5. Electrolyte and Acid/Base Disturbances in Postobstructive Diuresis

Blood Chemistry	Changes Observed in Postobstructive Diuresis	Mechanism
Sodium	Increased	Water and salt excretion are increased after obstruction is relieved. If urine output is not adequately matched in the setting of postobstructive diuresis, hypernatremia may ensue. However, if there is excessive repletion of urine output with hypotonic solution, hyponatremia results.
Potassium	Decreased	Polyuria is associated with increase in potassium excretion.
Magnesium	Decreased	Polyuria is associated with increase in magnesium excretion.
Bicarbonate	Decreased	Defective urinary acidification.

Table 6. Medications and Procedures to Avoid in AKI

Low-molecular-weight heparin	Patients with AKI or creatinine clearance < 30 mL/min have elevated anti-Xa, placing them at higher risk for major bleeding events.[10]
Phosphate-containing laxatives or enemas	Calcium phosphate deposits have been associated with acute phosphate nephropathy in certain patients (AKI and deaths are reported).[11]
Meperidine	The accumulation of a metabolite (normeperidine) in renal impairment lowers the seizure threshold in patients with AKI.[12] Hydromorphone is the preferred narcotic in AKI or CKD.[13]
NSAIDS	Renal vasoconstriction induced by NSAIDS reduces GFR
Metformin	Discontinue in patients with AKI or creatinine clearance < 60–70 mL/min, men with serum creatinine > 1.5 mg/dL, or women with serum creatinine > 1.4 mg/dL.[14]

(*Continued*)

Table 6. (*Continued*)

Peripherally inserted central venous catheters (PICCs)	PICCs will sclerose the entire length of the vein in which it is inserted. Since there is a chance that a patient with AKI can progress to CKD, preserving the integrity of veins is important for possible future arteriovenous access for dialysis. Hickman catheters (inserted in the internal jugular vein) are preferred if long term intravenous access is required.
Subclavian vein central lines	Subclavian lines can cause central venous stenosis, rendering all veins distal to this site inadequate for future AV fistula use. Internal jugular lines are preferred.
CT with intravenous contrast	See section on CIN.
MRI with gadolinium	Gadolinium in patients with AKI or creatinine clearance <30 mL/min is contraindicated, owing to the possibility of nephrogenic systemic fibrosis, which has been associated with reported fatalities.[15]

biopsy is warranted, and assess the indications for and the timing of dialysis initiation if there is no recovery.

References

1. Thadhani R, Pascual M, Bonventre J. (1996) Acute renal failure. *New Engl J Med* **334**: 1448–1460.
2. Carvounis C, Nisar S, Guro-Razuman S. (2002) Significance of the fractional excretion of urea in the differential diagnosis of acute renal failure. *Kidney Int* **62**: 2223–2229.
3. Katholi R, Woods W Jr, Taylor G, *et al.* (1998) Oxygen free radicals and contrast nephropathy. *Am J Kidney Dis* **32**: 64–71.
4. Tepel M, Van der Geit M, Schwartzfeld C, *et al.* (2000) Prevention of radiographic-contrast-agent–induced reductions in renal function by acetylcysteine. *New Engl J Med* **343**: 180–184.
5. Rudnick M, Berns J, Cohen R, Goldfarb S. (1994) Nephrotoxic risks of renal angiography: Contrast-media associated nephrotoxicity

and atheroembolism — A critical review. *Am J Kidney Dis* **24**: 713–727.
6. Merten G, Burgess W, Gray L, *et al.* (2004) Prevention of contrast-induced nephropathy with sodium bicarbonate: A randomized controlled trial. *JAMA* **291**(19): 2329–2334.
7. Sankar D, Navaneethan, Singh S, Appasamy S, *et al.* (2009) Sodium bicarbonate therapy for prevention of contrast-induced nephropathy: A systematic review and meta-analysis. *Am J Kid Dis* **54**: 617–627.
8. Barnett J, Parfrey P. (2006) Preventing nephropathy induced by contrast medium. *New Engl J Med* **354**: 379–386.
9. Zeidel M, Pirtskhalaishvili G. (2004) Urinary tract obstruction. In: Brenner B (ed.), *Brenner and Rector's The Kidney* Saunders, Philadelphia, pp. 1880–1885.
10. Lim W, Dentali F, Eikelboom J, Crowther M. (2006) Meta-analysis: Low-molecular-weight heparin and bleeding in patients with severe renal insufficiency. *Ann Intern Med* **144**: 673–684.
11. Markowitz G, Perazella M. (2009) Acute phosphate nephropathy. *Kidney Int* **76**: 1027–1034.
12. Davies G, Kingswood C, Street M. (1996) Pharmocokinetics of opioids in renal dysfunction. *Clin Pharmacokinet* **31**: 410–412.
13. Murphy E. (2005) Acute pain management pharmacology for the patient with concurrent renal or hepatic disease. *Anaesth Intensive Care* **33**: 311–325.
14. DeFronzo R. (1999) Pharmacologic therapy for type 2 diabetes mellitus. *Ann Intern Med* **131**: 281–303.
15. Kuo P, Kanal E, Abu-Alfa A, Cowper S. (2007) Gadolinium-based MR contrast agents and nephrogenic systemic fibrosis. *Radiology* **242**: 647.

Chapter 36

A Practical Approach to Acid-Base Disturbances

*Jaime Uribarri**

Key Pearls

- At least two of three components in the Henderson-Hasselbalch equation (pH, pCO_2 and HCO_3) need to be known to make an accurate diagnosis of a primary acid-base disorder. A low HCO_3 in the serum chemistry profile alone does not allow making the diagnosis of primary metabolic acidosis.
- A set of blood-gas and electrolyte results cannot be interpreted independent of the clinical details and knowledge of the condition being diagnosed — a normal blood gas may represent perfectly compensated metabolic alkalosis and acidosis in a renal failure patient who is vomiting.
- The urinary anion gap is useful to differentiate between gastrointestinal (GI) and renal causes of a hyperchloremic metabolic acidosis. A negative urinary anion gap suggests GI loss of bicarbonate (e.g. diarrhea), while a positive urinary anion gap suggests impaired renal distal acidification (e.g. distal renal tubular acidosis).
- Serum osmolal gap of $\geq$ 25 mOsm/kg, in the absence of obvious causes, such as alcohol intake, strongly suggests methanol or ethylene glycol intoxication.
- The most common cause of an increased anion gap is errors in measurements of sodium, chloride or total CO_2.

*Mount Sinai School of Medicine, New York, NY, USA.

Initial Considerations

Arterial blood gas is not a routine blood test and can be replaced by venous blood gas when only assessing acid-base balance. The arterial blood gas machine usually has electrodes for direct measurement of pH, PCO_2 and PO_2 and the HCO_3 is estimated from the first two using the Henderson-Hasselbalch equation.

The HCO_3 from serum chemistries is actually total CO_2 and is therefore slightly higher than true HCO_3 by about 1 mEq/l. Because of this reason and the fact that actual HCO_3 is slightly higher in venous than arterial blood, the total CO_2 obtained from venous blood (serum chemistry profile) is expected to be about 2 mEq/l higher than the actual HCO_3 estimated from arterial blood.

A common misconception is that total $CO_{2,}$ because it is measured directly, is more reliable than HCO_3 estimated from arterial blood gas. There is no *a priori* reason to justify this statement. If pH and pCO_2 are measured correctly, the estimated HCO_3 should be very reliable. Moreover, there are many potential mistakes in measuring venous total CO_2 including: difficulty obtaining blood requiring use of tourniquet and local increase of CO_2, small amount of blood in the vacuum tube which may be left uncovered with gas CO_2 escaping before actual measurement, etc.

Metabolic Acidosis

Definition: Blood pH < 7.35 with serum $HCO_3 < 22$ mEq/L

Causes

1. Extrarenal:

   - Endogenous generation of acids: DKA, lactic acidosis
   - GI HCO_3 loss (diarrhea, enteric fistula, etc.)
   - Administration of acid (NH_4Cl, cholestyramineHCL, sevelamerHCL, hyperalimentation solutions containing arginine HCl or lysine HCl)

2. Renal:
   - Renal HCO_3 loss (proximal RTA)
   - Failure to regenerate HCO_3 (uremia or type I and type IV RTA).

Classification of metabolic acidosis by anion gap:

AG = Na–(Cl + HCO_3) and is normally about 12 mEq/L

High AG acidosis (normochloremic):

- DKA
- Beta-hydroxybutyric acidosis
- Lactic acidosis
- D-lactic acidosis (suspect in short bowel syndrome with metabolic encephalopathy)
- Pyroglutamic acidosis (use of acetaminophen in critically ill patient)
- Uremic acidosis (serum creatinine ≥ 5 mg/dL)
- Ingestion of toxins: (a) ethylene glycol with antifreeze (urinary oxalate crystals); (b) methanol with bootlegged alcohol (ophthalmic neuritis); (c) salicylates (both metabolic acidosis and respiratory alkalosis)

Normal AG acidosis (hyperchloremic):

- Renal tubular acidosis (RTA)
- GI HCO_3 loss
- Use of carbonic anhydrase inhibitors such as acetazolamide (Diamox)
- Early uremic acidosis
- Urinary diversion procedures: ureterosigmoidostomy, ileal conduit
- Dilutional acidosis
- Acidosis following respiratory alkalosis
- Administration of chloride-containing acids: NH_4Cl, sevelamer-HCl

Clinical Manifestations

They are variable depending on the severity and chronicity of the acidosis. Acute severe acidosis can lead to cardiovascular collapse with hypotension and shock. Chronically, acidosis induces protein breakdown, osteomalacia and in children, failure to grow.

Compensatory Mechanisms

Compensation is achieved by hyperventilation that reduces pCO_2 according to the following formula: $\Delta pCO_2 = \Delta HCO_3 \times 1.2 \pm 2$

Diagnosis

The diagnosis is suggested by a low total CO_2 in the blood chemistry profile together with the clinical picture, but has to be confirmed with blood gas measurement (low HCO_3 and low pH). Next, the AG is calculated and the patient is assessed for the conditions listed above.

Treatment

In extrarenal acidosis the emphasis is on therapy of the underlying cause of acidosis, such as lactic acidosis. In renal acidosis, therapy with $NaHCO_3$ 650 mg po tid should be initiated and titrated upwards. In acute severe acidosis (in general, pH $\leq$7.2), intravenous alkali administration is indicated, starting with 2 ampoules of $NaHCO_3$ (44.6 mEq/ampoule) and repeating pH measurement; the goal should be to raise the blood pH to just above 7.20 while the underlying problem is corrected.

Metabolic Alkalosis

Definition: Blood pH > 7.45, with serum HCO_3 > 26 mEq/L

Causes:

Metabolic alkalosis requires simultaneously a mechanism to raise serum HCO_3 concentration as well as a mechanism to maintain the high serum HCO_3 concentration.

Causes of high serum HCO_3 concentration:

- Excessive endogenous production of HCO_3: GI H^+ loss (vomiting, nasogastric suction), renal H^+ loss (K depletion), intracellular H^+ shift

(K depletion), conversion of organic anions (ketones, lactate) to HCO_3 (recovery phase of organic acidosis).

- Ingestion of HCO_3 or its precursors (citrate, etc.)
- Contraction alkalosis (sudden decrease in extracellular fluid volume caused by loop diuretics).

Mechanisms maintaining high serum HCO_3 concentration:

- Low effective arterial volume
- K^+ depletion
- Hypercalcemia
- Hypoparathyroidism
- Severe renal failure

Clinical Manifestations

Clinical manifestations commonly include tetany and increased neuromuscular irritability, but metabolic alkalosis may also lead to metabolic encephalopathy with confusion or even coma.

Compensatory Mechanisms

Compensation is achieved by hypoventilation that results in high pCO_2 according to the formula: $\Delta pCO_2 = \Delta HCO_3 \times 0.7 \pm 5$.

Partly because of the hypoxemia that follows hypoventilation, compensation in metabolic alkalosis is very ineffective and incomplete.

Diagnosis

The diagnosis is suggested by a high total CO_2 in the blood chemistry profile together with the clinical picture, but it has to be confirmed with blood gas measurement (high HCO_3 and high pH). The next step should be assessing the patient for a cause of increased serum HCO_3 and what keeps it high.

Treatment

- Clinically, the most common factors sustaining metabolic alkalosis are K depletion and low effective arterial volume. Thus, administration of K and fluids is usually very effective in correcting metabolic alkalosis.
- Acetazolamide. Increased urinary excretion of HCO_3 can be obtained by using carbonic anhydrase inhibitors such as acetazolamide (250 mg po or intravenously bid), with close follow up of serum K levels.
- Administration of acid. In cases of severe alkalosis (pH >7.55 and serum HCO_3 >40), especially in conditions such as cardiac arrythmias, hepatic encephalopathy, IV administration of an acid could effectively reduce serum HCO_3 (arginine-HCl, lysine-HCl or dilute HCl acid [0.1N HCl] at a rate of about 0.2 mEq/kg/hr with frequent titration of arterial blood gases).

Respiratory Acidosis

Definition: Blood pH <7.35 (can be normal with good compensation) and pCO_2 >40 mmHg.

Causes — any factor causing inadequate ventilation leading to CO_2 retention:

1. Pharmacological CNS suppression: Drugs
2. Neuromuscular problem affecting breathing
3. Trauma or disease of the thoracic cage
4. Primary alveolar hypoventilation
5. Airway obstruction
6. Acute or chronic lung diseases.

Clinical Manifestations

Respiratory acidosis may be asymptomatic, if well compensated. There may be symptoms due to hypoxemia. Acute pCO_2 elevation produces a metabolic encephalopathy with confusion, asterixis and even coma.

Compensatory Mechanisms

Normal compensation raises HCO_3 by tissue buffering (very fast, within seconds by the formula: $\Delta HCO_3 = \Delta pCO_2 \times 0.07 \pm 1.5$), and then by increased renal excretion of acid (in many hours or days; formula: $\Delta HCO_3 = \Delta pCO_2 \times 0.4 \pm 3$).

Diagnosis

The diagnosis is usually suspected based on a clinical presentation, but should be confirmed by blood gas measurement (low pH and high pCO_2).

Treatment

Treatment of the underlying process causing CO_2 retention will correct respiratory acidosis. Acutely, the patient may require intubation and mechanical ventilation, regardless of the cause.

Respiratory Alkalosis

Definition: Blood pH >7.45 (but it could be normal with good compensation) and pCO_2 <40 mmHg.

Causes (anything that produces hyperventilation leading to low pCO_2):

- Hypoxia: High altitude, ventilation/perfusion abnormalities, alveolar capillary block
- CNS disorders such as stroke, infection
- Drugs that stimulate the respiratory center: Salicylates, progesterone
- Psychogenic hyperventilation
- Reflex stimulation of the respiratory center by any process causing lung stiffness such as pneumonia or congestion
- Hepatic failure
- Early gram-negative sepsis.

Clinical Manifestations

Chronic respiratory alkalosis tends to be asymptomatic, but acute alkalosis produces symptoms of dizziness, nervousness, paresthesias, tetany and altered level of consciousness.

Compensatory Mechanisms

Normal compensation lowers HCO_3 by tissue buffering (very fast, within seconds by the formula: $\Delta HCO_3 = \Delta pCO_2 \times 0.2 \pm 2.5$), and then by decreased renal excretion of acid (in many hours or days; formula: $\Delta HCO_3 = \Delta pCO_2 \times 0.2 \pm 2.5$).

Diagnosis

The diagnosis is usually suspected based on clinical presentation, but should be confirmed by blood gas measurement (high or normal pH, low pCO_2 and low serum HCO_3). Once the diagnosis of respiratory alkalosis is confirmed, the patient should be assessed taking into consideration the conditions listed above in relation to the clinical picture.

Treatment

- Correction of underlying disorder whenever possible
- Rebreathing bag. Breathing into a paper bag may be used for suppression of symptoms in acute alkalosis
- Sedation. This is particularly effective in psychogenic hyperventilation
- Pharmacological paralysis of respiratory muscles and mechanical ventilation. This may be necessary in cases of severe alkalosis when its cause cannot be rapidly eliminated.

Mixed Acid-Base Disorders

This is a clinical condition in which two or more primary acid-base disorders coexist. For example, the following acid-base disorders may

Table 1. Common Causes of Mixed Acid-Base Disorders

Mixed Acid-Base Disorder	Examples
1) Metabolic acidosis and respiratory acidosis	a) Respiratory failure with anoxia
2) Metabolic alkalosis and respiratory alkalosis	a) Congestive heart failure and vomiting b) Diuretic therapy and hepatic failure c) Diuretic therapy and pneumonia
3) Metabolic alkalosis and respiratory acidosis	a) Diuretic therapy and chronic obstructive airway disease b) Vomiting and chronic obstructive airway disease
4) Metabolic acidosis and respiratory alkalosis	a) Salicylate overdose b) Septic shock c) Sepsis and renal failure d) Congestive heart failure and renal disease failure
5) Metabolic alkalosis and metabolic acidosis	a) Diuretic therapy and ketoacidosis b) Vomiting and renal failure c) Vomiting and lactic acidosis or ketoacidosis

present together: respiratory alkalosis with metabolic acidosis; respiratory alkalosis with metabolic alkalosis; metabolic acidosis with respiratory acidosis; metabolic alkalosis with respiratory acidosis or metabolic acidosis with metabolic alkalosis.

A mixed acid-base disorder should be suspected in the following situations:

- Clinical background that suggests a combined mechanism; for example, a known CO_2 retainer who now develops severe diarrhea with expected GI HCO_3 loss;
- Whenever blood pH approaches normal despite abnormal PCO_2 and HCO_3;
- When the blood gas shows ΔPCO or ΔHCO_3 outside the predicted range using the formulas above.

Interpretation of Blood Gas Measurements

Determine the primary problem:

Step 1: Assess the pH to determine whether it is within the normal rage (7.35–7.45), low (acidemia) or high (alkalemia).
Step 2. If the pH is abnormal, assess the pCO_2 level to determine whether it is primarily a respiratory or metabolic problem. If the pH and pCO_2 are moving in opposite directions (e.g. pH rises while pCO_2 falls), the problem is primarily respiratory in nature.
Step 3. Just to confirm, now assess the serum HCO_3. If the pH and HCO_3 are moving in the same direction, the problem is primarily metabolic in nature.
Step 4. Check the compensatory response. If the observed compensation is not the expected compensation, it is likely than more than one acid-base disorder is present.

In general, a normal pH accompanied by an abnormal pCO_2 or HCO_3 indicates a mixed metabolic-respiratory disorder. Over- or undercompensation does not occur and is only indicative of another primary acid-base disorder. Any combination of acid-base disorder can occur, except for respiratory acidosis and respiratory alkalosis. For example, patients with a metabolic acidosis (acidemia plus a low plasma HCO_3), whose calculated pCO_2 is less than the measured value, have, in addition, an underlying respiratory alkalosis. Conversely, patients with a calculated value greater than the measured value have a primary respiratory acidosis in addition to the metabolic acidosis (provided the disorder has been present for more than a few hours).

In another example, a patient with metabolic alkalosis and a measured pCO_2 greater than 60 mmHg, or significantly greater than the value calculated from the compensation equation, is considered to have an additional underlying primary respiratory acidosis, whereas the patient with a pCO_2 less than the calculated value (provided the condition has been present for more than a few hours) has an additional respiratory alkalosis. In mixed acid-base disorders, therapeutic decisions should be based on the pH level.

References

1. Mitchell L, Halperin, Marc B, *et al. Fluid, Electrolyte & Acid-base Physiology. A Problem-based Approach*, 4th ed. Saunders, Elsevier.
2. Rose B. *Clinical Physiology of Acid-Base and Electrolyte Disorders*, 5th ed. McGraw-Hill.
3. Robert W. Schrier. *Renal and Electrolyte Disorders*, 7th ed. Kluwer/ Lippincot, Williams and Wilkins.

Chapter 37

Hyponatremia and Hypernatremia

Zygimantas C. Alsauskas[†] *and Michael J. Ross**

Key Pearls

- Hyponatremia and hypernatremia are usually caused by abnormal water balance.
- Neurologic symptoms of hyponatremia and hypernatremia are caused by changes in effective plasma osmolality.
- Assessment of volume status is key in evaluation of both hyponatremia and hypernatremia.
- Overly rapid correction of chronic hyponatremia and hypernatremia can cause central pontine myelinolysis and cerebral edema, respectively.
- Prediction equations should only be a rough guide for estimating the fluid administration rates. Frequent plasma sodium monitoring is essential in order to prevent overcorrection.

General Concepts

In most disorders of serum sodium concentration (SNa^+), the primary disturbance is abnormal handling of water.[1,2] SNa^+ reflects the ratio of sodium to water and has no relationship to the total body sodium content. Changes in SNa^+ can alter effective plasma osmolarity, leading to transcellular water shifts and potentially serious neurologic sequelae.

*Mount Sinai School of Medicine, New York, NY, USA.
[†]University of Louisville, Louisville, KY, USA.

The normal plasma osmolarity (Posm) is 275–290 mOsm/L. Urea is an ineffective osmole, i.e. it does not contribute to transcellular water shifts. Therefore, if BUN is elevated, *effective Posm* must be used when dealing with sodium disorders (effective Posm = Posm — BUN/2.8). Rising effective Posm stimulates hypothalamic osmoreceptors, causing increased ADH production in the hypothalamus (supraoptic and paraventricular nuclei) and secretion in the posterior pituitary. ADH, acting via V2 receptors, promotes insertion of water channels (aquaporin 2) into luminal membranes of collecting tubule principal cells. As a result, water is passively absorbed into hypertonic renal interstitium, promoting excretion of concentrated urine. Hypertonicity also stimulates thirst (hypothalamic receptors), leading to increased free water intake. Conversely, as effective Posm decreases, ADH secretion ceases, collecting tubules become impermeable to water, and free water is excreted in dilute urine. Hypovolemia is a powerful stimulus for ADH secretion, regardless of Posm.

Hyponatremia

Hyponatremia is defined as SNa^+ <135 mEq/L. A practical way to classify it is based on the effective Posm and volume status (see Fig. 1).

Hypertonic hyponatremia occurs due to translocation of water out of cells caused by increased concentration of extracellular osmoles (e.g. hyperglycemia, hypertonic mannitol infusion). SNa^+ decreases by about 2.4 mEq/L for each 100 mg/dL rise in glucose above normal.

Isotonic hyponatremia occurs due to absorption of large volumes of (near) isotonic solutions of glycine, sorbitol, or mannitol solutions used in transurethral prostate procedures.

Pseudohyponatremia is a lab artifact caused by severe hyperproteinemia (e.g. multiple myeloma) or severe hyperlipidemia.[3] Since Na^+ is present only in the aqueous portion of plasma, increasing the nonaqueous plasma components (protein or lipid, which normally constitutes 7% of plasma

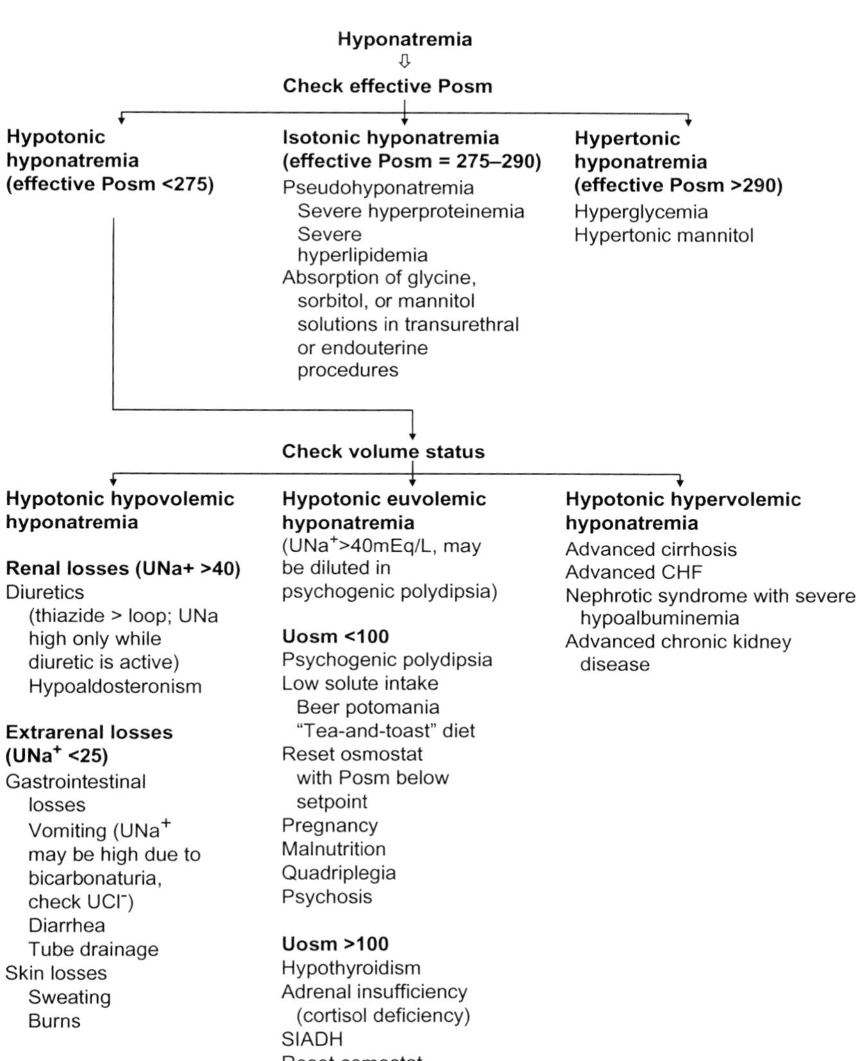

Fig. 1. Approach to hyponatremia.

volume) can factitiously lower the measured SNa^+. The use of ion-selective electrodes and direct potentiometry can control for this artifact.

Hypotonic hypovolemic hyponatremia occurs when volume-depleted persons replace fluid losses with electrolyte-free water. In this setting, decreased Posm cannot suppress ADH secretion due to the overriding effect of hypovolemia. Hyponatremia ensues due to impaired free water excretion by the kidneys.

Hypotonic euvolemic hyponatremia can occur in hypothyroidism or adrenal insufficiency, and these conditions must be excluded before diagnosing SIADH.[4] Excessive pituitary or ectopic ADH in the absence of physiologic stimuli for its secretion (hypovolemia or hyperosmolarity) causes SIADH (see Table 1). In a reset osmostat, osmotic regulation of ADH secretion occurs at a lower Posm, causing mild stable hyponatremia (125–135 mEq/L).

When ADH is suppressed, persons with normal renal function and diet can excrete large volumes of free water in the urine. For example, a person with a typical solute intake (900 mOsm/day) who dilutes urine to the minimum attainable value (50 mOsm/L) can excrete ≤18 L/day [(900 mOsm/day)/(50 mOsm/L)] of free water. Ingestion of massive quantities of fluid (e.g. psychogenic polydipsia) can overwhelm the kidneys' capacity to excrete water. When solute intake is low, e.g. 250 mOsm/day (beer potomania, tea-and-toast diet), hyponatremia may develop after drinking only ≥5 L/day [(250 mOsm/day)/(50 mOsm/L)] of fluid.

Hypotonic hypervolemic hyponatremia can occur in disease states characterized by signs of volume overload, but decreased effective arterial blood volume (EABV), including nephrotic syndrome with severe hypoalbuminemia, advanced cirrhosis, and congestive heart failure. Low EAVB activates baroreceptors and causes nonosmotic secretion of ADH. Hyponatremia is a poor prognostic factor, underscoring the severity of heart or liver disease. Free water excretion is also impaired in late stages of CKD.

In hypotonic hyponatremia, water enters brain cells, thereby increasing brain volume. When acute, it can cause neurologic symptoms, such as headache, seizures, coma, and even fatal brainstem herniation in the most

Table 1. Common Causes of SIADH

CNS or Psychiatric	Lung Diseases
• Meningitis • Encephalitis • Stroke • Intracranial hemorrhage • Brain neoplasms • Trauma • Psychosis	• Pneumonia • Acute respiratory failure • Asthma • Pneumothorax
Medications	**Miscellaneous**
• Carbamazepine • Cyclophosphamide (IV high-dose therapy) • Selective serotonin reuptake inhibitors (fluoxetine, sertraline) • Phenothiazines (thioridazine, thiothixene) • Haloperidol • Amitriptyline • Vasopressin, dDAVP • Oxytocin	• Ectopic production by carcinomas (e.g. small cell lung cancer, duodenal cancer, or pancreatic cancer) • Postoperative state • Severe nausea

extreme cases. Acute hyponatremia may become symptomatic when SNa^+ decreases to <125 mEq/L. Chronic hyponatremia, unless severe, is usually asymptomatic due to osmotic adaptation (efflux of osmolytes from brain cells, decreasing brain volume to normal).

Workup *(also see Fig. 1)*

History

- Symptoms of hyponatremia: malaise, nausea/vomiting, headache, lethargy, seizures, and coma.
- Clues to etiology in history: hypovolemia (weakness, postural dizziness, muscle cramps, diarrhea, vomiting, diuretics), volume overload (CHF, cirrhosis, nephrotic syndrome, ascites, edema, dyspnea), underlying causes of SIADH, etc.

Physical exam

- Assessment of volume status: weight changes, blood pressure, orthostatic hypotension, decreased skin turgor, dry mucous membranes, jugulovenous distension, respiratory rales, dependent edema, and ascites.

Labs

- Posm (effective Posm = Posm – BUN/2.8)
- Serum sodium, potassium, bicarbonate, BUN, creatinine, and glucose
- Uosm (indicates ADH action in the kidney)
- UNa^+

Treatment

Treatment of *hypotonic hyponatremia* should be aimed at correcting the underlying condition and normalizing SNa^+. The increase in SNa^+ must be limited to <10 mEq/L/24 hr. More rapid correction, especially in the case of chronic hyponatremia (>2 days), may cause central pontine myelinolysis, an often devastating and irreversible syndrome, manifesting as paraparesis or quadriparesis, dysphagia, dysarthria, lethargy, or coma.[5] When hyponatremia is severely symptomatic (e.g. seizures), a more rapid initial correction is appropriate, e.g. 1–2 mEq/L/hr for 2–3hr, or until symptoms abate.

In *hypotonic hypovolemic hyponatremia*, SNa^+ normalizes with volume repletion (IV 0.9% saline, oral NaCl solutions). Once the hypovolemic stimulus for ADH secretion is reversed, rapid excretion of free water ensues. Care must be taken to avoid an overly rapid rise in SNa^+, especially if the hyponatremia is chronic.

Hypotonic hypervolemic hyponatremia is treated with free water restriction in addition to optimizing therapy for underlying disease (CHF, cirrhosis). Vasopressin receptor antagonists (tolvaptan) may have a limited role in cirrhosis and CHF.[6–9]

Adrogué-Madias formula can be used to estimate the initial rate for the infusion of intravenous fluids to treat hyponatremia or hypernatremia:

$$\Delta SNa^{+} \text{ with1 L infusion} = \frac{\text{Infusate } Na^{+} + \text{InfusateK}^{+} - SNa^{+}}{TBW + 1}$$

Hyponatremia	**Hypernatremia**
A 40 year-old man (weight = 70 kg) with small cell lung cancer develops headache and somnolence, and is found to have acute hyponatremia (SNa+=120 mEq/L). A diagnosis of SIADH is made. Estimate the initial rate of 3% saline infusion to raise SNa^{+} to 130 mEq/L over 24 hr.	A 77-year-old female nursing home patient (weight = 70 kg) has had diarrhea and decreased PO intake for one week. After volume repletion with normal saline, SNa^{+}=165 mEq/L. Estimate the rate of D5 W infusion to lower SNa+ to 155 mEq/L over 24hr.
TBW = 0.6 x 70 = 42 kg. 3% NaCl $[Na^{+}]$ = 512 mEq/L. ΔSNa^{+} with 1 L infusion=[512-120]/(42 + 1) = 9 mEq/L	TBW = 0.5 x 70 = 35 kg. ΔSNa^{+} with 1L infusion = [0-165]/(35+1)=-4.6mEq/L (sodium will decrease, hence the negative value).
If the goal is to raise SNa+ from 120 to 130 mEq/L, i.e. by 10 mEq/L over 24 hr, 10/9=1.11L 3% saline would have to be infused, which amounts to 1111/24 = 46.3 mL/hr.	If the goal is to decrease her SNa^{+} from 165 to 155mEq/L, i.e. by 10 mEq/L over 24 hr, 10/4.6 = 2.2 L D5W would have to be infused, which amounts to 2200/24 = 92 mL/h. In addition, insensible losses and any ongoing losses (e.g. diarrhea) must also be replaced.

Alternatively, free water deficit can be calculated in hypernatremia, and used to estimate the rate of free water administration:

$$\text{Free water deficit } = TBW \frac{SNa^{+} - 140}{140}$$

77 year-old female, weight = 70 kg, SNa^{+} = 165 mEq/L.
Free water deficit = 0.5 x 70 x (165-140)/140 = 6.25 L.

Fig. 2. Estimating the initial rate of infusion of intravenous fluids to treat hyponatremia or hypernatremia.

SIADH is treated with free water restriction to less than 1–1.2 L/day. If hyponatremia is symptomatic or severe, more rapid correction with hypertonic (3%) saline may be required. A formula can be used to estimate the initial rate of infusion of hypertonic saline (see Fig. 2). However, it does not take into account ongoing renal and extrarenal losses water and solutes. Close monitoring of SNa^{+} is key to preventing undesirable overcorrection.

Table 2. Intravenous Solutions Used for Treatment of Sodium Disorders

D5W — dextrose (5% in water) Dextrose 5 g/100 mL Total osm 278 mOsm/L (consider this as a source of free water, as dextrose is rapidly taken up by cells and metabolized)	**½ NS — 0.45% Saline** NaCl 0.45 g/100 mL Na^+ 77 mEq/L Cl^- 77 mEq/L Total osm 154 mOsm/L
NS — 0.9% Saline NaCl 0.9 g/100 mL Na^+ 154 mEq/L Cl^- 54 mEq/L Total osm 308 mOsm/L	**3% Saline** NaCl 3.0 g/100 mL Na^+ 513 mEq/L Cl^- 513 mEq/L Total osm 1026 mOsm/L

In SIADH, Uosm is inappropriately high for Posm and is relatively fixed. Only solutions with higher osmolarity than urine can raise SNa^+ (see Table 2). Thus, 0.9% saline will worsen hyponatremia if Uosm is greater than 308 mOsm/L and therefore has only a minor role in SIADH, except perhaps for the correction of coexisting volume depletion. Loop diuretics (e.g. furosemide) can be used in conjunction with 3% saline to lower Uosm and thus facilitate free water excretion. Intravenous (conivaptan) or oral (tolvaptan) vasopressin receptor antagonists are approved for and may have a role in the treatment of SIADH. Disadvantages of vaptan use include the potential for overly rapid correction of hyponatremia, increased thirst, and high cost. Demeclocycline and lithium can induce resistance to ADH and increase free water excretion, but are rarely used to treat SIADH.

Hypernatremia

Hypernatremia is defined as $SNa^+ > 145$ mEq/L. It develops due to loss of hypotonic fluid (loss of water in excess of sodium) or, less commonly, due to excessive gain of sodium.

Table 3. **Etiologies of Central and Nephrogenic Diabetes Insipidus**

Central Diabetes Insipidus		Nephrogenic Diabetes Insipidus	
• Idiopathic • Neurosurgery • Head trauma • Cerebral anoxia or ischemia	• Primary or metastatic brain tumors • Infiltrative disorders (sarcoidosis, histiocytosis X)	• Hereditary • Hypercalcemia • Hypokalemia • Lithium toxicity • Ifosfamide	• Sickle cell nephropathy • Sjögren's syndrome • Amyloidosis

Hypernatremia rarely develops in a mobile alert person with adequate access to water and an intact thirst mechanism. In contrast, patients with altered mental status, immobility, or no access to water are prone to hypernatremia (infants, critically ill or nursing home patients). Impairment of thirst (hypodipsia) is uncommon.

Extrarenal hypotonic fluid losses occur with osmotic diarrhea (secretory diarrhea causes isotonic fluid losses), increased sweating, and increased respiratory water loss (fever, mechanical ventilation).

Central diabetes insipidus (CDI) occurs due to a defect of ADH production or secretion, whereas nephrogenic diabetes insipidus (NDI) is characterized by renal resistance to the action of ADH. (See Table 3 for a list of etiologies of CDI and NDI.) In diabetes insipidus, urine cannot be appropriately concentrated in the setting of elevated effective Posm, resulting in free water loss. Depending on the severity of the concentrating defect, diabetes insipidus can be complete (Uosm <300 mOsm/L) or partial (Uosm = 300–800 mOsm/L). Renal hypotonic fluid loss causing hypernatremia can also occur with osmotic diuresis due to hyperglycemia or mannitol, or, less commonly, with loop diuretics.

Sodium overload is an uncommon cause of hypernatremia and may occur due to hypertonic sodium bicarbonate administration during cardiopulmonary resuscitation, inadvertent hypertonic saline infusion, or massive oral salt ingestion. Mineralocorticoid excess can cause mild hypernatremia (usually <150 mEq/L) by resetting the osmostat to cause ADH secretion at higher effective Posm.

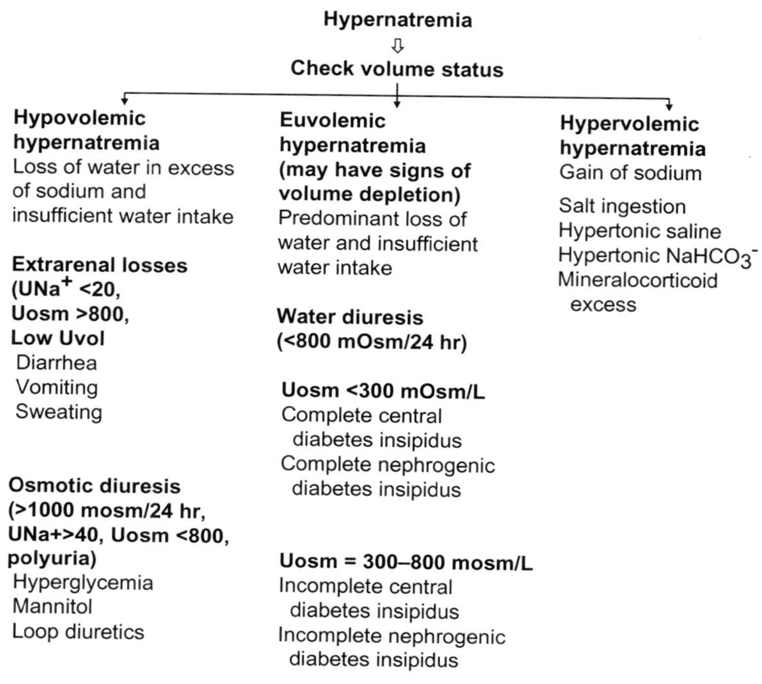

Fig. 3. Approach to hypernatremia.

Workup *(also see Fig. 3)*

History

- Symptoms of hypernatremia: weakness, lethargy, seizures, or coma.
- Clues to etiology in history: hypovolemia or volume overload, renal or extrarenal fluid losses, potential etiologies for CDI or NDI.
- Polyuria (without hyponatremia) in patients with diabetes insipidus and adequate water intake.

Physical exam

- Assessment of volume status (see section on hyponatremia).

Labs

- Uosm, UNa^+.
- Serum sodium, potassium, bicarbonate, urea nitrogen, creatinine, and glucose.
- The water restriction test may need to be performed in a consultation with a nephrologist to differentiate between psychogenic polydipsia, CDI and NDI.

Treatment

Treatment of *hypernatremia* should be aimed at correcting the underlying condition, restoring access to water, and normalizing SNa^+. The decrease in SNa^+ must be limited to <10 mEq/L/24 hr in order to avoid cerebral edema, especially if the hypernatremia is chronic (>2 days). More rapid correction may be appropriate if the hypernatremia causes severe symptoms.

In *renal* and *extrarenal hypotonic fluid losses*, treatment should be aimed at repleting the volume deficit and correcting the free water deficit. The volume deficit must be corrected quickly with 0.9% saline infusion, especially if it causes tissue hypoperfusion and organ dysfunction (e.g. hypotension, renal failure). Free water deficit can be slowly corrected by oral or intravenous free water administration (see Table 3 for available intravenous solutions). Formulas and sample calculations for estimating initial infusion rates are provided in Fig. 2. Note that these calculations do not always accurately predict the change in SNa^+ and do not take into account ongoing renal and extrarenal losses of water and solutes, and therefore close monitoring of SNa^+ is essential in order to prevent overcorrection.

Central diabetes insipidus is treated with oral or intranasal desmopressin (dDAVP). The lowest effective dose that controls polyuria is used to minimize the risk of SIADH and hyponatremia. *Nephrogenic diabetes insipidus* can be treated by inducing mild volume depletion with dietary sodium restriction and thiazide diuretics, hence increasing proximal tubular fluid absorption and minimizing distal delivery and water loss. A low protein diet decreases daily urinary osmole load (urea) and may improve polyuria. Amiloride can be used with thiazides to facilitate diuresis and prevent potassium depletion; it is uniquely useful in lithium-induced NDI by blocking its entry into tubular cells.

References

1. Adrogué HJ, Madias NE. (2000) Hyponatremia. *New Engl J Med* **342**(21): 1581–1589.
2. Adrogué HJ, Madias NE. (2000) Hypernatremia. *New Engl J Med* **342**(20): 1493–1499.
3. Nguyen MK, Ornekian V, Butch AW, Kurtz I. (2007) A new method for determining plasma water content: Application in pseudohyponatremia. *Am J Physiol Renal Physiol* **292**(5): F1652–F1656.
4. Ellison DH, Berl T. (2007) Clinical practice. The syndrome of inappropriate antidiuresis. *New Engl J Med* **356**(20): 2064–2072.
5. Brown WD. (2000) Osmotic demyelination disorders: Central pontine and extrapontinemyelinolysis. *Curr Opin Neurol* **13**(6): 691–697.
6. Decaux G, Soupart A, Vassart G. (2008) Non-peptide arginine-vasopressin antagonists: The vaptans. *Lancet* **371**: 1624–1632.
7. Schrier RW, Gross P, Gheorghiade M, *et al.* (2006) Tolvaptan, a selective oral vasopressin V2-receptor antagonist, for hyponatremia. *New Engl J Med* **355**(20): 2099–2112.
8. Gheorghiade M, Konstam MA, Burnett JC Jr, *et al.* (2007) Short-term clinical effects of tolvaptan, an oral vasopressin antagonist, in patients hospitalized for heart failure: The EVEREST Clinical Status Trials. *JAMA* **297**(12): 1332–1343.
9. Konstam MA, Gheorghiade M, Burnett JC Jr, *et al.* (2007) Effects of oral tolvaptan in patients hospitalized for worsening heart failure: The EVEREST Outcome Trial. *JAMA* **297**(12): 1319–1331.

Chapter 38

Disorders of Potassium Homeostasis

Raj K. Medapalli[†] *and Michael J. Ross**

Key Pearls

- When hyperkalemia develops in a nonoliguric patient with mild-to-moderate renal failure, renal failure is seldom the cause of hyperkalemia, and other concomitant causes should be sought.
- If ECG changes of hyperkalemia are present, emergent treatment is necessary and IV calcium should be given first to stabilize the cardiac cell membranes, in addition to interventions to lower the levels of plasma potassium.
- Hypomagnesemia is present in about 40% of patients with hypokalemia, and its correction minimizes urinary potassium losses and is a crucial component of the treatment for hypokalemia.
- Random urine potassium–creatinine ratio values greater than 25 mEq/g suggest inappropriately high renal potassium excretion in the setting of hypokalemia.
- Avoid administering intravenous potassium mixed in dextrose solutions (dextrose can lead to redistribution of potassium into cells) or in normal saline (the solution will become hypertonic). Use half-isotonic saline or sterile water for injection (SWI).

Introduction

The average dietary intake of potassium is 40–120 mEq/day.[1] The body handles this potassium load initially by transporting a portion of it

*Mount Sinai School of Medicine, New York, NY, USA.

into cells, which curtails the acute rise in the plasma potassium concentration, and subsequently by eliminating most of the potassium in the urine within 6–8 hr.[2]

Plasma concentrations of potassium, insulin and epinephrine are the major factors that promote entry of potassium into cells. An increase in plasma potassium or stimulation of insulin receptors or β_2 adrenergic receptors increases the activity of the sodium–potassium (Na–K)-ATPase pump.

The rate of potassium excretion in the urine is determined primarily by potassium secretion in the renal collecting tubule, as almost all of the filtered potassium is reabsorbed in the proximal tubule. Potassium secretion is regulated chiefly by the concentration of plasma potassium, the effect of aldosterone and the quantity of sodium and water delivered to the distal nephron.

Hyperkalemia

Hyperkalemia is defined as a plasma potassium concentration greater than 5.3 mEq/L.

Etiology

Hyperkalemia can develop due to increased potassium intake, impaired excretion of potassium, release of intracellular potassium or, often, due to a combination of these processes. It is important to note that potassium homeostasis is usually well-maintained even in patients with moderate renal failure because of an adaptive increase in Na–K-ATPase activity in the remaining functioning nephrons. Therefore, when hyperkalemia develops in a nonoliguric patient with mild-to-moderate renal failure, other concomitant causes of hyperkalemia should be sought. The causes of transcellular shifting of potassium and impaired excretion are outlined in Fig. 1.

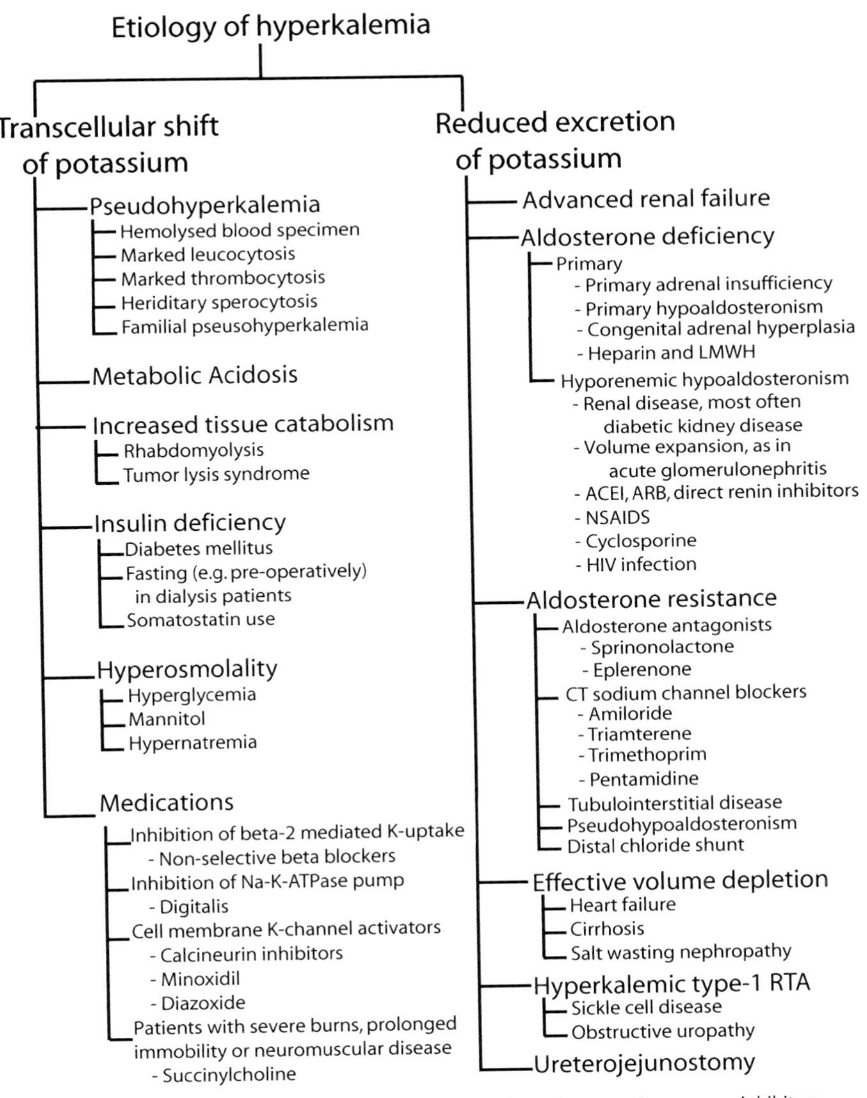
Etiology of hyperkalemia
Transcellular shift of potassium
Pseudohyperkalemia
Hemolysed blood specimen
Marked leucocytosis
Marked thrombocytosis
Heriditary sperocytosis
Familial pseusohyperkalemia
Metabolic Acidosis
Increased tissue catabolism
Rhabdomyolysis
Tumor lysis syndrome
Insulin deficiency
Diabetes mellitus
Fasting (e.g. pre-operatively) in dialysis patients
Somatostatin use
Hyperosmolality
Hyperglycemia
Mannitol
Hypernatremia
Medications
Inhibition of beta-2 mediated K-uptake
- Non-selective beta blockers
Inhibition of Na-K-ATPase pump
- Digitalis
Cell membrane K-channel activators
- Calcineurin inhibitors
- Minoxidil
- Diazoxide
Patients with severe burns, prolonged immobility or neuromuscular disease
- Succinylcholine
Reduced excretion of potassium
Advanced renal failure
Aldosterone deficiency
Primary
- Primary adrenal insufficiency
- Primary hypoaldosteronism
- Congenital adrenal hyperplasia
- Heparin and LMWH
Hyporenemic hypoaldosteronism
- Renal disease, most often diabetic kidney disease
- Volume expansion, as in acute glomerulonephritis
- ACEI, ARB, direct renin inhibitors
- NSAIDS
- Cyclosporine
- HIV infection
Aldosterone resistance
Aldosterone antagonists
- Sprinonolactone
- Eplerenone
CT sodium channel blockers
- Amiloride
- Triamterene
- Trimethoprim
- Pentamidine
Tubulointerstitial disease
Pseudohypoaldosteronism
Distal chloride shunt
Effective volume depletion
Heart failure
Cirrhosis
Salt wasting nephropathy
Hyperkalemic type-1 RTA
Sickle cell disease
Obstructive uropathy
Ureterojejunostomy
Key: LMWH: low molecular weight heparin, ACEI: angiotensin converting enzyme inhibitors, ARB: angiotensin receptor blockers, NSAIDS: non-steroidal anti-inflammatory drugs, CT: collecting tubule, RTA: renal tubular acidosis.

Fig. 1. Eitiologies of hyperkalemia organized by pathomechanism.

Clinical Manifestations

Signs and Symptoms

Symptoms of hyperkalemia are rare until the potassium concentration exceeds 6.5 mEq/L, unless the rise in the potassium concentration occurs very rapidly. When symptomatic, hyperkalemia manifests with muscle weakness and/or palpitations. Muscle weakness often develops in an ascending pattern and can progress to flaccid paralysis. Hyperkalemia can induce arrhythmias that can lead to cardiac arrest (see "ECG manifestations," below).

ECG Manifestations

The earliest ECG sign of hyperkalemia is tall, peaked T waves with a shortened QT interval, followed by progressive lengthening of the PR interval, widening of the QRS complex and eventual disappearance of the P wave. The widened QRS complex ultimately merges with the T wave to produce a sine-wave pattern, followed by ventricular fibrillation and, eventually, asystole. However, not all patients follow this classical progression and the initial ECG manifestation of hyperkalemia can be severe arrhythmia or cardiac arrest.

Workup

After ruling out fictitious causes of hyperkalemia (hemolysis during venipuncture, severe thrombocytosis, etc.), patients should be worked up to identify the underlying cause. The initial workup should include an assessment of the chronicity of hyperkalemia, an electrocardiogram and measurement of renal function. Any ongoing administration of potassium-containing medications (e.g. IV fluids and TPN solutions with potassium) should be discontinued. Conditions resulting in disturbances in the transcellular movement of potassium (Fig. 1) should be ruled out. If renal function is not severely impaired, the following additional tests should also be performed:

Transtubular potassium concentration gradient

The transtubular potassium concentration gradient (TTKG) estimates aldosterone activity by estimating the tubular fluid potassium concentration at the end of the cortical collecting tubule, where the majority of the potassium secretion occurs. It is derived using the following formula:

$$\text{TTKG} = [\text{urine potassium} \div (\text{urine osmolality/serum osmolality})] \div \text{serum potassium}$$

The TTKG is most accurate when the urine osmolality exceeds that of the plasma and the urine sodium concentration is above 25 mEq/L.

The TTKG in normal patients is 8–9 on a regular diet and above 11 after a potassium load. A value below 7 in a hyperkalemic patient is highly suggestive of hypoaldosteronism.[3]

Plasma Aldosterone Concentration and Plasma Renin Activity

Plasma aldosterone concentration (PAC) and Plasma renin activity (PRA) can be used in conjunction with the TTKG to narrow the differential diagnosis in hyperkalemic patients with normal renal function (see Fig. 2).

Treatment

Serum potassium concentration and ECG manifestations of hyperkalemia, if present, are the primary determinants of the choice of initial treatment (see Fig. 3). See Table 1 for information on dosing and pharmacodynamics of medications commonly used to treat hyperkalemia.

Emergent hemodialysis should be initiated in those patients who do not respond to medical therapy and/or if there is ongoing release of intracellular potassium, as in cases of rhabdomyolysis and tumor lysis syndrome.

In addition to instituting therapy to lower the potassium levels, the underlying cause of hyperkalemia should be sought and treated if possible. Volume status should be optimized and patients may require long-term dietary potassium restriction, treatment with loop or thiazide

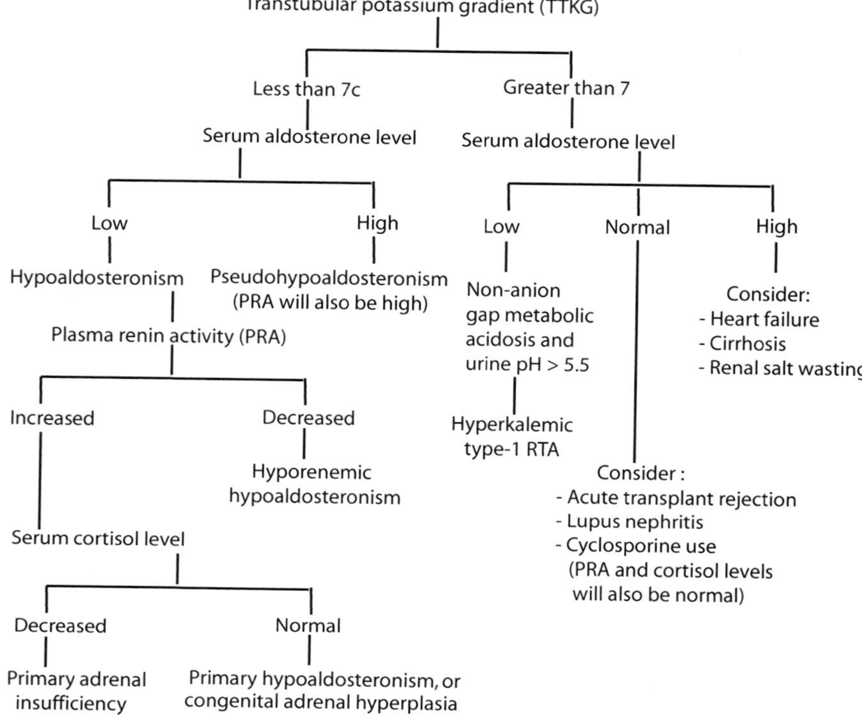

Fig. 2. Suggested approach for interpretation of transtubular potassium gradient in patients with hyperkalemia.

diuretics or, in rare circumstances, sodium polystyrene sulfate (SPS), depending on the cause of hyperkalemia.

Hypokalemia

Hypokalemia is defined as a serum potassium concentration less than 3.5 mEq/L.

Etiology

Hypokalemia is commonly encountered in hospitalized and ambulatory patients. Figure 4 shows the various causes of hypokalemia.

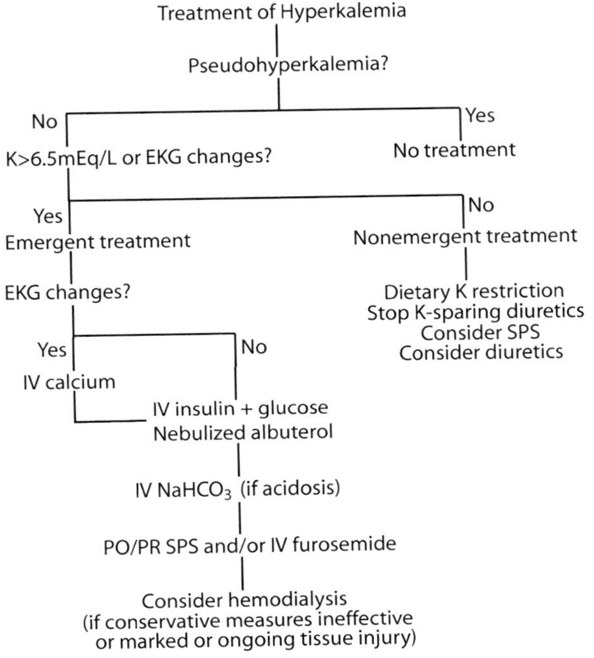

Fig. 3. Suggested approach to treatment of patients with hyperkalemia.

Decreased intake alone is rarely the culprit, as the kidney is able to lower potassium excretion to 5–25 mEq/day in the presence of hypokalemia.[4] However, decreased intake can exacerbate potassium depletion from another cause.

Hypokalemia is a common finding in alkalosis. This is often because the underlying disorder (e.g. diuretic treatment, vomiting and hyperaldosteronism) results in concomitant loss of both potassium and hydrogen ions. Alkalosis also contributes to hypokalemia, as intracellular hydrogen ions are exchanged for extracellular potassium ions to counteract the alkalosis and maintain electroneutrality.

In addition, alkalosis increases urinary potassium losses by increasing filtration of bicarbonate, exceeding the reabsorptive capacity of the proximal nephron, thereby increasing delivery of sodium and water to

Table 1. Medications Used in the Initial Treatment of Hyperkalemia

Drug	Dosage	Mechanism	Onset/Duration	Expected Effect	Comments
Calcium Gluconate or Calcium Chloride	IV: 1 amp (1 g; 10 mL of 10% solution) over 2–3 min. Can repeat once after 5 min.	Stabilizes cell membrane.	O: 5–10 min D: 30–60 min	EKG normalization	• Do not mix in bicarbonate solutions. • Central venous access required for $CaCl_2$. • $CaCl_2$ has 3 times more elemental Ca^{++}. • ↑ in Ca^{++} can cause digitalis toxicity.
Insulin + Glucose	IV: 10 units regular insulin + 1 amp D50W (50 mL of 50% glucose solution).	Drives K^+ into cells.	O: 15–20 min D: 4–6 hr	0.5–1.5 mEq/L ↓	• Use insulin alone in hyperglycemic patients.
Sodium bicarbonate	IV: 1 amp (45 mEq; 50 mL of 7.5% solution) over 5 min. Can repeat in 30 min.	Drives K into cells in exchange for H^+ ions.	O: 30–60 min D: 4–6 hr	Variable	• Most effective in patients with acidosis. • In patients with ↓Na^+, raises plasma Na^+ and counteracts EKG effects of ↑K^+.
Albuterol	INH: 10–20 mg in 4 mL Saline.	Drives K into cells.	O: 20–30 min D: 3–4 hr	0.5–1.5 mEq/L ↓	• Can cause tachycardia and angina in CAD patients.

(Continued)

Table 1. *(Continued)*

Drug	Dosage	Mechanism	Onset/Duration	Expected Effect	Comments
Furosemide	IV: ≥40 mg.	↑ delivery of Na^+ and H_2O to distal nephron, causing ↑ K^+ secretion	O: 30 min D: 2 hr	Variable	• Patients with chronic hyperkalemia typically have abnormality in renal K excretion and may not respond very much. • Large doses may be needed in renal failure.
Sodium polystyrene sulfate	PO: 15–30 g in 60–120 mL of 20% sorbitol. Repeat Q 4–6 hourly PRN. PR: 50 g in 150 mL of tap water. Retain for at least 60 min. Repeat Q 2–4 hourly PRN.	Binds K and releases Na in gut.	O: 1–2 hr (longer when given PR) D: 4–6 hr	Variable	• Avoid in the first week after surgery in postop patients and in patients with an illeus (risk of colonic necrosis). • Na^+ retention can lead to exacerbation of edema in susceptible patients.

O: onset of action; D: duration of action; CAD: coronary artery disease; IV: intravenous; INH: inhalation.

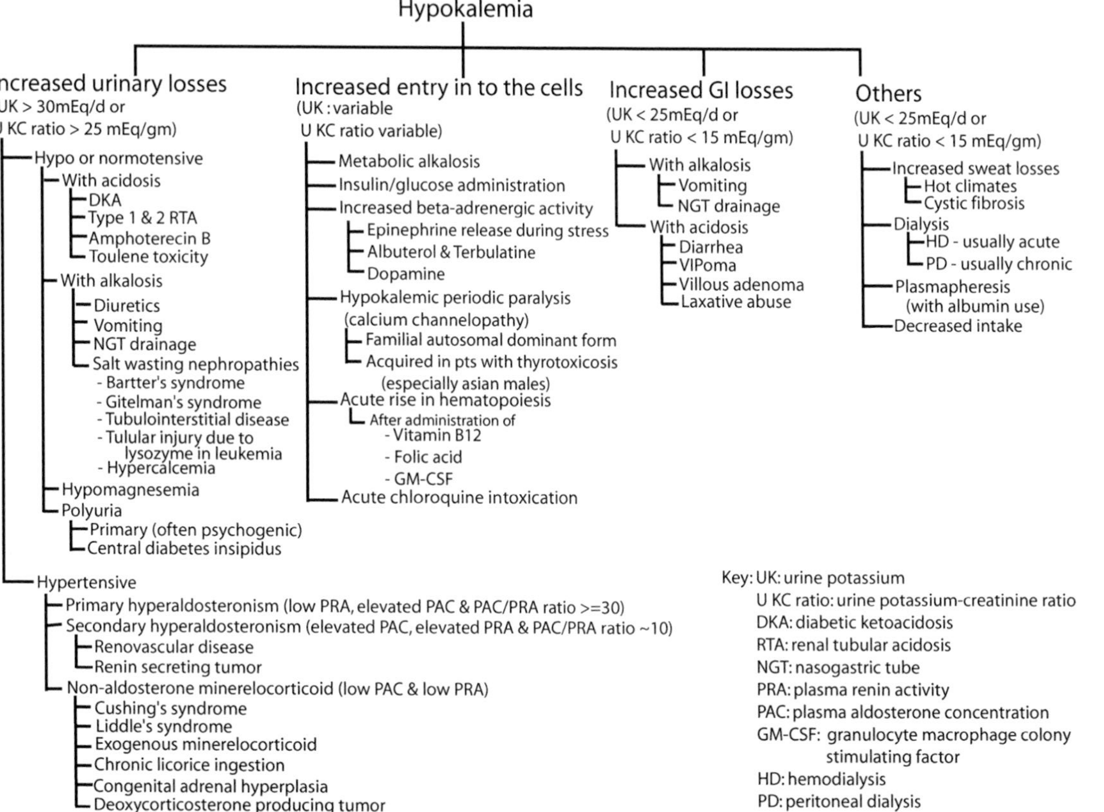

Fig. 4. Etiologies of hypokalemia organized by pathomechanism.

the collecting duct, where sodium is reabsorbed in exchange for tubular secretion of potassium and H^+.

Hypomagnesemia is present in about 40% of patients with hypokalemia, often because the underlying disorder (e.g. diuretics, vomiting, diarrhea, Bartter and Gitelman syndromes) leads to concurrent potassium and magnesium losses.[1] Though the mechanism by which hypomagnesemia increases urinary potassium excretion is incompletely understood, there is evidence that reduced intracellular magnesium increases potassium secretion by tubular cells into the tubular lumen.[5] Correction of hypomagnesemia therefore minimizes urinary potassium losses and is a crucial component of the treatment for hypokalemia in patients with concomitant hypomagnesemia.

Clinical Manifestations

Signs and Symptoms

Symptoms of hypokalemia are rare until the potassium concentration drops below 3 mEq/L, unless the plasma potassium falls rapidly or there is a predisposing factor for arrhythmias (digoxin, hypomagnesemia, coronary ischemia, drugs that prolong the QT interval and increased β-adrenergic activity). Symptomatic hypokalemia manifests with cardiac arrhythmias or muscle weakness, or both. The pattern of muscle weakness is similar to that found in hyperkalemia.

ECG Manifestations

U waves, which occur following T waves, are characteristic of hypokalemia and are most frequently seen in the lateral precordial leads (V4–V6). Hypokalemia is also associated with ST segment depression and T wave flattening.

Workup

The initial workup should include an assessment of the chronicity of hypokalemia, an electrocardiogram, arterial blood gas analysis and serum magnesium level. Conditions resulting in enhanced cellular uptake of potassium should be ruled out. Urinary potassium excretion should be assessed and, in cases where it is increased, measurement of blood pressure and acid base status can help identify the underlying cause (see Fig. 4).

Random Urine Potassium–Creatinine Ratio

The random urine potassium–creatinine ratio is usually less than 15 mEq/g creatinine when hypokalemia is caused by poor dietary intake, increased cellular uptake, or gastrointestinal losses.[6] Values greater than 25 mEq/g of creatinine suggest inappropriately high renal potassium excretion.[7]

24 hr Urinary Potassium Excretion

In patients with hypokalemia, excretion of greater than 30 mEq/day indicates excessive urinary potassium losses (except in oliguria).[1] In patients who excrete less than 15 mEq/day, renal losses are not the cause of the hypokalemia and the patient should be evaluated for extrarenal potassium losses or low intake.[1]

PAC, PRA and PAC/PRA Ratio

These tests aid in differentiating primary hyperaldosteronism, secondary hyperaldosteronism and other sources of mineralocorticoid excess (see Fig. 4).

The PAC/PRA ratio is typically calculated by measuring a morning (preferably 8 A.M.) ambulatory and paired PAC and PRA levels.[8]

ACE inhibitors, ARBs and direct renin inhibitors elevate the PRA and lower the PAC/PRA ratio. So, in a patient taking these drugs, a detectable PRA or a low PAC/PRA ratio does not exclude the diagnosis of primary hyperaldosteronism, but an undetectable PRA strongly suggests primary hyperaldosteronism.

Sprinonolactone and eplerenone should be discontinued for at least six weeks before prior testing. Amiloride and triamterene do not interfere

Table 2. Guide to Potassium Replacement

	Medication	Usual Dosing*	Comments
Oral	*Potassium chloride* Crystalline form (salt substitute): 50–65 mEq/level tsp Solution: 20 mEq/15 ml and 40 mEq/15 ml Slow release tablet: 8 mEq, 10 mEq, 15 mEq and 20 mEq.	If serum K 3.0–3.5 mEq/L: 10–20 mEq 2–4 times/day If serum K <3.0 mEq/L: 40–60 mEq 3–4 times/day. Continue until K is between 3.0 and 3.5 persistently; thereafter, reduce dose and/or frequency.	Crystalline form is the cheapest. Solution has a very bad taste. Slow-release preparation rarely causes ulcerative GI lesions. KCl preparations preferred in patients with metabolic alkalosis.
	Potassium citrate Solution: potassium citrate 1100 mg per 5 mL Powder: 3300 mg per packet	Solution: 15–30 mL QAC and HS Powder: 1 packet dissolved in water QAC and HS	Potassium citrate or bicarbonate preparations preferred for long-term use in patients with metabolic acidosis. Equivalent to 2 mEq of K and 2 mEq HCO_3 per mL. Adjust dose based on urinary pH.
	Potassium bicarbonate Tablet for oral solution: 25 mEq	25 mEq 2–4 times/day	Same as for potassium citrate.

(*Continued*)

Table 2. ***(Continued)***

	Medication	Usual Dosing*	Comments
Intravenous	*Potassium chloride* Available premixed solutions: 20 mEq in 1 L of half-isotonic saline Highly concentrated solutions in SWFI (sterile water for injection): 10 mEq, 20 mEq, 30 mEq and 40 mEq	Use in patients who cannot eat or as an adjunct to oral replacement in severe (K <3.0 mEq/L) or symptomatic hypokalemia: Max concentration through a peripheral vein: 40 mEq/L; Max concentration through a central line: 200 mEq/L; Max rate: 10–20 mEq/hr. Can use higher rates in life-threatening situations.	Avoid mixing in dextrose solutions as dextrose can lead to transient reduction in serum K^+ conc. (0.2–1.4 mEq/L) due to redistribution into cells. Avoid mixing in normal saline, as the solution will be hypertonic. Continuous EKG monitoring in patients receiving K >10–20 mEq/hr. Use concentrations >100 mEq/L only in severely symptomatic patients who cannot tolerate a large fluid load.

* Based on the assumption that there are no ongoing losses (e.g. diuretic therapy, GI losses) and that the patient does not have a chronic potassium wasting condition (e.g. diuretic therapy, primary aldosteronism, Gitelman's disease). For such patients the rate of replacement must be increased according to the rate of potassium loss.

unless the patient is on high doses. Most other antihypertensive medications can also be continued.[9]

Treatment

The initial treatment of hypokalemia is focused on normalizing the serum potassium levels, replacing magnesium (if low) and managing cardiac arrhythmias, (if present). See Table 2 for additional information on potassium replacement. The serum potassium concentration should be monitored periodically to ensure adequate repletion and to avoid hyperkalemia. Furthermore, the underlying cause of hypokalemia should be treated. Patients with ongoing losses will need chronic replacement with oral potassium preparations or the addition of a potassium-sparing diuretic.

References

1. Rose BD, Post TW. (2001) Hypokalemia. In: *Clinical Physiology of Acid-Base and Electrolyte Disorders*. McGraw-Hill, Columbus, OH, pp. 836–887.
2. Rennke HG, Denker BM (2007) Disorders of potassium balance. In: *Disorders of potassium balance*. In *Renal Pathophysiology: The essentials*. Lippincott Williams & Wilkins, Baltimore, MD, pp. 175–197.
3. Rose BD, Post TW. (2001) Hyperkalemia. In: *Clinical Physiology of Acid-Base and Electrolyte Disorders*. McGraw-Hill, Columbus, OH, pp. 888–930.
4. Rose BD, Post TW. (2001) Introduction to disorders of potassium balance. In: *Clinical Physiology of Acid-Base and Electrolyte Disorders*. McGraw-Hill, Columbus, OH, pp. 822–835.
5. Huang CL, Kuo E. (2007) Mechanism of hypokalemia in magnesium deficiency. *J Am Soc Nephrol* **18**(10): 2649–2652.
6. Groeneveld JH *et al.* (2005) An approach to the patient with severe hypokalaemia: The potassium quiz. *QJM* **98**(4): 305–316.
7. Lin SH *et al.* (2004) Laboratory tests to determine the cause of hypokalemia and paralysis. *Arch Intern Med* **164**(14): 1561–1156.

8. Weiner ID, Wingo CS. (1998) Hyperkalemia: A potential silent killer. *J Am Soc Nephrol* **9**(8): 1535–1543.
9. Gallay BJ *et al*. (2001) Screening for primary aldosteronism without discontinuing hypertensive medications: Plasma aldosterone–renin ratio. *Am J Kidney Dis* **37**(4): 699–705.

Gastrointestinal\Liver

Chapter 39

Acute Abdominal Pain in the Hospitalized Patient

Sarah Steinberg, Sita Chokhavatia* and Imuetinyan Asuen**

Key Pearls

- Acute abdomen is a surgical emergency. Early surgical consultation is mandated for the patient with abdominal rigidity and rebound tenderness, or if there is any indication of diverticulitis, cholecystitis or bowel ischemia.
- Abdominal contrast enhanced CT scan is the best initial imaging study for evaluating most patients with acute abdominal pain.
- Elderly patients often lack overt clinical findings and subacute presentations may lead to under diagnosis and treatment.
- Opiate pain management should be minimized in patients with inflammatory bowel disease (IBD), untreated *C. difficile* diarrhea, ileus and constipation.
- A pregnancy test is mandatory in all female patients of reproductive age who present with acute abdominal pain.

Acute abdominal pain accounts for 4–6% of Emergency Room visits with 24–27% of these patients being admitted to the hospital.[1,2] The first step in evaluation is identifying patients with acute abdomen, which is a surgical emergency. Presence of abdominal rigidity or rebound pain in association with nausea, vomiting, fever or leukocytosis suggests acute abdomen and

*Mount Sinai School of Medicine, New York, NY, USA.

Table 1. Differential Diagnosis of Abdominal Pain by Location

Quadrant	Right	Right, Left, Midline	Left
Upper	Cholecystitis/biliary colic Perforated duodenal ulcer Hepatic congestion/abcess	Herpes Zoster Lower lobe pneumonia Myocardial ischemia	Acute pancreatitis Splenic abscess/rupture
Lower	Appendicitis (late) Diverticulitis (Cecum, Meckel's)	Inflammatory bowel disease Gynecological Urological Incarcerated/strangulated hernia	Diverticulitis (Sigmoid)
Diffuse		Peritonitis Gastroenteritis Appendicitis (early) Mesenteric ischemia Bowel obstruction Sickle cell crisis	

demands expedited imaging tests and an immediate surgical consult. The best initial test for evaluating biliary disease is an ultrasound, and an abdominal X-ray when ileus, obstruction or perforation is suspected. CT scan is the best imaging modality for all other causes of acute abdominal pain, with the exception of bowel ischemia, which is diagnosed with MR or CT angiogram.[1] Early surgical consult should be obtained for suspected diverticulitis, cholecystitis, appendicitis or mesenteric ischemia.

Determining the location (Table 1), quality of pain and associated symptoms is essential to honing in on the correct diagnosis; age and gender further narrow the differential diagnosis. Cholecystitis, appendicitis, gynecological and urological etiologies are most common in adults <50-years old; diverticulitis in patients > 50-years old; and bowel ischemia in patients >65-years old. The most common causes of acute abdominal pain are discussed below. Small bowel obstruction, post-surgical pain, IBD, liver disease and acute GI bleeding will be addressed in subsequent chapters.

Appendicitis

Appendicitis is the most common GI cause of acute abdominal pain in18- to 50-year-old patients and constitutes 14–27% of acute abdominal pain patients seen in the Emergency Room.[1,2]

Clinical Presentation

Patients initially report periumbilical pain that later localizes to the right lower quadrant, and associated symptoms of nausea, vomiting and fever. Peritoneal signs of guarding and rebound tenderness may be elicited on examination.

Management

Initial management of suspected appendicitis should include supportive care, including intravenous fluids, pain management, and antibiotics. Early surgical consultation is required and a contrast enhanced CT can be done to confirm the diagnosis before surgery. CT criteria for acute appendicitis include an appendix larger than 6 mm and fat stranding.[1]

Acute Cholecystitis

Most commonly encountered in overweight/obese women of reproductive age and during pregnancy, acute cholecystitis also occurs in men with central obesity. Risk factors for gall bladder stones include cirrhosis, Crohn's disease, rapid weight loss, certain drugs (ceftriaxone, statins) and advanced age.[3] Elderly patients with cholecystitis are more likely to have subacute presentations and higher mortality than their younger counterparts.

Clinical Presentation

Patients rarely present with the classic clinical triad of right upper quadrant (RUQ) tenderness, fever and leukocytosis.[1] The Tokyo guidelines define three clinical criteria for cholecystitis: one local sign of inflammation (Murphy sign, mass or RUQ tenderness); one systemic sign of inflammation (fever, elevated C-reactive protein, elevated white blood cell count); and confirmatory imaging.[4]

Management

Abdominal RUQ ultrasound is the initial imaging study of choice for suspected cholecystitis. In the case of equivocal results or a study impaired by a patient's body habitus, an MRCP may be indicated, particularly if there is a suspicion of biliary obstruction. Initial management includes intravenous fluids, antibiotics, surgery and gastroenterology consultation. Ideally, cholecystectomy is done after the acute inflammation has subsided, but if the patient fails conservative management, either percutaneous drainage or cholecystostomy may be required.

Diverticulitis

Diverticulitis is a common cause of abdominal pain in patients 50 years and older. Approximately 90% of cases are left sided.[5,6]

Clinical Presentation

In addition to left lower quadrant pain, patients may report nausea, vomiting, constipation, diarrhea and urinary frequency. Peritoneal signs suggest perforation and systemic signs of inflammation such as fever and leukocytosis may be present.[6]

Management

Most patients respond to conservative management. CT scan or MRI can localize the site of inflammation. Colonoscopy is contraindicated due to risk of perforation. Surgery is indicated for recurrent diverticultis or diverticular disease complicated by perforation, abscess not amenable to percutaneous drainage or stricture causing colon obstruction. Diverticular bleeding rarely occurs with acute diverticulitis. Colonoscopy is indicated one to two months after resolution of inflammation as sigmoid colon cancer can present with symptoms similar to acute diverticulitis.[6]

Bowel Ischemia

Bowel ischemia is a rare but potentially fatal cause of acute abdominal pain in patients ≥65-years old. The majority of cases are colonic ischemia (75%), followed by acute mesenteric ischemia (25%), focal segmental ischemia (<5%) and chronic mesenteric ischemia (<5%).[5] Mesenteric ischemia is more likely to be occlusive and should be suspected in elderly patients with cardiovascular disease or younger patients with decreased blood flow to the mesentery secondary to vasculitis or a coagulation disorder.

Acute Mesenteric Ischemia

Clinical Presentation

Acute mesenteric ischemia of the small bowel presents as diffuse or focal abdominal pain with or without bloody diarrhea. The pain is often disproportionate to the physical exam. Leukocytosis, metabolic acidosis and elevated lactic acid indicate impending small bowel infarction, but are markers of advanced disease, so normal values cannot be used to rule out the diagnosis. Mesenteric ischemia may also present as a small bowel obstruction.

Management

CT or MR angiography can detect mesenteric vein obstructive emboli or thrombi but are not diagnostic for non-occlusive ischemia. All patients with suspected mesenteric ischemia should receive immediate fluid resuscitation, broad-spectrum antibiotic therapy and appropriate cardiac optimization. Although antibiotic treatment has not been well studied, it is an accepted component of standard care for mesenteric ischemia.[5]

Angiography, if performed early in a stable patient, can identify the location of ischemia, which will determine the surgical and therapeutic course. In critically ill patients who are too unstable for either angiography or surgery, diagnostic interventions are often deferred in favor of conservative management, including fluid resuscitation, antibiotic therapy and treatment of underlying illness. Thrombolytic therapy is controversial as a primary treatment but is commonly used in conjunction with embolectomy or arterial reconstruction.[5]

Colonic Ischemia

Clinical Presentation

Colonic ischemia presents with sudden onset left lower quadrant cramping pain followed by defecatory urgency and bloody diarrhea within 24 hours. Acute change in mental status is common in elderly patients.[5] The majority of colonic ischemia is secondary to hypoperfusion and usually resolves with supportive care and maintenance of hemodynamic stability.

Management

In patients with colonic ischemia, treatment of the underlying illness is key. Less common causes of colonic ischemia include acute pancreatitis, amyloidosis, coagulopathy, vasculitis, infection (*E. coli* 0157, parasites, hepatitis B, hepatitis C, cytomegalovirus), medications, surgical procedures and trauma.[5]

Iatrogenic Abdominal Pain

Abdominal pain due to iatrogenic causes can occur in all age groups. Prior surgery may be associated with the development of adhesions. Abdominal surgical scars should raise concern for adhesions and intestinal obstruction. Postoperative ileus or narcotic bowel syndrome can lead to constipation and increased abdominal pain. Patients requiring opioid analgesics should be treated prophylactically with stool softeners and laxatives. Osmotic laxatives such as lactulose can cause bloating and abdominal pain. A bowel regimen and appropriate low gas diet should be included in the systematic checklist for every hospitalized patient. Inpatients with abdominal pain should be put on a soft lactose-free diet.

Urological/Renal or Gynecological Causes of Abdominal Pain

A detailed obstetric and gynecological history is essential in the workup of all women. A pregnancy test is mandatory in all women of childbearing age prior to radiologic evaluation. Abdominal pain may be the presenting symptom in women with ectopic or intrauterine pregnancy, ovarian cyst, endometriosis, mittleshmerz and fibroids.

Urinary tract infections and nephrolithiasis are common causes of abdominal pain in young women and men respectively, with obstructive uropathy being more common in older men. Initial studies include urine analysis and culture for UTI and non-contrast CT for nephrolithiasis. Relief of abdominal pain with catheterization resulting in significant urinary output supports a diagnosis of obstructive uropathy.

General Concerns

Pain Management

Treatment with opiates can mask worsening pain or evolution of an acute abdomen, but as there is no difference in mortality when administered judiciously, opioid analgesics need not be withheld from patients requiring them for pain control.[7] Opiates should always be given with an aggressive bowel regimen to prevent ileus or constipation that may lead to further abdominal pain. Pre-existing ileus and severe constipation should deter initiation of opioid analgesics. Opiates should also be avoided in patients with untreated *C. difficile colitis* and inflammatory bowel disease as they are at high risk of developing toxic megacolon and perforation.

Geriatric Patients

Ischemic colitis and abdominal aortic aneurysm are among the most serious causes of acute abdominal pain in the elderly population. Acute cholecystitis, more common in younger patients, accounts for 25–41% of acute abdominal pain in the elderly. Biliary tract disease is the most common indication for surgery in this age group.[8] Although acute abdominal events in the elderly patient may have a subacute presentation, they often present with acute pain resulting from benign conditions such as constipation and polypharmacy.[9] The high mortality resulting from missed or delayed diagnoses underscores the importance of addressing a broad differential diagnosis in the elderly patients.[8,9]

Abdominal Pain of Unclear Etiology

Despite the wide array of diagnostic tools available, the underlying cause of acute abdominal pain is often elusive. Of all patients admitted for abdominal pain, the diagnosis remains unclear in 25% of cases on disposition from the ER and 9% of cases on discharge from the hospital, with higher rates (38% ER, 10% dicharge) for elderly patients.[10] The majority of non-specific diagnoses are later attributed to gynecological, urological, cardiac, or vascular causes. Additional diagnoses to consider include metabolic disorders (diabetic ketoacidosis adrenal insufficiency, acute intermittent porphyria), herpes zoster, muscle strain, inguinal or ventral hernia, and medication induced abdominal pain. Medication lists should be reviewed carefully. Common offenders[8] are:

- non-steroidal anti-inflammatory drugs
- antibiotics, potassium, iron
- colchicines
- oral hypoglycemics (including metformin)
- digoxin
- theophylline.

References

1. Stoker J, *et al.* (2009) Imaging patients with acute abdominal pain. *Radiology* **253**(1): 31–46.
2. Hastings RS, *et al.* (2010) Abdominal pain in the ED: A 35 year retrospective. *Am J Emerg Med* Apr 30 [Epub ahead of print].
3. Shaffer E. (2006) Epidemiology of gallbladder stone disease. *Best Pract Res Clin Gastro* **20**(6): 981–996.
4. Hirota, *et al.* (2007) Diagnostic criteria and severity assessment of acute cholecystitis: Tokyo guidelines. *J Hepatobil Pancreat Surg* **14**(1): 78–82.
5. Feldman M, Friedman LS and Brandt LJ. (2010) *Sleisenger and Fordtran's Gastrointestinal and Liver Disease*, 9th ed. Elsevier 2010.
6. Ferzoco, *et al.* (1998) Acute diverticulitis. *NEJM* **338**: 1521–1526.
7. Manterola C, *et al.* (2007) Analgesia in patients with acute abdominal pain. *Cochrane Database Syst Rev* **18**(3): CD005660.
8. Ching-Chih, *et al.* (2007) Acute abdominal pain in the elderly. *Int J Gerontol* **1**(2): 77–82.
9. Yeh EL, *et al.* (2007) Abdominal pain. *Clin Geriatr Med* **23**(2): 255–270.
10. Kizer KW and Vassar MJ. (1998) Emergency department diagnosis of abdominal disorders in the elderly. *Am J Emerg Med* **16**: 357–362.

Chapter 40

Acute Gastrointestinal Bleeding

*Jonathan Potack**

Key Pearls

- Acute gastrointestinal bleeding is a major source or morbidity and hospital admissions. The mortality from severe upper GI bleeding is 5–10%.
- Prognostic indices for patients with upper GI bleeding should be utilized early and guide triage decisions.
- Aggressive resuscitation with fluids and blood products is essential. Patients must be satisfactorily resuscitated prior to endoscopy.
- High dose acid suppression with IV bolus and continuous infusion of a proton pump inhibitor is indicated for patients who undergo endoscopic therapy for bleeding peptic ulcers.
- Early endoscopy is crucial in the management of GI Bleeding. Endoscopic therapy of peptic ulcer is guided by the appearance of the underlying lesion.

Introduction

Acute gastrointestinal bleeding (GIB) is major source of morbidity and mortality. Each year it accounts for approximately 1,000,000 hospitalizations.[1] GIB has historically been divided into upper GI bleeding (UGIB)

*Mount Sinai School of Medicine, New York, NY, USA.

when the source is proximal to the ligament of Trietz, and lower GI bleeding (LGIB) for sources distal to the ligament of Trietz. The key principles in the management of GIB are resuscitation, differentiation of upper versus lower bleeding, risk stratification and appropriate triage, medical management and definitive therapy — usually by way of endoscopy. Despite significant advances in hospital care and endoscopic therapy, mortality from severe UGIB remains at 5–10%. This chapter will address nonportal hypertension related GIB.

Clinical Presentation and Initial Assessment

Patients will present with hematemesis, melena or the passage of bright red blood per rectum (BRBPR). Hematemesis indicates an upper GI source. Melena may be due either an upper or lower source — but generally represents a small bowel or right colon lesion if the source is lower. BRBPR almost always signifies LGIB except in the patient with hemodynamic instability in which a brisk UGIB needs to be considered. Several pieces of information from the initial history can point toward a possible source of bleeding. These include risk factors for peptic ulcer, including NSAID use and *Helicobacter pylori* infection; history of chronic liver disease, which suggests portal hypertension related bleeding; and non-bloody emesis followed by hematemesis suggesting a Mallory Weiss tear. Painless BRBPR is suggestive of diverticular disease or bleeding from an AVM. The presence of abdominal pain suggests ischemia or inflammatory bowel disease. The use of anti-platelet agents or anticoagulation should be ascertained as they may lead to increased bleeding.

Vital signs including orthostatics should be obtained on all patients. All patients should be evaluated for stigmata of chronic liver disease. A digital rectal examination to classify stool color is mandatory for all patients.

Minimal laboratory examinations should include complete blood count (CBC), metabolic panel, liver function tests, PT/aPTT and a cross-match for transfusion.

Resuscitation

One to two large bore (at least 16 gauge) IVs are recommended. Crystalloid should be infused to maintain a normal systolic blood pressure and pulse. Packed red blood cells should be transfused if the hemoglobin is less than 8mg/dL; the threshold to transfuse may be lower in patients with cardiovascular disease. The decision to withhold or reverse anti-platelet agents or anticiagulation is complex and should be individualized after weighing the risks of ongoing bleeding versus the risk of thrombosis if the agent is held or reversed. Consultation with the patient's cardiologist or hematologist should be obtained in these scenarios. For patients with ongoing hematemesis and/or altered mental status, the trachea may be intubated for airway protection.[2]

Differentiation of Upper and Lower GI Bleeding

Appropriate differentiation between upper and lower bleeding has significant implications for risk stratification, medical therapy and choice of endoscopic investigation. The history and physical examination allow for determination of upper or lower GI bleeding in most cases. The placement of a nasogastric tube (NGT) is controversial. A return of fresh blood in the NG tube signifies a UGIB. However, clear or even bilious return in the NGT can be present in up to 20% of UGIB. Thus a clear or bilious return from the NGT should not preclude upper endoscopy if the clinical suspicion for an UGIB is high. There is no role for occult blood testing of NGT aspirates.

Etiology of Bleeding

The most common causes of non-variceal UGIB are peptic ulcer, esophagitis, upper GI tract malignancy, angioectasias and Mallory-Weiss tears. The most common causes of LGIB are diverticulosis, colonic neoplasia, and ischemic colitis (Table 1).

Risk Stratification

Mortality from GIB remains 5–10%. Mortality almost always occurs in patients who have ongoing bleeding despite therapy or early rebleeding

Table 1. Common Causes of GI Bleeding

Upper GI Lesions	Lower GI Lesions
Peptic Ulcer	Diverticulosis
Gastroesophageal Varices	Angioectasia
Esophagitis	Ischemic Colitis
Neoplasia	Hemorrhoids
Mallory Weiss Tear	Post Polypectomy
Angioectasia	Hemorrhoids
Gastritis	Rectal Ulcer
	Inflammatory Bowel Disease

after therapy. Risk stratification for UGIB should be performed prior to and after endoscopy. Several scoring systems have been created to predict mortality and rebleeding from nonvariceal UGIB. The Rockall score (Table 2)[3] is the most widely used and predicts mortality and rebleeding. It can be computed prior to endoscopy — clinical Rockall score and after endoscopic variables are assessed — complete Rockall score. The Forrest classification is an endoscopic risk stratification score that predicts rebleeding after endoscopy and will be discussed later.

Risk stratification for LGIB is less well defined. Risk factors for severe bleeding or recurrent bleeding include age > 65, abnormal vital signs at presentation, a non-tender abdomen, aspirin or NSAID use and 2 or more co-morbid illnesses.

Patients with a prediction score suggesting a worse outcome, ongoing overt bleeding, significant transfusion requirements or hemodynamic instability should be triaged accordingly. Generally, these patients should be managed in an ICU.

Medical Management

The main role for medical therapy in non-portal hypertension related GIB is in the treatment of peptic ulcer bleeding. Acid suppression has been the cornerstone of medical therapy of bleeding peptic ulcers. There

Table 2. Rockall Score

Variable	Points			
	0	1	2	3
Age	< 60	60–79	>80	N/A
Pulse	< 100	> 100	N/A	N/A
Systolic BP	Normal	> 100	<100	N/A
Co-Morbidities	None	N/A	CAD, CHF	Renal/liver failure Metastatic cancer
Diagnosis	Normal/ MWT	All other	Malignant	N/A
Endoscopic Findings	Clean Ulcer Flat Spot	N/A	AC, VV, AB	N/A

CAD = Coronary Artery Disease
CHF = Congestive Heart Failure
MWT= Mallory Weiss Tear
AC =Adherent Clot
VV = Visible Vessel
AB = Active Bleeding

Rockall TA, Logan RF, Devlin HB *et al.* (1996) Selection of patients for early discharge or outpatient care after upper gastrointestinal haemorrhage. National Audit of Acute Upper Gastrointestinal Haemorrhage. Lancet;**347**: 1138–40.

is significant evidence that therapy with proton pump inhibitors (PPI) reduces risk of rebleeding and need for surgery.[4] This data is most robust for patients with high-risk endoscopic lesions according to the Forrest classification and in patients who undergo endoscopic hemostasis (see next section). Therefore, the most accepted scenario for PPI usage is after a patient has undergone endoscopic evaluation and therapy. In clinical practice, most patients with suspected UGIB are started on PPI therapy during the initial evaluation prior to endoscopy. Some evidence suggests that PPI therapy prior to endoscopy may reduce the need for endoscopic therapy but has no effect on rebleeding rates, transfusion requirements, the need for surgery or mortality.[5] The optimal dose and route of administration of PPI therapy is unclear although an IV dosing loading dose and continuous infusion for 72 hours is the suggested protocol for patients with high-risk endoscopic lesions and those undergoing endoscopic therapy.

Endoscopic Management

Early endoscopic evaluation after appropriate resuscitation is a key component in the management of GIB. Endoscopic management of upper and lower GI bleeding sources are discussed separately.

Upper GI Bleeding

Peptic ulcer disease is the most common cause of UGIB and its endoscopic management has been extensively studied. Endoscopic therapy is guided by the appearance of the ulcer on its initial endoscopic visualization. The Forrest classification (Table 3) divides ulcers in five categories. These five categories predict the risk of rebleeding and guide the need for endoscopic therapy. Endoscopic therapy is recommended for high risk Forrest lesion — actively bleeding ulcer and a visible vessel. An adherent clot should be removed and therapy based on the underlying ulcer appearance. Low risk lesions do not require therapy.[2] Endoscopic therapy consists of injection therapy — mainly with epinephrine, thermal therapy with either monopolar or bipolar cauterization devices, or mechanical therapy with metallic clips. In general, evidence has shown cauterization therapy to be an equivalent mechanical therapy.[6] Thermal or mechanical therapy can be combined with injection therapy or used as monotherapy. There is no clear advantage to combination therapy. Monotherapy with epinephrine injections is inferior to either thermal or mechanical therapy and its use cannot be recommended.[7] The choice of endoscopic modality is usually based on available equipment and preference of the endoscopist. All patients undergoing endoscopic therapy should receive IV PPI therapy for 72 hours after endoscopy.

Table 3. Forrest Classification — Endoscopic Evaluation of Peptic Ulcer Bleeding

Endoscopic Classification	Frequency (%)	Rebleeding (%) Pre Treatment	Rebleeding (%) Post Treatment
High Risk			
Active Bleeding	12	90	15–30
Visible Vessel	22	50	15–30
Adherent Clot	10	33	0–5
Oozing	14	10	0–5
Low Risk			
Flat Spot	10	7	NA
Clean Based Ulcer	32	3	NA

Adopted from Feldman M, Friedman L, Brandt L. (2009) Sleisinger and Fordtrans Gastrointestinal and Liver Disease. Saunders Elsevier, Philadelphia. (Reprinted with permission.)

Other upper GI tract lesions that commonly require endoscopic therapy include Mallory Weiss tears (MWT), arteriovenous malformations (AVMS) and gastric antral vascular ectasia (GAVE). An MWT is a mucosal tear at the GE junction that occurs in the setting of severe retching and vomiting. It can be treated endoscopically with either thermal or mechanical therapy with adjunctive injection therapy if needed. Both AVMS and GAVE are superficial vascular lesions that are treated with thermal therapies. Argon plasma coagulation (APC) is a thermal modality that provides superficial cauterization and is well suited to the treatment of both AVMs and GAVE.

Lower GI Bleeding

The ability to isolate a solitary lesion that is amenable to endoscopic therapy is significantly less common in LGIB than UGIB. The most common lower GI lesions that are amenable to endoscopic therapy include diverticulosis, AVMs, post-polypectomy bleeding and hemorrhoids. Diverticulosis is a very common cause of LGIB but it is rare to isolate the exact bleeding site. When a diverticular bleeding site can be identified, either thermal or mechanical therapy can be utilized.[8] AVMS should be treated with thermal therapy. Bleeding hemorrhoids can be treated with sclerotherapy, band ligation, cryotherapy or infrared coagulation.

Refractory Bleeding

Bleeding that persists despite medical and endoscopic therapy especially when accompanied by significant transfusion requirements and hemodynamic instability warrant urgent consultation with an interventional radiologist and surgeon. Tagged red blood cell scans may be useful in localizing the source of LGIB. Angiography can be useful for both diagnosis and therapy of refractory bleeding. Angiography is often utilized prior to surgery.

Obscure GI Bleeding

Approximately 10% of patients presenting with GIB will not have a source localized after upper and lower endoscopic evaluations. These patients are classified as having obscure GIB. Wireless capsule endoscopy (WCE) is the most sensitive modality in detecting a bleeding source and should be pursued in all patients.[9] A positive finding on WCE should prompt a small bowel enteroscopy for definitive treatment.

References

1. Feldman M, Freidman L, Brandt L. (2010) *Sleisinger and Fordtrans Gastrointestinal and Liver Disease*. Saunders/Elsevier, Philadelphia.
2. Rockall TA, Logan RF, Devlin HB, *et al.* (1996) Selection of patients for early discharge or outpatient care after acute upper gastrointestinal haemorrhage. National Audit of Acute Upper Gastrointestinal Haemorrhage. *Lancet* **347**: 1138–40.
3. Gralnek IM, Barkun AN, Bardou M. (2008) Management of acute bleeding from a peptic ulcer. *N Engl J Med* **359**: 928–37.
4. Lau JY, Sung JJ, Lee KK, *et al.* (2002) Effect of intravenous omeprazole on recurrent bleeding after endoscopic treatment of bleeding peptic ulcers. *N Engl J Med* **343**: 310–6.

5. Lau, J, Leung WK, Wu JC *et al.* (2007) Omeprazole before endoscopy in patients with gastrointestinal bleeding. *N Engl J Med* **356**: 1631–40.
6. Saltzman JR, Strate LL, Disena V *et al.* (2005) Prospective trail of endoscopic clips versus combination therapy in upper GI bleeding. *Am J Gastroenterol* **100**: 1503–8.
7. Chung SS, Lau JY, Sung JJ, *et al.* (1997) Randomized comparison between adrenaline injection alone and adrenaline injection plus heat probe treatment for actively bleeding ulcers. *BMJ* **314**: 1307–11.
8. Jensen DM, Machicado GA, Jutabha R, *et al.* (2000). Urgent colonoscopy for the diagnosis and treatment of severe diverticular hemorrhage. *N Engl J Med* **342**: 78–82.
9. DeLeusse A, Vahedi K, Edery J, *et al.* (2008) Capsule endoscopy or push enteroscopy for first line exploration of obscure gastrointestinal bleeding? *Gastroenterology* **132**: 855–62.

Chapter 41

Inpatient Management of Inflammatory Bowel Disease

*Thomas A. Ullman**

Key Pearls

- Communicate effectively with the team. Gastroenterologists, surgeons, internists, nutritionists, nurses and others play key roles in the inpatient care of IBD patients.
- Think short-term: A plan to induce remission is an essential part of IBD care.
- Think long-term: Every short-term plan MUST be accompanied by a long-term strategy for the maintenance of remission and restoration of an excellent quality of life.
- Consider medication toxicity early and often. The medications used in IBD have numerous idiosyncratic side effects.
- Surgery is treatment and not the failure of treatment. Fibrostenotic Crohn's disease will not improve with medical therapy, and penetrating complications may also require surgery. Surgeons should be brought into management early.

Introduction

Ulcerative colitis (UC) and Crohn's disease are chronic inflammatory diseases of the gastrointestinal tract of uncertain etiology. While numerous

*Mount Sinai Medical Center, New York, NY, USA.

theories abound, most experts agree that dysregulation of innate and adaptive immunity, genetic factors, and environmental signal lead to an abnormal immune response to normal gut flora with subsequent mucosal damage in the gastrointestinal tract. While we usually classify inflammatory bowel diseases (IBDs) as either UC or Crohn's disease, a different nomenclature based on our knowledge of specific immune, genetic or environmental triggers will one day appear. In addition to our inability to understand the etiology of these diseases, we are currently limited in our ability to understand the triggers for flares, accurately prognosticate the future of our patients with these disease, and prevent a number of complications. Nevertheless, there have been substantial advances in imaging, medical therapy, and surgical therapy.

Ulcerative Colitis Inpatient Management

Communicate Effectively with Patient's Gastroenterologist

One of the most important aspects of IBD inpatient management, as well as that of most chronic illnesses, is the appropriate and timely communication of key features of key current and past issues in a patient's care. Often referred to as the "hand-off," the exchange of information about a patient's previous medical therapy of their colitis, the results of recent colonoscopic testing, laboratory testing, and any imaging must be communicated between treating physicians and healthcare professionals. Repeating expensive and invasive tests (including X-ray exposure and colonoscopic testing) offer little therapeutic value and can potentially harm patients. Also, determining the key reasons for admission is essential. These include:

- Is it a flare?
- Is it for a lack of response to oral medications?
- Is it to try a new medication for the patient (such as infliximab or cyclosporine)?
- Is it for possible surgery?

Table 1. American College of Gastroenterology Definitions of UC Severity

Severity	Characteristics
Mild	< 4 stools per day ± blood, normal ESR, no signs of toxicity
Moderate	≥ 4 stools per day, minimal signs of toxicity
Severe	> 6 stools per day with fever, tachycardia, anemia, or elevated ESR
Fulminant	> 10 stools per day, continuous bleeding, toxicity, abdominal tenderness/ distension, transfusion requirement, colonic dilation on X-ray

- For a complication such as dysplasia or colorectal cancer?
- For an extra-intestinal manifestation such as painful pyoderma gangrenosum or deep venous thrombosis from hypercoagulability?

Early and frequent communication with referring and treating physicians is an essential component of care.

Assess for Infection

Patients with ulcerative colitis can have periodic flares leading to hospital admission, but they can also have infections that either mimic a flare or are superimposed on one that is being treated. The emerging threat of *C. difficile* colitis is a particular problem in ulcerative colitis patients, and must be entertained in the differential diagnosis. *C. difficile* toxin assay should be ordered at admission for a flare in a UC patient.

If the flare is significant (i.e. the patient has severe disease, see Table 1), empiric therapy for *C. difficile* with intravenous metronidazole might additionally be helpful in treating bacteroides and other anaerobic bacteria that are more able to translocate across a compromised bowel. Gram negative coverage with a fluoroquinolone or other antibiotic should be considered as well.

In addition to considering *C. difficile* and normal gut bacterial pathogens, cytomegalovirus (CMV) super-infection appears to be an important process in patients on immunosuppressive medications, particularly those on glucocorticosteroids. Ruling out CMV generally involves sigmoidoscopy with biopsy, which is useful in assessing the mucosal severity of disease, and can be useful in picking up pseudomembranous colitis, though the absence of pseudomembranes does not rule out *C. difficile*.

Assess Toxicity

Assessing patients for toxicity of their colitis is an important part of inpatient evaluation and management of UC. The reflexive aphorism that "vital signs are vital" is as true in UC management as it is in that of sepsis, myocardial infarction, and others. True toxicity with fever, tachycardia, or hypotension should prompt urgent attention to intravascular volume status and surgical evaluation. Checking the vital signs frequently is essential. As in any gastroenterologic condition, frequent abdominal examinations are critical, with immediate surgical evaluation prompted by peritoneal signs, keeping in mind that glucocorticosteroids can mask peritoneal signs, as can narcotic analgesics. Narcotics and anti-cholinergics should be avoided in these patients. The presence of a dilated colon or a fixed column air often heralds free perforation, and should also result in surgical consultation.

Medical Therapy: Reduce Inflammatory Load

The goal of medical therapy for active ulcerative colitis is to reduce inflammation to restore colonic and therefore overall health. Therapy of mild disease is usually achieved by the administration of oral and rectal mesalamine medications (sulfasalazine, mesalamine, balsalazide, or olsalazine). Glucocorticosteroids and anti-tumor necrosis factor alpha therapies are the mainstays of therapy for moderate or severe disease and the latter has the added benefit of demonstrable effect in the maintenance of remission.[1]

Steroids should be allowed a modicum of time to result in an improvement before abandonment; usually 3–5 days is appropriate. Due to the myriad adverse effects of steroids, thiopurines (azathioprine or 6-mercaptopurine) or anti-TNF therapy should be considered whenever glucocorticosteroids are administered, particularly in steroid-dependent or steroid refractory patients. Cyclosporine has been demonstrated to result in colectomy avoidance in glucocorticosteroid-refractory patients, and is bridged to thiopurine therapy for long-term maintenance given its lack of effectiveness long-term.[2] Cyclosporine as a rescue therapy for patients who have recently failed anti-TNF therapy or vice versa should probably be avoided due to heightened toxicity, particularly infections. Whether given concomitantly with corticosteroids or as monotherapy as an inductive agent, cyclosporine is administered intravenously for seven days prior to conversion to oral therapy, and should be given that amount of time to result in clinical improvement. The time course of response to infliximab, currently the only FDA-approved anti-TNF for ulcerative colitis treatment, in the acute setting, is not well understood.

Monitor for Side Effects

Many of the medications used have serious short-term and long-term potential for adverse events. Infectious risks are a key consideration for anti-TNF therapy, particularly reactivation of tuberculosis, Histoplasmosis, Coccidiomycosis, and bacterial pathogens. Patients should be counseled as to these possibilities, and pre-treatment standards should be adhered to. It is important to consider these aspects of care at the time of admission to avoid delay in treatment. For example, a PPD test to assess prior TB exposure may be needed, and takes a minimum of 48 hours to be read.

Infectious risks are also possible with corticosteroids, cyclosporine, and thiopurines; such risks have been demonstrated to increase with combination therapies of these medicines. Other medication-induced adverse events are always of concern, particularly with corticosteroids, including:

- Bone and joint loss
- Psychosis
- Acne
- Hyperglycemia
- Hypertension

Common side-effects of cyclosporine in addition to infection include:

- Tremor
- Seizure
- Hypertension
- Renal insufficiency

When starting anti-TNF therapy or thiopurines, long-term risks of malignancy, such as lymphoma, particularly hepatosplenic T-cell lymphoma for both of these agents and non-melanoma skin cancers with thiopurines, should be reviewed with the patient.

Involve a Surgeon Early

While toxic and fulminant colitis are often indications for surgery, inpatients with more moderate flares in which medical therapy is underway should also have a surgical evaluation. Surgery is not the failure of treatment in IBD, it *is* treatment. It is best to educate patients about this possibility, and surgeons prefer to meet patients well in advance of any planned or emergent surgery when at all possible.

Think Long-term, not Just Short-term

While a hospitalization is a difficult event for any patient and a care team, ulcerative colitis is a disease of a lifetime, not of a few days or weeks. Careful consideration of long-term consequences of the disease and its therapy must be considered at every encounter, whether in the office or the hospital. The initiation of steroids warrants consideration of the initiation of a steroid-sparing agent (anti-TNF therapy or thiopurine therapy), even with the first course of steroids. Colorectal cancer screening and surveillance should also be considered. Importantly, because this is a life-long illness, clinicians should be judicious in performing X-ray tests as recent reports have noted the increase in Crohn's patients' exposure to ionizing radiation, the long-term effects of which are poorly understood.[3]

Miscellaneous Considerations

DVT prophylaxis with heparin is imperative in hospitalized IBD patients owing to their high rate of thromboembolic events due to a hypercoagulable state associated with these illnesses. Evaluation for extraintestinal manifestations (uveitis/scleritis, arthritis, pyoderma gangrenosum, erythema nodosum, primary sclerosing cholangitis, and others) is also an essential part of the care of all IBD patients. Hemorrhage from ulceration into medium-sized vessels is an indication for surgery, although endoscopic evaluation should be attempted unless the bleeding is life-threatening.

Crohn's Disease Inpatient Management

While often thought of as a separate entity from ulcerative colitis, and certainly a more complex disease in many respects, many of the same principles of care that apply to ulcerative colitis similarly apply to the care of Crohn's patients. It is imperative to communicate early and often with the gastroenterologist who best knows the patient; to rule out infection; to involve a surgeon early; to consider long-term issues while managing short-term problems; to institute DVT prophylaxis, guard against hemorrhage, and to evaluate for possible extraintestinal complications. Special considerations in Crohn's disease include the following:

1. Is there a penetrating complication?

Unlike ulcerative colitis, the transmural inflammation of Crohn's disease can result in the development of fistula, abscesses, and sinus tracts. A comprehensive and detailed rectal exam to exclude the presence of perianal fistulas is an important part of the evaluation of Crohn's patients in every setting. Intra-abdominal abscess, enetero-enteric fistula, enterocutaneous fistula, and fistula to the genitourinary tract should be considered in the appropriate situation — abdominal pain, fullness, or fever, diarrhea, drainage across the skin, or fecauluria or vaginal expression fecal contents, respectively.

A peri-rectal abscess with perianal pain, erythema, and/or swelling requires prompt attention and drainage by a colorectal surgeon.

Examination under anesthesia, rectal ultrasound, and pelvic MRI are the best methods for evaluating the perianal anatomy for planning and performing appropriate drainage of purulent material. Short-term therapeutic options, in addition to drainage of purulent material, include systemic antibiotics and anti-TNF therapies. Glucocorticoids are frequently used in this situation, but may paradoxically keep a fistula or other penetrating manifestation open. There is no defined role for mesalamine-based agents for these complications. Immunomodulator therapy with thiopurines may prove helpful over the long-term; calcineurin inhibitors (cyclosporine or tacrolimus) may prove helpful in the short-term.

2. Is there an obstruction?

Pain that is crampy in quality and associated with either distension or vomiting should prompt consideration for an obstructive process. Obstructive symptoms typically arise when there is a fibrostenotic lesion blocking the forward progression of peristalsis, or when there is sufficient luminal narrowing from inflammation. Current technologies for assessing the small intestinal lumen (barium X-rays, CT enterography, MR enterography, and video capsule endoscopy, and ileocolonoscopy) are not accurate at determining what proportion of a narrowed segment is from scarring and how much is from active inflammation.

Therapy for obstruction is usually a combination of nasogastric tube suction for those with persistent vomiting, nothing by mouth (NPO) with IV fluid, and possibly parenteral nutritional support. Often, dietary indiscretion in the form of ingestion of fibrous foods or nuts is responsible for the acute obstruction. Anti-inflammatory therapy has not been demonstrated to hasten resolution. An unrelieved obstruction over days is an indication for surgery and may herald a diagnosis of a malignancy.

3. Is the disease purely inflammatory?

If so, reducing active inflammation as in ulcerative colitis is the therapy of choice. Systemic corticosteroids or ileal release budesonide for ileal or right colonic disease may prove helpful. Anti-TNF therapy with infliximab, adalimumab, or certolizumab pegol may also be considered. As in ulcerative colitis, patients who undergo therapy with steroids should be advised as to the need for steroid-free maintenance agents.

Supportive Care

In the treatment of all chronic inflammatory disease, careful monitoring of fluid and electrolyte status, nutritional management, and psychosocial support are essential aspects of the care of patients with ulcerative colitis and Crohn's disease. A team-based approach with doctors, nurses, nutritionists, social workers, and other healthcare professionals is critical for the successful hospitalization, discharge, and transition to outpatient care of patients.

The inflammatory bowel diseases can be quite challenging to manage based on the many considerations and therapeutic options available to clinicians. Fortunately, outcomes are usually excellent when the appropriate evaluation and management strategies are utilized.

References

1. Rutgeerts P, Sandborn WJ, Feagan BG, *et al.* (2005) Infliximab for induction and maintenance therapy for ulcerative colitis. *N Engl J Med* **353**: 2462–76.
2. Moskovitz DN, Van Assche G, Maenhout B, *et al.* (2006) Incidence of colectomy during long-term follow-up after cyclosporine-induced remission of severe ulcerative colitis. *Clin Gastroenterol Hepatol* **4**: 760–5.
3. Desmond AN, O'Regan K, Curran C, *et al.* (2008) Crohn's disease: Factors associated with exposure to high levels of diagnostic radiation. *Gut* **57**: 1524–9.

Chapter 42

Pancreatitis

*Reza Akhtar**

Key Pearls

- Identify patients at risk for severe disease (organ failure, local, or systemic complications) and elevate their level of care and monitoring.
- Initiate early, aggressive intravenous fluid resuscitation with bolus isotonic fluid followed by maintenance of 250–300 mL/hour.
- Use CT when there is a question in the diagnosis, a complication of disease is suspected (abscess, necrosis, pseudocyst), or when the clinical course worsens.
- Enteral nutrition is safe and effective in certain patients.
- Gastroenterology and/or surgery should be consulted when there is a diagnosis of gallstone pancreatitis, a lack of clinical improvement, or development of complications.

Epidemiology

Pancreatitis accounts for over 200,000 hospitalizations each year.[1] The incidence of acute pancreatitis is on the rise globally.[2] Whether this trend is due to increased awareness and better diagnostic techniques versus a true increase in disease occurrence is debatable.

*Mount Sinai School of Medicine, New York, NY, USA.

Etiology

Gallstone disease remains the primary cause of acute pancreatitis, but only a minority of patients with gallstone disease develop pancreatitis. Gallstone pancreatitis occurs with greater frequency among females than males, particularly those over the age of 60. Alcohol is also a common cause. Tobacco dependence is another independent risk factors for an attack.[3] Other less common causes include: obstructive pancreatitis as in the case of malignancy or pancreas divisum, hypertriglyceridemia (>1000 mg/dL), medications (e.g. thiazide diuretics, anti-epileptics, antimetabolites in IBD), trauma and burn injury, infection, and autoimmune etiologies. Twenty percent of cases remain idiopathic.

Clinical Presentation

Symptom Complex

Although 80–90% of acute pancreatitis is self-limiting, recognition of typical symptoms at presentation is vital in initiating early management to halt disease progression. These symptoms include abdominal pain predominantly in the epigastrium radiating to the back, nausea, and vomiting.

Physical exam can reveal:

- Epigastric tenderness or fullness
- Signs of a severe inflammatory response syndrome such as fever, tachycardia, and leukocytosis

Important findings indicating more severe disease include:

- Shock
- Erythematous skin nodules due to subcutaneous fat necrosis
- Basilar rales with pleural effusions
- Rigid abdomen with lack of bowel sounds
- Periumbilical bruising due to hemoperitoneum (*Cullen's sign*)
- Flank discoloration due to tissue catabolism of hemoglobin (*Turner's sign*).

The clinical diagnosis is made based upon the presence of typical symptoms along with serum elevation of pancreatic enzymes (amylase and lipase).

Symptoms of chronic pancreatitis can overlap with those in acute disease, particularly epigastric pain. Additionally, patients may suffer from pancreatic insufficiency due to atrophy and chronic, irreversible inflammatory damage to the pancreatic parenchyma. This occurs late in the course of the disease. Without pancreatic enzyme replacement, carbohydrate, fat, and protein metabolism suffers greatly, resulting in a malabsorptive diarrhea. Patients may report loose stools with a foul odor that characteristically float in water due to their higher than normal fat content (*steatorrhea*). Endocrine disorder parallels exocrine malfunction and can lead to the development of diabetes.[4] Glucagon secretion is also altered putting patients at risk for severe hypoglycemia. Secondary effects of malabsorption such as vitamin D deficiency leading to a decrease in bone mineral density can also occur.

Labs

Amylase levels will elevate (>3× upper limit normal) and resolve (48–72 hours) prior to the respective peak and resolution of lipase. Levels *do not* correlate with severity of disease. Other laboratory anomalies may include: hypocalcemia, leukocytosis, and abnormal liver function tests (bilirubin, AST, alkaline phosphatase). In the chronic phase of disease, once the majority of the pancreatic parenchyma has been wiped out, amylase and lipase may no longer be secreted, negating serum detection in the setting of acute flares.

Pitfalls in Diagnosis

Lipase is produced anywhere lipolysis occus in the body. These sites include the small bowel, liver, and stomach among others. Therefore, it is not surprising that elevations in lipase can be seen with pathology in these organs such as small bowel obstruction, gastroparesis, and peptic ulcer disease. Salivary amylase may also be present in high levels, particularly in patients suffering from alcohol dependence; a distinction from pancreatic amylase is not made by most assays. Finally, decreased glomerular filtration may reduce clearance of amylase and lipase resulting in falsely elevated serum enzyme activity.[5] Heparin use during dialysis may also directly affect these levels.

Imaging

Though it is not necessary for diagnosis, radiologic evaluation of pancreatitis may help determine its etiology, demonstrate complications such as pseuodocysts, and risk stratify patients for a severe course of disease.

Abdominal X-ray is insensitive for diagnosis, but may assist in ruling out intestinal perforation by demonstrating a lack of free air. Ileus may be seen in association with acute pancreatitis; upper abdominal calcifications with chronic disease. Ultrasound can demonstrate gallstones, biliary sludge, dilation of the proximal bile duct, and pseudocysts, though the pancreas is often obscured by overlying bowel gas.

CT or MRI can confirm the diagnosis, evaluate the distal bile duct for filling defects, and demonstrate complications of disease such as pseudocysts and necrosis. Contrast-enhanced imaging is needed to demonstrate necrosis, taking advantage of the differential contrast uptake between the healthy and necrotic parenchyma. The damage to the pancreas is graded, and this finding, along with the presence or absence of necrosis, can predict those at risk for a severe disease course. These patients necessitate a higher level of inpatient care in an intermediate or intensive care unit.

Prognosis

Acute pancreatitis occurs across a spectrum of severity with most being mild to moderate. Severe pancreatitis has been reported to occur in up to 25% of patients with acute pancreatitis.[8] At a certain point, the inflammatory cascade responsible for multiorgan failure becomes advanced and significant morbidity and mortality is inevitable. Most deaths that occur within the first 1–2 weeks of disease are a result of multiorgan failure. Early recognition of those at the highest risk and aggressive intervention can prevent progression along this pathway.

Many scoring systems have been proposed to predict the severity of disease and mortality risk.[1] These systems take into account the presence or absence of organ failure:

- Systemic dysfunction determined by labs
    - Ranson criteria
    - APACHE II criteria
- Local complications determined by CT
    - abscess, pseudocyst, sterile or infected necrosis

Despite early treatment, however, necrotizing pancreatitis will develop in 10–20% of patients. Mortality is higher in this group, with 30–40% developing infected necrosis.[9]

Treatment

Fluids

Initial management is focused on aggressive resuscitation at presentation. This treatment should begin in the emergency room and continue on the medical floor. Intravenous fluid should be run at a maintenance speed of 250–300 mL/hour after initial bolus resuscitation with isotonic fluid.

Concerns often arise in those with impaired cardiac or renal function in regards to their ability to handle large amounts of intravenous fluid. Cautious patient observation and balance of inputs and outputs should be taken in this situation to avoid pulmonary edema and worsening of cardiac function. Though fluid resuscitation must be carefully monitored to decrease the risk of acute congestive heart failure, poor initial resuscitation and slow resolution of acute pancreatitis as a result can also lead to adverse cardiac outcomes in susceptible patients.

Nutrition

Enteral feeding in pancreatitis is often debated. Traditional teaching mandates complete bowel rest in an attempt to relieve the pancreas of its exocrine and endocrine functions. More recent studies suggests enteral feeding may pacify the inflammatory response and improve intestinal epithelial health. However, no randomized comparison exists between enteral and parenteral nutritional supplementation in this setting.[10] Several studies have demonstrated the safety of gastric and jejunal feedings. Some literature suggests the latter may be associated with less pain and complications.[11] Overall, total parenteral nutrition (TPN) may be as efficacious and safe as enteral feeding, but the cost, need for central venous access, and infectious complications of TPN need to be considered. Given the lack of clear evidence, it is prudent to initially withhold all oral intake and start feeding when symptoms have begun to subside and the abdominal exam is improved.

Endoscopy and Surgery

In acute biliary pancreatitis, endoscopic retrograde cholangiopancreatography (ERCP) can relieve persistent biliary obstruction. Its use is primarily indicated only with concomitant acute cholangitis. In pancreatitis without cholangitis, early ERCP (within 72 hours) may reduce complications of severe pancreatitis, but not for mild to moderate disease.[12] Early ERCP has not been shown to decrease mortality.[13] In the setting of severe pancreatitis, the risk of any invasive procedure needs to be strongly considered. Endoscopic ultrasound (EUS) or MRCP may be considered to evaluate the common bile duct for persistent obstruction or dilation in this setting.[14,15] Without obvious pathology, ERCP can then be avoided to prevent unnecessary errant pancreatic duct cannulation, sphincterotomy, and possible post-ERCP pancreatitis.

Surgery should be consulted early in the course of disease to plan for cholecystectomy during the same hospital admission. Surgical consultation should also be sought with necrotizing pancreatitis as surgical debridement may be necessary.

Antibiotics

Prophylactic antibiotics in patients with pancreatic necrosis remains controversial, having not been validated and confirmed in randomized trials. Diagnosing infected pancreatic necrosis can be difficult as fever and leukocytosis may already be present as part of the inflammatory response. CT may demonstrate gas bubbles within the necrotic tissue, aiding in this diagnosis.[16] EUS or CT-guided aspiration of necrotic tissue can be performed for microbiologic study. If the tissue is sterile, however, as it remains in most cases, instrumentation may introduce infection and increase mortality. In general, empiric antibiotics should be reserved for patients with fever or who appear toxic. When antibiotics are instituted, agents with activity against gram negative bacteria should be chosen, such as a carbapenem.

In the case of an obvious precipitant such as alcohol or medication, the offending agent should be removed. In viral infectious pancreatitis, infectious disease consultation should be sought to guide therapy if indicated. Finally, steroid therapy is indicated for autoimmune pancreatitis. The diagnosis should be made in conjunction with a gastroenterologist, however, as erroneous use of steroids may have deleterious consequences.

Discharge Planning

Once patients are able to tolerate oral feeding and there is a resolution of pain without the use of narcotics, it is safe to discharge with appropriate follow up. Even in mild cases, rehospitalization among Medicare beneficiaries is a costly and widespread problem approaching $18 billion.[6] Early readmission for acute pancreatitis is determined by use of alcohol, discharge with persistent gastrointestinal symptoms, or discharge on less than a solid diet.[7]

References

1. Whitcomb, David. (2006) Acute pancreatitis. *N Engl J Med* **354**: 2142–2150.

2. Yadav D, Lowenfels AB. (2006) Trends in the epidemiology of the first attack of acute pancreatitis: A systematic review. *Pancreas* **34**(1): 174.
3. Talukdar R, Vege SS. (2009) Recent developments in acute pancreatitis. *Clin Gastroenterol Hepatol* **7**(11 Suppl):S3–S9.
4. Hammer HF. (2010) Pancreatic exocrine insufficiency: Diagnostic evaluation and replacement therapy with pancreatic enzymes. *Dig Dis* **28**(2): 339–343).
5. Collen MJ, Ansher AF, Chapman AB, *et al.* (1990) Serum amylase in patients with renal insufficiency and renal failure. *Am J Gastroenterol* **85**(10):1377–1380.
6. Jencks SF, Williams MV, Coleman EA. (2009) Rehospitalizations among patients in the medicare fee-for-service program. *N Engl J Med* **360**(14): 1418–1428.
7. Whitlock TL, Repas K, Tignor A *et al.* (2010) Early Readmission acute pancreatitis: Incidence and risk factors. *Am J Gastroenterol* [Epub ahead of print].
8. Beger HG, Rau BM. (2007) Severe acute pancreatitis: Clinical course and management. *World J Gastroenterol* **13**(38): 5043–5051.
9. Sekimoto M, Takada T, Kawarada Y, *et al*. (2006) JPN Guidelines for the management of acute pancreatitis: Epidemiology, etiology, natural history, and outcome predictors in acute pancreatitis. *J Hepatobiliary Pancreat Surg*. **13**(1): 10–24.
10. Marik PE, Zaloga GP. (2004) Meta-analysis of parenteral nutrition versus enteral nutrition in patients with acute pancreatitis. *BMJ* **328**: 1407–1407.
11. Banks P, Conwell D, Toskes P. (2010) The management of acute and chronic pancreatitis. *Gastroenterol Hepatol (NY)* **6**(2_Suppl): 1–16.
12. Ayub K, Imada R, Slavin J. (2004) Endoscopic retrograde cholangiopancreatography in gallstone-associated acute pancreatitis. *Cochrane Database Syst Rev* (4):CD003630.
13. Petrov MS, van Santvoort HC, Besselink MG, *et al.* (2008) Early endoscopic retrograde cholangiopancreatography versus conservative

management in acute biliary pancreatitis without cholangitis: A meta-analysis of randomized trials. *Ann Surg* **247**(2): 250–257.

14. Liu CL, Fan ST, Lo CM. (2005) Comparison of early endoscopic ultrasonography and endoscopic retrograde cholangiopancreatography in the management of acute biliary pancreatitis: A prospective randomized study. *Clin Gastroenterol Hepatol* **3**(12):1238–1244.
15. Lévy P, Boruchowicz A, Hastier P, *et al.* (2005) Diagnostic criteria in predicting a biliary origin of acute pancreatitis in the era of endoscopic ultrasound: Multicentered prospective evaluation of 213 patients. *Pancreatology* **5**: 450–456.
16. Fauci AS, Langford CA. (2005) *Pancreatitis. Harrison's Manual of Medicine*, 16th ed., pp. 753–756.

Chapter 43

Small Bowel Obstruction

Kerri E. B. El-Sabrout and Celia M. Divino**

Key Pearls

- The most common causes are postoperative ileus and adhesion formation from previous surgeries, peritoneal dialysis, or prior peritoneal infection.
- Any complete obstruction carries the risk of vascular compromise, gangrene, and perforation.
- Ask the patient specifically about a history of abdominal surgery, malignancy, endocrine disorders, previous episodes of SBO or peritonitis, or inflammatory disorders including Crohn's disease.
- SBO warrants immediate surgical consultation, though 70% of patients with SBO can be successfully managed nonoperatively.
- Management includes avoiding all oral intake (NPO), aggressive fluid resuscitation, and nasogastric tube decompression.

Bowel obstruction is defined as the interruption of normal passage of bowel contents. If bowel contents, including air, are able to pass the point of obstruction, then it is described as partial; the more worrisome inability of contents to pass at all is defined as complete. In any case of obstruction, the bowel proximal to the point of blockage eventually becomes dilated, with hypersecretion and bacterial overgrowth, while the bowel distal to the blockage collapses. Small bowel obstruction (SBO) can be classified into two categories: non-mechanical and mechanical.

*The Mount Sinai Hospital, New York, NY, USA.

Non-mechanical Obstruction

An ileus, or intestinal paralysis, is characterized by complete atony of the gastrointestinal system. Ileus in the postoperative setting is the most common, and typically resolves within three days. Treatment should include early and frequent ambulation and narcotic minimization. Non-narcotic pain management, such as regional anesthesia and NSAIDS, should be used when possible in order to avoid a prolonged course of narcotics. It is rare for an ileus to arise in a non-postoperative setting, and is usually caused by medications or electrolyte abnormalities. Identifying and treating the cause are the goals of management.

Dysmotility, or impaired bowel peristalsis, can be caused by medications (opiates, anticholinergics, antipsychotics), hypothyroidsm, or electrolyte abnormalities (hypokalemia).

Although relatively common in the colon, a pseudo-obstruction of small bowel is a very rare phenomenon. This is usually caused by enteric nervous system disorders related to an imbalance between sympathetic and parasympathetic effects on bowel motility.

Mechanical Obstruction

A mechanical obstruction is defined as a structural abnormality or physical barrier to the progression of bowel contents. This abnormality can be caused by an intraluminal, intramural, or extraluminal source. The most common causes are adhesion formation from previous surgeries, peritoneal dialysis, or a previous peritoneal infection (peritonitis). Other causes are presented in Table 1. Peritoneal adhesions account for up to 85% of SBO admissions[1].

Any complete obstruction, potentially from cecal volvulus, incarcerated hernia, or a closed-loop segment, carries the dangerous risk of vascular compromise, leading to the progression of obstruction and to strangulation, followed by gangrene and perforation.

Table 1. Common Causes of SBO

Category	**Causes**
Inflammatory diseases (acute enteritis)	Inflammation, edema, fibrosis Crohn's disease Radiation enteritis Small bowel diverticulitis
Incarcerated hernias	Abdominal wall hernias (inguinal, ventral, umbilical, femoral, incisional) Internal hernias
Volvulus	Rotation of bowel around a single point Cecal Sigmoid Colon
Postoperative	Bowel edema Anesthesia/narcotics causing decreased bowel mobility
Malignancy	Intrinsic small bowel tumors Metastatic abdominal disease Desmoplastic reaction causing scarring Large intra-abdominal tumors causing extrinsic compression
Gallstones	Intraluminal obstruction, usually at ileocecal valve
Peritonitis	Spontaneous bacterial peritonitis
Foreign body ingestion	Intraluminal blockage by foreign body
Intussusception (especially in children)	Invagination of one bowel loop into another Luminal narrowing Bowel edema Intraluminal mass in adults
Intra-abdominal hematoma or abscess	Extrinsic compression on bowel Intramural small bowel hematoma with anticoagulation
Superior mesenteric artery syndrome	Compression of the 3rd portion of the duodenum, between the aorta and superior mesenteric artery

Clinical Presentation

History

Patients with SBO most often report abdominal pain, distention, obstipation, nausea and vomiting. The color and frequency of the emesis may suggest the location and severity of the blockage. It is essential to ask about the patient's last bowel movement and flatus.

Along with taking a complete history, it is important to ask the patient specifically about a history of abdominal malignancy, endocrine disorders, previous episodes of SBO or peritonitis, or inflammatory disorders including Crohn's disease, pancreatitis, and pelvic inflammatory disease. Any past surgical history, especially any previous intraperitoneal or pelvic procedures, or recent anesthesia, is pertinent.

Reviewing the patient's complete medication history, current and recent, is essential. Special attention must be paid to use of opiates, anticholinergics, and anticoagulants.

Physical Exam

Fever can suggest an infectious etiology for the SBO, such as an intra-abdominal abscess. Hypotension, especially when accompanied by tachycardia, often suggests dehydration and under-resuscitation, and can be a sign of sepsis.

It is important to do a complete physical exam. Patients may become dyspneic and tachypneic due to abdominal distension or pain.

When examining the abdomen, observe the degree of distention, and inspect for any abdominal scars. Auscultation may reveal high-pitched tones, tingles, and rushes with associated crampy abdominal pain, which would imply an obstructive process. A patient with absent bowel sounds may have intestinal paralysis or intestinal fatigue after a prolonged obstructive course.

Symmetric tenderness is present in approximately 70% of patients with SBO.[2] Less common are rebound tenderness, guarding, or rigidity, which are present in less than 50% of these patients.[2] Abdominal dullness on percussion can suggest an intra-abdominal mass, and tympany can be elicited over a distended bowel. A patient presenting with concomitant jaundice or icteric sclera could suggest a gallstone ileus or metastatic cancer with hepatic involvement.

It is crucial to evaluate for any hernias (inguinal, femoral, umbilical, incisional) and characterize any hernia as reducible or non-reducible, tender, or with associated skin changes. A rectal exam should be routine to examine for masses or fecal impaction. For any patient with a colostomy or ileostomy, a digital probe of the stoma should be performed to assess for obstruction at the level of the fascia.

Laboratory Findings

In early SBO, laboratory findings may be normal. But with progression of obstruction, hemoconcentration, leukocytosis, and electrolyte abnormalities, including hypokalemia and elevation of serum amylase and liver function tests, may all be present. Laboratory abnormalities depend on the extent of the disease progress. Although laboratory studies may not directly aide in diagnosis, results may assist in appreciating the extent of complications such as dehydration, strangulation, and sepsis.

Imaging Studies

The first-line radiological testing for all patients with suspected SBO should be chest and plain abdominal radiographs.[3] These can reveal dilated loops of small bowel, a dilated stomach, air/fluid levels within the bowel, or an obstructing foreign body or intraluminal gallstone. Radiographs can also aid in establishing the approximate level or location of the obstruction. Importantly, they can also identify promptly the more ominous process of perforation (with free air) or complete obstruction (with the lack of luminal air in the distal bowel).

All patients with inconclusive plain films for complete or high-grade obstruction should have a CT scan,[3] as it carries a 94% sensitivity and specificity for diagnosing SBO.[4,5] It is the modality of choice to identify a closed loop obstruction, which can be difficult to diagnose on plain radiographs, as the problematic loop may contain fluid and very little air. CT scanning can also detect hernias, free peritoneal fluid or air, inflammatory processes, and intra-abdominal masses or collections. It is more accurate than radiography in identifying the level of obstruction.

Oral contrast choice in CT scanning is significant. Water-insoluble solutions of barium provide clearer images, but can have catastrophic consequences in cases of perforation, causing severe peritonitis. Moreover, if imminent surgery is to be considered, intraluminal barium can make bowel resection and anastomosis difficult. Using instead a water-soluble solution (gastrograffin, hypaque) can provide both a diagnostic and therapeutic benefit in cases of partial obstruction. Water-soluble solutions are hyperosmotic and facilitate fluid translocation into the bowel lumen. Several studies have shown improved recovery from a partial obstruction with the administration of water-soluble solutions.[6,7]

Other imaging modalities, including ultrasonography and enteroclysis, are unlikely to provide any further diagnostic benefit, and may, in fact, delay early recognition and treatment.

Treatment

All cases of SBO warrant immediate surgical consultation, as the extent and progression of the disease are difficult to predict. Initial management of all patients should begin with barring any oral intake (NPO) and the placement of a large bore IV for immediate fluid and electrolyte replacement. Aggressive fluid resuscitation can be done with the administration of normal saline or isotonic Ringers solutions. Electrolyte replacement should be based on laboratory results.

Nasogastric tube decompression is almost always warranted, providing gastric decompression and reducing the risk of aspiration. A 16F or 18F sump tube (double lumen with a ventilation port) is optimal, placed to low or medium continuous wall suction. It is important to note the volume and character of output, as the output can suggest the extent and level of obstruction. Clear fluid suggests gastric outlet obstruction; bilious output

Table 2. Radiographic Presentations of SBO

	Abdominal Radiographs	CT Scan
Ileus	• Generalized or diffuse abnormal gas pattern with usually mild distention of the SB, colon, and rectum • Air/fluid levels may be seen in SB in upright position	• Diffuse SB and colonic dilatation without a discrete transition zone or identifiable mechanical cause
Partial SBO	• Dilated stomach and SB (>3 cm diameter) proximal to affected loop • Diminished air in distal SB and colon	• Dilated fluid- and air-filled loops of SB • Beak-like narrowing of affected SB loop • Collapsed distal SB loops • Oral contrast distal to point of obstruction
Closed loop obstruction	• Affected loop may contain fluid and very little gas, thus barely visible • A minimally dilated sentinel loop that is unchanged on multiple views and positions • Oval mass in the abdomen, known as the "pseudotumor" sign • If early presentation, distended proximal loops of SB may not be present	• U-shaped or C-shaped dilated bowel loop with a radial distribution of mesenteric vessels converging toward a torsion point • "Whorl" sign of tightly twisted mesentery seen with volvulus • Collapsed distal SB loops
High-grade or complete SBO	• Severely distended SB loops proximal to site of obstruction • Air/fluid levels within SB lumen, sometimes at differing heights within the same loop • Collapsed loops of SB distal to site of obstruction • Small bubbles of gas trapped between folds in dilated, fluid-filled loops producing the "string of pearls" sign • Lack of colonic air	• Severely distended proximal SB loops • Discrete transition zone to collapsed distal SB and colon • Particulate feculent matter mixed with gas bubbles is seen within dilated SB • Mesenteric edema or vascular engorgement • Intestinal wall thickening >2cm • Pneumatosis • Lack of colonic air • Oral contrast traverse only proximal to point of obstruction

SB = Small bowel

suggests medial to proximal small bowel obstruction; and feculent output suggests distal small bowel obstruction. Nasogastric tubes must be flushed frequently with normal saline or tap water, especially when the output is thick or contains particulate matter. The ventilation lumen must likewise be kept patent for optimal therapy, and should be flushed with air frequently.

An indwelling urinary catheter is indicated for acute fluid status assessment. Analgesics can be used, but the avoidance or minimization of opiates is crucial in aiding recovery. In cases of prolonged bowel obstruction or dysfunction, parenteral nutrition should be considered.

Antibiotic therapy in nonoperative management remains controversial. Antibiotics are routinely used to treat bacterial translocation in bowel obstruction,[8] but data supporting their use is lacking.[3] If initiating antibiotic therapy, a broad-spectrum therapy is essential; and, for those patients requiring surgery, antibiotic administration will reduce the risk of wound infection and abdominal sepsis. Therapy should include adequate coverage of gram-negative aerobes and anaerobes. This can be achieved with a second-generation cephalosporin, or a combination of a first generation cephalosporin or fluoroquinolone and metronidazole.

Frequent reassessment of patients with SBO is vital. Repeat abdominal radiography six to twelve hours after gastric decompression can reveal improvement or progression of the obstruction. Frequent abdominal exams, ideally by the same clinician, can identify any deterioration of the patient's clinical status.

Published studies have demonstrated that up to 70% of patients with SBO can be successfully managed nonoperatively[1]. However, in cases of high-grade SBO without strangulation, only 46% of patients can be managed nonoperatively.[9]

Surgical Treatment

Indications for surgical exploration include pneumoperitoneum, peritonitis, complete obstruction, strangulation, incarcerated hernia, internal hernia, or closed loop obstruction. However, in all cases of disease progression or failure to improve after 24–48 hours of conservative management, surgery should be considered. This can be characterized by increasing abdominal pain, distension or tenderness, increasing small bowel distention on X-ray, hemodynamic instability, worsening fever, or a decline in mental status.

Resolution of Obstruction

In cases if ileus, clinical improvement is first noted by resumption of bowel sounds. In SBO, a decrease in nasogastric output, decreasing abdominal distension and pain, and the passing of flatus or stool signal an improving clinical picture. Hospital discharge can occur only once bowel function has returned and the patient is able to tolerate oral fluids and diet.

References

1. Foster NM, McGory ML, Zingmond DS, Ko CY. (2006) Small bowel obstruction: A population-based appraisal. *J Am Coll Surg* **203**: 170–176.
2. Eskelinen M, Ikonen J, Lipponen P. (1994) Contributions of history-taking, physical examination, and computer assistance to diagnosis of acute small-bowel obstruction : A prospective study of 1333 patients with acute abdominal pain. *Scand J Gastroenterol* **29**: 715.
3. Diaz JJ Jr, Bokhari F, Mowery NT, *et al.* (2008) Guidelines for management of small bowel obstruction. *J Trauma* **64**: 1651–1664.
4. Megibow A. (1994) Bowel obstruction: Evaluation with CT. *Radiol Clin North Am* **32**: 861.
5. Balthazar E. (1994) CT of small-bowel obstruction. *AJR Am J Roentgenol* **162**: 255.
6. Assalia A, Schein M, Kopelman D, *et al.* (1994) Therapeutic effect of oral Gastrografin in adhesive, partial small-bowel obstruction: A prospective randomized trial. *Surgery* **115**: 433–437.
7. Choi HK, Chu KW, Law WL. (2002) Therapeutic value of Gastrografin in adhesive small bowel obstruction after unsuccessful conservative treatment: A prospective randomized trial. *Ann Surg* **236**: 1–6.

8. Deitch EA. (1989) Simple intestinal obstruction causes bacterial translocation in man. *Arch Surg* **124**: 699–701.
9. Rocha FG, Theman TA, Matros E, *et al*. (2009) Nonoperative management of patients with a diagnosis of high-grade small bowel obstruction by computed tomography. *Arch Surg* **144**: 1000–1004.

Chapter 44

Management of the Cirrhotic Patient

*Carmen M. Stanca and Douglas T. Dieterich**

Key Pearls

- Diagnostic paracentesis is recommended in all patients presenting with ascites. Clinicians need to have a high index of suspicion of spontaneous bacterial peritonitis in any cirrhotic patient with unexplained encephalopathy, fever or abdominal pain.
- Treatment of hepatic encephalopathy is aimed at correcting the precipitating factors (infection, hypokalemia, gastrointestinal bleeding, dyselectrolytemia).
- Esophagogastroduodenoscopy is the gold standard for diagnosis of varices and should be performed at the time the patient is diagnosed with cirrhosis.
- Patients with cirrhosis who develop any of the complications below should be referred for liver transplantation evaluation.
- Vaccinations for hepatitis A and B are vital to the care of all liver patients, whether hospitalized or not.

Hospital management of cirrhosis is like war. Ninety-five percent of the time it is sheer boredom, but 5 % of the time it is sheer terror for the team in-charge.

*Mount Sinai School of Medicine, New York, NY, USA.

The goals are to stabilize the extremely ill patient, prevent complications and begin treatment of the underlying liver disease. Contrary to popular opinion, even some decompensated cirrhosis is reversible when the offending agent is removed. That is particularly true for hepatitis B and alcoholic liver disease.[1] We will review the basic management of the common complications of cirrhosis in further detail below.

Ascites

Ascites consists of fluid accumulation in the peritoneal cavity and represents the most common complication of cirrhosis. Its pathogenesis includes portal hypertension, vasodilatation of the splanchnic arteries resulting in secondary hyperaldosteronism and sodium retention, and hypoalbuminemia. **Diagnosis** is based on clinical exam (distended abdomen; fluid wave; shifting dullness) and imaging (ultrasound or CT scan). Diagnostic paracentesis is recommended in patients presenting with ascites. Fresh frozen plasma or platelet transfusion is not recommended to correct coagulopathy before paracentesis. The serum-albumin-to-ascites gradient (SAAG) is >1.1 in patients with portal hypertension, as in cirrhosis. A low level of albumin in ascites correlates with increased risk of spontaneous bacterial peritonitis.

Treatment. Ascites in liver disease due to alcohol or hepatitis B responds to treatment addressing the cause (alcohol abstinence, hepatitis B treatment respectively.)

Diet. It is recommended that patients with ascites follow a diet with less than 2 g of sodium daily.

Diuretics. Treatment starts with spironolactone 100 mg daily and furosemide 40 mg daily; the dose can be increased simultaneously every 3–5 days based on weight loss (goal: 1 lb. daily weight loss after edema resolved) and natriuresis, up to a maximum of 400 mg spironolactone and 160 mg furosemide daily.[2] Amiloride, triamterene, metolazone and hydrocholothiazide are less studied alternatives.

Patients whose ascites cannot be managed with increased doses of diuretics due to adverse events (encephalopathy, hyponatremia <120 mEq/L; creatinine >2 mg/dL) benefit from large volume paracentesis. More than 5 liters of ascites can be removed safely if albumin (8 g/L of ascites removed) is infused simultaneously.[3]

Hyponatremia (serum Na level <130 mEq/L) develops in about 30% of cirrhotic patients and may play a role in the pathogenesis of hepatic encephalopathy. It is asymptomatic in most cases, although patients may complain of nausea, vomiting, and lethargy. Fluid restriction is rarely necessary and can be initiated at a Na level around 120–125 mEq/L, although there are no data to support a certain cut-off value. Vasopressin receptor antagonists (conivaptan and tolvaptan) have been used in patients with cirrhosis; more studies are needed to evaluate the efficacy and safety profile in this population.[4,5]

TIPS (*transjugular intrahepatic portosystemic shunt*). When ascites is refractory to treatment, patients may benefit from TIPS (transjugular intrahepatic porto-systemic shunt) placement, usually done by radiologists (see below).

Peritoneovenous shunts are nearly abandoned due to complications, increased risk of occlusion, and no survival advantage over medical therapy. They can be performed in patients with diuretic-resistant ascites who do not benefit, for various reasons, from the other treatment modalities mentioned above.

Development of refractory ascites is associated with poor prognosis and should prompt referral for ***liver transplantation***.

Spontaneous bacterial peritonitis (SBP) represents infection of the ascites without an obvious abdominal source of infection; the presumed mechanism is bacterial translocation from the gut into the peritoneal cavity. Clinicians need to have a high index of suspicion for SBP in any cirrhotic patient with unexplained encephalopathy, fever or abdominal pain.

Diagnosis is made by paracentesis showing an absolute PMN count >250/mm^3 in ascites, at which point treatment should be instituted without awaiting the Gram stain and culture results. Empiric antibiotic treatment with 3rd generation cephalosporin (cefotaxime, ceftriaxone, ceftazidime) provides good coverage until sensitivities are known. Intravenous followed by oral ciprofloxacin is an alternative in hospitalized patients unless they have vomiting, shock, hepatic encephalopathy grade II or higher, serum creatinine >3 mg/dL or have been on prophylaxis with fluoroquionolones (which raises suspicion for resistance to the drug class). Once culture results are back, the antibiotic spectrum can be narrowed. A five-day antibiotic treatment was shown to be as effective as a 10-day antibiotic treatment.[6]

Intravenous albumin (1.5 g/kg on day 1 and 1 g/kg on day 3) was shown to improve survival in patients with SBP,[7] although patients with a serum creatinine >1 mg/dL, blood urea nitrogen >30 mg/dL, or total bilirubin >4 mg/dL might benefit the most.[8]

Prophylaxis is recommended with norfloxacin 400 mg PO daily, bactrim DS daily 5 days/week, or ciprofloxacin 750 mg PO weekly in patients with ascites.

Development of SBP is associated with decreased survival and should prompt **referral for liver transplantation**.

Esophageal and Gastric Varices

Portal hypertension occurs due to an increased resistance to flow in the cirrhotic liver associated with intrahepatic vasoconstriction and elevated portal vein flow due to splanchnic vasodilatation. Gastric and esophageal varices occur when the hepatic venous pressure gradient reaches at least 10–12 mmHg. Esophagogastroduodenoscopy is the gold standard for diagnosis of varices and should be performed at the time the patient is diagnosed with cirrhosis; the size of varices, red signs (red wale marks, red spots) on the varix, and Child's class (C>B>A for gastric varices) are predictors of bleeding. Compliance with the practice guidelines in the diagnosis and treatment of esophageal varices was associated with a reduction in the first esophageal varices bleeding in the first two years.[9]

Treatment of acute variceal bleeding. Patients with variceal hemorrhage need to be admitted to an intensive care unit. Tracheal intubation may be needed for airway protection. Resuscitation is aimed at reaching hemodynamic stability; the target hemoglobin level is around 8 g/dL; care should be taken not to precipitate or worsen a variceal bleeding by aggressive fluid administration or blood transfusion which can increase the portal pressure. Coagulopathy can be corrected with fresh frozen plasma and/or platelet transfusion. Pharmacological therapy with octreotide (50 µg IV bolus, followed by 50 µg/hr infusion) should be started when variceal hemorrhage is suspected and continued for 3–5 days. Prophylactic antibiotic therapy (ceftriaxone 1 g daily or ciprofloxacin 400 mg IV every 12 hours or norfloxacin 400 mg PO every 12 hours for 7 days) was shown to decrease infections and prolong survival.

Esophagogastroduodenoscopy should be performed as soon as possible for diagnosis and treatment — endoscopic variceal ligation (EVL). TIPS can be performed if bleeding cannot be controlled. Balloon tamponade can be attempted as a temporizing measure when bleeding cannot be controlled, while preparing for TIPS.

Beta-blockers should not be used in acute bleeding.

Primary prophylaxis. Patients with cirrhosis without varices need to repeat EGD in 2–3 years; treatment with beta-blockers does not prevent development of varices. Patients with small varices, Child B or C cirrhosis and red marks on varices benefit from primary prophylaxis with nonselective beta-blockers (propranolol, nadolol). EVL is an alternative for primary prophylaxis in large (grade 3–4) varices. Sclerotherapy is not recommended for primary prophylaxis.

Secondary prophylaxis should be initiated in all the patients with non-selective beta-blockers (with or without nitrates) and EVL.[10]

Patients with variceal bleeding should be referred for transplant evaluation.

TIPS (transjugular intrahepatic portosystemic shunt)
TIPS is indicated in secondary prophylaxis of variceal bleeding and management of refractory ascites, due to its ability to reduce the pressure in the portal venous system. It can also be used in bleeding esophageal varices not controlled by medical or endoscopical therapy, and rebleeding esophageal or gastric varices. TIPS is not recommended in primary prophylaxis of variceal bleeding. Absolute contraindications are: congestive heart failure, severe tricuspid regurgitation, and severe pulmonary hypertension. Imaging for portal system patency and to exclude liver masses needs to be done prior to the procedure. The most common complications include: dysfunction (due to thrombosis or pseudointimal hyperplasia) and hepatic encephalopathy (which usually responds to therapy).[11]

Hepatic Encephalopathy

Hepatic encephalopathy is an alteration in mental status associated with liver failure. Precipitating factors are: infection, hypokalemia, GI bleeding, and dyselectrolytemia. The diagnosis is clinical (confusion, sleepiness, change in personality; asterixis is often present). The ammonia level may be elevated but is not necessary for the diagnosis; it does not correlate with the severity of encephalopathy. Treatment is aimed at correcting the precipitating factors mentioned above. Patients with ascites who become encephalopathic should have a diagnostic paracentesis, and other sources of infection should be sought. Lactulose (a non-absorbable disaccharide) is administered in doses starting with 15–30 mL for 2–4 times a day and adjusted to obtain 2–3 soft stools per day. Lactulose enema can also be used. Rifaximin (550 mg PO twice a day) reduces the risk of hospitalization due to hepatic encephalopathy and is effective in maintaining remission.[12] Zinc supplementation (220 mg PO 3 times a day) is also helpful in the treatment of hepatic encephalopathy.

Hepatorenal Syndrome

HRS is defined as lack of improvement in serum creatinine levels after two days of albumin infusion while off diuretics in a patient with cirrhosis, ascites and creatinine >1.5 mg/dL, in the absence of shock, treatment with nephrotoxic drugs, kidney disease and abnormal ultrasound.

Patients with HRS type I (rapid progression with doubling of serum creatinine level to above 1.5 mg/dL or a 50% decrease in creatinine clearance to below 20 mL/min within two weeks) might benefit from albumin infusion (10–20 g per day for 20 days) associated with midodrine (up to 12.5 mg PO three times a day to increase MAP by 15 mm Hg) and octreotide (200 μg subcutaneously three times a day).[13] HRS type II does not progress rapidly but leads to death in cirrhotic patients. Hemodialysis or continuous venovenous hemodialysis may be used in patients with HRS as a bridge to liver transplantation, which is effective in treating this condition.

Liver Transplantation

Patients with cirrhosis have an increased risk of developing hepatocellular carcinoma. Their life expectancy is reduced even in the absence of cancer. The MELD score is a mathematical model which uses bilirubin, creatinine and INR levels to predict survival in the absence of liver transplantation. Patients with cirrhosis who develop any of the above complications should be referred for liver transplantation evaluation.

References

1. Veldt BJ, Laine F, Guillogomarc'h A, *et al.* (2002) Indication of liver transplantation in severe alcoholic liver cirrhosis: Quantitative evaluation and optimal timing. *J Hepatol* **36**: 93–98.

2. Runyon BA; AASLD Practice Guidelines Committee. (2009) Management of adult patients with ascites due to cirrhosis: An update. *Hepatology* **49**(6): 2087–107.
3. Titó L, Ginès P, Arroyo V, *et al.* (1990) Total paracentesis associated with intravenous albumin management of patients with cirrhosis and ascites. *Gastroenterology* **98**(1): 146–51.
4. Wong F, Blei AT, Blendis LM, Thulavath PJ. (2003) A vasopressin receptor antagonist (VPA-985) improves serum sodium concentration in patients with hyponatremia: A multicenter, randomized, placebo-controlled trial. *Hepatology* **37**: 182–191.
5. Schrier RW, Gross P, Gheorghiade M, *et al.* (2006) Tolvaptan, a selective oral vasopressin V2-receptor antagonist, for hyponatremia. *N Engl J Med* **355**: 2099–2112.
6. Runyon BA, McHutchison JG, Antillon MR, *et al.* (1991) Short-course vs long-course antibiotic treatment of spontaneous bacterial peritonitis: A randomized controlled trial of 100 patients. *Gastroenterology* **100**: 1737–1742.
7. Sort P, Navasa M, Arroyo V, *et al.* (1999) Effect of intravenous albumin on renal impairment and mortality in patients with cirrhosis and spontaneous bacterial peritonitis. *N Engl J Med* **341**: 403–409.
8. Sigal SH, Stanca CM, Fernandez J, *et al.* (2007) Restricted use of albumin for spontaneous bacterial peritonitis. *Gut* **56**: 597–599.
9. Moodley J, Lopez R, Carey W. (2010) Compliance with practice guidelines and risk of a first esophageal variceal hemorrhage in patients with cirrhosis. *Clin Gastroenterol Hepatol* **8**(8): 703–708.
10. Garcia-Tsao G, Sanyal AJ, Grace ND, Carey W. (2007) Prevention and management of gastroesophageal varices and variceal hemorrhage in cirrhosis. Practice Guidelines Committee of the American Association for the Study of Liver Diseases; Practice Parameters Committee of the American College of Gastroenterology. *Hepatology* **46**(3): 922–38.
11. Boyer TD, Haskal ZJ. (2010) The Role of Transjugular Intrahepatic Portosystemic Shunt (TIPS) in the Management of Portal Hypertension: Update 2009. American Association for the Study of Liver Diseases. *Hepatology* **51**(1): 306.

12. Bass NM, Mullen KD, Sanyal A, *et al.* (2010) Rifaximin treatment in hepatic encephalopathy. *N Engl J Med* **362**: 1071–81.
13. Angeli P, Volpin R, Gerunda G, *et al.* (1999) Reversal of type I hepatorenal syndrome with the administration of midodrine and octreotide. *Hepatology* **29**: 1690–1697.

Chapter 45

Approach to the Hospitalized Patient with Abnormal Liver Function Tests

*Kalpesh K. Patel**

Key Pearls

- Abnormal LFTs in a hospitalized patient may reflect acute injury, chronic liver disease or a combination of both.
- Careful history taking and physical exam will contribute key clues to the etiology of abnormal LFTs.
- Medication side effects and abnormal hemodynamic states are the most common reason for acute elevations in LFTs in hospitalized patients.
- The majority of abnormal LFTs will improve after correction of the underlying cause; however, prompt recognition of impending acute liver failure is essential.
- Early request for GI/hepatology consultation is appropriate in cases of unexplained, severe, or prolonged elevations of LFTs.

Introduction

Abnormal liver function tests (LFTs) are a common finding in hospitalized patients. These abnormalities may relate to the primary reason for

*Baylor College of Medicine, Division of Gastroenterology and Hepatology, Houston, TX, USA.

admission, reflect chronic underlying liver disease, represent a de novo injury, or a combination of these factors.[1,2] Unlike ambulatory patients, who generally present with mild elevations in isolated LFTs, hospitalized patients often have significant elevations in single or multiple LFTs. Determination of the etiology and severity of liver injury and recognition of related complications are discussed in this chapter.

Definition of Abnormal LFTs

Liver function tests (or a hepatic panel) typically include measurements of:

1) Serum aminotransferases (alanine aminotransferase/ALT, and aspartate aminotransferase/AST)
2) Total and direct bilirubin
3) Alkaline phosphatase (AP) and gamma glutamyl transpeptidase (GGTP)
4) Albumin

Abnormal values are classified as those which are 2 standard deviations above the mean value (as measured in a healthy population). Additional laboratory markers of liver function include prothrombin time (PT) and platelet count.

Patient Evaluation

History

A careful taking of the medical history is crucial to determining the acuity and possible etiology of abnormal LFTs. The patient should be questioned specifically for the presence of known underlying liver disease, as well as for common risk factors (i.e. alcohol use, intravenous drug use, blood transfusion, unprotected sexual activity, foreign travel). Symptoms to assess include the presence or absence of itching, changes in urine or stool color, right upper quadrant abdominal pain, nausea/vomiting, fever, and features of systemic illness (i.e. heart failure, infection). Most importantly, a detailed medication history (prescription, over-the-counter, and herbal), including the precise timing of initiation of medication, should be obtained.[3]

Physical Examination

Careful examination of the liver bed can provide important etiologic clues. The size, firmness and presence of nodularity and/or tenderness should be noted. Evidence of right-sided heart failure, including jugular venous distension, tricuspid regurgitation murmur, and lower extremity edema should also be noted. Signs of chronic liver disease should be noted, including splenomegaly, spider angiomas, palmar erythema, ascites, gynecomastia, and caput medusa.

Laboratory Evaluation

Liver Function Tests

An isolated elevation in a liver test should be confirmed to be hepatic in origin. AST enzymes are found in cardiac/skeletal muscle, erythrocytes, kidneys, brain, and lungs. Alkaline phosphatase can be released from bone and intestine. Albumin can be lowered due to poor nutrition or protein losing states. Determination of hepatic origin is based on clinical evaluation of other illnesses, and use of isoenzyme fractionation when available.

Once a hepatic origin is confirmed, the pattern of elevation of the LFTs should be assessed. The most common patterns are those of a predominantly hepatocellular or cholestatic process. In a hepatocellular pattern, the AST and ALT levels are predominantly elevated in comparison to the alkaline phosphatase and GGTP. A cholestatic pattern presents as predominant elevations in AP and GGTP. Overlap between patterns may occur. The serum bilirubin can be elevated in either pattern, and thus is not necessarily helpful in differentiating the processes. An infiltrative process, such as a primary or metastatic neoplasm, may present with mild-moderate elevations in all LFTs. The pattern of LFT abnormalities can help generate a differential diagnosis and guide further evaluation (Table 1).

The prothrombin time may be elevated in the setting of prolonged biliary obstruction or severe hepatocellular injury. The serum albumin may be decreased during chronic liver disease. Reduced platelet counts may reflect portal hypertension and chronic liver disease. The timing of the

Table 1. Typical Patterns of Liver Function Tests During Injury

	Hepatocellular			Cholestatic		Infiltration
	Ischemia & Toxins	**Viral Hepatitis**	**Alcohol**	**Complete**	**Partial**	**Infiltrative Disease**
Aminotransferases	50–100×	5–50×	2–5×	1–5×	1–5×	1–3×
Alk phos/GGTP	1–3×	1–3×	1–10×	2–20×	2–10×	1–20×
Bilirubin	1–5×	1–30×	1–30×	1–30×	1–5×	1–5×
Prothrombin time	Prolonged; unresponsive to vitamin K in severe disease		Responsive to vitamin K			Usually nl Usually nl
Albumin	Decreased chronic disease		Usually nl			Usually nl
Platelet count	Decrease suggests stage III/IV					Usually nl

nl = Normal

elevation of LFTs should be carefully noted, in order to link to specific inciting or associated factors, i.e. onset of new medications, altered hemodynamics, abdominal pain, etc.

Directed Laboratory Testing

The following serologic testing should be performed in the initial evaluation in an effort to further refine the diagnostic possibilities (Table 2).

Further Evaluation

Imaging Studies

Radiologic testing is advised to supplement blood testing. A transabdominal ultrasound is the usual initial imaging study. The ultrasound can provide details regarding the size of the liver, biliary dilation, cholelithiasis, and hepatic masses. Computed tomography scanning (with intravenous contrast) provides a more detailed evaluation of the hepatic parenchyma, as well as information regarding other abdominal organs. If biliary obstruction is suspected, MRCP provides superior demonstration of both the intra- and extra-hepatic biliary system.

Table 2. Directed Laboratory Testing

Toxicology	Viral
Urine/serum drug toxicology	Hepatitis A IgM
Serum acetaminophen level	Hepatitis B surface Ag, Core Ab, Surface Ab
	Hepatitis C Ab
	HBV viral DNA or HCV viral RNA PCR if above screen is positive
	If immunosuppressed, add: CMV, EBV and HSV IgM Abs
Auto Antibodies	**Metabolic**
Anti-nuclear antibody — Autoimmune hepatitis	Serum ceruloplasmin — Wilson Disease
Anti smooth muscle antibody — Autoimmune hepatitis	Serum ferritin, iron, total iron binding capacity — Hereditary hemochromatosis
Anti mitochondrial antibody — Primary biliary cirrhosis	Fasting insulin, lipid profile — NASH
P-ANCA antibody — Primary sclerosing cholangitis	

Features of Common Conditions

Hepatocellular Injuries

Drug Induced Liver Injury

Pre-hospitalization exposure to prescription, over the counter, or herbal preparations may be responsible for abnormal LFTs noted upon admission. The most common culprit is acetaminophen, which causes a rapid, dose dependent injury, which can result in acute liver failure in 5–10% of cases.[4] In-hospital exposures are the most common anti-microbials. This association is usually confirmed after the offending agent is stopped, and the LFTs gradually return to normal.

Ischemia

Ischemic hepatitis generally presents as rapid elevation of the transaminases to levels >2000 U/L. Typically, this is seen in patients with significant cardiovascular disease, with resultant hepatic hypoperfusion and in patients with profound hypotension due to heart failure or sepsis.[5] The PT may be elevated as well, with a rapid return to normal values. An underlying chronic liver disease predisposes to ischemic injury, even in the setting of mild cardiac or hemodynamic dysfunction.

Alcohol

Mild to moderate elevations of the transaminases (typically with AST: ALT ratio of >2) may be seen in patients with chronic alcohol abuse.[6] More severe elevations, associated with elevated bilirubin and prothrombin time may represent an acute alcoholic hepatitis in the appropriate setting.

Viral Hepatitis

Although increasingly less common in developed countries, acute viral hepatitis should be considered in the setting of transaminases >1000 U/L.[7] Hepatitis A, via fecal-oral transmission, is the most common cause of acute symptomatic viral hepatitis. De novo or reactivation of hepatitis B remains common among certain, at-risk populations. Other viral hepatidities are rare causes of acute LFT elevations.

Cholestatic Injury

Cholestatic injury can be divided into intra- vs. extrahepatic causes of biliary obstruction. Common causes of intrahepatic cholestasis include medication effect, granulomatous disease, primary biliary cirrhosis, sepsis and malignant infiltration of the liver. Extrahepatic causes include choledocholithiasis, benign or malignant biliary strictures, and primary sclerosing cholangitis. Differentiation of these patterns can usually be made based on careful imaging of the biliary system with ultrasound or MRCP. Extrahepatic obstruction can usually be treated by endoscopic or percutaneous biliary drainage.

Patient Outcomes and Role of GI/Hepatology Consultation

The majority of hospitalized patients with abnormal LFTs will experience improvement once the underlying condition is corrected. This is typically true in patients with drug induced (in-hospital) or ischemic hepatitis, as well as extrahepatic biliary obstruction who undergo drainage. Patients with underlying chronic liver disease or a primary liver injury (i.e. viral hepatitis, acetaminophen toxicity) may be at risk for progressive injury and ultimately liver failure. Therefore, early identification of the etiology of abnormal LFTs and underlying patient risk factors is essential. In the case of unexplained, severe, or prolonged/worsening injury, early consultation with a GI/hepatology specialist may greatly aid in the management of these complex patients.

References

1. Aijaz A, Keeffe EB. (2006) Liver chemistry and function tests. In: Feldman, Friedman, Brandt (eds), *Sleisenger & Fordtran's Gastrointestinal and Liver Disease*, 8th ed. Saunders Elsevier: Philadelphia, pp. 1575–1586.
2. O'Brien CB. (2009) The hospitalized patient with abnormal liver function tests. *Clin Liver Dis* **13**(2): 179–192.
3. Agarwal VK, McHutchison JG, Hoofnagle JH. (2010) Drug-induced liver injury network. Important elements for the diagnosis of drug-induced liver injury. *Clin Gastroenterol Hepatol* **8**(5): 463–470.
4. Chun LJ, Tong MJ, Busuttil RW, Hiatt JR. (2009) Acetaminophen hepatotoxicity and acute liver failure. *J Clin Gastroenterol* **43**(4): 342–349.
5. Giallourakis CC, Rosenberg PM, Friedman LS. (2002) The liver in heart failure. *Clin Liver Dis* **6**(4): 947–967.
6. O'Shea RS, Dasarathy S, McCullough AJ. (2010) Practice Guidelines Committee of the American Association for the Study of Liver

Diseases; Practice Parameters Committee of the American College of Gastroenterology. Alcoholic liver disease. *Hepatology* **51**(1): 307–328.

7. Degertekin B, Lok AS. (2009) Update on viral hepatitis: 2008. *Curr Opin Gastroenterol* **25**(3): 180–185.

Endocrine

Chapter 46

Management of Diabetes and Hyperglycemia in Hospitalized Patients

*Maria Skamagas**

Key Pearls

- Blood glucose goals for medical and surgical ward patients are 100–140 mg/dL before meals and 100–180 mg/dL at other times (i.e. bedtime, postprandial).
- Oral medications should be discontinued in acutely ill patients.
- Insulin should be individualized to cover basal, mealtime, and correction requirements. There is a spectrum of insulin requirements in type 2 diabetes: correction insulin only; basal and correction insulin; or basal, mealtime, and correction insulin.
- Type 1 diabetics require basal insulin at all times, even when taking "nothing by mouth"(NPO).
- A hypoglycemia protocol should be in place to manage hypoglycemia in patients receiving insulin or oral diabetes medication.

Introduction

Diabetes Admissions to the Hospital

Diabetes ranks among the top three diagnoses for admission to US hospitals. Ten percent of all hospital admissions involve diabetes as the primary

*Mount Sinai School of Medicine, New York, NY, USA.

diagnosis.[1] In 2006, 5.2 million individuals with diabetes were discharged from a US hospital.[2] Such admissions are either directly related to diabetes, such as diabetic ketoacidosis, hyperosmolar hyperglycemic syndrome, coronary events, cerebrovascular events, lower extremity conditions, and hypoglycemia, or are due to an unrelated condition, such as surgery, injury, or psychiatric disease. The average hospital length of stay for individuals with diabetes is five days.[3] Given the ever-growing diabetes epidemic finding its way into the hospital system, practitioners will encounter patients with diabetes in all sectors of the hospital on a regular basis. Practitioners must become familiar with managing these patients in the hospital setting with the aim of maintaining blood glucose (BG) at goal while avoiding detrimental hypoglycemia and hyperglycemia. The recommendations herein will serve as a guide for the hospital practitioner in managing individuals with diabetes, and are based largely on consensus statement,[4] expert reviews, and the author's experience. Clinical judgment and individualization of care must be applied in each situation.

Glycemic Goals and Outcomes on the General Wards

Hospitalized patients with uncontrolled BG suffer more infections, prolonged length of stay, and increased mortality. Overly aggressive control can also be detrimental, as hypoglycemia is associated with increased length of stay and mortality in hospitalized patients.[5] There are no randomized control studies of glucose control in patients on general medical and surgical wards. During hospitalization, multiple variables contribute to either increased BG (acute illness, surgery, glucocorticoids, enteral and parenteral nutrition) or decreased BG (reduced oral intake, renal failure), making it more challenging to predict exact requirements and achieve tight glucose control. BG goals according to the ADA/AACE are 100–140 mg/dL before meals and 100–180 mg/dL at other times (Table 1). As BG levels trend to less than 100 mg/dL, consideration should be made to adjust the diabetes regimen. Attempting to achieve even lower glucose targets in all patients will result in more hypoglycemia, especially in a hospitalized population, who by definition have more comorbidities

Table 1. Inpatient Glucose Goals[4]

Population	BG Goals (mg/dL)
Ward	Premeal: 100–140 Random: 100–180
ICU	140–180

Ward patient: if BG < 100 mg/dL, consider adjusting diabetes regimen;
if BG < 70 mg/dL, adjust diabetes regimen.

which predispose to hypoglycemia. Glycemic goals may be individualized for each patient i.e. "tighter" or lower goals for a patient with an infection, and "looser" or higher goals for a frail elderly patient who cannot report hypoglycemic symptoms.

Differentiating Type 1 and Type 2 Diabetes[6]

Individuals with type 1 diabetes (DM 1) constitute 10% of all individuals with diabetes. They do not make insulin, and thus require basal insulin injections (long-acting insulin) to avoid diabetic ketoacidosis (DKA) and hyperglycemia even when NPO. Basal insulin provides 24 hr of blood insulin levels which suppress hepatic glucose production and lipolysis, thus preventing hyperglycemia in the fasting state and ketoacid formation (DKA). Examples of basal insulins are glargine once daily, detemir twice daily, and NPH twice daily. When type 1 diabetics eat carbohydrates, rapid-acting insulin is required to control BG elevations after the meal. Illness and infection result in increased circulating catecholamines, cortisol, and other counterregulatory hormones which increase BG and lipolysis, and raise the risk of DKA if the patient has not received basal insulin.

The characteristics of individuals with DM 1 include: diagnosis in youth (usually less than 30 years of age); initial presentation with DKA or symptomatic hyperglycemia and insulinopenia (weight loss, polyuria, polydipsia, polyphagia); lean body mass at diagnosis; and requiring insulin since diagnosis. Occasionally, individuals are diagnosed with DM 1 at an advanced age. Type 1 diabetics can also be overweight/obese if they lead an unhealthy lifestyle; this may translate into increased insulin resistance.

Individuals with type 2 diabetes (DM 2) constitute about 85%–90% of all individuals with diabetes. They suffer from both reduced insulin secretion and increased insulin resistance (difficulty in using the insulin that is made by beta cells). DM 2 is managed with diet, physical activity, oral medications, and/or insulin. In type 2 diabetics who require insulin injections, some need only basal insulin to control glucose, while others require both basal and mealtime insulin. The majority of people with DM 2 produce enough endogenous insulin to avoid DKA. However, some have little capacity for insulin secretion, i.e. long-standing diabetes requiring multiple insulin injections, and in the setting of severe stress or illness these individuals are vulnerable to DKA. Reduced PO intake and NPO status result in reduced basal insulin requirements. This is likely related to a reduction in hepatic glycogen stores,[7] and possibly improved insulin action[8] and insulin secretion. It is important to keep this in mind for the hospitalized patient who is eating a carbohydrate/calorie-controlled diet and less food than is eaten at home, as the insulin requirements may be less.

The characteristics of individuals with DM 2 include: overweight/obesity or increased abdominal adiposity/waist circumference, family history of diabetes, high risk ethnicity (non-Caucasians), and acanthosis nigricans. Although DM 2 is more common with advancing age, it is being diagnosed in obese younger individuals, including children and teenagers.

Insulin

In managing BG in a hospitalized patient, it is crucial to know the names and doses of diabetes medications that the patient is taking at home, and whether the patient is adherent to the regimen (always, sometimes, or infrequently). Diabetes medications include insulins (see Table 2), oral medications, and other injectable endocrine hormones (see Table 3). Oral diabetes medications should be discontinued in acutely ill, hospitalized patients for multiple reasons, including increased risk for hypoglycemia, reduced PO intake, and increased risk for contraindications to the oral medications

Table 2. Pharmacokinetic Profiles of Insulins (SC)

Class	Name (Brand)	Onset	Peak	Duration	Typical Use
Long-acting (basal)	Glargine (Lantus®) Detemir (Levemir®)	2 hr	None	24 hr 18–20 hr	• Basal — give at same time of day • Levemir — use twice daily in DM1
Rapid-acting	Aspart (Novolog®) Lispro (Humalog®) Glulisine (Apidra®)	5–15 min	1–2 hr	4–6 hr	• Mealtime • Corrrection
Short-acting	Human Regular (Humulin R®, Novolin R®)	30–60 min	2–4 hr	6–10 hr	• Insulin IV infusion • Enteral/tube feeds • Mealtime
Intermediate-acting	Human NPH (Humulin N®, Novolin N®)	2–4 hr	4–10 hr	12–20 hr	• Enteral/tube feeds • Steroid-induced hyperglycemia
Pre-mixed*	70/30 NPH/regular (Humulin N®, Novolin N®) 75/25 protaminated lispro & lispro (Humalog Mix®) 70/30 protaminated aspart & aspart (Novolog Mix®)	Variable	Variable	Variable	• Before meals: breakfast and dinner (do not use if NPO or poor intake)

*Premixed insulins: the two values refer to the percentage makeup of the mixture by intermediate-acting and short/rapid-acting insulin, in that order.

Table 3. Oral Diabetes Medications and Injectable Endocrine Hormones

Class of Medications	Names of Medications (brand in parentheses)
Biguanide	
• Reduces hepatic gluconeogenesis	Metformin (Glucophage®) Metformin extended release (Glucophage XR®, Fortamet®, Glumetza®)
Sulfonylureas	
• Long-acting insulin secretagogues	Glimepiride (Amaryl®) Glipizide (Glucotrol®, Glucotrol XL®) Glyburide (Micronase®, DiaBeta®)
Thiazolidinediones	
• Insulin sensitizers	Pioglitazone (Actos®) Rosiglitazone (Avandia®)
Meglitinides	
• Short-acting insulin secretagogues • Used at mealtimes	Repaglinide (Prandin®) Nateglinide (Starlix®)
Alpha-glucosidase inhibitors	
• Used at mealtimes	Acarbose (Precose®) Miglitol (Glyset®)
DPP-4 inhibitors	Sitagliptin (Januvia®) Saxagliptin (Onglyza®)
Injectable endocrine agents	
• GLP-1 receptor agonists	Exenatide (Byetta®), liraglutide (Victoza®)
• Amylin analog	Pramlintide (Symlin®)

(e.g. alteration in renal function). Metformin should be discontinued in ill patients with the following conditions: creatinine ≥ 1.5 mg/dL (males) and ≥1.4 mg/dL (females); congestive heart failure; severe liver disease; lung disease/hypoxemia; and for iodinated contrast or surgery. Sulfonylureas (e.g. glimepiride, glipizide, glyburide) and short-acting meglitinides (e.g. repaglinide, nateglinide), which all cause an increase in insulin secretion, should be held if the patient is NPO or has reduced PO intake (which is the case with many hospitalized patients), and used with caution in patients with renal insuffiency. Pioglitazone should be held in cases of volume overload, cardiovascular event, or congestive heart failure.

Insulin is the safest and most efficacious means of managing BG in hospitalized patients. There are weight-based guidelines for initiating insulin in type 2 and type 1 diabetes, and for titrating insulin (see Fig. 1 and Fig. 2). In regard to type 1 diabetes, all patients must receive basal insulin, even when NPO, to avoid ketoacidosis. Type 1 diabetes patients tend to be more insulin-sensitive. Matching mealtime rapid-acting insulin to carbohydrates eaten is important for preventing postprandial hyper- and hypoglycemia. In regard to type 2 diabetes, patients who have good glycemic control on oral medications at home may need only correction insulin scales (see Table 4) in the hospital. Type 2 diabetics who

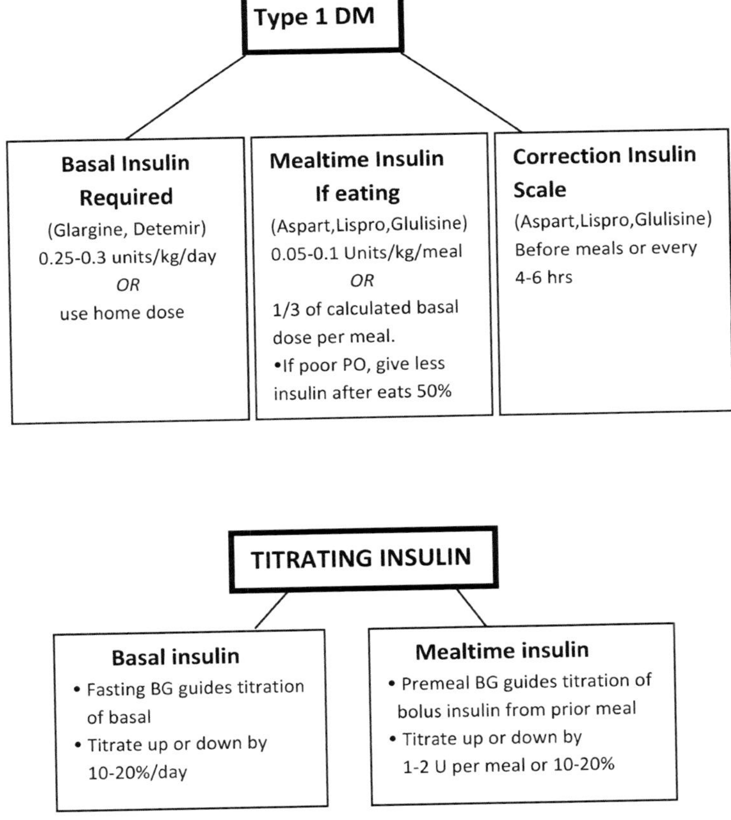

Fig. 1. Management of Type 1 Diabetes in Hospitalized Patients.

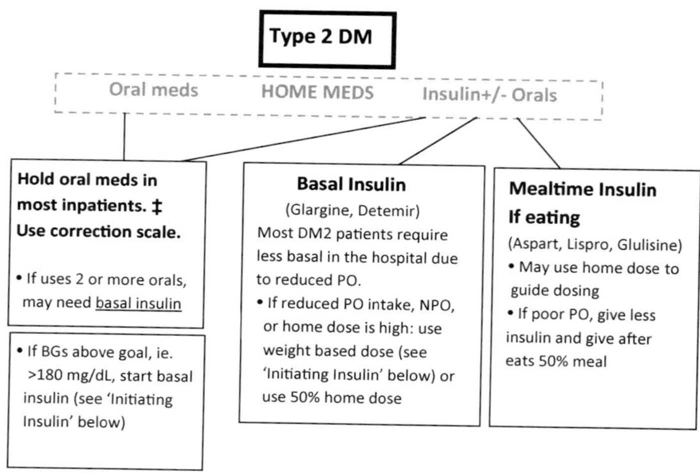

‡ DM 2 on oral meds: some require correction insulin only, some basal insulin only, others basal insulin and mealtime insulin.

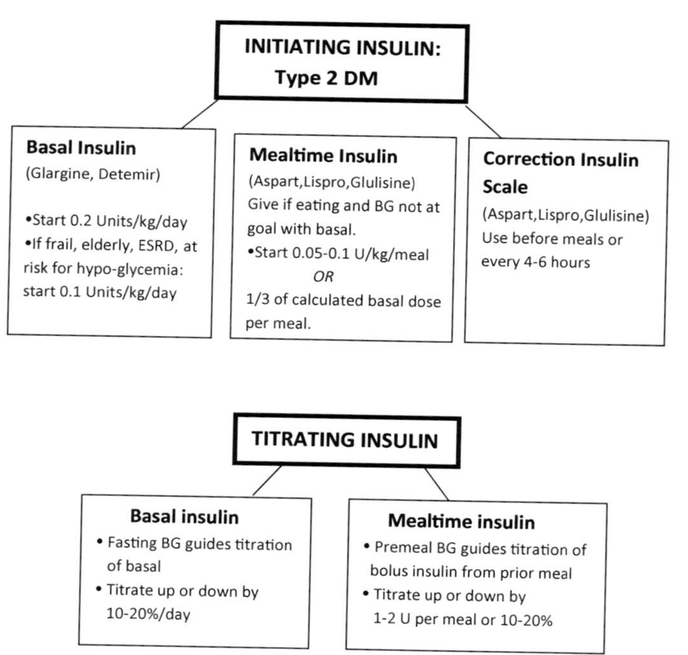

Fig. 2. Management of Type 2 Diabetes in Hospitalized Patients.

Table 4. Correction Insulin Scales

- Use every 4–6 hr SC to correct high blood glucose.
- Rapid-acting insulins are preferred. Ex.: lispro, aspart, glulisine.

Insulin Sensitive Patient		**Insulin-Resistant Patient**	
Use if: • Total daily insulin <30 units • DM type 1 • At risk for hypoglycemia (frail, ESRD, ESLD)		Use if: • Total daily insulin >30 units	
Insulin Dose (units)	**Blood Glucose (mg/dL)**	**Insulin Dose (units)**	**Blood Glucose (mg/dL)**
0	<180	0	<180
1	180–220	2	180–220
2	221–260	3	221–260
3	261–300	4	261–300
4	301–340	6	301–340
5	341–400	8	341–370
6	>400*	10	371–400
		12	>400*

*If blood glucose >400 mg/dL, call MD and measure urine ketones.

use two or more oral medications at home may require basal insulin in addition to correction insulin while in the hospital. It is important to recognize that mealtime carbohydrate and caloric portions in the hospital are controlled and may be less than what a patient eats at home. Therefore, a type 2 diabetic patient may require less basal and less prandial medication in the hospital, and patients who use large doses of basal insulin (e.g. glargine, detemir, NPH) at home may require lower doses in the hospital.

Hypoglycemia

Hypoglycemia is generally defined by BG < 70 mg/dL. Individuals who are at risk for hypoglycemia include those with prior hypoglycemia, hypoglycemia unawareness, poor PO intake, advanced age, frailty, renal insufficiency, advanced liver disease, mealtime insulin not administered at the appropriate time before a meal, and pancreatic disease/history pancreatectomy. The signs and symptoms include the initial adrenergic constellation of sweating, tremor, tachycardia/palpitations, and weakness, and the later neuroglycopenic signs of altered mental status, seizure, and coma.

Treat hypoglycemia immediately with glucose and repeat BG in 15 min. Retreat until BG >100 mg/dL. In patients who are unable to take PO, use intravenous (IV) dextrose, and in those without IV access, use intramuscular (IM) glucagon (see Table 5).

Table 5. Hypoglycemia Management

BG (mg/dL)	PO Status and Mental Status	Treatment
50–70	Awake, able to take PO	4 oz fruit juice, glucose gel (1 tube), or 4 glucose tabs
50–70	Unable to take PO, altered mental status	½ amp of D50% IV push
<50		1 amp of D50% IV push
<70	No IV access, unable to take PO glucose	Glucagon 1 mg IM, establish IV access

Prevention of hypoglycemia begins with identifying individuals at risk and adjusting glucose goals in those who are at high risk. A daily review of BG levels and BG patterns may uncover a patient who is approaching the hypoglycemia range. Common causes of hypoglycemia include the following: a large dose of basal insulin used at home is continued in the hospital but the patient is not eating as much as he or she ate at home; mealtime insulin is given and the patient does not eat the meal; elevated BG is corrected with high dose rapid-acting insulin; rapid acting insulin doses are given frequently or "stacked" and blood levels of insulin rise rapidly. Adjustment of the insulin regimen when BG < 100 mg/dL, and certainly when BG <70 mg/dL, is appropriate. If the PO intake is variable, administer rapid-acting insulin immediately after a certain amount of the meal is eaten (for example, give lispro after the patient eats 50% of a meal). Avoid sulfonylureas and rapid-acting secretagogues (repaglinide, nateglinide) in patients with variable PO intake.

Special Situations

Steroid-Induced Hyperglycemia

Glucocorticoids are used to manage various conditions of hospitalized patients, including asthma, transplant rejection, rheumatologic disease, hematologic malignancy, and CNS inflammation/tumors. They often result in exacerbation of BG in patients with pre-existing DM, but may also cause "steroid hyperglycemia" in individuals without diabetes. They primarily affect postprandial BG but may also raise fasting BG, especially in pre-existing diabetes.[9] Management of the hyperglycemia depends on the severity of BG elevations, pattern of BG elevation, and dose of glucocorticoids. Insulin is the primary therapy when BG exceeds the goal. Prednisone dosed in the morning tends to elevate the afternoon and evening BG, with improvement by the morning BG.

If BG is mildly elevated, such as 140–180 mg/dL, a diabetic diet and a correction insulin scale may be used. If BG is very elevated, such as >180–200 mg/dL, then standing insulin may be appropriate. A diabetic diet with no concentrated sweets should be ordered. It is important to proactively adjust insulin doses as steroids are tapered.

Examples

(1) Prednisone given in the morning elevates afternoon/evening BG: consider NPH insulin 0.1 units/kg/day, given at the same time as prednisone.
(2) Pre-existing DM, all BG elevated >200 mg/dL with glucocorticoids: consider NPH (dosed at the same time as the steroid) and mealtime rapid-acting insulin, or basal glargine and mealtime rapid-acting insulin.
(3) High dose steroids (such as methylprednisolone 1 g daily for three days for rejection or autoimmune disease, or dexamethasone for neurosurgical conditions) may cause severe hyperglycemia. IV insulin infusions may be necessary in order to control BG in this setting.

NPO (for Procedure/Imaging Study/Surgery)

(1) Hold all oral agents and mealtime insulin.
(2) *Type 1 DM*: Minor procedure/imaging study: give 80% of the basal insulin dose. Major surgery: insulin drip and D5 1/2NS.
(3) *Type 2 DM*: give 50%–80% of the basal insulin dose. If NPO >24 hr, give only 50%, or give 50% weight based dose = 0.1 units/kg/day.
(4) May use a correction insulin scale every 6 hr.

Nutritional Support

Enteral feeds and hyperglycemia. For continuous tube feeds, use NPH every 6–8 hr. Start low dose 0.05–0.1 units/kg NPH SC every 6–8 hr, and titrate. Hold the dose if tube feeds are held; if insulin is given and feeds are stopped, then infuse D10% to avoid hypoglycemia. For bolus feeds, use rapid-acting insulin or regular insulin before the feed.

Parenteral nutrition and hyperglycemia. Use 0.1 units insulin/g carbohydrate in parenteral nutrition. If the patient remains hyperglycemic, titrate insulin in the parenteral nutrition bag or use subcutaneous insulin.

Insulin Pumps[10]

Many patients with DM 1 use insulin pumps with continuous subcutaneous insulin infusions to provide basal insulin and mealtime insulin. If the hospitalized patient is awake, alert, and capable of actively managing the insulin pump, then it may be continued. The nurse staff should record fingerstick glucose as usual. Hospitals should have guidelines in place for glucose monitoring, documentation of insulin pump doses, and criteria for insulin pump discontinuation.

Situations in which insulin pumps should be disconnected and subcutaneous insulin injections administered include:

- General anesthesia
- Prolonged procedure >2–3 hr

- The patient is unable to actively manage the insulin pump: impaired alertness, receiving sedatives/analgesia, psychiatric instability
- Critical illness

Such patients require SC basal insulin (or IV insulin). There must be overlap between the subcutaneous basal insulin injection and discontinuation of the pump infusion, so that the basal insulin may reach adequate blood levels (i.e. if glargine is injected SC, wait 2 hr prior to disconnecting the insulin pump).

Pregnant Patient[11]

Goal glucoses in gestational diabetes are premeal ≤ 95 mg/dL and 2-hr postprandial ≤ 120 mg/dL. Glucose goals in pregnant women with pre-existing diabetes are premeal 60–99 mg/dL and postprandial 100–129 mg/dL. Insulins used in pregnancy include NPH (basal insulin), aspart, and lispro (meal time and correction insulin).

Labor and delivery requires significant energy expenditure, so insulin requirements are low. Dextrose infusion and low dose insulin drip 0.5–1 units/hr should be initiated and titrated to goal glucose 80–120 mg/dL.

Discharging Home

If A1c is at goal and home glucoses are at goal, continue the prehospital regimen. If A1c is not at goal or home glucoses are uncontrolled (hypoglycemia and hyperglycemia), adjust the regimen and inform the patient and the patient's physician of the change. Avoiding hypoglycemia should be a priority.

Survival Skills

(1) *Glucose goals (ADA)*: fasting: 70–130 mg/dL, postprandial 2 hr: <180 mg/dL. Individualize these goals.

(2) *Glucose monitoring*:

- Once daily if on oral meds or basal insulin
- Before each meal and bedtime if on multiple injections/day

(3) *Hypoglycemia management*: signs/symptoms/treatment
(4) *Basic meal planning*
(5) *Insulin administration and storage*

Prescriptions that a diabetic patient may need include:

(1) Insulin

— pens and pen needles (convenient)
— vials and syringes (cheaper)
— alcohol pads

(2) Glucometer supplies: lancets and test strips
(3) Oral medications

References

1. Data Source: Centers for Disease Control and Prevention (CDC), National Center for Health Statistics, Division of Health Care Statistics; data from the National Hospital Discharge Survey. Data computed by personnel in CDC's Division of Diabetes Translation, National Center for Chronic Disease Prevention and Health Promotion. Distribution of First Listed Diagnoses Among Hospital Discharges with Diabetes as Any Listed Diagnosis, Adults Age 18 Years or Older, United States, 2006. http://www.cdc.gov/diabetes/statistics/hosp/adulttable1.htm
2. Data Source: Centers for Disease Control and Prevention (CDC), National Center for Health Statistics, Division of Health Care Statistics; data from the National Hospital Discharge Survey and Division of Health Interview Statistics, data from the National Health Interview Survey. U.S. Bureau of the Census; census of the population and population estimates and National Center for Health Statistics, CDC, bridged-race population estimates. Data computed by personnel in the CDC's Division of Diabetes Translation, National Center for Chronic Disease Prevention and Health Promotion. http://www.cdc.gov/diabetes/statistics/dmany/fig1.htm

3. Data Source: Centers for Disease Control and Prevention (CDC), National Center for Health Statistics, Division of Health Care Statistics; data from the National Hospital Discharge Survey and Division of Health Interview Statistics, data from the National Health Interview Survey. U.S. Bureau of the Census; census of the population and population estimates and National Center for Health Statistics, CDC, bridged-race population estimates. Data computed by personnel in the Division of Diabetes Translation, National Center for Chronic Disease Prevention and Health Promotion, CDC. http://www.cdc.gov/diabetes/statistics/dmany/fig2.htm
4. Moghissi ES, Korytkowski MT, DiNardo M, *et al.* (2009) American Association of Clinical Endocrinologists and American Diabetes Association consensus statement on inpatient glycemic control. *Endocr Pract* **15**: 353–369.
5. Turchin A, Matheny ME, Shubina M, *et al.* (2009) Hypoglycemia and clinical outcomes in patients with diabetes hospitalized in the general ward. *Diabetes Care* **32**: 1153–1157.
6. American Diabetes Association. (2009) Diagnosis and classification of diabetes mellitus. *Diabetes Care* **32**(Suppl 1): S62–S67.
7. Exton JH, Corbin JG, Harper SC. (1972) Control of gluconeogenesis in liver. V. Effects of fasting, diabetes, and glucagon in lactate and endogenous metabolism in the perfused rat liver. *J Biol Chem* **247**: 4996–5003.
8. Halberg N, Henriksen M, Söderhamn N, *et al.* (2005) Effect of intermittent fasting and refeeding on insulin action in healthy men. *J Appl Physiol* **99**: 2128–2136.
9. Clore, JN, Thurby-Hay L. (2009) Glucocorticoid-induced hyperglycemia. *Endocr Pract* **15**: 469–474.
10. Bailon RM, Partlow BJ, Miller-Cage V, *et al.* (2009) Continuous subcutaneous insulin infusion (insulin pump) therapy can be safely used in the hospital in select patients. *Endocr Pract* **15**: 24–29.
11. Standards of Medical Care in Diabetes (2012). *Diabetes Care* **35**(Suppl 1): S11–S63.

Chapter 47

Diabetic Ketoacidosis (DKA) and Hyperglycemic Hyperosmolar State (HHS): Diabetes Emergencies

Maria Skamagas and Erin Rule**

Key Pearls

- DKA is characterized by ketoacidosis and hyperglycemia, while HHS is characterized by hyperosmolality and hyperglycemia.
- Anion gap = $Na^+ - (Cl^- + HCO3^-)$.
- Effective serum osmolality = [2 * measured Na^+ (mEq/L)] + [glucose (mg/dL) ÷ 18].
- Management includes volume resuscitation, correcting ketoacidosis in DKA, correcting serum osmolality in HHS, correcting hyperglycemia, replacing electrolyte deficits, frequent monitoring, and identifying and treating the precipitator.
- Transition to subcutaneous insulin should involve overlap with IV insulin to prevent relapse into DKA or HHS.

Diabetic ketoacidosis (DKA) and hyperglycemic hyperosmolar state (HHS) are acute decompensated diabetic states which must be recognized immediately and managed appropriately in order to achieve the best clinical outcome. DKA is a state of severe insulin deficiency and excess counterregulatory hormones, resulting in metabolic acidosis, hyperglycemia, and subsequent volume and electrolyte depletion. Lack of

*Mount Sinai School of Medicine, New York, NY, USA.

insulin and high levels of glucagon and cortisol generate unrestrained hepatic glucose output, reduced peripheral utilization of glucose, unrestrained lipolysis, and conversion of fatty acids to ketone bodies in the liver. DKA usually occurs in type 1 diabetes, but may also develop in type 2 diabetes with severe illness or in ketosis-prone type 2 diabetes. HHS is a state with less severe insulin deficiency than DKA, without ketoacidosis, but with more profound dehydration, hyperglycemia, hyperosmolality, and altered mental status. Electrolyte depletion also ensues in HHS. It usually occurs in elderly individuals with type 2 DM who have limited access to free water and/or a diminished thirst drive. Infection and omission of insulin are common precipitators of DKA and HHS[1] (Table 2).

Physical signs and symptoms of DKA and HHS include volume depletion (tachycardia, dry mucosa, orthostasis, and hypotension) and signs of hyperglycemia and insulinopenia (polyuria, polydipsia, and weight loss). The onset of DKA tends to be rapid, while that of HHS is more insidious. Individuals with DKA are more likely to report abdominal complaints (pain, nausea, vomiting) which are related to the severity of acidosis,[2] and to demonstrate hyperventilation as an attempt to compensate for metabolic acidosis. If abdominal complaints persist after acidosis is cleared, further evaluation is required. Altered mental status is more common in HHS than in DKA, and correlates with the degree of hyperosmolality[3]; mental status deterioration occurs at effective serum osmolality greater than 320 mOsm/kg. The laboratory diagnosis of DKA and HHS is presented in Table 1. Ketoacidosis is the key feature of DKA, and hyperosmolality is the main feature of HHS. Thirty percent of patients exhibit laboratory features of both DKA and HHS, i.e. DKA with elevated serum osmolality.

Management of DKA and HHS (Tables 5 and 6) includes volume resuscitation, correcting ketoacidosis in DKA, correcting serum osmolality in HHS, correcting hyperglycemia, replacing electrolyte deficits (Table 4), frequent monitoring, and identifying and treating the precipitator (Table 2). Standardized protocols have been shown to correct anion gap acidosis more rapidly and to reduce the length of hospital stay and ICU stay.[4] Patients should be admitted to a monitored setting for frequent evaluation

Table 1. Laboratory/Diagnostic Criteria for DKA and HHS

	DKA	HHS
Plasma glucose (mg/dL)	>250	>600
Arterial pH	≤7.3	>7.3
Serum acetone	Positive	Negative/small
Serum bicarbonate (mEq/L)	<18	>18
Anion gap	>12	Variable
Urine ketones	Positive	Negative/small
Effective serum osmolality (mOsm/kg)	Variable	>320
Mental status	Alert, drowsy, or stupor	Stupor/coma

Mild DKA: pH = 7.25–7.3; bicarbonate 15–18.
Moderate DKA: pH = 7.00–7.24; bicarbonate 10 to < 15; mental status — alert/drowsy.
Severe DKA: pH < 7.00; bicarbonate < 10; mental status — stupor/coma.

Table 2. Precipitators of DKA and HHS

New presentation of DM 1 and 2, respectively
Omission of insulin
Infection: UTI, pneumonia, sepsis
Ischemia: MI, CVA, PE
Intra-abdominal process: pancreatitis, appendicitis, etc.
Medications: 2nd generation antipsychotics, glucocorticoids
Trauma
Surgery
Endocrine disease: thyrotoxicosis, acromegaly
Pregnancy (DKA)
Drugs: cocaine

of vital signs, urine output, mental status, fingerstick glucose, and electrolytes, and for treatment with intravenous (IV) fluids and IV insulin. If the patient is severely ill, i.e. with hypotension not responsive to IV fluids, severe acidosis, severe electrolye derangements, severe mental status changes from baseline, or organ failure (cardiac, pulmonary, or renal), admission to the intensive care unit (ICU) is warranted.

Table 3. Initial Data Evaluation of the Acutely Ill Diabetic Patient

Glucose
Basic metabolic panel (K^+, creatinine)
Anion gap
Urinalysis (acetone)
Serum acetone
Blood gas, pH (venous or arterial)
Lactic acid
Effective serum osmolality
Calcium, magnesium, phosphorus
CBC
Liver function panel, amylase, lipase
Chest X-ray
EKG
Cultures (as appropriate)
Pregnancy test (as appropriate)
Hemoglobin A1c
TSH

Anion gap (AG) = $Na^+ - (Cl^- + HCO3^-)$.
Effective serum osmolality (mOsm/kg) = [2 * measured Na^+ (meq/L)] + [glucose (mg/dL) ÷ 18].

In DKA, transition to subcutaneous (SC) basal insulin (glargine, detemir) is appropriate when the anion gap acidosis is cleared, the blood glucose is less than 200 mg/dL, and the patient is clinically stable. In HHS, transition to SC basal insulin is appropriate when the effective serum osmolality is <315 mOsm/kg, the blood glucose is improved, and the mental status is improved. There must be overlap between the injection of SC basal insulin and the IV insulin by 2 hrs to ensure adequate blood levels of insulin prior to discontinuing the IV insulin infusion; otherwise, the patient is at risk for relapse into DKA and HHS. Mealtime rapid-acting insulin may be initiated when the patient is eating. Correction insulin may be used before meals or every 6 hrs if the patient is not eating.

In preparation for discharge, it is obligatory to educate the patient and the patient's family and caregivers regarding basic diabetes survival skills. These include blood glucose monitoring, glucose goals, insulin administration and storage, meal planning, hypoglycemia management, sick day management, and when to call the physician. Followup appointments with the outpatient physician should be made within 1–2 weeks of discharge.

Table 4. Typical Deficits of Total Body Water and Electrolytes in DKA and HHS[6]

	DKA	HHS
Total Body Water (L)	6	9
Sodium (Na^+) (mEq/kg)	7–10	5–13
Potassium (K^+) (mEq/kg)	3–5	4–6
Phosphorus (PO^4) (mmol/kg)	5–7	3–7
Magnesium (Mg^{++}) (mEq/kg)	1–2	1–2

Table 5. Guidelines for Management of DKA[5–8]

DKA Diagnosis:

Glucose >250 mg/dL	(Diabetic)
+ Serum acetone	(Keto)
pH ≤7.3, $HCO3^-$ <18, AG >12	(Acidosis)

Caveats: Other acid base disorders can affect $HCO3^-$ and pH.
Prior insulin treatment "in the field" may create "euglycemic DKA."
Anion gap acidosis: if acetone is negative, look for other causes, e.g. lactic acidosis.

Goals of Treatment:

— Volume-resuscitate;
— Correct anion gap acidosis;
— Correct glucose to 150–200 mg/dL;
— Replete electrolytes: K^+, Mg^{++}, Phos;$^-$
— Identify and treat precipitator (Table 2);
— Frequent monitoring (volume status, mental status, labs).

(Continued)

Table 5. Guidelines for Management of DKA (*Continued*)

FLUIDS

Goal: Normalize blood pressure and hemodynamic status (immediately);
Replete fluid deficit over 24 hrs (usually ~ 6 L).

Rx: 1–1.5 L normal saline (NS) over 1st hr

Then 250–500 mL/hr NS x 2 L, followed by 150–250 mL/hr NS or ½ NS (depending on hydration status and serum Na^+).

If hypovolemic shock, then use more aggressive IVF.

When glucose <250 mg/dL, start D5 ½ NS at 150–250 mL/hr.

Caution with IVF in patients at risk for volume overload (CHF, ESRD).

INSULIN

If K^+ <3.3 mEq/L, hold insulin until actively correcting K^+ and K^+ >3.3 mEq/L.

Initial Rx: regular insulin IV bolus 0.1 units/kg, then insulin drip 0.1 units/kg/hr

Ex.: 60 kg person requires 6 units IV push, followed by 6 units/hr.

Initial Goal: ↓ glucose by 50–75 mg/dL/hr

If glucose not decreasing by ≥50 mg/dL in 1st hour → increase/double IV insulin rate; ensure adequate volume repletion and ensure insulin in bag.

If glucose is decreasing by >75 mg/dL/hr → reduce IV insulin rate.

Check FS glucose every 1 hr. MD adjusts insulin drip rate.

When glucose <200–250 mg/dL

Start D5 ½ NS at 150–250 mL/hr

↓ insulin drip to 0.02–0.05 units/kg/hr. *Ex.: 60 kg person: 1–3 units/hr.*

Glucose goal = 150–200 mg/dL (buffer against hypoglycemia while treating ketoacidosis).

Titrate insulin drip and/or dextrose infusion to maintain glucose.

POTASSIUM/ELECTROLYTES:

Goal K^+ = 4–5 mEq/L.

Expect K^+ to decrease during treatment of DKA (insulin causes intracellular shifting of K^+). Be proactive and replete.

If renal failure and urine output <50 cc/hr → caution with electrolyte repletion.

K^+ < 3.3: give 10–20 mEq IV KCl/hr until K^+ >3.3. Cardiac monitoring.
Check K^+ every 1–2 hr until K^+ >3.3.

K^+ = 3.3–4: give KCl 40 mEq/L of IVF administered.

K^+ = 4.1–5: give KCl 20 mEq/L of IVF administered.

Can administer KCl separately from IVF.

Adjust potassium administration based on repeat K^+ levels.

(*Continued*)

Table 5. Guidelines for Management of DKA (*Continued*)

Mg^{++} <1.5 mg/dL: give 2 g IV magnesium sulfate.
Phosphorus <1 mg/dL: give 0.24 mmol/kg IV potassium phosphate in 250 cc fluid over 6 hr; monitor calcium level, which can decrease with IV phosphorus.
Ex.: 70 kg person: give ~15 mmol KPhos.
Bicarbonate use is controversial; consider using bicarbonate *Only if* pH <7.

CLINICAL CHECKS: Vital signs, urine output, mental status
LAB CHECKS:
- ✓ Glucose every 1 hr
- ✓ At 2 hr after initial treatment: Chem 7 (K^+) and pH (venous)
- ✓ Chem 7, Mg^{++}, $Phos^-$ every 4 hr until anion gap closed and lytes normal

RESOLUTION OF DKA: AG <12, $HCO3^-$ >18 mEq/L, glucose <200 mg/dL, patient clinically stable.
Expected time to clearance of anion gap acidosis is 12–20 hr.

TRANSITION TO SUBCUTANEOUS INSULIN
Administer basal insulin SC, and discontinue insulin drip 2 hr after SC dose. Also discontinue dextrose IVF.
Calculation of insulin doses:
(1) Basal insulin = 0.25–0.3 units/kg/day.
Use glargine daily or detemir divided twice daily.
(2) Mealtime insulin = 0.25 units/kg/day ÷ 3.
Use rapid-acting lispro, aspart, glulisine.
Start mealtime insulin only if patient is eating. If PO intake is variable, give smaller doses of mealtime insulin after patient eats meal (to avoid hypoglycemia).
Ex.: give 50% of calculated dose after patient eats 50% meal.
(3) Correction insulin scale (rapid-acting) before meals.
*Ex.: Patient weight = 60 kg. Basal insulin = 60 * 0.25 = 15 units. Mealtime insulin = 15 ÷ 3 = 5 units.*

Prior diagnosis of DM: start insulin as above, or restart home insulin basal and mealtime insulin if patient was adherent, controlled, and with no major hypoglycemia.

Hypoglycemia orders: see Chapter 46 "Management of Diabetes and Hyperglycemia in Hospitalized Patients," section on Hypoglycemia.

Diet orders: NPO while on insulin drip.
After transition to SC insulin: diabetes diet 2100–2400 kcal/day, no concentrated sweets.

(*Continued*)

Table 5. Guidelines for Management of DKA (*Continued*)

Diabetes education of patient and family:
— Glucose monitoring
— Glucose goals
— Insulin administration and storage
— Basic meal planning
— Hypoglycemia management: signs/symptoms/treatment
— Sick day management: sugar-free liquids, glucose and urine ketone monitoring, use of basal insulin and correction insulin scale
— When to call physician (including hyperglycemia and hypoglycemia thresholds)
— Followup appointments with medical providers

Table 6. Guidelines for Management of HHS[5,6]

HHS Diagnosis
Glucose >600 mg/dL
Effective serum osmolality >320 mOsm/kg
Altered mental status (usually)
Urine ketones / serum acetone negative or small
pH >7.3

Effective serum osmolality = [2 * measured Na^+ (mEq/L)] + [glucose (mg/dL) ÷ 18]
Caveats: Acidosis and anion gap may be present and due to other conditions, i.e. lactic acidosis.

Goals of Treatment
— Volume resuscitate;
— Correct hyperosmolar state (goal osm <315 mOsm/kg) & correct glucose;
— Improvement in mental status;
— Replete Electrolytes: K^+, Mg^{++}, $Phos^{-}$
— Identify & treat precipitator (Table 2);
— Frequent monitoring (volume status, mental status, and labs).

FLUIDS
Assess volume status. Total body water deficit may be up to 8–10 L.
Goal: correct estimated fluid deficits in 24 hr.
Use caution in patients at risk for volume overload (CHF, ESRD).

Rx: 1–1.5 L normal saline (NS = 0.9% NaCl) over 1 hr
Then 250–500 mL/hr NS × 2 L, followed by 150–250 mL/hr NS or ½ NS (depending on hydration status and serum Na^+).
If hypovolemic shock, then use more aggressive IVF.

When glucose <300 mg/dL, start D5 ½ NS at 150–250 mL/hr.

(Continued)

Table 6. Guidelines for Management of HHS (*Continued*)

INSULIN If K^+ <3.3 mEq/L, hold insulin until actively correcting K^+ and K^+ >3.3 mEq/L.
Initial Rx: regular insulin IV bolus 0.1 unit/kg, then insulin drip 0.1 unit/kg/hr
Initial Goal: ↓ Glucose by 50–75 mg/dL/ hr

If glucose not decreasing by ≥50 mg/dL in 1st hour → increase/double IV insulin rate; ensure adequate volume repletion and ensure insulin in bag.
If glucose is decreasing by >75 mg/dL/hr → reduce IV insulin rate.
Check FS glucose every 1 hr. MD adjusts insulin drip rate.

When glucose <300 mg/dL:

Start D5 ½ NS at 150– 250 mL/hr.
↓ insulin drip to 0.02–0.05 unit/kg/hr. *Ex.: 70 kg person: 1.5–3.5 unit/hr.*
Glucose goal = 200–300 mg/dL, until mental status improves and osm < 315 mOsm/kg.
Titrate insulin drip and/or dextrose infusion to maintain glucose 200–300 mg/dL.

POTASSIUM/ELECTROLYTES: see Table 5.

CLINICAL CHECKS: Vital signs, urine output, mental status, volume status
LAB CHECKS:
✓ Glucose every 1 hr
✓ Chem 7, Mg^{++}, $Phos^-$ every 4 hr until HHS resolved and electrolytes normal

RESOLUTION OF HHS: plasma osmolality <315 mOsm/kg, mental status improved, and glucose improved.

TRANSITION TO SUBCUTANEOUS INSULIN
Administer basal insulin SC, and discontinue insulin drip 2 hr after SC dose. Also discontinue dextrose IVF.
Calculation of insulin doses: these are starting doses which may need to be titrated. Patients with significant insulin resistance will need higher doses.

(1) Basal insulin = 0.2 units/kg/day.
Use glargine daily or detemir divided twice daily.
(2) Mealtime insulin = 0.2 units/kg/day ÷ 3.
Use rapid-acting lispro, aspart, glulisine.
Start mealtime insulin only if patient is eating. If PO intake is variable, give smaller doses of mealtime insulin after patient eats meal (to avoid hypoglycemia).
Ex.: give 50% of calculated dose after patients eats 50% meal
(3) Correction insulin scale (rapid-acting) before meals.

(*Continued*)

Table 6. Guidelines for Management of HHS (*Continued*)

Hypoglycemia orders: see Chapter 46 "Management of Diabetes and Hyperglycemia in Hospitalized Patients," section on Hypoglycemia.

Diet orders: NPO while on insulin drip.
After transition to SC insulin: diabetes diet 2100–2400 kcal/day, no concentrated sweets.

Diabetes education of patient and family/caregivers:
- Ensure adequate hydration
- Ensure adherence to medications (oral diabetes meds and insulin)
- Glucose monitoring
- Glucose goals
- Insulin administration and storage
- Basic meal planning
- Hypoglycemia management: signs/symptoms/treatment
- Sick day management: sugar-free liquids, glucose and urine ketone monitoring, use of basal insulin and correction insulin scale
- When to call physician (including hyperglycemia and hypoglycemia thresholds)
- Followup appointments with medical providers

References

1. Kitabchi AE, Umpierrez GE, Miles JM, Fisher JN. (2009) Hyperglycemic crises in adult patients with diabetes. *Diabetes Care* **32**: 1335–1343.
2. Umpierrez G, Freire AX. (2002) Abdominal pain in patients with hyperglycemic crises. *J Crit Care* **17**: 63–67.
3. Daugirdas JT, Kronfol NO, Tzamaloukas AH, Ing TS. (1989) Hyperosmolar coma: Cellular dehydration and the serum sodium concentration. *Ann Intern Med* **110**: 855–857.
4. Bull SV, Douglas IS, Foster M, Albert RK. (2007) Mandatory protocol for treating adult patients with diabetic ketoacidosis decreases intensive care unit and hospital lengths of stay: Results of a nonrandomized trial. *Crit Care Med* **35**: 41–46.
5. Kitabchi AE, Nyenwe EA. (2006) Hyperglycemic crises in diabetes mellitus: Diabetic ketoacidosis and hyperglycemic hyperosmolar state. *Endocrinol Metab Clin N Am* **35**: 725–751.

6. Kitabchi AE, Umpierrez GE, Murphy MB, *et al*. (2001) Management of hyperglycemic crises in patients with diabetes. *Diabetes Care* **24**: 131–153.
7. Umpierrez GE, Jones S, Smiley D, *et al*. (2009) Insulin analogs versus human insulin in the treatment of patients with diabetic ketoacidosis: A randomized controlled trial. *Diabetes Care* **32**: 1164–1169.
8. Kitabchi AE, Murphy MB, Spencer J, *et al*. (2008) Is a priming dose of insulin necessary in a low-dose insulin protocol for the treatment of diabetic ketoacidosis? *Diabetes Care* **31**: 2081–2085.

Chapter 48

Diagnosis and Treatment of Thyroid Dysfunction

Noga C. Minsky and Richard S. Haber**

Key Pearls

- Serum TSH is a sensitive test for thyroid failure. An elevated TSH alone is usually sufficient to establish the diagnosis of hypothyroidism.
- In treating hypothyroidism, the average full replacement dose of levothyroxine is 1.6 μg/kg/day, but in older patients and those with heart disease, the initial dose should be lower (25–50 mcg) to avoid precipitating cardiac symptoms.
- TSH is an adequate screening test for hyperthyroidism, and is usually suppressed to less than 0.1 μU/L in clinically significant hyperthyroidism.
- In medical therapy for hyperthyroidism, methimazole is preferred over propylthiouracil because of the small risk of potentially fatal hepatocellular injury associated with propylthiouracil.
- In hospitalized patients with nonthyroidal illness (sick euthyroid syndrome), there are transient physiologic changes in thyroid function tests: Serum T3 is low, while TSH and Free T4 levels vary.

*Mount Sinai School of Medicine, New York, NY, USA.

Hypothyroidism

Hypothyroidism has a prevalence of 4.6% in the adult United States population,[1] and is frequently undiagnosed because associated symptoms can be nonspecific and insidious in onset. The most common cause is Hashimoto's (chronic autoimmune) thyroiditis, which is frequently familial, with a female to male ratio of 5:1. Iatrogenic causes of primary hypothyroidism are also common, including thyroid surgery, radioiodine treatment for hyperthyroidism, thyroidal exposure to external beam radiation, and medication use (e.g. lithium, α-interferon, and amiodarone). Central (or secondary) hypothyroidism due to insufficient thyroid stimulating hormone (TSH) is less common, occurring with pituitary and hypothalamic disease.

Clinical Manifestations

The most common symptoms of hypothyroidism are fatigue, weakness, lethargy, weight gain, impaired memory, cold intolerance, dry skin, constipation, paresthesias, hair loss, menstrual irregularity and depression. In severe hypothyroidism, the signs may include bradycardia, a raspy voice, edema, delayed relaxation of deep tendon reflexes, slow mentation, and cool, dry skin. A diffuse and firm goiter may be present in some patients with Hashimoto's thyroiditis.

Laboratory Evaluation

Serum TSH is a sensitive test for thyroid failure, and elevated TSH alone is usually sufficient to establish the diagnosis of hypothyroidism. If central hypothyroidism is a consideration, then serum thyroxine (T4) levels should be assessed as well. Low or inappropriately normal TSH in the presence of low T4 is consistent with central hypothyroidism. Laboratory findings associated with hypothyroidism may include hyponatremia, mild anemia, and elevated creatine kinase.

Management

The replacement dose of levothyroxine depends on the degree of hypothyroidism. The average full replacement dose is 1.6 μg/kg/day. In older patients with longstanding hypothyroidism and those with heart disease, the initial dose should be lower (25–50 mcg) to avoid precipitating cardiac symptoms.[2] To optimize intestinal absorption, levothyroxine should be taken on an empty stomach and not with other medications or nutritional supplements that interfere with its absorption (e.g. calcium and iron). If parenteral administration is required, 60% of the patient's oral dose of levothyroxine can be given intravenously.

The symptoms of hypothyroidism may begin to resolve after two to three weeks of levothyroxine therapy, but steady-state TSH concentrations are not achieved for about six weeks. Therefore, TSH is assessed after 6–8 weeks of therapy and the levothyroxine dose is adjusted to normalize the TSH levels, with smaller dose increments in the elderly (e.g. 12.5 to 25 μg). In central hypothyroidism, the goal is to normalize an index of free T4 after any associated central cortisol deficiency is corrected.

Myxedema Coma

Myxedema coma is a syndrome of severe hypothyroidism complicated by an altered mental status, hypothermia, hypoventilation, bradycardia, and gastric atony. Typical patients are elderly women with a previous history of long-standing untreated or inadequately treated hypothyroidism, and there is often a precipitating event or illness.[3] The condition is rare, but also dangerous, with up to a 20% mortality rate. Treatment requires hospitalization. Supportive measures include ventilatory support and gradual rewarming. If associated adrenal insufficiency is suspected because of hypotension, empiric therapy with corticosteroids is provided until adrenal insufficiency is ruled out. Initial thyroxine replacement is given intravenously, with a loading dose of levothyroxine 300–500 μg followed by daily replacement doses, with lower, more conservative dosing for elderly patients or those with cardiac disease.[4]

Hyperthyroidism

Graves' disease is the most common cause of hyperthyroidism, followed by solitary or multiple hyperfunctioning thyroid nodules. Transient forms of hyperthyroidism can be caused by various forms of thyroiditis, such as silent (lymphocytic), subacute (granulomatous), and medication-related (e.g. amiodarone).

Clinical Manifestations

The symptoms include weight loss, palpitations, heat intolerance, insomnia, tremor, increased frequency of defecation, proximal muscle weakness, irritability, and menstrual irregularity. Elderly patients sometimes lack these symptoms, and may present with weight loss or atrial fibrillation alone.[5] Associated signs include tachycardia, a diffuse or nodular goiter, tremor, hyperreflexia, and warm, moist skin. The presence of Graves' ophthalmopathy (proptosis, lid retraction, periorbital edema) or a thyroid bruit confirm the diagnosis of Graves' disease in hyperthyroid patients. Thyroid pain and tenderness suggest subacute thyroiditis.

Diagnostic Evaluation

TSH is an adequate screening test and is usually suppressed to less than 0.1 μU/L in clinically significant hyperthyroidism. If TSH is suppressed to below this level, serum triiodothyronine (T3) and thyroxine (T4) levels should be assessed to support the diagnosis of hyperthyroidism and determine its severity. If the underlying cause is unclear, the presence of TSH receptor antibodies can confirm the diagnosis of Graves' disease. Nodular thyroid disease can be detected by ultrasound examination, and hyperfunctioning nodules are verified with a radioiodine scan. Demonstration of low thyroidal radioiodine uptake can confirm the diagnosis of transient hyperthyroidism caused by various forms of thyroiditis.[6] Laboratory abnormalities associated with hyperthyroidism include anemia, elevated liver enzymes, and hypercalcemia.

Management

Hyperthyroidism may be effectively treated with three modalities, including antithyroid drugs, radioactive iodine, or thyroid surgery. Radioactive iodine is the most commonly used form of treatment in the United States and is especially preferred in older patients. Antithyroid drugs may be used in younger patients with mild Graves' hyperthyroidism and small goiters, in hopes of achieving remission after 12–18 months of therapy.[7] Hyperthyroidism due to hyperfunctioning nodules should be treated with radioactive iodine or surgery. In patients with transient hyperthyroidism due to thyroiditis, none of these therapies are indicated. Mild hyperthyroidism due to Graves' disease or hyperfunctioning nodules should be treated prior to administration of iodinated contrast for imaging studies, which can exacerbate an underlying hyperthyroidism.

Antithyroid drugs. Methimazole and propylthiouracil inhibit thyroid hormone biosynthesis. Methimazole is generally preferred because of the small risk of fatal hepatocellular injury associated with propylthiouracil. Initial doses of methimazole are 10–40 mg daily according to severity, and the doses of propylthiouracil are ten-fold higher and given in divided daily doses. If higher doses of antithyroid drugs are used initially, they should be reduced when the patient becomes euthyroid. Minor side effects occur in about 5% of patients and include rashes, urticaria, arthralgias, and gastrointestinal upset. Rare serious reactions include agranulocytosis (0.3%), vasculitis, and hepatitis (0.1–0.2%). Hepatitis occurring with methimazole use is cholestatic and completely reversible. Patients on antithyroid drugs presenting with fever, sore throat, or sepsis should have their medication held until agranulocytosis is ruled out.[8]

Radioactive Iodine. This treatment strategy is safe and effective, but leads to permanent hypothyroidism necessitating life-long thyroid hormone replacement in most patients. It is contraindicated in women who are pregnant or breast-feeding. There is evidence that radioiodine therapy may be associated with worsening of Graves' ophthalmopathy.[9] Individuals at risk for developing cardiac complications may be pretreated with antithyroid drugs prior to radioactive iodine therapy, especially if hyperthyroidism is severe. Antithyroid drugs, when used, should be discontinued for 3–7 days before radioiodine therapy. Response to radioactive iodine usually occurs within 6–18 weeks, after which time close monitoring for development of hypothyroidism is essential.

Surgery. Thyroidectomy may be indicated in patients who decline radioiodine treatment, or have hyperfunctioning nodules, or a large or obstructive goiter, or have coexisting thyroid cancer. Complications from thyroidectomy occur at a rate of up to 3%, and include hypoparathyroidism and damage to the laryngeal nerves.

Beta blockers. Beta blockers, such as atenolol (25–50 mg/day), are used to ameliorate the adrenergic effects of hyperthyroidism, such as tachycardia, tremors, and anxiety, until a euthyroid state is achieved.

Thyroid Storm

Thyroid storm is a rare, life-threatening condition characterized by severe hyperthyroidism, fever, and an altered mental status.[10] As this disorder progresses, congestive heart failure and coma can develop. It usually occurs in patients who have preexisting untreated or partially treated thyrotoxicosis and a superimposed precipitating factor, most commonly infection.

Management of Severe Hyperthyroidism and Thyroid Storm

Patients with thyroid storm or hyperthyroidism with cardiovascular instability are best treated as inpatients. Multiple agents are used to achieve a rapid reduction in thyroid hormone levels and target cardiovascular complications (see Table 1). Antithyroid drugs are the principal agents used. If oral or gastric tube administration is not possible, antithyroid drugs may be given rectally or intravenously with appropriate preparation

Table 1. Therapy for Severe Hyperthyroidism and Thyroid Storm

Medication Class	Specific Regimens
Antithyroid drugs	Methimazole 20 mg PO every 6 hr
	Propylthiouracil 200 mg PO every 6 hr
Iodine	SSKI (saturated solution of potassium iodine) 5 drops PO every 6 hr
	Lugol's Solution 10 drops PO every 8 hr
β-blockers	Esmolol IV drip: loading 250–500 μg/kg, maintenance 50–100 μg/kg/min
	Metoprolol 5–10 mg IVP every 4 hr
	Propranolol 20–80 mg PO every 8 hr
Glucocorticoids	Dexamethasone 2 mg IV every 6 hr
	Hydrocortisone 100 mg IV every 8 hr

(not commercially available).[11] Iodine is given enterally to block both thyroid hormone synthesis and release. Glucocorticoid therapy decreases peripheral conversion of T4 to T3. Beta blockers also decrease T4 to T3 conversion, and are indicated for severe tachycardia, but must be used with caution because of the risk of exacerbating congestive heart failure. Therapy is initiated with short acting beta blockers in a monitored setting. Supportive measures include cooling, cardiovascular support, fluid replacement, and oxygen therapy.

Effects of Nonthyroidal Illness on Thyroid Function Tests (Euthyroid Sick Syndrome)

Thyroid function test abnormalities are prevalent in hospitalized patients with acute and chronic nonthyroidal illness in the absence of thyroid disease. In seriously ill patients who are suspected to have thyroid disease, TSH is usually sufficient for screening. Most hospitalized patients without true thyroid disease have normal TSH levels. However, in some patients with nonthyroidal illness TSH may be reduced, but is usually not undetectable. When the patient is recovering, TSH may be transiently elevated to up to 25 μU/L.[12]

Many hospitalized patients have low T3 due to reduced peripheral conversion of T4 to T3. Total T4 is often normal, but can be low with more severe underlying illness. Free T4 concentrations vary.[13]

Since thyroid function test abnormalities in nonthyroidal illness are thought to be physiologic, thyroid hormone replacement is not indicated.[14]

Evaluation of Hospitalized Patients with Known Thyroid Disease

In patients receiving therapy for hypothyroidism, serum TSH alone is adequate for assessment of the replacement dose. In hyperthyroid patients, laboratory assessment should include serum TSH, T4 and T3 levels. However, these thyroid tests need to be interpreted in the context of the known confounding effects of nonthyroidal illness (see above).

References

1. Hollowell JG, Staehling NW, Flanders WD, *et al.* (2002) TSH, T4, and thyroid antibodies in the United States population (1988 to 1994): National Health and Nutrition Examination Survey (NHANES III). *J Clin Endocrinol Metab* **87**: 489–499.
2. McDermott MT. (2009) In the clinic. Hypothyroidism. *Ann Intern Med* **151**: ITC61.
3. Goldberg PA, Inzucchi SE. (2003) Critical issues in endocrinology. *Clin Chest Med* **24**: 583–606.
4. Yamamoto T, Fukuyama J, Fujiyoshi A. (1999) Factors associated with mortality of myxedema coma: Report of eight cases and literature survey. *Thyroid* **9**: 1167–1174.
5. Boelaert, K, Torlinska, B, Holder, RL, Franklyn, JA. (2010) Older subjects with hyperthyroidism present with a paucity of symptoms and signs: A large cross-sectional study. *J Clin Endocrinol Metab* **95**: 2715–2726.
6. Baskin HJ, Cobin RH, Duick DS, *et al.* (2002) American Association of Clinical Endocrinologists. American Association of Clinical

Endocrinologists medical guidelines for clinical practice for the evaluation and treatment of hyperthyroidism and hypothyroidism. *Endocr Pract* **8**: 457–69.

7. Brent GA. (2008) Clinical practice. Graves' disease. *N Engl J Med* **358**: 2594–2605.
8. Cooper DS. (2005) Antithyroid drugs. *N Engl J Med* **352**: 905–917.
9. Bartalena L, Marcocci C, Bogazzi F, *et al.* (1998) Relation between therapy for hyperthyroidism and the course of Graves' ophthalmopathy. *N Engl J Med* **338**: 73–78.
10. Singer PA, Cooper DS, Levy EG, *et al.* (1995) Treatment guidelines for patients with hyperthyroidism and hypothyroidism. *JAMA* **273**: 808–812.
11. Nayak, B, Burman, K. (2006) Thyrotoxicosis and thyroid storm. *Endocrinol Metab Clin North Am* **35**: 663.
12. Adler SM and Wartofsky L. (2007) The nonthyroidal illness syndrome. *Endocrinol Metabl Clin N Am* **36**: 657–672.
13. Chopra IJ. (1996) Nonthyroidal illness syndrome or euthyroid sick syndrome? *Endocr Pract* **2**: 45–52.
14. Klemperer JD, Klein I, Gomez M, *et al.* (1995) Thyroid hormone treatment after coronary-artery bypass surgery. *N Engl J Med* **333**: 1522–1527.

Chapter 49

Adrenal Insufficiency

Maria E. Lamothe, Robert Yanagisawa* and Alice C. Levine**

Key Pearls

- Primary adrenal insufficiency (Addison's disease) presents with signs and symptoms of both mineralocorticoid and glucocorticoid deficiency and requires replacement of both, whereas secondary adrenal insufficiency only requires glucocorticoid replacement.
- Secondary adrenal insufficiency is defined as deficient production of cortisol from the adrenal cortex due to a lack of ACTH stimulation from the pituitary gland (mineralocorticoid and androgen levels are not impaired).
- The main sign of acute adrenal insufficiency (adrenal crisis) is persistent hypotension or shock out of proportion to the current illness.
- In a stress situation, if adrenal insufficiency is suspected, send a random cortisol and ACTH level and treat with 150 mg of intravenous hydrocortisone or its equivalent for 24 hours.
- A morning cortisol level <3 mcg/dL in a non-stressed patient and <15 mcg/dL in a stressed patient warrants treatment with steroids.

Adrenal insufficiency (AI) is a potentially life-threatening disorder of impaired adrenocortical function. The adrenal cortex consists of three layers: the glomerulosa which produces mineralocorticoids (aldosterone); the

*Hilda and J. Lester Gabrilove Division of Endocrinology, Diabetes and Bone Diseases of the Mount Sinai School of Medicine, New York, NY 10029, USA.

fasciculata which produces glucocorticoids (cortisol); and the reticularis which produces adrenal androgens (testosterone and DHEA). Production of cortisol is regulated by pituitary adrenocorticotropin hormone (ACTH), which is regulated by the hypothalamic corticotrophin-releasing hormone (CRH). Insufficient production of cortisol may be due either to primary failure of the adrenal cortex (primary adrenal insufficiency), or to failure of the pituitary gland to secrete ACTH (secondary adrenal insufficiency). In this chapter, we will discuss the etiology, diagnosis and management of adrenal insufficiency.[1,2]

Clinical Signs and Symptoms of Adrenal Insufficiency (Table 1)

Primary Adrenal Insufficiency

Primary adrenal insufficiency (Addison's disease) is a deficiency in production of all hormones from the adrenal cortex. Patients with primary AI may have symptoms of glucocorticoid deficiency including weakness, fatigue and anorexia in addition to signs of mineralocorticoid deficiency such as orthostatic hypotension. The mineralocorticoid deficiency causes clinical signs that are unique to primary adrenal insufficiency such as hyponatremia and hyperkalemia. Primary adrenal insufficiency may also cause hyperpigmentation of the skin and mucous membranes due to the elevated levels of ACTH.[2,3]

Secondary Adrenal Insufficiency

Secondary adrenal insufficiency is defined as deficient production of cortisol from the adrenal cortex due to a lack of ACTH stimulation from the pituitary gland. Mineralocorticoid production and adrenal androgen production are not deficient in secondary AI.[3] Even though patients with secondary AI produce aldosterone, they can develop hypotension when stressed, due to deficiency of cortisol, which is necessary for increasing vascular responsiveness to vasoconstrictive hormones such as angiotensin II and norepinephrine.[3]

Acute Adrenal Insufficiency

The main sign of acute adrenal insufficiency (adrenal crisis) is persistent hypotension or shock out of proportion to the current illness. Other presenting features include fever, abdominal pain, altered mental status and electrolyte disturbances, but these symptoms are nonspecific. If adrenal crisis is suspected in an unstable patient, immediate initiation of stress dose steroids is necessary.[1]

Table 1. Features of Primary and Secondary Adrenal Insufficiency

	Primary Adrenal Insufficiency	Secondary Adrenal Insufficiency	Acute Adrenal Insufficiency
Clinical Symptoms			
Weakness	Yes	Yes	Yes
Fatigue	Yes	Yes	Yes
Anorexia	Yes	Yes	Yes
Nausea/vomiting	Yes	Yes	vomiting
Salt craving	Yes	No	n/a
Orthostatic hypotension	Yes	Yes (less common)	Yes
Psychiatric changes	Yes	Yes	altered mental status
Abdominal pain	Yes	Yes	Yes
Clinical Signs			
Weight loss	Yes	Yes	n/a
Hyperpigmentation	Yes	No	Yes
Hypotension	Yes	Yes (less common)	shock
Hypoglycemia	Yes	Yes (more common)	Yes
Laboratory Data			
Hyponatremia	Yes	Yes (less common)	Yes
Hyperkalemia	Yes	No	Yes
Hypercalcemia	Yes (rare)	No	Yes

Source: *Williams Textbook of Endocrinology*, 11th ed. 2008.

Etiology of Adrenal Insufficiency (Table 2)

Primary Adrenal Insufficiency

Autoimmune destruction of the adrenal cortex is the most common cause of primary AI in developed countries. Autoimmune adrenalitis can occur either alone or in association with other autoimmune disorders such as in autoimmune polyglandular syndromes type 1 and 2. Infectious causes, such as TB, are more common in underdeveloped countries, but adrenal destruction due to HIV-related causes is becoming more prevalent in developed countries.[2,4] Although many diseases and infections can cause adrenal insufficiency, by far the most common cause of AI in developed countries is iatrogenic (i.e. drugs).

Secondary Adrenal Insufficiency

Any drug or condition that causes prolonged suppression of ACTH production from the pituitary gland can cause atrophy of the zona fasciculata and therefore induce secondary adrenal insufficiency.[3] The most common cause of secondary adrenal insufficiency is abrupt cessation of prolonged, exogenous steroids. Steroid doses greater than a total daily dose of prednisone 5 mg or equivalent for longer than three weeks can cause atrophy of the zona fasciculata and secondary AI.[4] There are other classes of drugs that can indirectly induce AI through increased cortisol metabolism, decreased cortisol synthesis and increased glucocorticoid resistance peripherally.[5]

ESTABLISHING THE DIAGNOSIS OF ADRENAL INSUFFICIENCY

Unstressed State

Cortisol is secreted in a circadian rhythm with peak levels in the early morning (between 06:00 h and 08:00 h) and the lowest levels around midnight (24:00 h).[7] Cortisol circulates in the serum bound to the proteins cortisol binding globulin (CBG) and albumin and only the free fraction of cortisol in the serum is biologically active.[6] There are factors that can cause

Table 2. Etiology of Adrenal Insufficiency

Primary Adrenal Insufficiency	Secondary Adrenal Insufficiency
Autoimmune	**Pituitary Lesions**
• Autoimmune polyglandular syndrome 1	• Trauma/Surgery
• Autoimmune polyglandular syndrome 2	• Hemorrhage (apoplexy)
	• Tumors
Infectious	• Inflammation
• TB	• Infectious
• AIDS (CMV)	• Granulomatous Infiltration
• Fungal	• Radiation
	• Congenital (aplasia/hypoplasia)
Infiltrative	**Drugs:**
• Sarcoidosis	*Suppression of CRH/ACTH*
• Amyloidosis	• Glucocorticoid therapy
• Hemachromatosis	• Megestrol acetate
Metastatic neoplasia	• Medroxyprogesterone
Bilateral adrenal hemorrhage	• Ketorolac
Bilateral adrenal vein thrombosis	• Opiates
Bilateral adrenalectomy	
Congential	
• Congenital adrenal hyperplasia	*Secondary increase in endogenous cortisol levels through decreased metabolism*
• Congenital adrenal hypoplasia	
• Adrenoleukodystrophy	
Drugs:	• Ritonavir
Impair steroid synthesis	• Itraconazole
• Aminoglutethimide	• Fluoxetine
• Etomidate*	• Diltiazem
• Ketoconazole	• Cimetidine
• Metyrapone	• Arepitant
Enhances steroid metabolism	*Peripheral Glucocorticoid resistance*
• Rifampicin	• Mifepristone
• Phenytoin	• Chlorpromazine
• pioglitizone	• Imipramine

Source: [5,6]*Etomidate has been reported to cause adrenal insufficiency for up to 48 hrs after a single bolus in some cases.

variability in cortisol levels such as age, low serum protein levels (cortisol binding globulin/albumin) and stress. Many drugs can cause suppression of steroid levels without overt signs or symptoms of adrenal insufficiency in the unstressed patient that may be uncovered in the hospitalized setting.[5]

A baseline morning cortisol level drawn between 06:00 h and 08:00 h may be used as an initial screening test for an unstressed patient. See Fig. 1 for values.

The cosyntropin stimulation test is the most widely used test for diagnosis of adrenal insufficiency. This test uses synthetic ACTH injected intravenously to stimulate the adrenal gland to produce cortisol. Peak cortisol levels occur between 30 and 60 minutes after ACTH injection. The test can be performed at any time of day and is generally easy and safe.[2,3] See Fig. 1 for values.

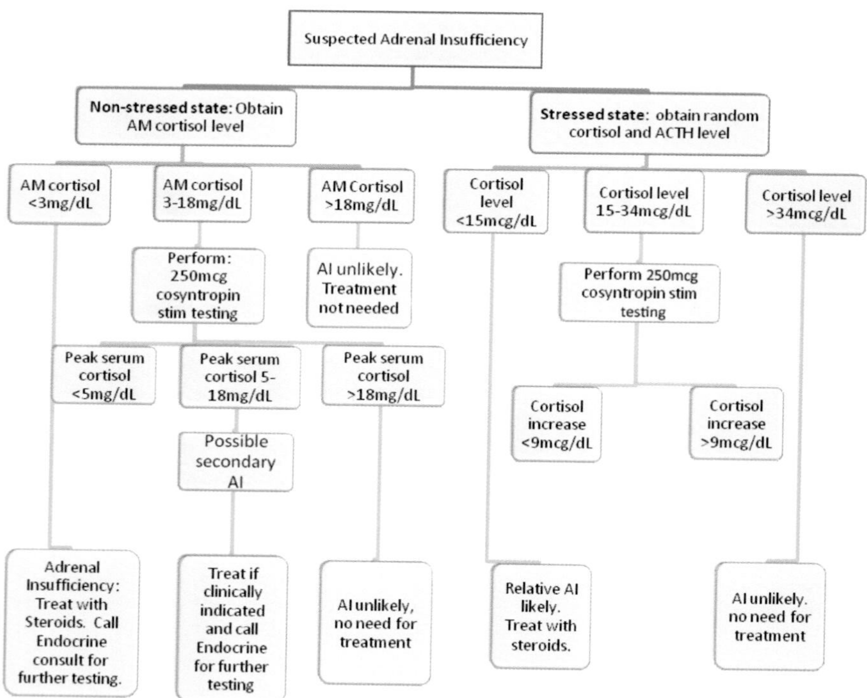

Figure 1. Algorythm for establishing the diagnosis of adrenal insufficiency.
Source: Refs. 2 and 4.

Stressed State

Any patient in a stressed state who is suspected of having adrenal insufficiency should have a random cortisol level and immediate initiation of stress dose steroids. A random cortisol level less than 15 mcg/dL in a stressed patient likely indicates adrenal insufficiency, and stress dose steroids should be continued. Cortisol levels between 15–34 mcg/dL are indeterminate and a cosyntropin stimulation test is the next step to make the diagnosis.[4]

Distinguishing primary AI versus secondary AI can be difficult but in general, patients with primary AI will have high levels of ACTH and low levels of the mineralocorticoid aldosterone. Patients with secondary AI generally have low or inappropriately normal levels of ACTH with no aldosterone deficiency.

Treatment of Adrenal Insufficiency

Acute Adrenal Insufficiency

Acute adrenal insufficiency is potentially life-threatening and stress dose steroids should be initiated immediately if it is suspected. Hydrocortisone intravenously at an initial dosage of 50 mg q6–8 hr is the preferred treatment because of its mineralocorticoid activity when given at high doses. If a steroid is chosen which does not have mineralocorticoid activity such as dexamethasone, then fludrocortisones at 50 mcg daily should also be given in cases of primary AI. Clinical improvement should be seen in within 4–6 hr after administration of stress dose steroids.[5,6]

Chronic Treatment of Primary and Secondary Adrenal Insufficiency

Patients with primary AI require administration of both glucocorticoid and mineralocorticoid replacement, whereas patients with secondary AI only require glucocorticoid replacement. Patients are followed clinically for signs and symptoms of either cortisol deficiency or excess, and steroid dosages are tailored to the individual patient's needs.

Table 3. Dosage and Tapering Schedule for Steroids in *Acute Adrenal Insufficiency*

Steroid	Route	Initial Dose	Taper	Relative Glucocorticoid Activity	Relative Mineralocorticoid Activity
Hydrocortisone (preferred)	IV	50 mg q6 hr	Taper over 7 days	1	1
Dexamethasone	IV	2 mg q6 hr	2 mg q8 hr	25–30	0
Methylprednisolone (solumedrol)	IV	10 mg q6 hr	10 mg q8 hr	5	0.5

Source: Ref. 4

Table 4. Dosages For Steroids in Primary and Secondary Adrenal Insufficiency in *Non-Stressed State*

Chronic Adrenal Insufficiency					
Hydrocortisone	PO	15–30 mg	TID:10 mg/5 mg/5 mg BID:15 mg/10 mg	1	1
Dexamethasone	PO	1–1.5 mg	BID: 1 mg/0.5 mg	25–30	0
Prednisone	PO	5–7.5 mg	Dosed qam	3.5	0.8
*Fluticasone (mineralocorticoid)	PO	0.05–0.2 mg/day			
Moderate illness/ minor surgery	PO/IV/IM	Increase dose 3x baseline	Decrease back to baseline 24 hr after resolution		
Major illness/major surgery	IV/IM	Stress dose levels	Taper to normal by 50% per day		

Source: Ref. 4,7 and 8

**Note*: All patients with primary AI need fluticasone in conjunction with glucocorticoid replacement. Patients with documented secondary AI do not need mineralocorticoid supplementation and generally require lower daily doses of glucocorticoid.[2]

In cases of moderate illness such as fever, minor trauma or minor injuries, the steroid dose should be increased by 3× the normal dose until 24 hr after resolution of the illness. In cases of severe illness or major surgery, the patient will require stress dose steroids as above, but this can be tapered back to their normal dose by 50% per day once the illness has resolved.[4]

References

1. Chakravarthy MV, (2009) Adrenal Insufficiency. In: *Endocrinology Subspecialty Consult,* 2nd ed., Lippincott Williams & Wilkins, Washington, pp. 70–75.
2. Neary N, Nieman L (2010) Adrenal insufficiency: Etiology, diagnosis and treatment. *Curr Opin Endocrinol Diabetes Obes* **17**(3): 217–223.
3. Kronenberg HM, (2008) Glucocorticoid deficiency. In: *Williams Textbook of Endocrinology,* 11th ed. Saunders Elsevier, Philadelphia.
4. Cooper MS, Stewart PM. (2003) Corticosteroid insufficiency in acutely ill patients. *N Engl J Med* **348**(8): 727–734.
5. Bornstein SR. (2009) Predisposing factors for adrenal insufficiency. *N Engl J Med* **360**(22): 2328–2339.
6. Maxime V, Lesur O, Annane D. (2009) Adrenal insufficiency in septic shock. *Clin Chest Med* **30**(1): 17–27, vii.
7. Lennernas H, Skrtic S, Johannsson G. (2008) Replacement therapy of oral hydrocortisone in adrenal insufficiency: The influence of gastrointestinal factors. *Expert Opin Drug Metab Toxicol* **4**(6): 749–758.
8. Stefanie H, Bruno Allolio M. (2009) Therapeutic management of adrenal insufficiency. In: *Clinical Endocrinology and Metabolism.* Elsevier, Zurich, pp. 167–179.

Chapter 50

Malnutrition

Jeffrey I. Mechanick, Elise M. Brett**

Key Pearls

- *Cachexia* is the loss of body cell mass in the setting of a persistent cytokine-mediated inflammatory process. *Protein energy undernutrition* is characterized by a decrease in visceral protein stores associated with a reduction in protein and energy intake, and *marasmus* is loss of body weight due to pure starvation.
- Every hospitalized patient requires a formal nutritional assessment, which at the minimum consists of height, weight, and identification of risk factors for malnutrition, such as recent weight loss, change in dietary habits, recent surgery, NPO >3 days, inability to chew or swallow, and malignancy.
- Total caloric requirements are generally 20–25 kcal/kg/day for critically ill patients and 30–35 kcal/kg/day for noncritically ill patients. Protein requirements are generally 1.2–1.5 g/kg/day for critically ill patients and 1.0–1.2 g/kg/day for all others.
- Enteral nutrition should be initiated if there is a functional GI tract, no contraindications to intestinal feeding, and no oral nutrition for

*Mount Sinai School of Medicine, New York, NY, USA.

at least 1–3 days in the intensive care unit (ICU) or 5–7 days elsewhere in the hospital.

- Observe patients receiving nutritional support for refeeding syndrome, characterized by hypophosphatemia and cardiac complications.

What is Malnutrition?

The role of nutritional medicine in both routine and specialized management of hospitalized patients has garnered increased attention over recent years. This is primarily due to a better understanding of the biology of disease as well as the emergence of higher quality scientific evidence. Nutrition can be conceptualized as the interaction between dietetics (the environment) and metabolism (the patient). In order to understand and competently implement principles of nutritional medicine, the physician must learn about the nutrient content of foods and other chemicals delivered to a patient as well as the relevant physiology governing a response.

Malnutrition describes any physiological state where the interaction between dietetics and metabolism deviates from normal. Specifically, undernutrition is a state of negative energy and/or protein balance, and overnutrition is a state of positive energy and/or protein balance. A malnourished state develops over weeks to years as result of reduced protein and calorie intake and/or inflammation. This leads to changes in body composition; altered body cell mass, fat mass, and extracellular water; and, ultimately, loss of function. Micronutrients may also be deficient.

The term "malnutrition" is a vague one. Several more precise terms communicate information about a patient's nutritional status more specifically, even if there is considerable overlap and less than unanimous consensus regarding their use. One way to categorize malnutrition in hospitalized patients is as follows.[1] *Cachexia* is defined as loss of body cell mass in the setting of an underlying, persistent cytokine-mediated inflammatory process. Patients with cachexia exhibit reductions in visceral proteins and increases in extracellular fluid (ECF). Body weight is usually unchanged, but there can be some loss or gain. Examples of disease states that can result in cachexia are cancer, heart failure, liver failure, and renal failure. *Protein energy undernutrition* or PEU (otherwise known as mixed marasmus–kwashiorkor overlap syndrome) is characterized by a decrease in visceral protein stores, which is often associated with a reduction in protein and energy intake. ECF may be increased and may mask weight loss. An underlying inflammatory state is present. Examples are exploratory laparotomy, closed head injury, infection, and burns. *Marasmus* is loss of body weight due to pure starvation. Protein and energy intakes are reduced. Inflammation and edema are not typically present. Visceral protein stores are preserved until the late stages. Examples are anorexia nervosa and esophageal stricture.

Detection of the presence or absence of inflammation helps identify patients at nutritional risk and predict the response to nutrition support. Low serum albumin and prealbumin are indicators of an inflammatory state and abnormal body composition. Malnutrition states due to cachexia and adult PEU are irreversible and muscle wasting is not preventable with nutrition support. However, adequate feeding may help limit lean tissue mass losses and improve outcomes. The nutritional status will improve with treatment of the underlying disease state.

Malnutrition can be further classified as "mild" [serum albumin 3.1–3.4 g/L; usual body weight (UBW) loss 10%–15%; BMI 18–18.9], "moderate" (albumin 2.4–3.0 g/L, UBW loss 15%–25%, BMI 16–17.9), or "severe" (albumin< 2.4 g/L, UBW loss > 25%; BMI < 16). The usefulness of detecting and describing malnutrition in a hospitalized patient is related to the impact nutritional status has on the overall prognosis for many clinical conditions (Table 1) as well as coding for enhanced third party reimbursement.

Nutritional Evaluation and Management

Nutritional Assessment

Every hospitalized patient requires a formal nutritional assessment (Joint Commission on Accreditation of Health Care Organizations — JCAHO).[2] Minimal requirements consist of height, weight, and identification of

Table 1. Complications of Nutritional Status in Prognosis of Clinical Conditions

Clinical Condition	Nutritional Status	Impact/Complications
Cancer	Undernutrition	Chemotherapy toxicity Radiotherapy toxicity
	Cachexia	Survival
Critical illness	Undernutrition	Nosocomial infections ICU length of stay Time on ventilator
	Cachexia	Survival
Depression	Undernutrition	Decreased response
Inflammatory bowel disease	Undernutrition	Response to medical therapy Surgical risks
Perioperative	Undernutrition	Complications Mortality
Transplantation	Undernutrition	Rejection
Wound care	Undernutrition	Wound healing

specific risk factors for malnutrition, such as recent weight loss, change in dietary habits, or medical conditions (e.g. nonhealing pressure ulcers, carcinoma, anorexia, gastrointestinal disease, chronic kidney disease, or diabetes), recent surgery, NPO >3 days, inability to chew or swallow, or psychiatric disorder. Other conditions that are part of the three-tiered patient priority system include use of an MAO inhibitor or anticonvulsive drug therapy, life-threatening food allergy, sensitivity, or intolerance, albumin <2.5–3.0 g/dL, total lymphocyte count <800–1199 mm^3, hemoglobin <10–12 g/100 mL (male) or <8–10 g/100 mL (female), pregnancy, HIV, edema, and tube feeding. *Sarcopenia*, the involuntary loss of muscle mass that occurs with normal aging, may also be noted and identify patients at increased nutritional risk. A registered dietitian (RD) should evaluate any patient at nutritional risk. Specific dietetic issues are routinely addressed by the RD. They include determination of appropriate diet and meal supplements, calorie and protein counting in cases of borderline intake, and assessments of whether nutrition support is indicated. Patients with prolonged hospitalizations may require repeated evaluations over time.

A body mass index (BMI; defined as weight in kilograms divided by height squared in meters squared) must be computed for each patient to screen for underweight (BMI <18.5 kg/m^2), overweight (25.0–29.9 kg/m^2), and obesity (≥30 kg/m^2). When physical examination and biochemical findings are evaluated, specific malnutrition diagnoses can be assigned and levels of nutritional risk determined. In addition, there are several nutritional risk assessment tools that correlate with clinical outcomes (Table 2). When these tools are applied correctly, appropriate nutritional interventions can be designed to optimize disease-specific clinical outcomes.

Table 2. Nutritional Risk Assessment Tools

Tool	Description
Nutrition risk index (NRI)[8]	NRI = (% usual body weight × 0.417) + (albumin g/dL × 15.19); normal >100, mild risk 90–100, moderate risk 83.5–90, severe risk <83.5; instrument used in VA Cooperative Trial for perioperative PN[9]; note — another "nutrition risk index".[10] is based on 16 multifactorial items but is too laborious for routine use.
Nutrition risk score[11]	Validated multifactorial instrument based on weight change, BMI, appetite, ability to eat and retain food, stress factor.
Prognostic nutritional index (PNI)[12]	PNI (% risk) = 158 − 16.6 (Alb) − 0.78 (TSF) − 0.20 (TFN) − 5.8 (DH); validated to predict clinical outcomes.
Subjective global assessment (SGA)[13]	Validated multifactorial instrument based on weight change, dietary intake, GI symptoms, metabolic demand, fat/muscle/edema on exam.
Body mass index[14]	Weight (kg)/height (m^2); normal 18.5–25, increased risk due to undernutrition with lower BMI.
Visceral protein stores	Albumin (half-life 20 days; insensitive and nonspecific for nutritional status but sensitive for metabolic stress); prealbumin (half-life 1–2 days; more sensitive for nutritional status but still nonspecific); others include retinol-binding protein and transferrin.

Abbreviations: TSF — triceps skinfold; TFN — transferrin; DH — delayed hypersensitivity.

Status of the Gastrointestinal Tract

Once the type of malnutrition is identified, a formal assessment of the gastrointestinal (GI) tract is performed. This includes evaluation of accessibility (oral, nasogastric tube, nasoenteric tube, percutaneous gastrostomy or jejunostomy, or surgical gastrostomy or jejunostomy tube, structural integrity (obstruction, fistula, or perforation), functional impairment (dysphagia, dysmotility), or malabsorption. The clinical history and physical examination may be all that is necessary. Sometimes radiologic/nuclear studies or special testing such as D-xylose or fecal fat measurements must be performed. Gastroenterology or surgical consultative services may also be useful. Speech pathologists are invaluable in assessing swallowing difficulties and aspiration risk with oral feeding. Thus, the GI tract may be accessible or inaccessible, functional or nonfunctional, or the function may be "uncertain." Patients with dysphagia or pulmonary intubation but a functional GI tract are typically candidates for *enteral nutrition* (EN) support, whereas patients with abnormal GI function (uncertain or nonfunctional) may be appropriate for *parenteral nutrition* (PN) support. In patients with normal GI function but an inaccessible GI tract, PN may be "unavoidable." For example, this may occur with severe malnutrition, inadequate oral nutrition, or the patient refuses EN, or if the patient is receiving bilevel positive airway pressure (BiPAP) and NGT placement or other forms of enteral access are not possible.

Nutrition Support

General Statements

Patients who are malnourished or at risk of malnutrition but have a functional GI tract and can take food orally can be managed with oral nutritional supplements. These are ready-made liquid supplements that are calorically dense and typically balanced in macronutrients while also providing adequate micronutrients (i.e. Ensure®, Boost®). They come in different palatable flavors, such as chocolate, vanilla, and strawberry. They have the consistency of a milkshake but most are lactose-free. Some supplements are fat-free, usually in fruit flavors, and are designed for those patients requiring only clear liquids or a fat-free diet (i.e. Resource Breeze®, Enlive®). A variety of disease-specific supplements, such as for diabetes and kidney disease, are also available (i.e. Boost DM®, Nepro®). Supplements can be taken in place of meals or between meals to provide extra calories.

EN is defined as provision of nutrients employing the small intestine through the use of an enteral access device. PN is defined as provision of nutrients through the veins. It may be provided through peripheral intravenous access (peripheral parenteral nutrition — PPN) or central intravenous access (central parenteral nutrition — CPN). The use of the term "total parenteral nutrition" (TPN) has historically referred to CPN but can be confusing. First, "total" nutrition (meeting the protein, energy, and micronutrient needs of the patient) can be achieved in some cases using a peripheral IV (i.e. patients with large volume requirements and small body weight so that the osmolarity of the PPN is acceptable). Second, total nutrition may not always be provided with CPN, especially in patients who are critically ill, have volume restrictions as with cardiac, renal, or hepatic insufficiency, or have other clinicobiochemical abnormalities. Thus, the term "*parenteral nutrition support*" is best for describing the use of PN, regardless of the access route.

Indications

Hospitalized patients who are at significantly increased nutrition risk, and unable to meet their needs with oral nutrition, should be considered for nutrition support. EN should be initiated if there is:

- A functional GI tract;
- No contraindications to intestinal feeding;
- No oral nutrition (actual or anticipated) for at least 1–3 days in the intensive care unit (ICU) or 5–7 days otherwise (depending on the level of nutrition risk).

NG intubation should be performed to commence EN. If EN is required for a longer duration (usually a few weeks), then a PEG may be the best option. If the patient has gastroparesis, postgastrectomy, or a partial gastric outlet obstruction, then a PEJ should be considered. If a PEG or PEJ cannot be performed, then open (surgical) gastrostomy or jejunostomy tube placement should be performed.

PN is indicated in hospitalized patients who are at significantly high nutritional risk and are unable (or anticipated to be unable) to meet their needs with intestinal feeding according to the same time interval parameters as above with EN. In other words, EN and PN are *not* mutually exclusive. Logistically, EN should be considered, and if possible, attempted first, based on its ease of use, safety, and cost compared with PN. If PN is believed to be needed for less than 14 days and there is adequate peripheral intravenous access, then peripheral PN is preferable. However, in particularly high-risk patients, those with volume restrictions, or those with poor peripheral access, earlier central PN is often necessary.

Several clinical practice guidelines have provided specific recommendations on the use of EN and PN. Clinicians should utilize them with caution, as they are general guidelines rather than hard rules. Also, many of the guidelines are not consistent with each other due to different patient populations, experiences of the primary writing committees, and emerging scientific data.[4,5]

Formulation

Once enteral access is achieved, EN may be started. Some GI endoscopists and surgeons prefer waiting 24 hr after placement before starting the EN. The head should be elevated approximately 40° with NG or PEG feeds, but this is less important with postpyloric feeds. There are three broad categories of tube feeding formulas: intact protein, semielemental/elemental protein (hydrolysates / free amino acids, respectively), and disease-specific (renal impairment, liver failure, diabetes, pulmonary disease, and critical illness). Hospitalists can consult an RD in their institution for a list of the available formulas. Total caloric (energy) requirements are generally 20–25 kcal/kg/day for critically ill patients and 30–35 kcal/kg/day for noncritically ill patients. For obese patients, an adjusted body weight {([actual BW – ideal BW] x 0.25) + ideal BW} may be used. Higher or lower amounts may be necessary, depending on other clinical or biochemical factors. Protein requirements are generally 1.2–1.5 g/kg/day for critically ill patients and 1.0–1.2 g/kg/day for all others, again with deviations depending on other clinical or biochemical factors. Volume requirements are 30–40 cc/kg/day (more for younger, less for older patients), and the difference between requirements and the free water provided in the tube feed (70%–80% volume of tube feed per day) is provided as water or saline flushes in 3–4 divided doses. Saline flushes may be safer than free water for patients receiving jejunal feeding, especially if the patient is at risk for ischemic bowel.

PN is formulated based on the same caloric, protein, and volume requirements as for EN.[6] A "3-in-1" admixture contains amino acids, dextrose, and lipid emulsion all in the same bag. A "2-in-1" PN contains amino acids and dextrose in one bag, and the lipid as a separate intravenous piggyback. Most patients should receive lipids as a source of calories and to prevent an essential fatty acid deficiency. Lipids may be omitted in cases of severe liver failure, very high infection risk, and patients receiving propofol as a sedative at amounts that meet lipid needs. Lipids should not exceed a dose of 1 g/kg/day. Dextrose is provided as a calorie source and to limit gluconeogenesis. Amino acids serve as the protein source. Electrolytes are provided with sodium content approximating the usual tonicity requirements, where a half normal saline solution is 77 mEq/L. Acetate may be required to buffer metabolic acidosis when the patient is catabolic; more is needed with worse acidosis, and less is needed with alkalosis, such as with NG suction or glucocorticoid use. Other electrolytes can be adjusted from the default amounts provided on a standard PN form. Standard multivitamins and trace elements are also provided except in cases of hepatobiliary disease where copper and manganese must be omitted to avoid toxicity. Certain trace elements and vitamins, such as selenium, chromium, copper, vitamin B12, iodine, vitamin C, thiamine, and folic acid, can be added separately as needed. Other compatible additives include insulin, famotidine or ranitidine, and carnitine. Iron should not be added to a standard PN formula. In the hospital, PN is most commonly infused over 24 hr but may also be cycled over 12–18 hr to allow for time off the pump. To calculate the infusion rate, divide the total PN volume by the number of desired hours in the cycle minus one; one-half of this number is the rate for the first and the last hour of the cycle, and the full number is the rate for the other infusion hours.

Monitoring Nutrition Support

Refeeding Syndrome

Patients with severe or chronic malnutrition, anorexia nervosa, alcoholism, pregnancy, postbariatric surgery, hemodialysis, and other medical conditions are at risk for acute electrolyte and volume status changes with refeeding.[3] The hallmark of *refeeding syndrome* is hypophosphatemia. In addition, significant cardiac insufficiency can ensue. At-risk patients require gradual introduction of calories with micronutrient and electrolyte support.

EN

Patients receiving EN should be interviewed regularly regarding the presence of abdominal pain, diarrhea, nausea, or vomiting. The abdomen should be examined for signs of distension or tenderness. In patients who are unable to verbalize symptoms, it is essential that nurses report episodes of vomiting or persistent diarrhea. Patients should be monitored for fever and the access device site inspected on a regular basis for signs of erythema or warmth. Sinusitis is a rare cause of fever in patients with long-term NG feeding. Serum sodium should be monitored regularly and water flushes adjusted accordingly. Sometimes changes in serum sodium warrant a change to a more or less concentrated formula. Hyperglycemia is common in patients receiving EN even without a prior diagnosis of diabetes. Patients who develop it may benefit from a change to a lower-carbohydrate formula. Furthermore, reductions in the glomerular filtration rate may necessitate a change to an electrolyte-restricted formula. In hospitalized patients, diarrhea frequently results from bacterial overgrowth when antibiotics are used, or from the incidental use of sorbitol-containing medications. When diarrhea occurs with EN, some empiric treatments may help: adding bismuth subsalicylate (Pepto-Bismol®) 10–30 cc per 500 cc bag of feeds, cholestyramine, probiotics, and/or changing from an intact protein to a semielemental/elemental feed.

PN

In patients receiving PN, the intravenous catheter site should be inspected regularly for erythema or swelling, which may be signs of infection or a thrombus. Fever and chills are typically the first indication of catheter-related infections. Lungs should be auscultated and the presence of worsening edema assessed for signs of volume overload. Heart sounds should be auscultated for the development of tachycardia or new murmurs. Rarely, a reaction to the lipid component of PN is reported at the start of an infusion manifested by acute chest pain, back pain, dyspnea, sweats, or flushing. Capillary and whole blood glucose determinations are indicated in patients with, or at risk for, hyperglycemia. Routine electrolytes should be checked daily until they are stable and then 2–3 times a week as appropriate in the hospital. Liver function should be checked initially, and weekly thereafter, with more frequent testing when there are significant abnormalities. The CBC should also be monitored at appropriate intervals, as patients with malnutrition are frequently anemic and those on PN may develop leukocytosis indicating infection. For all patients receiving nutrition support, periodic monitoring of body weight, serum albumin or prealbumin, and calculations of nitrogen balance may be helpful in guiding the nutritional prescription.

Hyperglycemia and Nutrition Support

Hyperglycemia is extremely common among hospitalized patients, with a prevalence of approximately 38%. In the hospital it may be due to established type 1 or type 2 diabetes, undiagnosed type 2 diabetes, or stress hyperglycemia in response to severe injury or inflammation, typically seen in critically ill patients. Patients with stress hyperglycemia are

Table 3. Synchronizing Glycemic Control Interventions with Nutrition

Type of Nutrition	Glycemic Control Intervention		
	T1DM non-ICU	T2DM or stress, non-ICU	ICU
NPO	Basal + correction insulin	Basal insulin for FBG >110 mg/dL + correction insulin	IV insulin to correct to ICU target
PO	Basal, prandial, and correction insulin	Oral agents and/or insulin to achieve fasting/prandial targets	IV insulin to correct to ICU target Prandial sq insulin as needed
Continuous TF	Q 12–24 hr glargine or determir, or q 6–8 hr NPH, + correction insulin	Q 12–24 hr glargine or determir, or q 6–8 hr NPH, + correction insulin	IV insulin to correct to ICU target
Cycled TF	Rapid-acting insulin at start NPH at start and 8–12 hr later if needed Correction insulin	Rapid-acting insulin at start NPH at start and 8–12 hr later if needed Correction insulin	IV insulin to correct to ICU target
Bolus TF	Rapid-acting insulin prebolus HS glargine or detemir (0.3 units/kg initially) Correction insulin	Rapid-acting insulin prebolus HS glargine or detemir (for FBG >110 mg/dL) Correction insulin	Rapid-acting (sq) insulin prebolus IV insulin as needed to correct to ICU target
PN	Insulin R (0.1 units per g dextrose in PN) Basal sq insulin (0.3 units/kg) as glargine or detemir Correction insulin	Insulin R (0.1 units per g dextrose in PN) — more if known to have significant insulin resistance Correction insulin	Insulin R (0.1 units per g dextrose in PN) Separate IV insulin drip to correct to ICU target

Abbreviations: T1DM — type 1 diabetes; T2DM — type 2 diabetes; NPO — nil per os; FBG — fasting blood glucose; TF — tube feed.

treated the same as those with type 2 diabetes. Current glycemic targets for patients with diabetes are <110 mg/dL fasting and <180 mg/dL post-prandial for noncritically ill patients, and no higher than 140–180 mg/dL for ICU patients. In non-ICU patients receiving PN, insulin in the PN should be titrated to a target range of 100–140 mg/dL. Tighter glycemic control as low as 80–110 mg/dL may be appropriate for certain critically ill patient populations when these targets can be achieved safely using nurse-driven intensive insulin therapy protocols under direct physician supervision. Interventions to achieve these targets must be synchronized with nutrition (Table 3).[7] Consultation with endocrinology may be necessary if glycemic control is not easily achieved.

References

1. Jenson GL, Bistrian B, Roubenoff R, *et al.* (2009) Malnutrition syndromes: A conundrum vs continuum. *P Parent Enteral Nutr* **33**: 710–716.
2. Joint Commission on Accreditation of Health Care Organizations. JCAHO Standards: Environment of care. List of Standards TX.4. Nutritional assessment. http://www.nyspi.org/jcho/NYSPI/nutritionsrv/nutritass.htm (accessed on June 12, 2010).
3. Boateng AA, Sriram K, Meguid MM, *et al.* (2010) Refeeding syndrome: Treatment considerations based on collective analysis of literature case reports. *Nutrition* 26: 156–167.
4. McClave SA, Martindale RG, Vanek VW, *et al.* (2009) Guidelines for the Provision and Assessment of Nutrition Support Therapy in the Adult Critically Ill Patient: Society of Critical Care Medicine (SCCM) and American Society for Parenteral and Enteral Nutrition (ASPEN). *J Parenter Enteral Nutr* **33**: 277–316.
5. Bozzetti F, Forbes A. (2009) The ESPEN Clinical Practice Guidelines on Parenteral Nutrition: Present status and perspectives for future research. *Clin Nutr* **28**: 359–364.
6. Mechanick JI. (1996) Parenteral nutrition formulation: An integral part of the endocrinologist's metabolic support consultation service. *Endocr Pract* **2**: 197–203.

7. Brett EM. (2006) Nutrition support and hyperglycemia. In: Mechanick JI, Brett EM, *Nutritional Strategies for the Diabetic and Prediabetic Patient*. Taylor & Francis, New York, pp. 171–192.
8. Kyle UG, Schneider SM, Pirlich M, *et al*. (2005) Does nutritional risk, as assessed by nutritional risk index, increase during hospital stay? A multinational population-based study. *Clin Nutr* **24**: 516–524.
9. The Veterans Affairs Total Parenteral Nutrition Cooperative Study Group. (1991) Perioperative total parenteral nutrition in surgical patients. *N Engl J Med* **325**: 525–532.
10. Wolinsky FD, Coe RM, McIntosh WMA, *et al*. (1990) Progress in the development of a nutritional risk index. *J Nutr* **120**: 1549–1553.
11. Reilly HM, Marineau JK, Moran A, *et al*. (1995) Nutritional screening — Evaluation and implementation of a simple nutrition risk score. *Clin Nutr* **14**: 269–273.
12. Dempsy DT, Buzby GP, Mullen JL. (1983) Nutritional assessment in the seriously ill patient. *J Am Coll Nutr* **2**: 15–22.
13. Detsky AS, McLaughlin JR, Baker JP, *et al*. (1987) What is subjective global assessment of nutritional status? *J Parent Enteral Nutr* **11**: 8–13.
14. van Venrooij LMW, de Vos R, Borgmeijer MMMJ, *et al*. (2008) Preoperative unintended weight loss and low body mass index in relation to complications and length of stay after cardiac surgery. *Am J Clin Nutr* **87**: 1656–1661.

Infections Disease

Chapter 51

Hospital-Acquired Fever

*Maria A. A. Reyna**

Key Pearls

- The most common infectious causes of hospital-acquired fever are urinary tract infection, pneumonia, sinusitis and bloodstream infection.
- The most common noninfectious causes are related to procedures, ischemic conditions and malignancy.
- Neither the presence of significant bacteruria nor of pyuria is reliably predictive of infection in catheterized patients.
- Routine stool cultures and examination for ova and parasites are rarely positive when used to evaluate diarrhea that began during hospitalization.
- Empiric antibiotics may be withheld in stable, nonseptic patients until culture results come back.

Introduction

Approximately one-third of medical patients will become febrile during their hospitalization. Physicians who care for these patients are faced with the daunting task of determining the source of the fever and deciding whether to begin treatment before severe morbidity occurs. This chapter offers a pragmatic approach to diagnosing and managing hospital-acquired fever, defined as fever that occurs at least 24–48 hr after admission of an

*Mount Sinai School of Medicine, New York, NY, USA.

immunocompetent patient for a nonfebrile illness. Specific disease entities and their definitive treatment are elucidated elsewhere in this book.

Definition

The definition of fever is arbitrary. In an attempt to establish a standard temperature for critically ill adult patients, a joint task force of the American College of Critical Care Medicine and the Infectious Disease Society of America defined fever as a body temperature that is 38.3°C or higher and is considered a reasonable trigger for investigation.[1] This threshold should, however, be lowered in elderly and immunocompromised patients.

Incidence and Etiology

In a systematic review, the incidence of hospital acquired fever ranged from 2% to 17%. Infection was the cause of fever in 3%–74% of patients, and 3%–54% had a noninfectious etiology.[2] The common infectious causes included urinary tract infection, pneumonia, sinusitis and bloodstream infection (Table 1). The most common noninfectious causes were related to procedures, ischemic conditions and malignancy (Table 2).

Infectious Causes

Clostridium Difficile Infection

C. diff should be suspected in any patient with fever or leukocytosis and diarrhea who received an antibacterial agent or chemotherapy within 60 days before the onset of diarrhea. Although diarrhea is the cardinal symptom in *C. diff*, some patients may present with or develop constipation, which should alert physicians to consider intestinal ileus and toxic megacolon.[3]

Catheter-related Bacteremia

The presence of erythema, induration and tenderness along the catheter insertion site and difficulty in drawing or infusing through the catheter are signs of catheter-related bacteremia. However, in the majority of cases

Table 1. Infectious Causes of Fever

Site	Potential Causes of Fever
Urinary tract	Catheter related UTI Postinstrumentation
Respiratory tract	Hospital/Ventilator-Acquired pneumonia Aspiration pneumonia Empyema Sinusitis
Bloodstream	Primary bacteremia Catheter-related Transfusion-related bacteremia
Gastrointestinal	*Clostridium difficile* Abscess Cholangitis
Cardiovascular	Endocarditis Mediastinitis
Skin, soft tissue	Cellulitis Necrotizing fasciitis
Central nervous system	Meningitis
Surgical site	Wound infection Prosthetic device infection Thrombophlebitis

these are absent and the diagnosis can be difficult. Catheter-related bacteremia should be considered in all febrile patients with central venous catheter in-site for more than 48 hr.

Catheter-related Urinary Tract Infection

Urinary catheters that are functioning properly infrequently cause bloodstream infection and fever.[4] The presence of fever and bacteruria/pyuria does not necessarily indicate urosepsis. Urosepsis should be strongly considered, however, if the patient has urinary obstruction, has undergone recent genitourinary instrumentation or is neutropenic.

Table 2. Non-infectious Causes of Fever

Etiologies	Specific Causes
Postprocedure/Postoperative	Surgery Endoscopy Trauma Transfusion reaction
Tissue ischemia/infarction/inflammation	MI Venous thromboembolism Cerebrovascular accident/subarachnoid hemorrhage Hematoma Heterotopic ossification Infusion-related phlebitis/chemical injury Pancreatitis Ischemic colitis Renal/splenic infarct Acalculous cholecystitis Malignancy Gout/pseudogout Flare of rheumatoid disease
Autonomic/endocrine dysfunction	Delirium tremens/alcohol withdrawal Thyrotoxicosis Addison's disease Central/spinal cord fever
Drugs/biological agents	Drug fever Drug overdose (anticholinergics) Neuroleptic malignant syndrome

Sinusitis

Acute nosocomial sinusitis does not manifest the typical clinical findings of sinus disease. Sinusitis should be suspected in patients with prolonged endotracheal/nasotracheal/nasogastric tube and patients with maxillofacial trauma.

Noninfectious Causes

Postop Fever

Fever within the first 48 hr of surgery is usually noninfectious in origin and is caused by release of endogenous pyrogens into the bloodstream. Once the patient is >96 hr postop, fever is likely to represent infection. Exceptions most commonly occur if there was a breach in the sterile technique or pulmonary aspiration perioperatively including development of necrotizing wound infection due to streptococci or clostridia, which often present within the first 48 hr and anastomotic leakage/dehiscence, which can occur at any time postop.[5] A high level of suspicion should also be maintained for thromboembolic events and superficial thrombophlebitis.

Drug Fever

The diagnosis of drug fever is difficult and is usually a diagnosis made after excluding other causes, due to the nonspecific signs and symptoms. The median time between initiating a drug and fever appearance is estimated to be 7–10 days. The degree of pyrexia is commonly between 38.8°C and 40°C.[6] There is usually a lack of appropriate pulse rate response and relative bradycardia in the absence of sinoatrial disease or beta adrenergic blockade. A generalized maculopapular rash occurs in 18%–29% of patients and may be urticarial. Leukocytosis with or without left shift, eosinophilia and elevation in ESR, hepatic transaminase and lactic dehydrogenase levels may occur. However, normal values do not preclude the diagnosis.[7] A definitive diagnosis can be made only when the fever resolves after removal of the implicated agent, usually within 72 hr and no infectious cause is found. Table 3 lists common medications that have been found to cause drug fever.

Approach to Fever in the Hospitalized Patient

The presence of new fever should trigger a clinical assessment rather than a routine battery of laboratory and radiographic tests. Ordering multiple

Table 3. Drugs Reported in the Literature to Cause Drug Fever

Category	Drug
Antimicrobials	**Penicillins:** penicillin, nafcillin, oxacillin, cloxacillin, ampicillin, piperacillin, ticarcillin **Cephalosporins:** cefazolin, cephalexin, cefotaxime, ceftazidime **Tetracyclines:** minocycline, tetracycline, declomycin, oxytetracycline **Antiviral**: acyclovir **Antituberculous:** isoniazid, rifampin **Antifungal**: amphotericin B **Miscellaneous**: erythromycin, vancomycin, streptomycin, novobiocin, trimethoprim-sulfamethoxazole, nitrofurantoin, quinidine, chloramphenicol
Antineoplastic agents	**Cytotoxic antibiotic:** bleomycin **Alkylating agents:** cisplatin, procarbazine, chlorambucil, streptozocin, cyclophosphamide **Antimetabolites:** hydroxyurea, cytarabine, 6-mercaptopurine **Miscellaneous:** cytosine arabinoside, daunorubicin, interferon, L-asparaginase, vincristine
Cardiovascular agents	**Antiarrhythmics:** procainamide, quinidine **Diuretics:** furosemide, triameterene, hydrochlorothiazide **Adrenergic agonists:** dobutamine, methyldopa **Calcium channel blockers:** nifedipine, diltiazem **Beta blocker:** labetalol **Miscellaneous:** clofibrate, heparin, hydralazine, captopril
Immunosuppressants	Azathioprine, mycophenolate mofetil, sirolimus
Symphathomimetic and hallucinogenic agents	Amphetamine, cocaine, lysergic acid, methamphetamine, 3, 4 methylene dioxymethamphetamine
Antiseizure	Carbamazepine, phenytoin, phenobarbital, primidone
Antiemetics	Metoclopramide, antihistamines, phenothiazine, butyrophenone
Antidepressants	SSRI
Analgesics	**NSAIDS:** aspirin, naproxen, sulindac, ibuprofen **Opiod:** meperidine
Anesthetic agents	Halothane, isoflurane, enflurane
Other	Propylthiouracil, thyroxine, iodide, mebendazole, allopurinol, cimetidine, folate, prostaglandin, ritodrine, sulfasalazine, theophylline, haloperidol

tests indiscriminately increases patient care costs and leads to a high rate of false positive cultures and subsequent inappropriate use of antibiotics. An algorithmic approach to fever in the hospitalized patient is presented in Fig. 1.

Evaluation of the febrile hospitalized patient begins with a comprehensive history and physical exam, as well as a thorough review of the patient's hospital course, medications and previous studies. In most instances, febrile medical patients will have an obvious infectious or noninfectious cause for the fever on initial evaluation. Focused, directed diagnostic testing should be performed based on the apparent source of the fever. In evaluating febrile nosocomial diarrhea, aside from *C. diff* toxin assay, routine stool cultures and examination for ova and parasites to search for other enteric pathogens are not indicated unless the patient has at least one of the following risk factors: An elderly patient (over 65 years old) with pre-existing comorbidity, a suspected nosocomial outbreak, suspected nondiarrheal manifestations of enteric infection (e.g. acalculous cholecystitis, fever of unknown origin, polyarthritis), HIV infection or neutropenia.[8] The management of HIV patients is described in another chapter.

If the febrile patient lacks localizing signs and symptoms or if there is no clear etiology for the fever, it is reasonable to empirically consider septic syndrome due to common infectious causes of hospital-acquired fever. Obtaining blood cultures is mandatory in this subset of patients, as mortality in undetected septicemia is high. A chest X-ray may be indicated in febrile patients who are noted to have purulent sputum, have had a decline in oxygenation, are debilitated, intubated, or have risk factors for aspiration. Urinalysis and urine cultures should be sent for patients with indwelling urinary catheters or who have undergone urological instrumentation. However, the results of these tests should be interpreted with caution, as it is difficult to distinguish between true urinary tract infection and asymptomatic bacteruria due to colonization. Determination of the WBCs with differential can help exclude neutropenia. The presence of eosinophilia is a specific but insensitive indicator of drug reaction. Leukocytosis with left shift in the myeloid series is highly

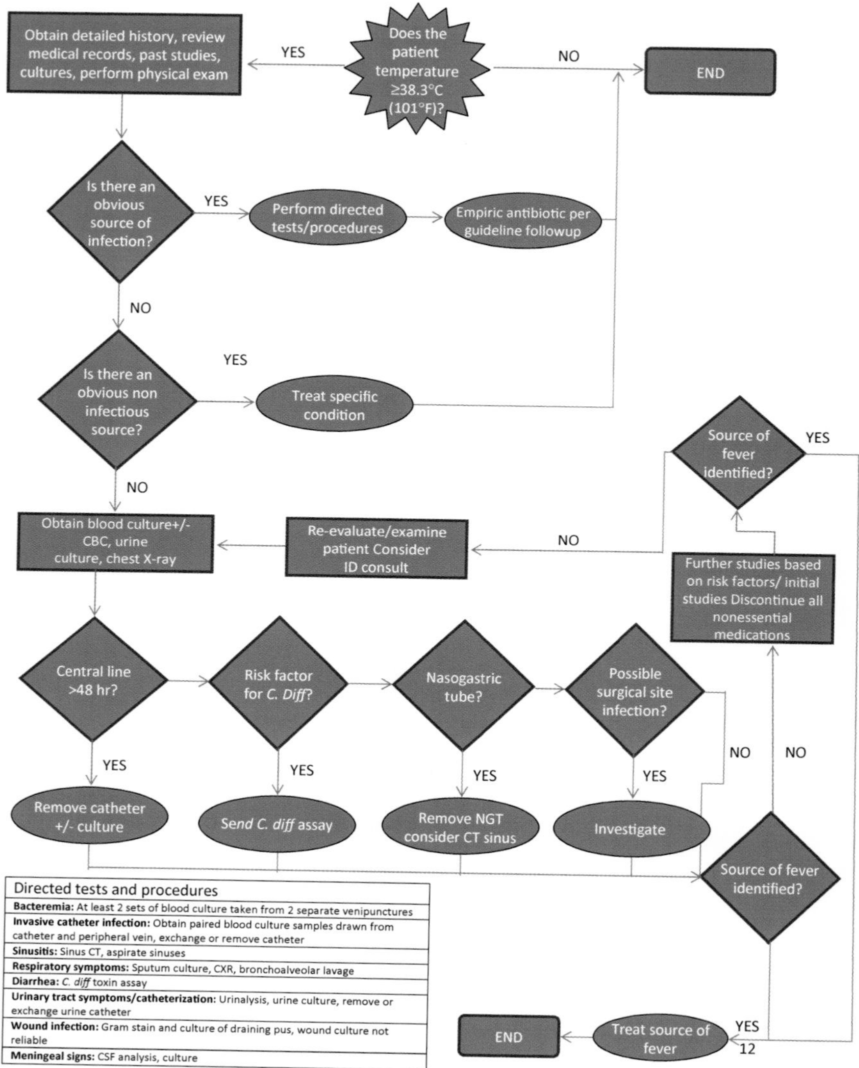

Fig. 1. Approach to fever in the hospitalized patient.

suggestive of bacterial infection. Patients with a central venous catheter *in situ* for more than 48 hr with no apparent cause of fever should have the catheter removed. A peripheral venous catheter should be routinely changed every 72 hr. Patients with a nasogastric tube should have it removed if possible. Patients with risk factors for *C. diff* should be tested.

If the patient remains febrile and there is still uncertainty about the etiology of the fever despite focused evaluation, more invasive studies can be undertaken based on the patient's risk factor for developing certain diseases, clinical suspicion of the physician, and results of the initial studies. In immobilized patients, venous Doppler ultrasound can be done to rule out deep venous thrombosis. Patients who have had recent abdominal surgery may have an intra-abdominal abscess or hematoma and may require abdominal CT.

It is also important to discontinue all potential causative medications, if possible, to rule out a drug-induced fever. Persistence of fever beyond 72 hr after the suspected drug has been removed indicates that the drug was not the cause of the fever.[9]

If the fever persists despite an extensive evaluation, an infectious disease consultation should be obtained.

Approach to Empiric Antibiotic Therapy

The first step when considering antibiotic treatment is to determine if the patient is clinically unstable or is septic (Fig. 2). Septic patients should generally be started on antibiotic therapy after appropriate cultures are obtained. Ideally, antibiotics should be started within 1 hr of recognition of severe sepsis.[10]

Clinically stable patients with no obvious cause of fever on initial exam can generally be observed without antibiotic treatment until culture results come back or after other diagnostic tests and procedures are done. Physicians may consider empiric antibiotics for patients who have multiple risk factors that predispose them to bacterial infection. These include diabetes mellitus, length of stay to fever onset of >10 days, maximal

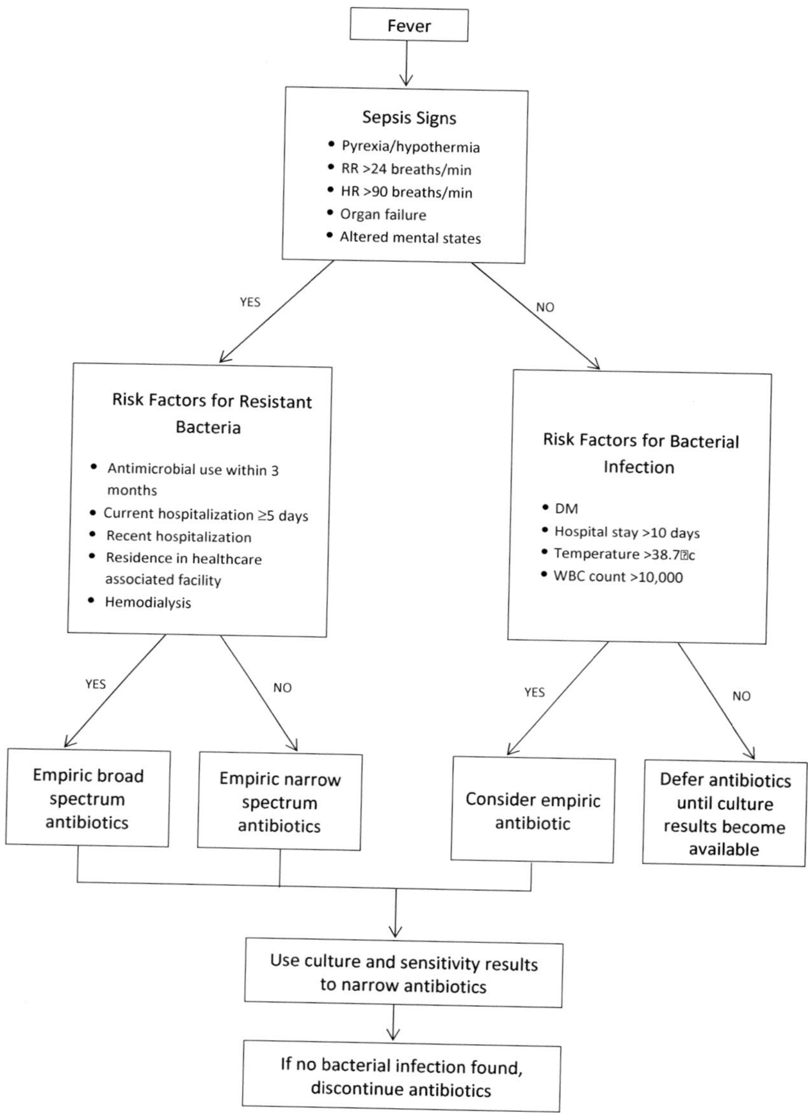

Fig. 2. Approach to empiric antibiotics.

Table 4. Empiric Antibiotic Choice*

Likely Source	Etiologies	Suggested Antibiotic	Notes
Complicated UTI catheter-related	Enterococci, *Pseudomonas aeruginosa*, *enterobacteriaceae*, *Staphylococcus* aureus	Ampicillin + gentamycin or PIP-TZ/TC-CL or imipenem/meropenem	• Alternative: intravenous floroquinolone, ceftazidime, cefepime • Treat for 2–3 weeks.
HAP/HCAP/VAP	***No risk factor for MDR bacteria***: *Streptococcus pneumoniae Haemophilus influenzae* Methicillin-sensitive *S. aureus* *Escherichia coli* *Klebsiella pneumoniae* *Enterobacter* species *Proteus* species *Serratia marcescens*	Ceftriaxone or levofloxacin/moxifloxaxin/ciprofloxacin or ampicillin sulbactam or ertapenem	
	With risk factors for MDR Bacteria: *Pseudomonas* *Klebsiella pneumoniae* *Acinetobacter* species Methicillin-resistant *S. aureus (MRSA)* *Legionella pneumophila*	Antipseudomonal cephalosporin (cefepime, ceftazidime) or Antipseudomonal carbepenem (imipenem or meropenem) or ß-lactam/ß-lactamase inhibittor (Pip-Tazo) + Antipseudomonal fluoroquinolone (cipro/levofloxacin) or	

(Continued)

Table 4. (*Continued*)

Likely Source	**Etiologies**	**Suggested Antibiotic**	**Notes**
		aminoglycoside (amikacin, tobramycin, gentamycin) + linezolid or vancomycin	
Catheter-related bacteremia	*S. epidermidis*, *S. aureus*	Vancomycin	Alternative: daptomycin
Sinusitis (hospitalized with nasotracheal or NGT tube)	*Pseudomonas*, *Acinetobacter*, *E. coli*, *S. aureus*, Yeast. 80% polymicrobial	Imipenem/meropenem Add vancomycin if MRSA is likely.	• Alternative: ceftazidime or cefepime with vancomycin • It is recommended that sinus aspiration for culture be done prior to empiric therapy.
Postoperative wound infection (not involving GI tract)		**Without sepsis:** TMP-SMX DS or clindamycin **With sepsis:** Vancomycin	
C. difficile		**Mild:** metronidazole 500 mg po TID x 10–14 days **Moderate:** vancomycin 125 mg po qid x 10–14 days **Severe:** metronidazole 500 mg IV q 6 hr + vancomycin 500 mg po q 6 hr	

(*Continued*)

Table 4. (*Continued*)

Likely Source	Etiologies	Suggested Antibiotic	Notes
Sepsis, unknown source		***Pseudomonas* unlikely:** Vancomycin + one of the following: (a) Cephalosporin, 3rd or 4th generation (b) Beta-lactam/beta-lactamase inhibitor (c) Carbapenem ***Pseudomonas* likely:** Vancomycin + two of the following: [+] (a) Antipseudomonal cephalosporin (e.g. ceftazidime, cefepime) (b) Antipseudomonal carbapenem (e.g. imipenem, meropenem) (c) Antipseudomonal beta-lactam/ beta-lactamase inhibitor (e.g. piperacillin-tazobactam, ticarcillin-clavulanate) (d) Fluoroquinolone with good antipseudomonal activity (e) Aminoglycoside (e.g. gentamicin, amikacin), (f) Monobactam (e.g. aztreonam)	• If intra-abdominal source is suspected, add metronidazole. • Start antibiotics within 1 hr of recognition of sepsis or septic shock.

*Choice of antibiotic should consider patient's history, past culture results and local resistance patterns.

*Blood cultures should be obtained prior to giving antibiotics.

[†]Selection of two agents from the same class should be avoided.

temperature of >38.7°C, leukocyte count >10 × 10^9/L and number of invasive procedures performed have been found to be independent predictors of bacterial infection.[11]

When selecting antibiotics for empiric therapy for unstable or septic patients, an assessment for risk of infection with multidrug-resistant organisms must be made. Risk factors include[12]:

- Antimicrobial use within the past three months
- Recent hospitalization
- Residence in a healthcare associated facility
- Current hospitalization more than five days
- Hemodialysis

Controversy surrounds the use of combination antibiotics for treatment of gram-negative infection. A recent meta-analysis comparing beta lactam monotherapy to a beta lactam plus an aminoglycoside for sepsis found that double coverage conferred no advantage over single coverage even when gram-negative and *Pseudomonas* infection were analyzed separately.[13] In addition, nephrotoxicity was more frequent in the double coverage group. Current clinical evidence does not support the routine use of combination antimicrobial therapy for treatment of gram-negative infections except in patients with severe sepsis or septic shock or when there is a high level of antibiotic resistance among common gram-negative bacteria in the hospital, as the use of inappropriate initial antibiotic therapy for these situations is associated with increased mortality.[14]

If double coverage is initiated in patients suspected to have MDR gram-negative infection, de-escalation to monotherapy is recommended once susceptibilities are determined.

For patients in whom empiric antibiotic therapy is initiated, the regimen should be reassessed and tailored when culture and sensitivity results become available. Antibiotics should be discontinued if no infection is found and the patient improves.

References

1. O'Grady N, Barie P, *et al.* (2008) Guidelines for evaluation of new fever in critically ill adult patients: 2008 update from the American College of Critical Care Medicine and the Infectious Diseases Society of America. *Crit Care Med* **36**: 1330–1349.
2. Kaul D, Flanders S, *et al.* (2006) Brief report: Incidence, etiology, risk factors and outcomes of hospital-acquired fever. *J Gen Intern Med* **21**: 1184–1187.
3. Cohen S, Gerding D, *et al.* (2010) Clinical practice guidelines for *Clostridium difficile* infection in adults: 2010 update by the Society for Healthcare Epidemiology of America (SHEA) and the Infectious Diseases Society of America (IDSA). *Infect Control Hosp Epidemiol* **31**: 431–455.
4. Tambyah PA, Maki DG, *et al.* (2000) Catheter-associated urinary tract infection is rarely symptomatic: A prospective study of 1497 catheterized patients. *Arch Intern Med* **160**: 678–682.
5. Schwartz D, Weinstein R. (1999) Fever in the hospitalized patient. In: Root R (ed), *Clinical Infectious Diseases: A Practical Approach* Oxford University Press, New York, pp. 449–458.
6. Dimopoulos G, Falagas M. (2009) Approach to the febrile patient in the ICU. *Infect Dis Clin N Am* **23**: 471–484.
7. Patel RA. (2010) Drug fever. *Pharmacotherapy* **30**: 57–69.
8. Bauer TM, Lalvani A, Fehrenbach J, *et al.* (2001) Derivation and validation of guidelines for stool cultures for enteropathogenic bacteria other than *Clostridium difficile* in hospitalized patients. *JAMA* **285**: 313–319.
9. Mourad O, Palda V, *et al.* (2003) A comprehensive evidence-based approach to fever of unknown origin. *Arch Intern Med* **163**: 545–551.
10. Dellinger P, Levy M, *et al.* (2008) Surviving sepsis campaign: International guidelines for management of severe sepsis and septic shock. *Crit Care Med* **36**: 296–327.
11. Arbo MJ, Fine MJ, *et al.* (1993) Fever of nosocomial origin: Etiology, risk factors and outcomes. *Am J Med* **95**: 505–512.

12. Morrell M, Micek, S, *et al.* (2009) The management of severe sepsis and septic shock. *Infect Dis Clin Morth Am* **23**: 485–501.
13. Paul M, Silbiger I, *et al.* (2006) Beta lactam antibiotic monotherapy versus beta lactam-aminoglycoside antibiotic therapy for sepsis. *Cochrane Database Systematic Reviews*, Issue 1. Art. No: CD003344.
14. Kang CI, Kim SH, *et al.* (2005) Bloodstream infections caused by antibiotic-resistant gram-negative bacilli: Risk factors for mortality and impact of inappropriate initial antimicrobial therapy on outcome. *Antimicrob Agents Chemother* **49**(2): 760.

Chapter 52

Community-Acquired and Healthcare/Hospital-Acquired Pneumonia

*Keith Sigel and Mikyung Lee**

Key Pearls

- Elderly patients frequently have atypical presentations of pneumonia.
- Clinical improvement in pneumonia may not be apparent for up to 72 hr after the initiation of antibiotic therapy. Patients who deteriorate or do not improve after 72 hr should be reassessed.
- Early empiric antimicrobial therapy should be initiated to decrease morbidity and mortality; treatment should be targeted according to clinical response and culture results.
- Simple scoring algorithms can identify high-risk pneumonia patients who may benefit from hospitalization and ICU monitoring.
- Patients with significant healthcare exposure or who are hospitalized are at risk for pneumonia caused by multi-drug resistant organisms.

Pneumonia

Pneumonia is a common diagnosis in hospitalized patients. It is useful to differentiate pneumonias into those acquired in the community — or community-acquired pneumonia (CAP) — and those acquired in the hospital (HAP), as well as those acquired in a healthcare setting (HCAP),

*Mount Sinai School of Medicine, New York, NY, USA.

as these conditions can potentially require different treatment and diagnostic strategies.

CAPs are seen in patients with no previous healthcare exposure and who have been hospitalized for less than 48 hr.

HAPs are those diagnosed 48 hours or later after the initiation of hospitalization and not incubating at the time of admission.

Healthcare associated pneumonia (HCAP) is a broader category that aims to identify patients at risk for infection with multidrug-resistant (MDR) organisms and includes patients with any of the following risk factors: hospitalization for at least 2 days during the previous 90 days, residence in a nursing home or extended care facility, receipt of home infusion therapy or chronic hemodialysis (HD), home wound care, exposure to a family member known to be colonized with an MDR pathogen, and presence of chronic immunosuppression.

Community-Acquired Pneumonia

Epidemiology

Forty-to-sixty percent of CAP patients are hospitalized, with 10% of these patients eventually requiring intensive care unit (ICU) admission and an overall mortality rate of 10%.[1] CAP is the most common infectious cause of death.

Several risk stratification tools have been derived for aiding in the management of CAP. CURB-65, a simple validation risk assessment tool, is useful for determining which patients should be admitted to the hospital and may require higher levels of care. ATS/IDSA guidelines propose a simple risk assessment tool for determining which patients should be admitted to the ICU (Table 2).[2]

The most commonly identified bacterial pathogen in CAP is *Streptococcus pneumoniae*, followed by *Haemophilus influenzae*. Atypical organisms, including *Legionella pneumophila*, *Chlamydia pneumoniae*, and *Mycoplasma* species, are also commonly identified (Table 1). *Staphylococcus aureus* pneumonia is an uncommon cause of CAP but, given the increasing prevalence of methicillin-resistant *Staphylococcus aureus* (MRSA), is worth considering in refractory cases of CAP.

Table 1. Most Common Bacterial Etiologies of CAP and HCAP in Order of Approximate Prevalence

HealthCare-Associated Pneumonia	Community-Acquired Pneumonia
MRSA	*Streptococcus pneumoniae*
Streptococcus pneumoniae	*Haemophilus* species
Pseudomonas aeruginosa	Mycoplasma species
MSSA	MSSA
Haemophilus species	MRSA
Enteric gram-negative rods	*Escherichia coli*
Klebsiella species	*Pseudomonas aeruginosa*
Escherichia coli	*Klebsiella* species
Legionella species	*Legionella* species
	Other enteric gram-negative rods

Table 2. Criteria for Severe CAP

Major Criteria	Minor Criteria
Invasive mechanical ventilation	Respiratory rate $\geq$30 breaths/min
Septic shock with the need for vasopressors	PaO_2/FiO_2 ratio $\leq$250
	Multilobar infiltrates
	Confusion/disorientation
	Uremia (BUN level $\geq$20 mg/dL)
	Leukopenia (WBC count $<$4000 cells/mm^3)
	Thrombocytopenia (platelet count $<$100,000 cells/mm^3)
	Hypothermia (core temperature $<$36°C)
	Hypotension requiring aggressive fluid resuscitation

ICU admission should be considered strongly when one major or three minor criteria are met. Other criteria to consider include hypoglycemia, alchohol withdrawal, hyponatremia, metabolic or lactic acidosis, advanced liver diseases, and asplenia.
Adapted from IDSA/ATS 2007 Guidelines.

Nonbacterial etiologies of pneumonia should always be considered. Influenza may cause pulmonary infiltrates and predispose patients to a bacterial superinfection; it also has important treatment and infection control issues. Patients should be assessed for risk factors for tuberculosis, including HIV or risk factors for HIV, history of incarceration, or travel to or origin from developing countries.

Clinical Presentation

Patients with CAP may present with a combination of fever, cough with sputum production, and/or pleuritic chest pain. However, these symptoms may be absent, especially in the elderly. Eldery patients can have atypical presentations of CAP, such as altered mental status, anorexia, and abdominal pain in the absence of classical symptoms. Other important historical factors in assessing pathogen-specific risks include occupational exposure, HIV risk factors, and travel history.

Physical exam may reveal rales or bronchial breath sounds. Chest imaging is mandatory in the evaluation of the patient with suspected CAP, and is more sensitive and specific than exam findings.[3]

Radiologic Evaluation

Chest radiographs (PA and lateral) are implicit in confirming the diagnosis of pneumonia and detecting potential complications.

Laboratory Testing

Leukocytosis greater than 15,000/mm^3 is commonly noted in CAP, but leukopenia may be present and is a poor prognostic sign. Blood and sputum culture have relatively low diagnostic yield in CAP, mainly due to low yield with blood culture and the difficulty of obtaining quality specimens with sputum culture.

Urine Antigens

Urine antigens tests are available for *Streptococcus pneumoniae* and *Legionella pneumophila*. Urine *Streptococcal* antigen tests have a sensitivity as high as 74% and a specificity as high as 94% in HIV-negative adults with pneumonia.[4] Urine *Legionella* antigen assays detect infections with *Legionella pneumophila* serotype 1, which is responsible for 90% of

Legionella pneumonias. A systematic review comparing the efficacy of these tests has estimated a pooled sensitivity of 74% and a pooled specificity of 99%.[5]

Although there is little evidence that routine culture or antigen testing improves outcomes in CAP, a Dutch randomized controlled trial comparing pathogen-directed treatment using culture and antigen testing decreased adverse events and benefited patients with severe CAP.[6] Therefore sputum culture, blood culture, urine streptococcal antigen testing, and urine *Legionella* testing should be strongly considered in patients with severe pneumonia, characterized by any of the following: ICU admission, failure of outpatient antibiotics, cavitary infiltrates, leucopenia, active alcohol abuse, chronic severe liver disease, severe COPD, asplenia, and a pleural effusion.[2]

Treatment

Prompt antibiotic therapy reduces mortality and length of stay for hospitalized patients.[7] Patients with CAP and illness severe enough to require hospital admission should be treated empirically with either a beta-lactam plus a macrolide or a respiratory fluoroquinolone. Patients with a penicillin allergy should be given flouroquinolones. Doxycycline can be used in patients who are intolerant to macrolides.[2] (Table 3).

Empiric treatment for *Pseudomonas* and methicillin-resistant *Staphylococcus aureus* should be considered in patients with certain risk factors. Patients with structural lung disease and/or a significant smoking history should be considered for empiric antipseudomonal therapy with piperacillin/tazobactam, cefepime, antipseudomonal respiratory quinolones, or imipenem. Patients at increased risk of MRSA include those with known obstructive lesions or a history of intravenous drug abuse, and empiric therapy with either vancomycin or linezolid should be considered in concert with standard CAP therapy.[2]

Treatment of CAP should be for 5–7 days. It can be completed in 5 days if the patient becomes afebrile within the first 48–72 hr, and is clinically stable. If a specific pathogen is identified, antibiotics should be refined to target this pathogen. Patients can be switched to oral

Table 3. Risk Factors for Multidrug-Resistant Pathogens in HAP/HCAP

Risk Factor
Antimicrobial therapy in preceding 90 days
Current hospitalization of 5 days or more
High frequency of antibiotic resistance in the community or in the specific hospital unit
Chronic indwelling device
Hospitalization for at least 2 days during the previous 90 days
Residence in a nursing home or extended care facility
Receipt of home infusion therapy or chronic hemodialysis (HD)
Home wound care
Exposure to a family member known to be colonized with an MDR pathogen
Advanced pulmonary disease
History of advanced liver disease or immunosuppression (chronic steroid use, hematologic malignancy, organ transplant, etc.)

antimicrobials within 48–72 hr of treatment initiation if they are clinically responding: they do not need to be observed as inpatients on oral therapy.[2] Oral regimens can include respiratory fluoroquinolones, oral cephalosporins, or amoxicillin/clavulinic acid.

Outcomes/Failure to Respond

Most physiologic abnormalities in CAP will resolve with treatment within 2–3 days but more severe cases may take longer. Radiographic abnormalities may persist for as long as 10 weeks, with the longest intervals found in patients with underlying lung disease.

Up to 15% of CAPs may not respond to initial antimicrobial therapy within 72 hr. Patients who deteriorate or fail to respond to treatment by 72 hr should be re-evaluated. Potential issues to consider include the presence of resistant or untreated organisms, metastatic foci of disease including intravascular lesions or effusions, or noninfectious etiologies of pulmonary disease. Further workup such as sputum culture or urine antigen testing (if not previously performed), chest CT scan, and/or bronchoscopy for a more definitive diagnosis may be beneficial in patients who are not responding.

Healthcare-Associated Pneumonia/ Hospital-Acquired Pneumonia

Epidemiology

HAP is the second-most-common nosocomial infection and is responsible for significant hospital-related morbidity and mortality, adding on average 7–9 days to length of stay (HAP/HCAP guidelines). The microbiology of HAP/HCAP differs from that of CAP, with *Staphyloccus aureus*, *Pseudomonas* and enteric gram-negative organisms being more prevalent (Table 1).

HCAP is a heterogeneous term and encompasses both hospitalized patients and other patients with healthcare exposure. Subgroups of HCAP include nursing home patients (NHAP), hemodialysis patients (HDAP), hospital-acquired pneumonia (HAP), and ventilator associated pneumonia (VAP). These patients are among those at risk for infection with MDR organisms (Table 3). Recent studies suggest that *Staphyloccus aureus*, *Pseudomonas*, and resistant gram-negative organisms are less common pathogens in NHAP and HDAP patients, and that empiric antibiotics in these patients can be similar to those used in CAP.

Clinical Presentation

Patients with HCAP and HAP are more likely to have atypical presentations of pneumonia, due to advanced age and the high prevalence of comorbid conditions and neurologic disorders in this risk group. Fever may be absent, and extrapulmonary symptoms may predominate in this group. HCAP in patients with multiple comorbidities may present as an acute exacerbation of a chronic condition, such as heart failure or COPD.[8]

Important physical findings in hospitalized patients that should raise the suspicion of HCAP include change in lung exam, evidence of new hypoxia, tachypnea, and altered mental status.

Radiologic Evaluation

As with CAP, PA and lateral chest radiographs are implicit in confirming the diagnosis of pneumonia and detecting potential complications.

Laboratory Evaluation

The laboratory evaluation of patients with suspected HCAP should include a complete blood cell count and chemistries. Blood cultures are indicated in patients with HAP and HCAP patients with illness severe enough to merit hospitalization.

Sputum culture is controversial but likely contributes to the management of HCAP. Lower respiratory tract sputum samples, indicated by a high proportion of neutrophils to epithelial cells on microscopic examination, are most likely to provide useful information. Respiratory cultures can also aid in identifying unrecognized resistant organisms or targeting antimicrobials against specific organisms. In addition, Sputum samples should be sent for viral culture and/or DFA for respiratory viruses.

Urine Antigens

Streptococcus pneumoniae and *Legionella pneumophilia* are frequent pathogens causing HCAP, and therefore urinary antigen testing for both is indicated, as early identification can help streamline antimicrobial therapy.

Treatment

Empiric antibiotics for treatment of HCAP or HAP are shown in Table 3. Delaying appropriate antimicrobial therapy leads to increased mortality, so recognition of potential pathogens and optimal antibiotic dosing are important.[9]

Patients with HAP or VAP should all be considered at risk for MDR pathogens, particularly patients who are later in their hospital course and who have been on previous antibiotics. Other patients with

HCAP should be assessed for risk of multidrug-resistant pathogens (Table 3); if the risk is low, they can be treated similarly to those with CAP (Table 4).

Antimicrobial regimens in patients at risk for MDR pathogens should include coverage for *Pseudomonas* and MRSA. If *Legionella* is suspected,

Table 4. Empiric Antibiotic Regimens for CAP and HAP/HCAP

Condition	Antibiotics	Duration	Comments
CAP or HCAP with no MDR risk factors	Beta-lactam (cefuroxime, ceftriaxone, ampicillin/sulbactam or ertapenem) *plus* a macrolide *or* respiratory fluoroquinolone (levofloxacin, moxifloxacin, gatifloxacin)[1]	5–7 days based on response	• PCN allergy: use respiratory quinolone.
HAP or HCAP with MDR risk factors	Antipseudomonal cephalosporin (cefepime, ceftazidime) *or* antipseudomonal carbapenem (imipenem, meropenem) *or* antipseudomonal penicillin (piperacillin-tazobactam) *plus* linezolid or vancomycin	7 days	• In patients at high risk of *Pseudomonas* infection, consider empiric second antipseudomonal agent (antipseudomonal fluoroquinolone or aminoglycoside). • PCN allergy: assess degree of allergy; consider 4th generation cephalosporin if not severe; if severe use respiratory quinolone.

empiric therapy should include a fluoroquinolone or macrolide. Patients with a significant penicillin allergy should be treated with a respiratory fluoroquinolone in combination with therapy for MRSA. Combination therapy is controversial and may be considered in patients at risk for *Pseudomonas* infection, such as those with severe structural lung disease.

The duration of antibiotic therapy for HAP/HCAP should be seven days if the patient is clinically responding. If during the course of therapy a likely pathogen is identified, the antibiotic spectrum can be narrowed to focus on the pathogen.

Outcomes/Failure

Response to appropriate antimicrobial therapy may not occur until 72 hr after initiation; failure of therapy should not be assigned during this time

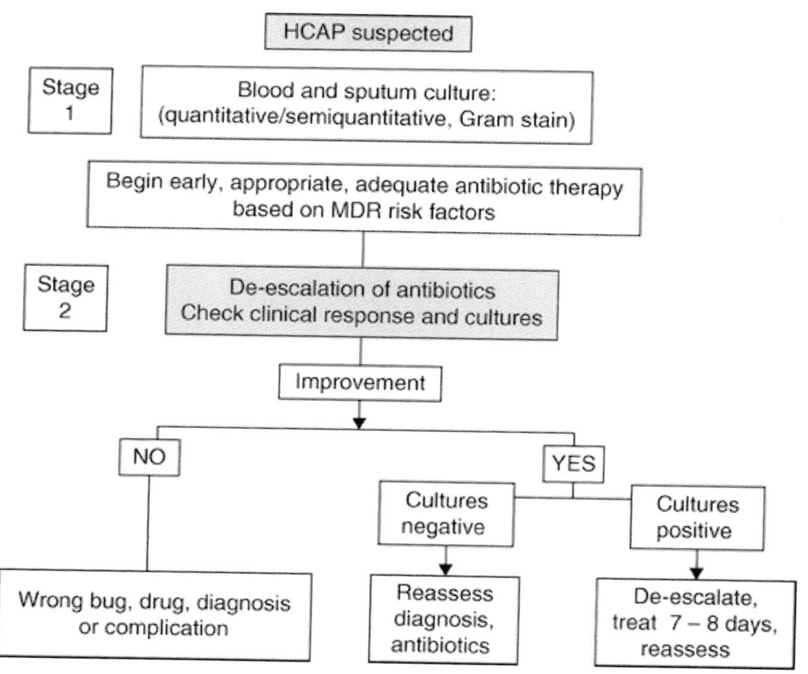

Fig. 1. Management of HCAP/HAP adapted from ATS/IDSA 2005 Guidelines.

period. If after 72 hr the HCAP patient has not clinically improved or has worsened, blood cultures and respiratory cultures should again be performed. CT scanning and bronchoscopy should be considered for a clearer diagnosis. A treatment schematic for a HCAP/HAP is seen in Fig. 1.

References

1. Torres A, Rello J. (2009) Update in community-acquired and nosocomial pneumonia 2009. *Am J Respir Crit Care Med* **181**(8): 782–787.
2. Mandell LA, *et al.* (2007) Infectious Diseases Society of America/American Thoracic Society consensus guidelines on the management of community-acquired pneumonia in adults. *Clin Infect Dis* **44**(Suppl 2): S27–S72.
3. Wipf JE, *et al.* (1999) Diagnosing pneumonia by physical examination: Relevant or relic? *Arch Intern Med* **159**(10): 1082–1087.
4. Klugman, KP, Madhi SA, Albrich WC. (2008) Novel approaches to the identification of *Streptococcus pneumoniae* as the cause of community-acquired pneumonia. *Clin Infect Dis* **47**(Suppl 3): S202–S206.
5. Metlay JP, Fine MJ. (2003) Testing strategies in the initial management of patients with community-acquired pneumonia. *Ann Intern Med* **138**(2): 109–118.
6. van der Eerden MM, *et al.* (2005) Comparison between pathogen directed antibiotic treatment and empirical broad spectrum antibiotic treatment in patients with community acquired pneumonia: A prospective randomised study. *Thorax* **60**(8): 672–678.
7. Houck PM, *et al.* (2004) Timing of antibiotic administration and outcomes for Medicare patients hospitalized with community-acquired pneumonia. *Arch Intern Med* **164**(6): 637–644.
8. Polverino E, Torres A. (2009) Diagnostic strategies for healthcare-associated pneumonia. *Semin Respir Crit Care Med* **30**(1): 36–45.
9. Iregui M, *et al.* (2002) Clinical importance of delays in the initiation of appropriate antibiotic treatment for ventilator-associated pneumonia. *Chest* **122**(1): 262–268.

Chapter 53

Skin and Soft Tissue Infections

*Maurice Policar**

Key Pearls

- *Group A Streptococcus* and *Staphylococcus aureus* continue to be the most common organisms involved in skin and soft tissue infections.
- Community-acquired methicillin-resistant *Staphylococcus aureus* is a frequent and possibly more virulent cause of purulent infections.
- Drainage of abscesses and debridement of deeper infections is crucial to optimal outcomes.
- In severely ill patients, or when there is progression despite therapy, a search for deeper infections may be warranted.
- Wound exploration and culture may be necessary when necrotizing soft tissue infections are suspected, as noninvasive tests cannot definitively exclude the diagnosis.

Introduction/Microbilogy

Skin and soft tissue infections (SSTIs) usually occur at a site of skin disruption often not found on examination. Risks include diabetes or malignancy, previous disruption of lymphatic tracts, surgery, trauma, burns, injection drug use and animal or human bites. *Streptococcus pyogenes* or *Group A Streptococcus* (GAS) and *Staphylococcus aureus* (SA) continue to be the major pathogens involved. There has been a shift in the predominance from GAS to SA in conditions such as impetigo and a sharp rise in

*Elmhurst Hospital Center, Elmhurst, NY, USA.

the incidence of community-acquired and hospital-acquired methicillin-resistant SA (MRSA). Community-acquired MRSA (CA-MRSA) is responsible for up to 60% of SSTIs treated in US emergency departments.[1] Abscesses and cellulitis with purulent draining are present in 90% of these cases. Infection with CA-MRSA may be more severe; animal models suggest that CA-MRSA strains are more virulent than nosocomial strains of SA.[2] When antistaphylococcal treatment is indicated, one must consider the incidence of MRSA in the community or hospital, comorbidities, and the severity of illness. When there is an inadequate response to treatment directed at sensitive SA, one should consider treatment of MRSA and/or other organisms, as well as possible surgical intervention. CA-MRSA infections cannot be clinically distinguished from other purulent SSTIs.

Criteria for Inpatient Management

Evaluation of the patient with a SSTI involves determination of the extent and depth of infection. Inpatient management should be considered for patients with comorbid conditions such as diabetes, cirrhosis, neutropenia or those receiving immunosuppressive treatment. Complicated SSTIs include those with evidence of systemic infection, surgical wound infections, animal or human bites and perineal infections, any of which may require inpatient management. When clues to deeper infections are present, or for those with rapidly advancing or life-threatening infections, urgent surgical referral is required.

Impetigo

Impetigo is a superficial skin infection historically associated with GAS that is now caused primarily by SA. The infection starts as a vesicle on the face or extremities, then changes to a pustule and ruptures, leaving golden crusted lesions without ulceration. Ten percent are bullous impetigo; vesicles evolve to flaccid bullae which rupture and leave light brown crusts. The lesions are painless; pruritis and mild lymphadenopathy are common. Management of limited disease involves soaking with soap and water, and applying mupirocin. Numerous lesions or lack of response should prompt treatment with oral antistaphylococcal antibiotics.[3] (see Table 1). When

Table 1. Antistaphylococcal Antibiotics

	First-line Therapy	Alternatives	Comments
Oral	Dicloxacillin 500 mg every 6 hr	Amoxicillin/Clavulanate 500–875 gm every 12 hr	
	Cefalexin 500 mg every 6 hr Cefadroxil 1 g daily or 500 mg twice daily		
β-Lactam allergy	Clindamycin 300–450 mg every 6–8 hr	Clarithromycin 500 mg twice daily Linezolid 600 mg every 12 hr	Regional US increase in macrolide resistance among SA & GAS
	TMP/SMX 2 DS tablets twice daily		TMP/SMX may be ineffective against GAS
IV	Nafcillin 1–2 g every 4–6 hr	Ampicillin/Sulbactam 1.5–3 g every 6 hr	
	Cefazolin 1 g every 6–8 hr		
β-Lactam allergy	Vancomycin 1 g every 12 hr	Linezolid 600 mg every 12 hr	Occasional cross-resistance to clindamycin with erythromycin-resistant strains
	Clindamycin 600 mg every 8 hr	Daptomycin 4 mg/kg every 24 hr	

Table 2. Treatment of MRSA

	First-line Therapy	Alternative	Comments
Oral	TMP/SMX 1–2 DS tablets twice daily	Clindamycin 300–450 mg every 6–8 hr	Occasional cross-resistance to clindamycin with erythromycin-resistant strains.
	Doxycycline 100 mg twice daily	Linezolid 600 mg every 12 hr	Inducible resistance to Clindamycin in MRSA.
IV	Vancomycin 1 g q12 hr	Linezolid 600 mg every 12 hr Daptomycin 4 mg/kg every 24 hr	

there is suboptimal response to antibiotics, empiric treatment of MRSA should be tried (see Table 2). Ecthyma is similar but causes a punched out ulcer with greenish yellow crusts and raised violacious margins. Treatment is the same as for impetigo.

Folliculitis

Folliculitis is an infection of hair follicles in the apocrine regions, consisting of erythematous papules often topped by a pustule. Treatment involves local measures such as saline compresses or topical antibiotics. *Pseudomonas aeruginosa* can occasionally cause a diffuse folliculitis associated with hot tub use that resolves spontaneously.[4]

Skin Abscesses, Furuncles and Carbuncles

A skin abscess is a collection of pus within the dermis and deeper skin tissues. A furuncle or boil is an abscess extending into the subcutaneous tissue, while a carbuncle is a collection of abscesses that coalesce and drain via multiple hair follicles. These infections usually develop on the neck, face, axillae and buttocks. Affected areas are firm, tender and fluctuant. Patients may have fever, malaise and leukocytosis, and at times can be acutely ill. Lesions are sometimes complicated by cellulitis or bacteremia. Spontaneous drainage is common and can be facilitated by moist heat. When drainage does not occur, incision and drainage may be necessary. Although drainage alone may be curative, treatment with oral antistaphylococcal antibiotics should be considered in immunocompromised patients or diabetics; for infections caused by MRSA, when associated with surrounding cellulitis or fever, and for lesions along the upper lip or around the nose to prevent possible spread to cavernous sinus. If signs of systemic toxicity exist, consider parenteral therapy.

Erysipelas

Erysipelas is a superficial cellulitis with prominent lymphatic involvement, most often caused by GAS, rarely by SA. Infection is commonly on the lower extremities with involvement of the face in less than 20%. Lesions consist of fiery red plaques with well-demarcated raised borders. Fever and leukocytosis are common, and progression is rapid if untreated. Although erysipelas can be treated with penicillin, if the diagnosis is in doubt, treat as cellulitis.

Cellulitis

Cellulitis involves the skin, dermis and subcutaneous tissue. It is often caused by strep species and typically unassociated with a defined focus or injury.[3] When cellulitis is associated with furuncles, carbuncles or abscesses, it is usually caused by SA. Other organisms should be considered when cellulitis is associated with human or animal bites or exposure to salt water or contaminated fresh water (see "Necrotizing Soft Tissue Infections"). Those with disruption of lymphatic drainage from surgery or radiation are at increased risk of developing cellulitis. An episode of cellulitis can result in lymphatic obstruction, further predisposing a patient to recurrence. Cellulitis is manifest by rapidly spreading areas of erythema, edema and warmth, at times with lymphangitis and regional lymphadenopathy. Vesicles, bullae, petechiae or echymosis may develop in inflamed areas. There is commonly local tenderness. Systemic symptoms are usually mild, but can at times be severe. White blood cell counts are usually elevated. Blood cultures are positive in less than 5%. Collecting culture material is warranted in patients not responding to empiric therapy or when there is unusual environmental exposure, trauma or human or animal bites.

Some suggest using penicillin when cellulitis is not associated with purulence,[5] but since the causative organism cannot be determined clinically, antistaphylococcal antibiotics should be used. Parenteral therapy should be considered in patients with systemic toxicity or significant comorbidities. Cellulitis in diabetics may be caused by a broader number of organisms; those who were previously treated or have more than mild infection may benefit from treatment with agents such as ampicillin-sulbactam or other combinations which treat anaerobes and gram negative aerobes. In patients who are more ill, use broad spectrum antibiotics and consider treatment for MRSA. Uncomplicated cellulitis can be treated with courses as short as five days.[5] Patients can be discharged when afebrile, if the cellulitis has stopped spreading and the WBC count is decreasing.

Necrotizing Soft Tissue Infections (NSTIs)

NSTIs include several conditions whose classification is based on location, depth of infection and microbial cause. Most often, the necrosis is limited to the subcutaneous tissue, but more serious infections occur with involvement of the fascia and muscle (fasciitis, myositis). Most infections are polymicrobial and involve the trunk and perineal areas in patients with comorbidities such as diabetes and peripheral vascular disease. Other risks include surgery or trauma, chronic renal failure and perforation of the GI tract, but quite often no risk factor is identified. In the immunocompetent host, monomicrobial infection can be caused by highly virulent organisms which produce exotoxins, and may cause rapidly spreading necrotizing infection.[6] These include GAS (alone or associated with SA), *Streptococcus agalactiae* or group B *Streptococcus* (GBS), CA-MRSA, and *Clostridium spp*. Other species associated with environmental exposures include *Pasteurella spp*. (animal bites), *Vibrio spp*. (shell fish or salt water exposure) and *Aeromonas hydrophila* (contaminated fresh water exposures).[6] GAS infections may be associated with toxic shock syndrome. *Vibrio vulnificus* infection usually occurs in the setting of liver disease, and is uniformly fatal if not promptly treated. *C. perfringens* is now a rare cause of NSTI, and is usually found in crush or burn injuries.[7]

Early diagnosis of NSTI is critical to achieving optimal outcomes. Clues include tense edema, grayish or other discolored wound drainage, vesicles or bullae, necrosis, ulcers or crepitus. Pain may be out of proportion to findings, or may be decreased with areas of anesthesia.[6] Laboratory values associated with NSTI include leukocytosis, thrombocytopenia, elevated creatinine or acidosis. Imaging may reveal subcutaneous gas. Fascial edema on CT is a frequent but non-specific finding. MRI findings can be sensitive but non-specific, and CT is usually more expeditious. Intravenous contrast may be of little benefit.[7] Clinical judgment is the most important element in diagnosis.[3] The gold standard for diagnosis of NSTI is tissue biopsy, usually obtained at the time of surgical exploration. With the exception of wound exploration and culture, negative results on other tests cannot exclude necrotizing infections.[8] Time to first debridement and its adequacy are predictors of survival.[6]

Since most of these infections are mixed infections, antimicrobial regimens should provide coverage for anaerobic, gram-positive, and enteric gram-negative organisms (see Table 3). Vancomycin or other MRSA antibiotic should be added until culture results become available. Antibiotic therapy may need to be altered when specific highly virulent organisms are suspected or confirmed: GAS, GBS, CA-MRSA, *Clostridium spp*. or *Vibrio spp*. Addition of antibiotics that inhibit protein synthesis is recommended to decrease toxin production: clindaymycin or linezolid for gram positive infections, and tetracyclines for Vibrio and aeromonas.[6]

Table 3. Treatment of Necrotizing Soft Tissue Infections

Antimicrobial Agent	Dosage	Patients with β Lactam Allergy
Mixed infection		
Vancomycin or other treatment for MRSA Plus		
• Imipenem-cilastatin	1 g every 6–8 hr	Clindamycin 600–900 mg every 8 hr **or**
• Meropenem	1 g every 8 hr	Metronidazole 500 mg every 8 hr **PLUS**
• Ertapenam	1 g daily	Ciprofloxaxin 500 mg every 12 hr **or**
• Pipercillin-tazobactam	3.37 g every 6–8 hr	An aminoglycoside
• Ticarcillin-clavulanate	3.1 g every 4–6 hr	
• Ceftazidime **PLUS** Clindamycin **or** Metronidazole	1–2 g every 8 hr 600–900 mg every 8 hr 500 mg every 8 hr	
***Streptococcus* infection**		
• Penicillin **PLUS** Clindamycin	2–4 million units every 4–6 hr 600–900 mg every 8 hr	Vancomycin 1 g every 12 hr **or** Daptomycin 4 mg/kg every 24 hr **or** Linezolid 600 mg every 12 hr **PLUS** Clindamycin 600–900 mg every 8 hr
***Staphylococcus* infection**		
• Nafcillin	1–2 g every 4 hr	Vancomycin 1 g every 12 hr **or**
• Cefazolin	2 g every 8 hr	Daptomycin 4 mg/kg every 24 hr **or**
• Vancomycin (MRSA)	1 g every 12 hr	Linezolid 600 mg every 12 hr
***Clostridium* infection**		
• Penicillin **PLUS** Clindamycin	2–4 MU every 4–6 hr 600–900 mg every 8 hr	Vancomycin 1 g every 12 h **or** Daptomycin 4 mg/kg every 24 h **or** Linezolid 600 mg every 12 h **PLUS** Clindamycin 600–900 mg every 8 hr

References

1. Breen JO. (2010) Skin and soft tissue infections in immunocompetent patients. *Am Fam Physician* **81**: 893–899.
2. DeLeo FR, Otto M, Kreisworth BN, *et al.* (2010) Community-associated methicillin-resistant *Staphylococcus aureus*. *Lancet* **375**: 1557–1567.
3. Stevens DL, Bisno AL, Chambers HF, *et al.* (2005) Practice guidelines for the diagnosis and management of skin and soft tissue infections. *Clin Infect Dis* **41**: 1373–1406.
4. Pasternak MS, Swartz MN. (2010) Cellulitis, necrotizing fasciitis, and subcutaneous tissue infections. In: GL Mandell, JE Bennet, R Dolin (eds), *Mandell, Douglas and Bennett's Principles and Practice of Infectious Diseases*. Churchill Livingstone, Philadelphia, PA, pp. 1289–1312.
5. Eron LJ. (2009) Cellulitis and soft-tissue infections. *Ann Intern Med* **150**: ITCI-1–ITCI-16.
6. May AK. (2009) Skin and soft tissue infections. *Surg Clin N Am* **89**: 403–420.
7. Sarani B, Strong M, Pascual J, Schwab CE. (2009) Necrotizing fasciitis: Current concepts and review of the literature. *J Am Coll Surg* **208**: 279–288.
8. Headley, AJ. (2003) Necrotizing soft tissue infections: A primary care review. *Am Fam Physician* **68**: 323–328.

Chapter 54

Urinary Tract Infections

Meenakshi M. Rana and David P. Calfee*[†]

Key Pearls

- Acute uncomplicated cystitis can usually be diagnosed in women with classical signs and symptoms of UTI and can be treated with three days of trimethoprim-sulfamethoxazole without a pre-treatment urine culture.
- For patients with pyelonephritis who cannot tolerate oral intake, have signs of sepsis or poor follow up, empiric therapy should be broad and include a third generation cephalosporin or a parenteral fluoroquinolone.
- Asymptomatic bacteriuria should not be treated except in the setting of pregnancy or patients about to undergo genitourinary procedures.
- In hospitalized patients with a urinary catheter, catheter-associated urinary tract infection (CAUTI) is diagnosed in patients with signs and symptoms of a urinary tract infection and a positive urine culture; diagnosis cannot be made based on foul-smelling or cloudy urine or pyuria alone.
- Urinary catheters should only be placed for appropriate indications and removed as soon as possible in order to prevent CAUTI.

Introduction and Epidemiology

Urinary tract infections (UTIs) are one of the most frequent bacterial infections encountered in the hospital setting. They account for over 7 million

*Mount Sinai School of Medicine, New York, NY, USA.
†Weill Cornell Medicial College, New York, NY USA.

office visits and over one million hospital admissions every year.[1] About 60% of women will have an episode of urinary tract infection in their lifetime. They carry not only significant clinical but also economic burden costing from $1.6 to $2.5 billion yearly.[2]

Diagnosis and management of UTI can be challenging. The clinical spectrum can vary from benign asymptomatic bacteriuria to urosepsis and septic shock. While appropriate antimicrobial management is important, inappropriate treatment can lead to further antimicrobial resistance and the development of nosocomial complications, including infection with *Clostridium difficile.* This chapter addresses pathogenesis, microbiology, clinical presentation, diagnosis and treatment of the various infectious urinary tract syndromes.

Pathogenesis

Urinary tract infections occur as a result of three different mechanisms by which bacteria invade the urinary tract: ascending, hematogenous and lymphatic. The ascending route of infection is the most important mechanism and accounts for the majority of urinary tract infections in women. Pathogens from the fecal flora colonize the vagina and periurethral area. Given that the female urethra is short, bacteria then easily ascend to the bladder, such as can occur after vaginal intercourse. The hematogenous route of infection is uncommon and involves seeding of the kidney in the setting of a bloodstream infection. The lymphatic route involves increased pressure in the bladder that causes lymphatic flow to be directed toward the kidney.[3]

In patients with a urinary catheter, development of a UTI occurs through a different mechanism. Microorganisms ascend on the extraluminal or the intraluminal surface of the catheter. This contamination of the catheter can occur during insertion, during manipulation of the catheter or drainage bag (including failure to maintain a closed drainage system), or resulting from the migration of bacteria present in the urethra or on the skin at the external urethral meatus. The formation of biofilm made up of microorganisms and extracellular matrix on the urinary catheter can complicate management and make antimicrobial penetration difficult if the catheter is left in place.[4]

Microbiology

Acute, uncomplicated cystitis is most often caused by *Escherichia coli*, which is isolated in 80–85% of episodes (Table 1). *Staphylococcus saprophyticus* is responsible for up to 5–10% of episodes of acute uncomplicated cystitis in

Table 1. Characteristic Pathogens and Empiric Treatment Regimens

Condition	Characteristic Pathogen	Recommended Empiric Treatment
Acute uncomplicated cystitis in women	*E. coli, S. saprophyticus*	Trimethoprim-sulfamethoxazole × 3 days; fluoroquinolone × 3 days or nitrofurantoin × 7 days.
Acute pyelonephritis	*E. coli, K. pneumoniae, P. mirabilis*	Parenteral ceftriaxone, fluoroquinolone or ampicillin-sulbactam or piperacillin-tazobactam in severely ill patients.
Complicated urinary tract infections:	*E. coli, Proteus, Klebsiella Pseudomonas, Serratia* spp, enterococci, staphylococci	
Men		Fluoroquinolone or trimethoprim-sulfamethoxazole × 7 days.
Pregnancy		Cephalexin or trimethoprim-sulfamethoxazole × 3 days (trimethoprim-sulfamethoxazole should be avoided in third trimester).
Hospitalized or catheter-associated		Parenteral fluoroquinolone or cefepime/piperacillin-tazobactam/carbapenems in patients with extended hospital stays.

young women in the outpatient setting. However, *Proteus, Pseudomonas, Klebsiella, Enterobacter spp.* and other gram negative organisms are more likely to be seen in patients who acquire hospital-associated infections and in patients with complicated UTI.[3] The most commonly seen gram positive organisms include enterococci and staphylococci. Since enterococci are part of the normal human fecal flora, enterococcal UTI is often from an endogenous source; however, vancomycin resistant enterococci (VRE) is more common in the inpatient population and is usually the result of exogenous acquisition in healthcare settings. Identification of VRE in the urine often represents colonization rather than symptomatic infection.[4] In addition, coagulase negative staphylococci is seen in patients with urinary catheters, whereas *Staphylococcus aureus* in the urine is usually seen in patients with bacteremia.

Candiduria is also common in the inpatient population and usually occurs in patients with urinary catheters, those receiving antimicrobial therapy or in patients with prior surgical procedures or diabetes. However, in most cases, candiduria represents asymptomatic colonization.[4]

Acute, Uncomplicated Cystitis in Women

Acute cystitis is an acute bacterial infection of the urinary bladder. The term uncomplicated refers to a structurally and neurologically normal urinary tract. This is most commonly seen in young women in the outpatient setting. Women present with characteristic symptoms of dysuria, urinary frequency or urgency, suprapubic pain, hematuria or fever. Pyuria or presence of LE on urine dipstick is a sensitive test. While traditionally 10^5 colony-forming units per milliliter (cfu/mL) is used to define a positive urinary culture, in women with typical symptoms, 10^3 cfu/mL is adequate for diagnosis. Given the expense, time consuming nature and predictability of the pathogens, urine culture is no longer routinely recommended in this population.[2]

Antimicrobial therapy is usually empiric and a three day course of trimethoprim-sulfamethoxazole (TMP-SMX) is recommended. Alternatives include a three day course of a fluoroquinolone or a seven-day course of nitrofurantoin. In women with recurrent urinary tract infection, urine culture should be done to make sure resistance is not a problem and the patient should be treated based on culture and susceptibility results. In patients with frequent recurrences, patient-initiated therapy or prophylaxis may be an option.

Acute Pyelonephritis

Pyelonephritis refers to infection of the kidney and renal pelvis. Patients usually present with fever, flank pain and tenderness and may also have dysuria, nausea/vomiting and abdominal pain. In some cases, this may progress to bacteremia and septic shock. The diagnosis is made clinically and urine and blood cultures should be done. Indications for hospital admission include[6]:

- Inability to tolerate oral intake
- Signs of sepsis including hypotension or tachycardia
- Inability of patients to seek follow-up care

In hospitalized patients, empiric therapy may include a parenteral fluoroquinolone or a third-generation cephalosporin such as ceftriaxone; other alternatives in seriously ill patients include ampicillin-sulbactam or piperacillin-tazobactam. If gram-positive organisms are suspected, empiric antimicrobial therapy should also be directed against enterococcus or staphyloccus. If there is no clinical improvement after 48 hours or if blood cultures remain positive despite appropriate therapy, imaging with ultrasound or CT scan should be considered to rule out obstruction or abscess. After clinical improvement, antimicrobial therapy can be completed with oral therapy based on urine culture and susceptiblility results for a period of fourteen days; in mild cases seven days of therapy with a highly active agent such as an oral fluoroquinolone is likely sufficient.[3]

Complicated Urinary Tract Infection

Complicated UTI refers to infection in a urinary tract that is not functionally or structurally normal, and traditionally includes all urinary tract infection in men, pregnant women, patients with indwelling urinary catheters, and calculi.[3] In general, men with urinary tract infection should have a pretreatment urine culture done and be treated with a seven day course of TMP-SMX or a fluoroquinolone. As complicated UTI encompasses a wide variety of topics, this review will primarily focus on catheter-associated urinary tract infection (CAUTI) as this is largely healthcare-associated.

Catheter-Associated Urinary Tract Infection (CAUTI)

Catheter-associated bacteriuria is the most common health care-associated infection worldwide, accounting for 40% of all hospital-acquired infections. 80% of nosocomial UTIs are catheter associated and approximately 12–16% of patients will have a urinary catheter placed during their inpatient stay. In addition, patients who remain catheterized have a 3–7% daily risk of developing bacteriuria. Of patients who become bacteriuric, 10–25% will go on to develop symptoms consistent with a urinary tract infection and 1–4% will become bacteremic.[7]

Despite the known risk of infection, catheter use remains widespread in many hospitals. Physicians should be aware of the appropriate indications for urinary catheterization. These are limited to[8]:

- Perioperative use for selected surgical procedures
- Monitoring urine output in a critically ill patient
- Management of acute urinary retention or obstruction
- Assistance in pressure ulcer healing in an incontinent patient and for the purpose of comfort care or per patient request.

Unfortunately, many physicians place catheters for inappropriate indications and these catheters are likely to become "forgotten."[9]

Hospital physicians should therefore be aware of which patients have urinary catheters and monitor for signs and symptoms of possible infection. The diagnosis of CAUTI can be challenging. Most catheterized patients with CAUTI do not usually manifest the classical symptoms of dysuria or frequent or urgent urination. In a prospective study of 1497 patients with a urinary catheter, there was no difference in patients with bacteriuria as compared to patients without bacteriuria with respect to signs and symptoms associated with a UTI (fever, dysuria, flank pain).[10] In addition, the foul smell of urine or cloudy urine in a catheterized patient alone should not be used as an indication for antimicrobial therapy or considered as diagnostic of CAUTI. Lastly, in patients with a urinary catheter, pyuria alone should not be used as a way to diagnose urinary tract infection. Unlike women with uncomplicated acute cystitis, pyuria is not sensitive for diagnosis of CA-bacteriuria. In a 761 newly catheterized patients, the sensitivity of pyuria for CA-bacteriuria was only 47% and the specificity was 90%. Therefore, the presence or absence of pyuria alone should not be used to differentiate asymptomatic bacteriuria from symptomatic urinary tract infection in a catheterized patient.[11]

According to recent IDSA guidelines, evaluation for CAUTI should be performed in patients with a urinary catheter who develop symptoms such as fever, suprapubic pain or costovertebral tenderness, acute hematuria or altered mental status with no other identified cause. These patients should have a single urine specimen sent for urine culture by sampling through the catheter port using aseptic technique or collecting urine specimen from a freshly placed catheter. Patients with these signs and symptoms who then have a urine culture with greater than 10^3 cfu/mL of one or more bacterial species are diagnosed with CAUTI. In patients who had a urinary catheter in place that was removed and then develop urinary symptoms, the diagnosis of CAUTI may still apply if the catheter was removed within 48 hours.[7]

Patients with a diagnosis of CAUTI should have the catheter discontinued if possible; if not possible, catheters in place greater than two weeks should have the catheter replaced because the presence of biofilm makes bacteria difficult to eradicate. As with other complicated UTI, CAUTI should be treated for 7–14 days with appropriate antimicrobial therapy. Asymptomatic bacteriuria should not be treated except in the setting of pregnancy or patients about to undergo genitourinary procedures.[12]

Prevention of catheter-associated urinary tract infections in hospitalized patients is important in reducing hospital length of stay as well as morbidity and mortality. Urinary catheters should only be placed when absolutely necessary and discontinued as soon as possible. Implementation of automatic stop-orders or electronic reminders in the hospital can help facilitate discontinuation of unnecessary catheters.[7] Evidence-based recommendations for prevention of CAUTI are listed in Table 2.[13]

Table 2. Prevention of Catheter-Associated Urinary Tract Infections in Hospitals

Recommendation	Comments
Insert urinary catheters only if an appropriate indication exists	Ensure that catheters are inserted only when necessary. Consider use of alternatives to indwelling urinary catheters (e.g. condom catheters) when appropriate.
Remove urinary catheters as soon as possible	Catheter necessity should be reviewed at least once each day. Consider "automatic stop orders" where catheters are routinely removed unless certain conditions, such as urinary obstruction, exist.
Use aseptic technique for catheter insertion	Aseptic technique includes: hand hygiene, use of sterile equipment (gloves, drapes, antiseptic or sterile solution for periurethral cleansing), insertion by staff who have been properly trained
Secure the catheter after insertion	Catheter securement may reduce catheter movement and urethral traction.
Maintain a closed drainage system	Replace the catheter and tubing if breaks in aseptic technique, disconnection of catheter tubing, or leakage of urine occurs.
Maintain an unobstructed flow of urine	Do not allow tubing to become kinked. Keep the drainage bag below the level of the bladder at all times.
Perform routine hygiene of the urethral meatus	Daily cleaning of the urethral meatus with antiseptic solutions is not routinely recommended.
Additional considerations	In certain situations, the use of antimicrobial- or antiseptic coated catheters may be considered.

References

1. Stamm WE, Hooton, TM. (1993) Management of urinary tract infections in adults. *NEJM* **329**(18): 1328–1334.
2. Drekonja DM, Johnson JR. (2008) Urinary tract infections. *Prim Care Clin Office Pract* **35**: 345–367.
3. Sobel JD, Kaye D. (2009) Urinary tract infections. In: Mandell, Bennett and Dolin's Principles and Practice of Infectious Disease, Philadelphia: Elsevier Churchill Livingston.
4. Shuman EK, Chenoweth CE. (2010) Recognition and prevention of healthcare-associated urinary tract infections in the intensive care unit. *Crit Care Med* **38**(8): S373–378.
5. Warren JW, Abrutyn E, Hebel R, *et al.* (1999) Guidelines for antimicrobial treatment of uncomplicated acute bacterial cystitis and acute pyelonephritis in women. *CID* **29**: 745–758.
6. Hooton TM, Stamm WE. (1997) Diagnosis and treatment of uncomplicated urinary tract infection. Infectious Disease Clinics of North America **11**(3): 551–581.
7. Hooton TM, Bradley SF, Cardenas DD, *et al.* (2010) Diagnosis, prevention and treatment of catheter-associated urinary tract infection in adults: 2009 International Clinical Practice Guidelines from the Infectious Diseases Society of America. *CID* **50**: 625–663.
8. Lo E, Nicolle L, Classen D, *et al.* (2008) Strategies to prevent catheter-associate urinary tract infections in acute care hospitals. *ICHE* **29S**: S41-S50.
9. Saint S, Wiese J, Amory JK, *et al.* (2000) Are Physicians aware of which of their patients have indwelling urinary catheters? *The American Journal Of Medicine*. **109**: 476–480.
10. Tambyah PA, Maki DG. (2000) Catheter-associated urinary tract infection is rarely symptomatic: A prospective study of 1497 catheterized patients. *Arch Intern Med* **160**: 678–672.
11. Tambyah PA, Maki DG. (2000) The relationship between pyuria and infection in patients with indwelling urinary catheters. *Ach Intern Med* **160**: 673–677.

12. Nicolle LE, Bradley S, Colgan R, *et al*. (2005) Infectious disease society of America guidelines for the diagnosis and treatment of asymptomatic bacteriuria in adults. *CID* **40**: 643–654.
13. Gould CV, Umscheid CA, Agarwal RK, Kuntz G, Pegues DA, and the Healthcare Infection Control Practices Advisory Committee (HICPAC). (2009) Guideline for Prevention of Catheter-Associated Urinary Tract Infections, 2009. http://www.cdc.gov/hicpac/pdf/CAUTI/CAUTIguideline2009final.pdf Accessed November 7, 2010.

Chapter 55

HIV for the Hospitalist

Richard MacKay and Beverly Forsyth**

Key Pearls

- All hospitalized patients between 13 and 64 years of age should be offered testing for HIV, regardless of perceived risk.
- The degree of immunosuppression (CD4 count) of the HIV+ patient determines the risk of opportunistic infections or malignancies.
- An understanding of interactions between HIV medications and other medications is crucial for the hospitalist.
- The HIV-infected population is aging and, in resource-rich settings, may be more likely to be admitted with expected comorbidities of an aging population than with opportunistic infections.
- Hospitalized patients newly diagnosed with HIV need appropriate counseling and should be linked to specialty care prior to discharge.

Causes of Hospitalization Among HIV-Infected Patients

In the United States, approximately 1.1 million people are living with HIV, of whom 21% are undiagnosed. Persons aged 50 and older account for 24% of people living with HIV. Hospitalization rates for persons infected with HIV have declined dramatically since the advent of comprehensive antiretroviral therapy, and discharge diagnoses have shifted from HIV-related opportunistic infections to the more common problems of an aging

*Mount Sinai School of Medicine, New York, NY, USA.

population with expected comorbidities. AIDS-defining conditions, including opportunistic infections and malignancies, are seen either in patients unaware of their HIV status or in those unable to engage in care due to ongoing substance abuse, psychiatric comorbidities or other barriers to care. Standards of care for non-HIV-related diagnoses are those of the general population; the major challenge for the hospitalist is to avoid therapies that interact with the patient's antiretroviral regimen.

The approach to diagnosing illness in patients with HIV is guided by knowledge of the degree of immunosuppression as measured by CD4 cell count (Table 1). Practitioners should be aware that certain conditions such as intercurrent illness, steroid use or chronic liver disease can produce spuriously low values. In these situations, the CD4 percentage may give a

Table 1. Common Diseases by Level of Immunosuppression[1]

CD4 Cell Count 200–500 cells/μL
Bacterial pneumonia, especially *Streptococcus pneumoniae* and *Haemophilus influenzae*
Pulmonary tuberculosis
B-cell and Hodgkin's lymphomas
HPV-related squamous cell carcinomas of anus and cervix
Idiopathic thrombocytopenic purpura
Kaposi's sarcoma
CD4 Cell Count < 200 cells/μL
Pneumocystis jiroveci pneumonia (PCP)
Disseminated and extrapulmonary tuberculosis
Geographic disseminated invasive fungal infections (e.g. histoplasmosis and coccidiodomycosis)
CD4 Cell Count < 100 cells/μL
Toxoplasma encephalitis
Cryptococcal meningitis
Candida esophagitis
Cryptosporidium chronic diarrhea and wasting
CD4 Cell Count < 50 cells/μL
Cytomegalovirus retinitis and encephalitis
Disseminated *Mycobacterium avium* complex
Primary CNS lymphoma

more accurate estimation of immune status, with CD4 percentage of 14% approximating a CD4 cell count of 200 cells/μL.

Diagnosing and Treating Common Infections in the HIV-Infected Patient[1,5]

Physicians caring for hospitalized AIDS patients should be aware that those with advanced immunosuppression often do not have a unifying diagnosis but may have multiple pathogens.

Bacterial Pneumonia

- Risk for pneumococcal disease occurs early in HIV, is much greater than in the general population, and persists to some extent even with immunologic recovery.
- If the presentation is acute and classic, treat as any community-acquired pneumonia (CAP).
- Low threshold for considering tuberculosis; in these patients airborne respiratory isolation, sputum collection for acid-fast bacilli (AFB) and avoidance of fluoroquinolones are recommended until CAP is confirmed by negative sputa and response to therapy.

Pneumocystis Pneumonia (PCP)

- Caused by the fungus *Pneumocystis jiroveii*
- Presents as a subacute respiratory illness with prominent dyspnea, nonproductive cough, and chest X-ray with symmetrical interstitial infiltrates which can progress to consolidation. Chest X-ray can be normal in early disease. Lactate dehydrogenase (LDH) is commonly elevated.
- Diagnosed by induced sputum for direct fluorescent antibody staining or selected stains for cysts and trophozoites. If sputum studies are negative, bronchoscopy with broncoalveolar lavage +/– biopsy is

indicated and much more sensitive. Routine expectorated sputa are insensitive and should not be used for diagnosis.

- Preferred treatment is trimethoprim-sulfamethoxazole, 5 mg/kg of trimethoprim, three times daily for 21 days.
- In patients with significant hypoxia, $PaO_2 < 70$ mmHg or A-a gradient > 35, add prednisone 40 mg bid for 5 days, then taper to 40 mg/day for 5 days and 20 mg/day for 11 days.
- Recovery is slow.
- If no response in 7 days, consider additional pathogens, drug toxicity or, rarely, treatment failure.
- For acute worsening, rule out pneumothorax.

Mycobacterium Tuberculosis

- The risk for reactivation of latent tuberculosis is exceptionally high in HIV-infected patients; the risk occurs early in the disease. Latent TB is diagnosed by PPD 5 mm or greater; however, false negatives are common with immunosuppression.
- Active tuberculosis in patients with CD4 > 350 cells/μL presents classically with fever, chronic cough, weight loss, sweats and upper lobe infiltrates.
- Diagnosis is made by collecting three sputa for stain and culture for mycobacterium.
- The highly immunocompromised patient is more likely to have an atypical clinical presentation of tuberculosis. Peritoneal, pleural, pericardial, lymphatic and meningeal involvement are common. chest X-ray may be normal or show noncavitating lower lobe infiltrates. Diagnosis is made by tissue or fluid sample, or by blood culture for AFB.
- Treatment is similar to that for the normal host and is often presumptive pending culture results. Drug therapy in the patient on antiretroviral therapy is particularly complex, due to potential drug–drug interactions and hepatotoxicity. Consultation with an infectious diseases specialist is recommended.

Cryptococcal Meningitis

- Cytococcal infection is the most common cause of meningitis in the AIDS patient.
- Presents as a subacute meningitis with headache, fever progressing to lethargy and obtundation late in the disease.
- Diagnosis is made by lumbar puncture and positive cryptococcal antigen, India ink prep or culture. CSF cell count and chemistry may be normal or show high protein with lymphocytic pleocytosis.
- CSF opening pressure should be measured and is frequently elevated.
- Serum cryptococcal antigen is most often positive; a positive serum antigen necessitates lumbar puncture even in the asymptomatic patient.
- Treatment is with liposomal amphotericin B +/– flucytosine for two weeks followed by fluconazole 400–800 mg/day.
- Control of increased intracranial pressure is essential for therapeutic success. Daily lumbar punctures to remove fluid and lower pressures may be required for up to two weeks. Mannitol, steroids and acetazolamide are ineffective.

Toxoplasma Encephalitis

- Focal encephalitis caused by reactivation of latent CNS infection with toxoplasma gondii.
- Presents with headache, fever, focal neurologic signs and seizures.
- Diagnosis is presumptive and suggested by one or more ring-enhancing lesions on MRI, positive serum anti-toxoplasma IgG antibody, and clinical and radiographic response to specific therapy within the first two weeks of treatment.
- Preferred treatment in patients over 60 kg is pyrimethamine 200 mg once, then 75 mg/day plus leucovorin 20 mg/day and sulfadiazine 1.5 g 4 times a day for 6 weeks followed by maintenence therapy.
- Failure to improve in two weeks or worsening after a week requires further diagnostic investigation with stereotactic brain biopsy, if feasible.

Candida Esophagitis

- Patients present with odynophagia, which can be severe. Generally thrush is visible on exam but absence does not preclude presumptive therapy targeted at *Candida* in the proper clinical setting.
- Preferred treatment in the hospitalized patient is with oral or IV fluconazole 200 mg/day.
- Failure to respond can occur with azole-resistant *Candida* species or alternate diagnoses, including herpes simplex virus (HSV) or cytomegalovirus (CMV) esophagitis or aphthous ulcers. If the patient with esophagitis has candida that fails to respond to fluconazole, therapy can be switched to an echinocandin.
- If the patient fails to respond to treatment, esophagoscopy with biopsy and culture is required for diagnosis and targeted alternate therapy.

CMV Retinitis

- Retinitis is the most common presentation for cytomegalovirus reactivation and occurs in advanced immunosuppression.
- Diagnosis is suggested by floaters, light flashes or visual loss, though patients may be asymptomatic early in disease.
- Fundoscopic exam with dilated pupil is required for diagnosis, preferably by a retina specialist with experience in HIV care.
- Patients admitted with CD4 count <50 cells/μL should have routine examination of the retina to diagnose early disease before visual loss occurs.
- Treatment is with intravenous ganciclovir or oral valganciclovir.

Disseminated *Mycobacterium Avian* Complex (dMAC)

- A common cause of fever of unknown origin in the AIDS patient with CD4 <50 cells/μL.
- Presents with fever, sweats, weight loss, severe anemia, elevated alkaline phosphatase, hepatosplenomegaly, and thoracic or abdominal lymphadenopathy.

- Diagnosis is confirmed by isolating MAC from AFB cultures of the blood, bone marrow biopsy, or biopsy of involved lymph nodes. Specific DNA probes are used for rapid lab identification of MAC.
- Treatment is with either clarithromycin or azithromycin plus ethambutol. In seriously ill patients amikacin, rifabutin or a fluoroquinolone can be added as a third or fourth drug.

Antiretroviral Treatment

Antiretroviral treatment is a complex topic and is usually performed in conjunction with an HIV specialist. However, a basic understanding of HIV treatment is essential for the hospitalist.[3]

Criteria for Starting Antiretroviral Medication (ARVs)

- Patient willing to start medications and able to comply with the regimen.
- All patients with a history of an AIDS-defining illness (infection or malignancy).
- CD4 <500 cells/μL. Some experts recommend treating at any CD4 count.
- Patient with an HIV-negative partner.
- All patients with the following conditions:
  - Pregnancy
  - Chronic hepatitis B (HBV)
  - Chronic hepatitis C (HCV)

Hospitalized patients who fall into one of the above categories and are not on treatment should be linked to HIV care and considered for treatment, with a goal of starting antiretroviral therapy within two weeks of their hospitalization.

Antiretroviral Therapy

The reverse transcriptase of the HIV virus has a high error rate, enabling it to escape both host defenses and ARVs. This ability to rapidly mutate can lead to medication resistance. To prevent resistance, the cornerstone of HIV treatment is the use of at least three active medications from at least two different classes of medications. Each class of medications interferes with replication at a different step in the replication pathway.

There are currently five different classes of antiretroviral medications (see Table 2). Nucleoside reverse transcriptase inhibitors except for abacavir are renally dosed. The protease inhibitors are generally "boosted"; that is, the drug level is increased in the bloodstream by adding a low dose of the protease inhibitor ritonavir, allowing for a reduced frequency of dosing. Ritonavir is always used in conjunction with another protease inhibitor. All protease inhibitors except for nelfinavir can or must be boosted with ritonavir. All medications are oral except for enfuvirtide, which is administered by subcutaneous injection. Some medications come in a liquid formulation.

Common first-line regimens for HIV treatment are listed in Fig. 1.

Toxicity from ARVs may be class toxicities or drug-specific (see Table 3).

Many of the HIV medications interact with other common medications (Table 4). All medications should be reviewed for their potential interaction with the patient's antiretroviral regimen.

In general, hospitalized patients should be continued on their ARVs except in these situations:

- Suspected toxicity from medication
- NPO

If ARVs are held, the entire regimen must be stopped, otherwise resistance may develop. However, caution must be used in patients with chronic HBV — holding medications that are also active against HBV risks reactivation of HBV and potentially fulminant hepatitis (for example, tenofovir, lamivudine, and emtricitabine).

Diagnosing HIV

Since 2006 the Center for Disease Control has advocated offering routine HIV testing to all hospitalized patients between 13 and 64 years of age,

Table 2. Antiretroviral Medications

Nucleoside/Nucleotide Reverse Transciptase Inhibitors (NRTIs)	Nonnucleoside Reverse Transcriptase Inhibitors (NNRTIs)	Protease Inhibitors (PIs)	Integrase Inhibitors	Entry Inhibitors
Abacavir	Efavirenz	Atazanavir	Raltegravir	*Enfuvirtide* (fusion inhibitor)
Emtricitabine	Nevirapine	Darunavir		Maraviroc (CCR5 entry inhibitor)
Lamivudine	Etravirine	Fosamprenavir		
Tenofovir	Rilpivirine	*Indinavir*		
Zidovudine		Lopi navir + ritonavir (Kaletra®)		
Didanosine	***Fixed-dose combinations*:**	*Nelfinavir*		
Stavudine	Efavirenz + emtricitabine + tenofovir (Atripla®)	*Saquinavir*		
***Fixed-dose combinations*:**	Rilpivirine + emtricitabine + tenofovir (Complera®)	Ritonavir: for boosting all PIs except for nelfinavir; no longer used in treatment doses		
Zidovudine + lamivudine (Combivir®)				
Abacavir + lamivudine (Epzicom®)				
Abacavir + zidovudine + lamivudine (Trizivir®)				
Tenofovir + emtricitabine (Truvada®)				

Note: Drugs in italics are rarely used now.

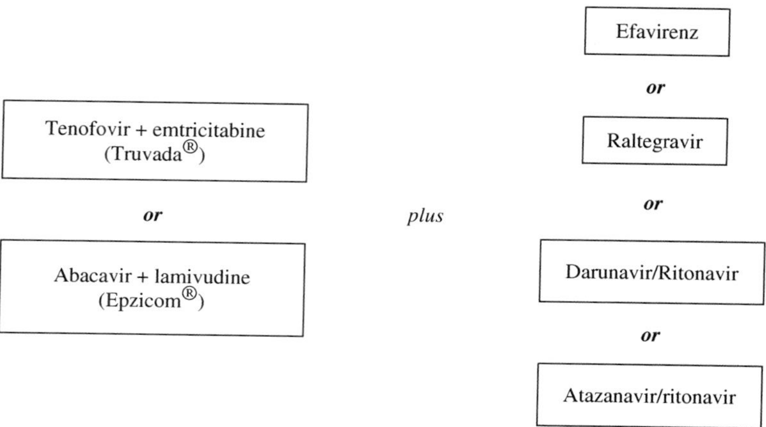

Fig. 1. Common first-line regimens for HIV treatment.

Table 3. Major Drug-Specific Toxicities[3]

Medication	Toxicity
Zidovudine	Macrocytic anemia
Stavudine, didanosine	Lactic acidosis, peripheral neuropathy pancreal
Abacavir	Hypersensitivity reaction
Nevirapine	Stevens–Johnson; hepatotoxicity
Tenofovir	Renal injury; Fanconi's syndrome
Tipranavir	Intracerebral bleed
Atazanavir	Indirect hyperbilirubinemia
Saquinavir	Prolonged QT interval

regardless of risk, in order to identify those unaware of their status and engage them in care. The patient should be given the opportunity to refuse testing.[2]

The diagnosis of HIV is made either by detection of circulating antibodies or, in early infection, by measurement of circulating virus. Screening tests include enzyme-linked immunosorbent assay (ELISA) and bedside rapid diagnostic tests (see Fig. 2). The current fourth generation ELISA can be positive as early as two weeks after infection; almost all patients test positive by six weeks after exposure. If either screening

Table 4. Important Drug–Drug Interactions[4]

ARV or Class	Medication(s)	Interaction/Recommendation
Ritonavir	Inhaled and injected steroids	Can lead to iatrogenic Cushing's syndrome.
NNRTIs or PIs	Voriconazole	Decreases voriconazole levels.
NNRTIs or PIs	Carbemazepine, phenobarbital and phenytoin	May effect level of anticonvulsants or ARV agent; monitor levels frequently if unable to switch anticonvulsants; avoid with raltegravir, as may reduce raltegravir concentration.
PIs	Rifampin	Can reduce PI concentration; use rifabutin with proper dose adjustment.
PIs	Clarithromycin	Alteration in clarithromycin levels; use azithromycin if possible.
Efavirenz	Methadone	Can induce methadone metabolism and withdrawal; may need to increase methadone dose.
PIs	Statins	Increase risk of myositis; simvastatin and lovastatin contraindicated; may use rovustatin, atorvastatin and pravastatin but start at low dose and titrate.
Atazanavir	Proton pump inhibitors	Can decrease levels of atazanavir; if needed, use H2 blocker instead and separate dose by 10 hr

method is positive, a confirmatory Western blot (WB) assay is necessary in order to confirm the diagnosis. The Western blot measures the presence of antibodies to a panel of HIV proteins and is reported as positive, negative or indeterminate. A positive WB confirms HIV infection and a negative result suggests a false positive screening test. An indeterminate test can reflect early infection before full seroconversion, late infection with seroreversion, or false positive serology.

Indeterminate WB test results require further investigation. If the patient has no risk factors for HIV, the test is most likely false negative.

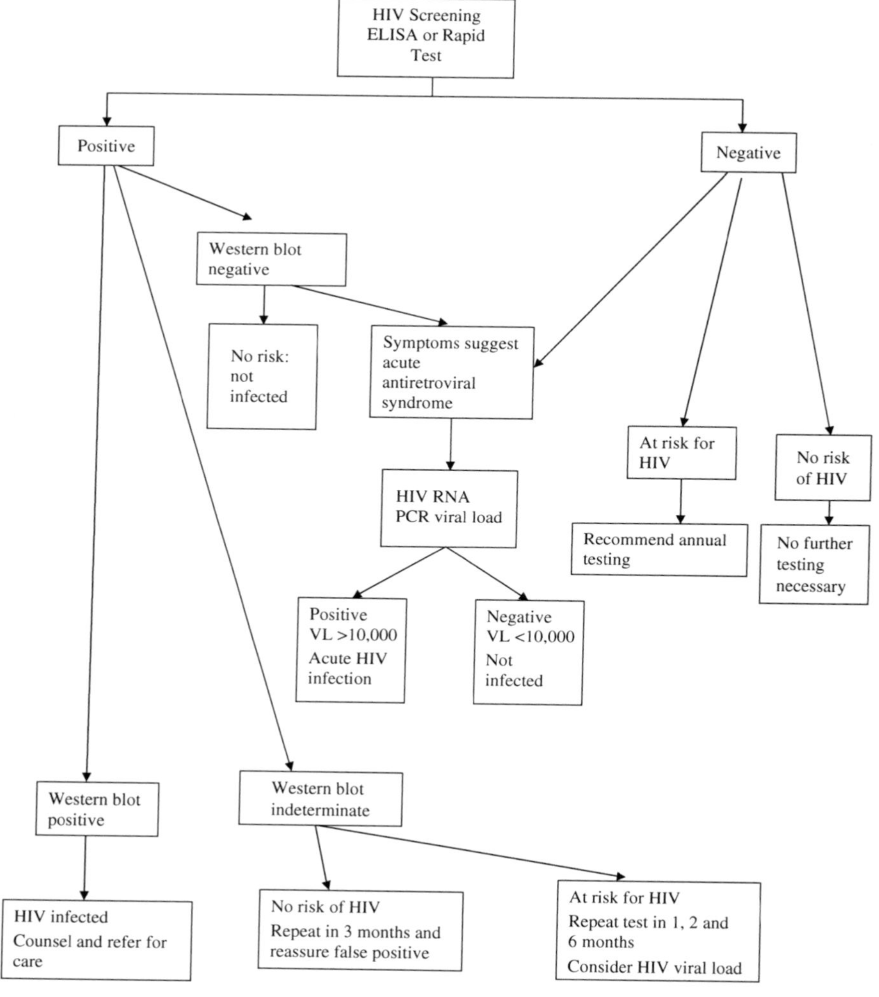

Fig. 2. Schema for HIV testing.

In this case, the patient should be reassured and the test repeated in three months. If the patient is at risk for HIV, then testing is repeated at one, two and six months, or if the clinical situation suggests acute HIV infection an HIV RNA PCR or viral load may confirm infection.

If the patient has identified risk factors for HIV and the screening test is negative, then repeat testing annually or more frequently is recommended.

Acute Retroviral Syndrome

A significant percentage of persons acutely infected with HIV experience a nonspecific flulike clinical syndrome characterized by fever, pharyngitis, lymphadenopathy, rash, diarrhea, headache and myalgias. Less commonly, patients may exhibit neurologic complications during primary infection, including aseptic meningitis, facial nerve palsy, Guillain–Barre and peripheral neuropathy. This syndrome occurs during the window period, a time during the first weeks of primary infection when there is a high circulating viral load but absence of antibody response. When primary infection is suspected, diagnostic testing is best accomplished by antibody screening and measuring circulating viral load. To avoid false positive results, viral load should be >10,000 copies/mL for a diagnosis of HIV.

Hospitalized patients newly diagnosed with HIV need to receive appropriate counseling and be linked to specialty care prior to discharge.

Occupational Exposure to HIV

Healthcare workers may be exposed to HIV via percutaneous injury with a device contaminated with blood or with bodily fluids that are bloody and potentially harbor the virus. Viral transmission may rarely occur when nonintact skin or mucous membranes are exposed to blood or other fluids. In needle-stick injuries risk of infection is increased by deep penetrating injuries, visible blood on the device, a device that was intravascular and a source patient with a high HIV viral load.

Limited human data and experimental data from animal studies show that the risk of infection can be significantly decreased by prompt admini-stration of postexposure prophylaxis with antiretroviral therapy. There is no broad consensus on specific choice of therapy.

All hospitals should have in place a clear protocol for responding to needle-stick injuries and mucocutaneous exposures. In general this should include:

- Careful documentation of the event and estimation of risk of infection
- 24 hr access to rapid HIV testing of the source patient
- Provision of antiretroviral therapy to the exposed person, ideally within 1–2 hr of exposure, and sufficient medications to complete a month of treatment
- Testing of the employee for HIV soon after exposure
- Ongoing counseling and testing of the employee, including consideration of other blood-borne pathogens
- Management of medication side effects
- Expert consultation if the source has a resistant virus

Examples of postexposure prophylaxis regimens are:

- Tenofovir 300 mg/day + emtricitabine 200 mg/day + rattegravir 400 mg twice a day
- Tenofovir 300 mg/day + emtricitabine 200 mg/day + atazanavir 300 mg/day + ritonavir 100 mg/day

Initiation of treatment should not be delayed by lack of test results from the source patient, as treatment can subsequently be terminated if no risk of HIV transmission becomes apparent.

References

1. Bartlett JG, Gallant JE, Pham PA. (2009) *Medical Management of HIV Infection (2009–2010).* Knowledge Source Solutions, LLC; Durham, NC.
2. Revised Guidelines for HIV Counseling, Testing, and Referral, http://www.cdc.gov/mmwr/pdf/rr/rr5019.pdf

3. Guidelines for the Use of Antiretroviral Agents in HIV-1 Infected Adults and Adolescents, http://www.aidsinfo.nih.gov/ContentFiles/AdultandAdolescentGL.pdf
4. HIV Drug–Drug Interactions, http://www.hivguidelines.org/clinical-guidelines/adults/hiv-drug-drug-interactions
5. Guidelines for the Prevention and Treatment of Opportunistic Infections in HIV-Infected Adults and Adolescents, http://www.aidsinfo.nih.gov/Guidelines/GuidelineDetail.aspx?MenuItem=Guidelines&Search=Off&GuidelineID=211&ClassID=4

Chapter 56

Influenza

*Nicole M. Bouvier**

Key Pearls

- Clinically significant influenza disease is caused by the influenza A and influenza B viruses.
- In typical flu seasons, influenza-related hospitalizations and deaths are more likely to occur in the elderly and in persons with chronic medical conditions.
- Primary viral pneumonia begins similarly to uncomplicated influenza, but the acute illness rapidly progresses and is accompanied by signs and symptoms of lower respiratory tract disease. Secondary bacterial pneumonia follows a biphasic course, with a period of clinical improvement followed by a recrudescence of systemic and lower respiratory symptoms consistent with bacterial pneumonia.
- Annual influenza vaccination is recommended for all persons aged six months or older, and it remains the best way to prevent illness and death associated with influenza virus infection.
- Neuraminidase inhibitors are effective when used as treatment or postexposure prophylaxis to prevent complications in patients at high risk for influenza-related morbidity and mortality.

*Mount Sinai Medical Center, New York, NY, USA.

Introduction

The influenza viruses are characterized by segmented, negative-strand RNA genomes. There are three *types* of influenza viruses, designated A, B, and C. Influenza A viruses are further classified by *subtype*, according to their surface glycoproteins, namely hemagglutinin (HA) and neuraminidase (NA). Many genetically distinct subtypes — 16 for HA and 9 for NA — have been isolated from domestic and wild birds, but only three HA (H1, H2, and H3) and two NA (N1 and N2) subtypes have caused human epidemics, as defined by person-to-person transmission.[1,2]

Epidemiology

Influenza-associated morbidity and mortality vary widely each year, depending on factors such as the predominant circulating type/subtype and the degree of the antigenic match between circulating strains and the annual vaccine. Between 1976 and 2006, anywhere from 3000 to 49,000 deaths per year are estimated to have been attributable to influenza. The rates of infection are highest in young children, whereas complications, including hospitalization and death, are highest among older adults. In a typical "flu season," approximately 90% of deaths occur in persons aged 65 years and older. Complications are also more likely to occur in persons with certain medical conditions, including chronic cardiovascular, pulmonary, kidney, and neurological disease; diabetes; congenital and acquired immunodeficiency states; and pregnancy.

During pandemics, influenza epidemiology shifts, with younger people disproportionately affected by complications like lower respiratory tract infections and death. The 2009 influenza A/H1N1 pandemic resulted in more than 12,000 influenza-related deaths in the United States; unlike in typical flu seasons, nearly 90% of deaths occurred among people younger than 65 years of age.[3–5]

Clinical Manifestations of Influenza

Within 1–2 days of infection with influenza virus, uncomplicated influenza typically begins with an acute onset of systemic and respiratory symptoms. Systemic symptoms, including fever and chills, headache, myalgia, lethargy, and anorexia, develop early in the course of illness. Fever generally ranges from 100°F to 104°F (38°C to 40°C), but may be as high as 106°F (41°C), with peak temperatures on the first day and decreasing over 3–8 days thereafter. Respiratory symptoms, including dry cough, pharyngeal pain, and nasal congestion and discharge, tend to persist longer than systemic symptoms; however, it is the presence of systemic symptoms and the abruptness of their onset that clinically distinguishes influenza from other viral diseases of the upper respiratory tract.

Pulmonary complications of influenza virus infection include primary viral pneumonia and secondary bacterial pneumonia. In seasonal influenza, primary viral pneumonia is rare; when it occurs, patients tend to be older, with chronic comorbidities. Clinically, primary viral pneumonia begins like typical uncomplicated influenza, but the acute illness rapidly progresses, accompanied by signs and symptoms of lower respiratory tract disease, such as dyspnea, hypoxemia and cyanosis, and occasionally hemoptysis. Chest radiography typically demonstrates diffuse, multilobar opacities. In contrast, the clinical course of secondary bacterial pneumonia is biphasic. Following a characteristic influenza illness, after a period of clinical improvement lasting 4–14 days, there is a recrudescence of systemic and lower respiratory symptoms consistent with bacterial pneumonia, such as fever and chills, dyspnea, pleuritic chest pain, and cough with bloody or prurulent sputum. In the pneumonic phase, chest imaging is also characteristic of a bacterial pneumonia, generally showing a focal lobar consolidation.[1,5]

Diagnosis of Influenza

In temperate climates of the Northern Hemisphere, the flu season typically extends from October to May, with peak activity in the mid-to-late-winter months. When influenza viruses are circulating in the community, the presence of characteristic influenza symptoms, particularly fever with cough, has a sensitivity of 63%–78% for the diagnosis of influenza.[6,7] Clinical diagnosis alone compares favorably with point-of-care rapid influenza antigen tests, which have sensitivities in the 60%–90% range.[8] Thus, for the diagnosis of uncomplicated influenza in otherwise healthy young and middle-aged adults during the flu season, rapid antigen testing adds little to clinical management.

Laboratory confirmation of suspected influenza may, however, alter management in certain clinical settings, particularly with elderly and immunosuppressed patients, who can present with atypical symptomatology, or with patients who present with influenza-like illness (ILI) outside of the flu season. Direct or indirect fluorescence antigen (DFA or IFA) assays generally have higher overall sensitivity than rapid antigen tests, but they require more technical expertise, and thus sensitivity varies among clinical laboratories. The highest sensitivity is achieved either with virus culture, in which virus is grown from a clinical specimen, or with nucleic acid testing, in which viral genomic RNA is detected through conventional or real-time reverse transcriptase–polymerase chain reaction (RT-PCR). However, like DFA/IFA, these assays require technical expertise, and actual sensitivities vary from lab to lab.[8]

Management of Influenza: Antiviral Medications

Two classes of antiviral drugs are clinically available for the treatment of influenza: M2 ion channel inhibitors (amantadine and rimantidine) and NA inhibitors (oseltamivir and zanamivir). Zanamivir is formulated as a powder delivered by an inhaler device; the other three drugs are administered orally. Due to the high prevalence of adamantane-resistant influenza viruses in the United States, in 2010–2011 the CDC recommended against the use of M2 inhibitors for influenza treatment or prophylaxis; periodic updates on antiviral recommendations are posted at www.cdc.gov.

Intravenous (IV) zanamivir, as well as a third NA inhibitor, the IV drug peramivir, are in clinical trials but are not yet approved by the U.S. Food and Drug Administration (FDA). Thus, parenteral antivirals are not readily available to patients who cannot take oral or inhaled medications. In some circumstances, IV oseltamivir, peramivir, and zanamivir may be available from the manufacturers under the FDA's Emergency Investigational New Drug (E-IND) application procedure; further information can be found at www.fda.gov.

When started within 48 hrs of the symptom onset, oseltamivir and zanamivir have been shown to modestly shorten the duration of symptoms in otherwise healthy adults.[9] However, influenza in these patients is generally a self-limited disease that requires only supportive care. In contrast, antiviral treatment should always be considered in hospitalized patients and in outpatients at high risk for complications. Two studies[10,11] have shown a survival benefit of antiviral treatment in hospitalized patients with laboratory confirmed influenza; importantly, both also demonstrated that the survival benefit persists even when antiviral treatment is delayed more than 48 hrs after the symptom onset.

Prevention of Influenza: Vaccination

Annual vaccination remains the best way to prevent influenza-attributable morbidity and mortality. Currently, the CDC's Advisory Committee on Immunization Practices (ACIP) recommends annual influenza vaccination for all persons aged 6 months or older. There are two vaccine formulations: trivalent inactivated influenza vaccine (TIV), administered intramuscularly by injection, and live attenuated influenza vaccine (LAIV), delivered as a nasal spray. Both preparations are trivalent, containing antigens from three influenza virus strains: an influenza A/H3N2 virus, an influenza A /H1N1 virus, and an influenza B virus. Because the elderly tend to have less robust antibody responses to standard influenza vaccines, a new TIV containing more HA antigen per dose (Fluzone High-Dose) has recently been approved for persons aged ≥65 years. Data suggest improved immunogenicity in this population, though it is unknown whether better antibody responses will translate into reduced morbidity or mortality.[12] LAIV is formulated from live viruses that are attenuated, or genetically altered to be less pathogenic. Thus, it stimulates an immune response but does not cause overt influenza illness; however, side effects can include rhinorrhea, nasal congestion, fever, or sore throat. LAIV is licensed for use among nonpregnant persons aged 2–49 years, but safety has not been established in persons with underlying medical conditions that confer a higher risk of influenza complications.[4]

Prevention of Influenza: Chemoprophylaxis and Nonpharmaceutical Interventions

Four prospective studies have shown NA inhibitors to be effective in preventing influenza in the household contacts of infected individuals.[9] Thus, postexposure prophylaxis (PEP) to prevent influenza in high-risk contacts of persons with ILI, in either households or healthcare settings, is recommended, if PEP can begin within 48 hrs of an exposure. However, because influenza is a self-limited illness in persons at low risk for complications, routine PEP in otherwise healthy contacts of suspected influenza cases is not necessarily required, and clinicians should individualize the risk of influenza complications when considering PEP.

There is limited evidence in favor of nonpharmaceutical interventions — handwashing, with or without adjunct antiseptics; barrier measures like gloves, gowns, and masks; and isolation of persons with suspected infection — to prevent the transmission of respiratory viruses, including influenza viruses.[13,14] In healthcare settings, the CDC recommends the use of standard and droplet precautions during the care of any patient suspected of having influenza virus infection. Standard precautions include the use of gloves and gowns, changed after each patient encounter, if contact with respiratory secretions or potentially contaminated surfaces is anticipated, and frequent handwashing or, if hands are not visibly soiled, use of alcohol-based hand rubs. Under droplet precautions, patients with suspected influenza virus infection should be isolated in private rooms or, if unavailable, cohorted with other suspected cases; healthcare workers and guests should wear disposable surgical masks when in the patient's room; and the patient should wear a surgical mask during transport or when otherwise out of isolation.[15]

References

1. Wright PF, Neumann G, Kawaoka Y. (2007) Orthomyxoviruses. In: Fields B N, Knipe DM, Howley PM (eds), *Fields Virology,* 5th ed. Wolters Kluwer Health/Lippincott Williams & Wilkins, Philadelphia, pp. 1692–1741.
2. Palese P, Shaw ML. (2007) Orthomyxoviridae: The viruses and their replication. In: Fields BN, Knipe DM, Howley PM (eds), *Fields Virology*, 5th ed. Wolters Kluwer Health/Lippincott Williams & Wilkins, Philadelphia, pp. 1647–1690.
3. Centers for Disease Control and Prevention (CDC). (2010) Seasonal influenza — key facts about influenza (flu) & flu vaccine. http://www.cdc.gov/flu/keyfacts.htm (accessed Mar. 2, 2011).
4. Fiore AE, Uyeki TM, Broder K, *et al.* (2010) Prevention and control of influenza with vaccines: Recommendations of the Advisory Committee on Immunization Practices (ACIP), 2010. *MMWR Recomm Rep* **59**: 1–62.
5. Treanor JJ. (2010) Influenza viruses, including avian influenza and swine influenza. In: Mandell GL, Bennett JE, Dolin R (eds), *Mandell, Douglas, and Bennett's Principles and Practice of Infectious Diseases* 7th ed. Churchill Livingstone/Elsevier, Philadelphia, PA, pp. 2265–2288.
6. Boivin G, Hardy I, Tellier G, Maziade J. (2000) Predicting influenza infections during epidemics with use of a clinical case definition. *Clin Infect Dis.* **31**: 1166–1169.
7. Monto AS, Gravenstein S, Elliott M, *et al.* (2000) Clinical signs and symptoms predicting influenza infection. *Arch Intern Med* **160**: 3243–3247.
8. Petric M, Comanor L, Petti CA. (2006) Role of the laboratory in diagnosis of influenza during seasonal epidemics and potential pandemics. *J Infect Dis* **194** (Suppl. 2): S98–S110.
9. Jefferson T, Jones M, Doshi P, *et al.* (2010) Neuraminidase inhibitors for preventing and treating influenza in healthy adults. *Cochrane Database Syst Rev* 2: CD001265.

10. Lee N, Choi KW, Chan PK, *et al.* (2010) Outcomes of adults hospitalised with severe influenza. *Thorax* **65**: 510–515.
11. McGeer A, Green KA, Plevneshi A, *et al.* (2007) Antiviral therapy and outcomes of influenza requiring hospitalization in Ontario, Canada. *Clin Infect Dis* **45**: 1568–1575.
12. Licensure of a high-dose inactivated influenza vaccine for persons aged ≥65 years (Fluzone High-Dose) and guidance for use — United States, 2010, *MMWR Morb Mortal Wkly Rep* **59**: 485–486.
13. Cowling BJ, Zhou Y, Ip DK, *et al.* (2010) Face masks to prevent transmission of influenza virus: A systematic review. *Epidemiol Infect* **138**: 449–456.
14. Jefferson T, Del Mar C, Dooley L. (2010) Physical interventions to interrupt or reduce the spread of respiratory viruses. *Cochrane Database Syst Rev* CD006207.
15. Centers for Disease Control and Prevention (CDC). (2010) Prevention strategies for seasonal influenza in healthcare settings. http://www.cdc.gov/flu/professionals/infectioncontrol/healthcare settings.htm (accessed Sep. 22, 2010).

Chapter 57

Multidrug-Resistant Organisms: Emerging Resistance and Therapeutic Options

*Gopi Patel**

Key Pearls

- Removal of the primary focus of infection (source control), like removing an infected central venous catheter or draining an abscess, is always recommended as adjunctive therapy when treating an infection.
- Serious infections with extended-spectrum β-lactamase (ESBL) — producing organisms should be treated with carbapenems.
- Gram-negative organisms are becoming increasingly resistant to carbapenems, and few antimicrobials are available for treating these infections.
- Early detection and infection control are important in preventing nosocomial spread of multidrug-resistant pathogens.
- Infectious disease consultation is recommended for the treatment of bloodstream infections with multidrug-resistant organisms, since treatment regimens are undefined and continue to evolve.

Introduction

With few agents in development, we may soon be approaching the end of the "antibiotic era."[1] Infections with multidrug-resistant organisms (MDROs)

*Mount Sinai School of Medicine, New York, NY, USA.

are associated with significant patient morbidity and mortality. MDROs of great concern include methicillin-resistant *Staphylococcus aureus* (MRSA), vancomycin-resistant *Enterococcus faecium* (VRE), extended-spectrum β-lactamase (ESBL)–producing *Enterobacteriaceae. Acinetobacter baumannii,* and carbapenemase-producing *Enterobacteriaceae.* Recognized risk factors for infections with these organisms are similar: prior carriage, antibiotic use, frequent and prolonged hospitalizations, residence in long term care facilities, ICU exposure, and invasive devices (e.g. central venous catheters, ventilators, urinary catheters). The increasing prevalence of MDROs is forcing practitioners to be creative with antibiotics including utilizing older drugs and employing approved agents for off-label indications (Table 1).

Methicillin-Resistant *Staphylococcus aureus*

MRSA remains the most commonly isolated MDRO in the United States.[2] The spectrum of clinical diseases ranges from skin infections to endocarditis. Although much dialogue previously focused on the distinction between community-associated and healthcare-associated MRSA, the clinical relevance of this differentiation is controversial.

Additional cited risk factors for MRSA include dialysis, intravenous drug use, HIV infection, and the presence of prosthetic devices. Despite some controversy, vancomycin remains the mainstay of MRSA therapy. Debate surrounding appropriate vancomycin dosing and therapeutic drug monitoring exists, but maintaining a minimum serum trough of 10–15 mg/L seems to be widely accepted.[3] Isolates with decreased susceptibility to vancomycin, vancomycin-intermediate *S. aureus* (VISA), can be difficult to detect. The presence of subpopulations of VISA is associated with clinical failures, especially in the presence of "suboptimal" vancomycin levels. Clinical isolation of vancomycin-resistant *S. aureus* remains rare.[4] Some experts favor the use of linezolid for MRSA pneumonia.[5]

Daptomycin is rapidly bactericidal against MRSA. It is approved for the treatment of complicated skin infections as well as bloodstream infections (BSIs). Inactivation by pulmonary surfactant prohibits its use

Table 1. Concerning Multidrug-Resistant Bacterial Pathogens

Pathogen	Reported Risk Factors	Potential Antibiotic Agents
Methicillin-resistant *Staphylococcus aureus* (MRSA)	• Nasal or skin colonization • Recent hospitalization • Intravenous drug use • Residence in long term care facility (LTCF) • HIV infection • Dialysis • Central venous catheters	• Vancomycin • Daptomycin[a] • Linezolid • Tigecycline[b]
Vancomycin-resistant *Enterococcus faecium* (VRE)	• Vancomycin exposure • Exposure to antimicrobials with anaerobic activity • Gut colonization • Solid organ or hematopoietic stem cell transplantation • Residence in LTCF • Central venous catheters	• Quinupristin/ dalfopristin • Daptomycin • Linezolid • Tigecycline
Extended-spectrum β-lactamase (ESBL)–producing *Enterobacteriaceae*	• Antibiotic exposure • Gut colonization • Prolonged hospitalization • Residence in LTCF • Central venous catheters • Dialysis • Urinary catheters • Increased severity of illness	• Carbapenems[c] • Tigecycline
Carbapenemase-producing *Enterobacteriaceae* (e.g. KPC, NDM-1)	• Antibiotic exposure • Prolonged hospitalization • Solid organ or hematopoietic stem cell transplantation • ICU stay • Mechanical ventilation • Recent healthcare exposure in an area of endemicity[d]	• Polymyxins • Tigecycline • Fosfomycin
Carbapenem resistant *Acinetobacter* species	• Carbapenem use • Prolonged hospitalization • Mechanical ventilation • ICU stay • Residence in LTCF	• Polymyxins • Sulbactam • Rarely tigecycline

[a] Not recommended for the treatment of pulmonary infections.
[b] Not recommended for the treatment of primary bloodstream infections.
[c] Include ertapenem, imipenem, meropenem, and doripenem.
[d] KPCs are considered endemic to the northeastern United States and Israel. NDM-1 is considered endemic to the Indian subcontinent and Pakistan.

in the treatment of pneumonia. Although considered non-inferior to traditional regimens for *S. aureus* BSIs, its utility in the treatment of left-sided endocarditis remains controversial.[6] Development of resistance has been reported both on and off daptomycin therapy. Daptomycin is rarely associated with rhabdomyolysis. Monitoring of serum creatine phosphokinase is recommended, especially in the setting of renal insufficiency or concurrent use of medications with similar side effect profiles (e.g. statins).

Source control (i.e. draining an abscess or removing an infected catheter) is as vital as appropriate antibiotics and evidence-based treatment recommendations continue to evolve.[7]

Vancomycin-resistant *Enterococcus faecium*

Although not as virulent, increasing isolation of VRE is worrisome. Most *E. faecium* isolated in ICUs are vancomycin-resistant and infections with VRE are challenging to treat.

In addition to the aforementioned common MDRO risk factors, the risk factors for VRE include vancomycin use, prior exposure to anti-anaerobic antimicrobials, and recent solid organ or hematopoietic stem cell transplantation.

The appropriate treatment for severe VRE infections remains undefined.[8] Agents with activity against VRE include quinopristin/dalfopristin, linezolid, and daptomycin. It should be noted that quinopristin/dalfopristin has no activity against *E. faecalis* and this agent is often used as salvage therapy.

Linezolid is arguably the most common agent employed to treat VRE. Due to equivalent bioavailability, it can be used to transition patients to oral therapy. Caution should be taken with concomitant use of antidepressants and some pain medications, due to the risks of serotonin syndrome. Prolonged linezolid use has been associated with rare but serious complications, including marrow suppression, lactic acidosis, and neurotoxicity. Close followup is strongly recommended (e.g. weekly serum chemistry and leukocyte and platelet counts).

Although not approved for this indication, daptomycin may be used to treat VRE infections when other agents are contraindicated. Resistance to both linezolid and daptomycin has been described.

Extended-Spectrum β-Lactamase-Producing *Enterobacteriaceae*

No discussion on Gram-negative resistance can begin without mention of ESBLs. Escalating use of third-generation cephalosporins coincided with increasing isolation of *Klebsiella pneumoniae* and *Escherichia coli* producing enzymes (β-lactamases) capable of hydrolyzing and inactivating penicillins, cephalosporins, and aztreonam.

ESBL production is concerning because of complicated resistance profiles. Most ESBL producers retain susceptibility to carbapenems (i.e. imipenem, meropenem, ertapenem, doripenem), making them the drugs of choice for treating serious infections with these organisms. *In vitro* susceptibility profiles can be misleading and clinical failures have been associated with the use of noncarbapenems despite contrary susceptibility profiles.[9]

The heavily antibiotic-experienced and patients with frequent healthcare exposures are considered at the highest risk for developing infections with these pathogens. Due to the increasing isolation of these organisms and the morbidity associated with delayed effective treatment, empiric use of carbapenems in the setting of sepsis may be appropriate until more data are available.

Acinetobacter baumannii

The emergence of carbapenem resistance in non-*Enterobacteriaceae*, notably *Acinetobacter* species, accompanied increasing carbapenem use. *A. baumannii* is environmentally resilient and is often linked with healthcare-associated pneumonias. According to US surveillance data, the proportion of ICU-associated pneumonias due to *Acinetobacter* increased from 4% in 1986 to 7% in 2003.[10] Of epidemiologic significance are the increased numbers of *A. baumannii* infections reported among civilian and military personnel returning from Afghanistan and the Middle East.[11]

Nosocomial *A. baumannii* isolates are often resistant to β-lactams, aminoglycosides, and fluoroquinolones. In hospitals with low carbapenem resistance rates, imipenem or meropenem monotherapy is usually effective. Previous carbapenem exposure and high institutional carbapenem use, however, is associated with the recovery of carbapenem-resistant strains.

Treatment of carbapenem-resistant *A. baumannii* is problematic.[12] Ampicillin-sulbactam, specifically sulbactam, and polymyxins can be used to treat these infections when susceptible. Early reports suggested that tigecycline was a potential treatment option for MDR *A. baumannii.* Unfortunately, breakthrough infections have been described, making tigecycline unreliable.[13]

Carbapenem Resistant *Enterobacteriaceae*

Carbapenem resistance among *Enterobacteriaceae*, specifically *K. pneumoniae*, is a relatively recent phenomenon. In a short period of time, these MDROs have expanded worldwide. Although various resistance mechanisms are described, of concern are infections with organisms producing carbapenemases, like *K. pneumoniae* carbapenemases (KPCs) or, more recently, the metallo-β-lactamase, NDM-1.[14] These resistance determinants often reside on transferrable plasmids, facilitating dissemination and cross-transmission.

KPCs can hydrolyze all β-lactam antibiotics, including carbapenems. Frequently, KPC-expressing *Enterobacteriaceae* (KPC-E) demonstrate concomitant fluoroquinolone and aminoglycoside resistance, thus severely handicapping practitioners treating these organisms. In 2007, the Centers for Disease Control and Prevention noted that 8.7% of all *K. pneumoniae* responsible for device-related infections were carbapenem-resistant, compared with less than 1% in 2000.[15] Suggested risk factors for KPC-E infection include immunosuppressing conditions such as transplantation and increased severity of illness.

NDM-1, the New Delhi metallo-β-lactamase, is considered endemic to the Indian subcontinent. Due to the conveniences of travel and medical tourism, NDM-1 has emerged as an international threat. It is now the most common resistance mechanism identified among submitted isolates of carbapenem-resistant *Enterobacteriaceae* in the United Kingdom, with many patients reporting previous healthcare exposure in India.[16]

The commercial development of more tolerable agents led to the dismissal of polymyxins (i.e. polymyxin B and colistin) from routine use. The resurrection of polymyxins paralleled the increasing resistance among Gram-negative pathogens. Unfortunately, polymyxin dosing regimens remain undefined and are complicated in the setting of renal insufficiency and dialysis. Some experts advocate the use of polymyxin-based combination therapy rather than monotherapy when treating KPC-E.[17]

Tigecycline is approved for the treatment of skin infections, pneumonias, and intra-abdominal infections. Its antimicrobial spectrum is broad, and includes Gram-positive organisms and ESBL-producing *Enterobacteriaceae*. Of note is that, tigecycline has no activity against *Pseudomonas*, *Proteus*, or *Providencia* species. Anecdotal reports on successful treatment of carbapenem-resistant Gram-negative infections exist, but despite tigecycline being commercially available only since 2005 resistance appears to be increasing. Use of tigecycline for primary BSIs and urinary tract infections is controversial. In rare cases, however, tigecycline may be the only "active" drug available.[18]

When susceptible, aminoglycosides have been used as unconventional monotherapy when no other agent exists. Fosfomycin can be used to treat uncomplicated urinary tract infections but susceptibility is not universal. No single commercially available agent serves as a "magic bullet." Pan-resistance in Gram-negative organisms is described and is associated with devastating outcomes.[19] Retrospective studies have shown that aggressive source control may be helpful in the treatment of infections with carbapenem-resistant organisms.[20]

Summary

MDRO rates vary between and within healthcare facilities. Knowledge of institution-specific flora and susceptibility patterns is crucial in the management, prevention, and control of serious healthcare-associated infections. When possible, abscesses should be drained and infected catheters removed. Practitioners are urged to discontinue unnecessary antibiotics and to narrow coverage when susceptibility profiles allow. In the setting of serious MDRO infections and infections with carbapenem-resistant Gram-negative pathogens, infectious disease consultation is advised as practice continues to evolve. Due to the paucity of drugs in development, emphasis should be placed on early detection and adherence to infection control practices.

References

1. Boucher HW, Talbot GH, Bradley JS, *et al.* (2009) Bad bugs, no drugs: No ESKAPE! An update from the Infectious Diseases Society of America. *Clin Infect Dis* **48**: 1–12.
2. Klevens RM, Morrison MA, Nadle J, *et al.* (2007) Invasive methicillin-resistant *Staphylococcus aureus* infections in the United States. *JAMA* **298**: 1763–1771.
3. Rybak M, Lomaestro B, Rotschafer JC, *et al.* (2009) Therapeutic monitoring of vancomycin in adult patients: A consensus review of the American Society of Health-System Pharmacists, the Infectious Diseases Society of America, and the Society of Infectious Diseases Pharmacists. *Am J Health Syst Pharm* **66**: 82–98.
4. Sievert DM, Rudrik JT, Patel JB, *et al.* (2008) Vancomycin-resistant *Staphylococcus aureus* in the United States, 2002–2006. *Clin Infect Dis* **46**: 668–674.
5. Wunderink RG, Niederman MS, Kollef MH *et al.* (2012) Linezolid in methicillin-resistant *Staphylococcus aureus* nosocomial pneumonia: a randomized, controlled study. *Clin Infect Dis* **54**: 621–629.
6. Fowler VG, Boucher HW, Corey GR, *et al.* (2006) Daptomycin versus standard therapy for bacteremia and endocarditis caused by *Staphylococcus aureus*. *New Engl J Med* **355**: 653–665.

7. Liu C, Bayer A, Cosgrove SE, *et al.* (2011) Clinical Practice Guidelines by the Infectious Diseases Society of America for the treatment of methicillin-resistant *Staphylococcus aureus* infections in adults and children. *Clin Infect Dis* **52**: 1–38.
8. Arias CA, Murray BE. (2008) Emergence and management of drug-resistant enterococcal infections. *Expert Rev of Anti Infect Ther* **6**: 637–655.
9. Hyle EP, Lipworth AD, Zaoutis TE, *et al.* (2005) Impact of inadequate initial antimicrobial therapy on mortality in infections due to extended-spectrum β-lactamase–producing *Enterobacteriaceae*: Variability by site of infection. *Arch Intern Med* **165**: 1375–1380.
10. Gaynes R, Edwards JR. (2005) Overview of nosocomial infections caused by Gram-negative bacilli. *Clin Infect Dis* **41**: 848–854.
11. Scott P, Deye G, Srinivasan A, *et al.* (2007) An outbreak of multidrug-resistant *Acinetobacter baumannii-calcoaceticus* complex infection in the US military health care system associated with military operations in Iraq. *Clin Infect Dis* **44**: 1577–1584.
12. Munoz-Price LS, Weinstein RA. (2008) *Acinetobacter* Infection. *New Engl J Med* **358**: 1271–1281.
13. Gordon NC, Wareham DW. (2009) A review of clinical and microbiological outcomes following treatment of infections involving multidrug-resistant *Acinetobacter baumannii* with tigecycline. *J Antimicrob Chemother* **63**: 775–780.
14. (2010) Detection of *Enterobacteriaceae* isolates carrying metallo-beta-lactamase — United States, 2010. *MMWR Morb Mortal Wkly Rep* **59**: 750.
15. Hidron AI, Edwards JR, Patel J, *et al.* (2008) NHSN annual update: Antimicrobial-resistant pathogens associated with healthcare-associated infections: Annual summary of data reported to the National Healthcare Safety Network at the Centers for Disease Control and Prevention, 2006–2007. *Infect Control Hosp Epidemiol* **29**: 996–1011.
16. Kumarasamy KK, Toleman MA, Walsh TR, *et al.* (2010) Emergence of a new antibiotic resistance mechanism in India, Pakistan, and the

UK: A molecular, biological, and epidemiological study. *Lancet Infect Dis* **10**: 597–602.

17. Hirsch EB, Tam VH. (2010) Detection and treatment options for *Klebsiella pneumoniae* carbapenemases (KPCs): An emerging cause of multidrug-resistant infection. *J Antimicrob Chemother* **65**: 1119–1125.
18. Anthony KB, Fishman NO, Linkin DR, *et al.* (2008) Clinical and microbiological outcomes of serious infections with multidrug-resistant Gram-negative organisms treated with tigecycline. *Clin Infect Dis* **46**: 567–570.
19. Elemam A, Rahimian J, Mandell W. Infection with panresistant *Klebsiella pneumoniae*: A report of 2 cases and a brief review of the literature. *Clin Infect Dis* **49**: 271–274.
20. Patel G, Huprikar S, Factor SH, *et al.* (2008) Outcomes of carbapenem-resistant *Klebsiella pneumoniae* infection and the impact of antimicrobial and adjunctive therapies. *Infect Control Hosp Epidemiol* **29**: 1099–1106.

Chapter 58

Tuberculosis

Joseph R. Masci

Key Pearls

- Clinical manifestations vary with the age and the degree of immune suppression of the host.
- The diagnosis of active TB is best made by isolation of the organism in culture for precise identification and subsequent sensitivity testing. Nucleic acid amplification tests on respiratory secretions are most useful for confirming the diagnosis rapidly.
- Sensitivity testing is essential for the identification of treatment regimens most likely to be effective.
- The treatment of extrapulmonary TB is similar to that for pulmonary TB.
- The hospitalized patient with active TB may be discharged when the conditions under "Discharge Planning" are met.

Introduction

Tuberculosis (TB), caused by *Mycobacterium tuberculosis* (M.Tb), remains a global health issue of vast proportions, although the global disease burden is gradually declining.[1] In recent decades the HIV epidemic has had a dramatic impact on the incidence, rates of transmission and mortality of this ancient infectious disease. Resistant strains of M.Tb have emerged and spread particularly throughout the developing world.

Department of Medicine, Elmhurst Hospital Center, Elmhurst. New York, USA.

Epidemiology

Worldwide, there were an estimated 9.27 million incident and 13.7 million prevalent cases of active TB in 2007, the most recent year for which adequate data have been published.[1] There were 1.3 million cases and 456,000 deaths among HIV-negative and HIV-positive individuals, respectively.

Clinical Manifestations

Pulmonary

The clinical manifestations of pulmonary TB vary with the age and the degree of immune suppression of the host. The most recognizable form presents with persistent fever, productive cough often with blood-streaked sputum, and sometimes such systemic signs of infection as weight loss and night sweats. The most characteristic roentgenographic pattern is the appearance of cavitating infiltrates in one or both lung apices. This pattern on a chest X-ray, however, is much less common among individuals with significant immune deficiency states, particularly advanced HIV infection. In such patients, lower low infiltrates, often bilateral without cavitation, are the rule. This atypical pattern may pose a special diagnostic challenge, since it may resemble other opportunistic infections associated with HIV infection.

Extrapulmonary

M. Tb may cause active disease in a variety of extrapulmonary sites. The most common of these sites are the pleura, lymph nodes, and bones and joints. Active infection may also present in the central nervous system, genitourinary tract, pericardium and gastrointestinal tract. The diagnosis of extrapulmonary TB typically poses challenges in excluding other diagnoses, particularly malignancy, and in obtaining adequate material for culture and sensitivity.

Diagnosis

Latent Tuberculosis

The diagnosis of latent TB is most often made, by means of the tuberculin skin test (TST), although interferon gamma release assays (IGRAs) have come into increasing use in the developed world. These blood tests have greater specificity for the diagnosis of latent TB than the TST. Regardless of the technique used to diagnose latent infection, it is incumbent on the practitioner to exclude active TB before beginning therapy.

Active Tuberculosis

The diagnosis of active TB is best made by isolation of the organism in culture for precise identification and subsequent sensitivity testing. Unfortunately, this is not possible in all cases, resulting in the need for empiric treatment and possible treatment failure due to drug resistance. Positive tests for latent TB, either the TST or IGRAs, cannot be used to establish a diagnosis of active TB, although negative results by IGRA may be taken as partial evidence against such a diagnosis of active TB in a patient with a high pretest probability of TB. Rapid tests utilizing nucleic acid amplification technology may hasten the identification of the organism in respiratory secretions, and studies utilizing polymerase chain reaction assays on other clinical specimens such as pleural fluid hold promise because of high specificity but are not yet established because of their relatively unpredictable sensitivity.

Sensitivity Testing

Sensitivity testing is essential for the identification of treatment regimens most likely to be effective. Although the incidence of multi-drug resistant TB (MDRTB) and extensively-drug resistant TB (XDRTB) is currently low in the United States and most other developed countries, much of the world is confronted by expanding outbreaks of these resistance patterns.[2]

Common Differential Diagnoses

Pulmonary tuberculosis: neoplasm, anerobic lung abscess, histoplasmosis, coccidioidomycosis, atypical mycobacterial infection.

Extrapulmonary tuberculosis: varies widely, depending on the site of disease; neoplasm most frequent.

Laboratory Testing

Routine laboratory testing of patients initiating therapy for TB should consist of a complete blood count, liver function tests and a basic metabolic panel including creatinine.

Treatment

General Principles

It has long been established that treatment of active TB requires combinations of agents to which the organism is sensitive. The treatment of extrapulmonary TB is similar to that for pulmonary TB. Strict adherence to the treatment regimen is of paramount importance. Directly observed therapy (DOT) is preferred and should be arranged whenever feasible.

Sensitive Tuberculosis

If M. Tb is isolated and found to be sensitive to all available agents, the combination of four drugs — isoniazid (INH), rifampin (RIF), pyrazinamide (PZA) and ethambutol (EMB) — should be initiated, or continued if it has been started empirically. EMB may be discontinued when sensitivity testing indicates that the organism is susceptible to INH and RIF. PZA can be discontinued after two months. INH and RIF should be continued to complete a six-month total course of therapy. Concerns have been raised regarding the effectiveness of these standard regimens among patients with HIV/TB coinfection.[3] and demonstrating lower relapse rates with regimens including at least eight months of rifampin or rifabutin.

Multidrug-Resistant Tuberculosis

Multidrug resistant tuberculosis (MDRTB) is defined as TB with resistance to at least INH and RIF. Effective therapy of MDRTB requires a complete knowledge of the sensitivity pattern of these strains of MTb, which by definition are resistant to the best-established first-line agents: INH and RIF. Therapeutic options should be dictated by sensitivity patterns, and the duration of therapy must be individualized.

Extensively Drug-Resistant Tuberculosis

Extensively drug-resistant tuberculosis (XDRTB) is defined as TB with resistance to at least INH and RIF as well as resistance to a fluroquinolone and a second-line injectable agent such as capreomycin or amikacin. Since therapeutic options are extremely limited and treatment failure likely, consultation with a specialist experienced in the management of drug-resistant TB is essential in the care of patients with XDRTB.

TB and HIV: The Importance of HIV Testing

Coinfection with HIV and M. Tb greatly increases the likelihood that latent TB will become active and is associated with higher rates of relapse and death. Pulmonary TB often presents with atypical features on a chest X-ray, including lower lobe involvement and rarely, a completely normal study. In addition, it has been demonstrated that initiation of effective antiretroviral therapy early in the course of TB therapy for coinfected individuals significantly enhances the likelihood of survival.[4] For this reason, early voluntary HIV testing is strongly recommended for patients with proven or suspected TB. In addition, TB has also been among the most frequent infections complicating rapid immune reconstitution in HIV-infected inviduals.[5]

Monitoring for Side Effects of Treatment

Patients receiving INH and/or RIF must be monitored closely for drug-induced hepatitis. Although transient elevations of liver enzymes are frequently seen, it is recommended that these agents, INH in particular, be discontinued if transaminase levels exceed 3–5 times normal. EMB may cause optic neuritis. PZA can cause arthralgias and hyperuricemia, and is contraindicated in pregnancy.

Indications for Hospitalization

Severity of Illness

In developed countries where hospitalization is readily available, patients who have possible or proven active TB, regardless of the severity, usually benefit from an inpatient stay to facilitate obtaining appropriate specimens for culture and sensitivity and, if possible, initiation of therapy. Patients with smear-positive, cavitary pulmonary infection pose a risk of transmission to close contacts, and hospitalization can be justified while appropriate arrangements are made for outpatient therapy, contact tracing and close followup of treatment. Patients with significant pulmonary compromise, substantial immune deficiency states, or proven or suspected infection involving the central nervous system or pericardium require close observation for disease progression, which is most easily provided in the inpatient setting.

Prevention of Nosocomial Transmission

Nosocomial transmission of pulmonary TB has been documented in both developed and developing countries. Ideally, patients with proven or suspected active pulmonary TB should be placed in single rooms under airborne precautions. These precautions include negative pressure within the room relative to the corridor, six air exchanges per hour with air vented to the outside after passage through a HEPA filter, and the use of N95 or N100 face masks by anyone entering the room.

Public Health Considerations

Individuals with active pulmonary TB, particularly those who are smear-positive and/or have cavitary lesions on chest X-rays, may readily transmit

TB to close contacts. Of greatest concern are children living in the same household. Those under five years of age are at high risk of developing symptomatic primary TB. All household contacts should be screened with the TST or IGRAs.

Discharge Planning

Several elements of the effective planning for hospital discharge are essential. Among them are thorough education of the patient regarding the need for prolonged therapy, and the potential signs of drug toxicity. DOT is optimal under all circumstances but not always readily available. In any case, specific arrangements must be in place for monitoring the response to therapy and possible medication side effects. Household contacts of patients with proven or possible pulmonary TB should be evaluated for latent and active infection and, in some instances, particularly among young children, provided with empiric therapy for latent infection pending close followup. In general, patients with multiple (three or more) negative specimens of adequate respiratory secretions may be discharged from the hospital. If appropriate arrangements for evaluation of the household, education of the patient regarding precautions to be taken at home and DOT can be made and if local public health laws permit, even patients with positive sputum acid-fast stains may be discharged from the hospital. The decision to discharge under these circumstances is best made with subspecialty and/or public health consultation.

Indications for Subspeciality Consultation

Because of the difficulties often encountered in the diagnosis of active TB, some of which have been highlighted above, it is advisable for subspeciality consultation to be sought whenever the primary provider does not have substantial experience in the management of TB and ready access to an outpatient system of care offering DOT. Individuals diagnosed with latent TB may also benefit from subspecialty consultation to facilitate monitoring of therapy. Patients with proven or suspected MDRTB or XDRTB should be managed by providers with specific experience in treating these complex patients.

References

1. World Health Organization. (2009) *Global Tuberculosis Control 2009: Epidemiology, Strategy, Financing.* World Health Organization, Geneva.
2. World Health Organization. (2008) *Anti-tuberculosis Drug Resistance in the World: Report No. 4.* World Health Organization, Geneva.
3. Khan FA, Minion J, Pal M, *et al.* (2010) Treatment of active tuberculosis in HIV-coinfected patients: A systematic review and meta-analysis. *Clin Infect Dis* **50**: 1288–1299.
4. Karim A, Naidoo K, Grobler A, *et al.* (2010) Timing of initiation of antiretroviral drugs during tuberculosis therapy. *N Engl J Med* **362**: 697–706.
5. Lawn SD, Wilkinson RJ, Lipman MC, Wood R. (2008) Immune reconstitution and "unmasking" of tuberculosis during antiretroviral therapy. *Am J Respir Crit Care Med* **177**: 680–685.

Chapter 59

Clostridium difficile Infection

*Sofia Novak, Lisa Hayes and Ekaterina Sokolova**

Key Pearls

- Presentation: Elderly patients with recent hospitalization on prior or current antibiotics who are presenting with diarrhea.
- Diagnosis: Check stool for *C. diff* toxin (EIA) × 2 to increase sensitivity.
- Treatment: Stop the offending antibiotic if possible. Empirically treat the severely ill. Use metronidazole and/or vancomycin based on disease severity. Do not treat asymptomatic carriers.
- Resolution: Monitor for clinical improvement. No need to check for test of cure.
- Prevention: Contact precautions.

Introduction

Clostridium difficile is a gram-positive, spore-forming and toxin-producing obligatory anaerobic rod. *C. difficile* toxins were identified to be a cause of pseudomembranous colitis in 1977.[1] It remains the most common cause of nosocomial diarrhea. Transmission occurs via the fecal–oral route. Spores can pass through the acidic environment of the stomach unharmed and convert to the vegetative form in the small bowel, leading to colonization of the colon. Colonization can result in the release of toxins that mediate diarrhea and colitis.[1,5]

*Mount Sinai Hospital of Queens, Long Island City, NY, USA.

C. difficile infection (CDI) can present as a wide spectrum ranging from asymptomatic carriage to mild-to-moderate diarrhea, all the way to fulminant, sometimes fatal disease.[2] It is defined by the latest SHEA–IDSA guidelines as "presence of symptoms (usually diarrhea) and either a stool test result positive for *C. difficile* toxins or toxigenic *C. difficile*, or colonoscopic findings demonstrating pseudomembranous colitis."[3]

Epidemiology

C. difficile can be found in about 20% of asymptomatic, hospitalized adults and in up to 50% of residents of long term care facilities.[4,26] CDI epidemiology has been changing rapidly, with increased numbers and severity of cases. The epidemic strain, NAP1/027, originally reported in 2003, has been associated with a higher incidence of disease and produces a larger amount of toxin.[5–7] Community-acquired CDI, defined as infection in patients who have not been hospitalized in the year prior to infection, is also on the rise.

Pathogenesis

CDI occurs as a result of *C. difficile* overgrowth by several key steps:

(1) Disruption of normal colonic flora by antibiotic or antineoplastic agents with antibacterial activity;
(2) Colonization with toxigenic *C. difficile*;
(3) Production of toxin A, toxin B, or both, which in turn increases intestinal permeability; a third toxin has been recognized, and it is known as binary toxin;
(4) Mucosal injury and inflammation.

Toxin B is the more potent of the two toxins and a higher toxin level is associated with greater severity of disease.[6,7] Patients at risk are listed in Table 1.[5,8,9]

Table 1. Risk factors for *C. difficile* Infection

Patients at Risk	Possible Risk Factors
• History of hospitalization (more than 72 hr) • Prior or current antibiotic use (up to 2 months prior, but seen as early as 1st day of antibiotics; usually seen after 5–10 days of antibiotic therapy) *Antibiotics that are most commonly implicated: fluoroquinolones, cephalosporins, clindamycin, penicillins* • Elderly, over 60–65 • Severity of underlying illnesses	• Gastric acid suppression • Enteral feeding • Gastrointestinal surgery • Cancer chemotherapy • Hematopoietic stem cell transplantation

Presentation

- Diarrhea +/– at-risk patient
- At-risk patient with either leukocytosis (50%–60% rate), fever (30%–50% rate) or abdominal pain or cramping (20%–33% rate).[5]

CDI should be considered in any at-risk patient presenting with loose or watery stools. Diarrhea can be brief and self-limited or cholera-like, resulting in more than 20 stools per day. The frequency of diarrhea may range widely and can be accompanied by leukocytosis, with a mean leukocytosis of 15,000–16,000, fecal leukocytosis, fever and abdominal pain. Abdominal pain may localize to lower quadrants. CDI progresses rapidly and leukocytosis should be routinely monitored. Paralytic ileus, megacolon and systemic toxicity can complicate CDI. Infrequently, CDI manifests without diarrhea, but it should be considered in at-risk patients who have abdominal pain with an acute abdomen or toxic megacolon. Toxic megacolon is suggested by a dilatation of the colon to a diameter greater than 6 cm, associated with systemic toxicity and without mechanical obstruction.

Differential Diagnosis

It is important to distinguish CDI from other infectious and noninfectious causes of diarrhea.[10]

Table 2. Differential Diagnosis

Bacterial	*Shigella*, *Campylobacter*, *Klebsiella*, *E. Coli* (enterotoxigenic or enterohemorrhagic), *S. aureus*, *B. cereus*, *C. perfringes*, *L. monocytogenes*
Viral	Norovirus, rotavirus
Fungal	*Candida* spp.
Protozoa	*Entamoeba histolytica*, *Giardia*, *Cryptosporidium*, *Cyclospora*
Vascular	Ischemic colitis
Malabsorptive syndromes	Lactose intolerance, celiac disease, chronic pancreatitis, bacterial overgrowth
Inflammatory bowel disease	Crohn's, ulcerative colitis
Other etiologies	Irritable bowel syndrome, microscopic colitis, drug-related

Pathology

CDI most commonly causes nonspecific colitis. However, pseudomembranous colitis can be seen, especially in more severe cases (see Fig. 1). This is described as raised, white or yellowish lesions adhering to the colonic mucosa with skip areas of normal mucosa. In severe disease, these lesions coalesce along the mucosa to form plaques.[5]

Diagnosis

- Based on clinical suspicion and supporting diagnostic evidence;
- Testing should be done on diarrheal (unformed) stool only;
- Current guidelines discourage repeat testing, due to its limited value.

Stool sample testing should be performed on patients for whom strong clinical suspicion of CDI exists. There are numerous modalities available for testing. Generally, an enzyme immunoassay (EIA) is used. It may be

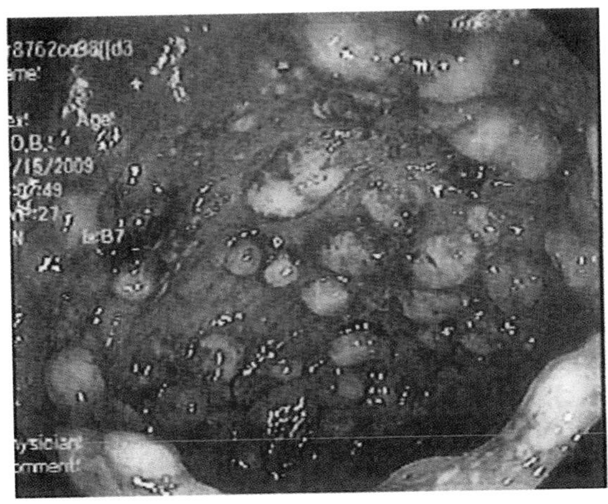

Fig. 1. Pseudomembranes in descending colon (photos courtesy of Dr. Sabino Augello).

done on two samples to increase test sensitivity. If the EIA comes back negative and the suspicion is still high, there should be consideration to send a tissue culture cytotoxicity assay and/or endoscopy for patients not responding to therapy. The cytotoxicity assay has been considered the gold standard for diagnosis.[5,6]

- Testing modalities:
  - EIA: Rapid. May be repeated × 1 to increase sensitivity.
  - Cytotoxicity assay: More sensitive than EIA. Slow turnaround time.
  - PCR: Rapid, sensitive and specific.
  - Culture: Most sensitive, but slow turnaround time.

Monitoring

- Abdominal pain
- Leukocytosis
- Electrolytes
- Lactate in severe cases
- Abdominal X-ray or CT scan if megacolon is suspected

CDI may progress rapidly to fulminant disease. It is imperative to monitor leukocytosis and lactate levels in severe cases, as they may serve as useful predictors of perioperative morbidity and mortality.[11]

Currently there is no accepted set of characteristics for defining disease severity. One study used a point system, giving one point for age >60 years, temperature >38.3°C, albumin level <2.5, WBC count >15,000 cells/mm^3, and two points for evidence of pseudomembranous colitis. Mild disease was defined as having <2 points.[12] Clinical judgment should be used.

Treatment

- Discontinue causative antibiotic(s), if possible.
- Supportive care: fluid and electrolyte repletion.
- Initiate therapy immediately if there is strong suspicion, or in the severely ill.
- Avoid antiperistalic and opiate-containing medications.
- Do not treat asymptomatic carriers.
- For the initial or first recurrence of mild-to-moderate CDI: metronidazole 500 mg orally three times per day for 10–14 days.
- For initial severe CDI or unresponsiveness or intolerance to metronidazole: vancomycin 125 mg orally four times per day for 10–14 days.
- For severe and complicated CDI: vancomycin 500 mg orally four times per day + vancomycin per rectum as a retention enema four times per day for ileus +/– metronidazole 500 mg IV three times per day for ileus.
- For severe CDI, consider colectomy.

CDI patients, like any other patients with diarrhea, require supportive care with IV hydration and electrolyte repletion. Stopping the offending agent, i.e. the antibiotic, is beneficial on its own in 20% of patients, but by itself this is not recommended.[13] Oral vancomycin is the only antibiotic FDA-approved for treatment of CDI.[13] However, metronidazole is the recommended initial treatment for mild-to-moderate CDI and its first recurrence. It is low-cost and its use decreases concern for development of vancomycin-resistant bacteria.[3]

Patients with ileus or megacolon are believed to have impaired gut motility, harming delivery of oral medications. Diarrhea may be absent in such patients. Intravenous metronidazole + vancomycin (orally or via nasogastric tube or via enema) should be considered.[3,5]

Recurrence Treatment

- The first recurrence may be treated with metronidazole 500 mg po q 8 hr.
- The second and further recurrences should be treated with vancomycin orally, with tapered or pulsed doses.

The CDI recurrence rate is about 20% within the first two weeks. Metronidazole may be used for the first and mild recurrence. However, therapy should be escalated if there is no response or if the disease is severe. For subsequent recurrence, oral vancomycin with tapered and pulsed doses should be used.[3]

Other Treatment Modalities

- Rifampin
- Rifaximin
- Probiotics
- IVIG
- Stool transplant
- Resins
- Nitazoxanide
- Monoclonal antibodies
- *C. difficile* toxoid vaccine

Rifampin may be used in combination with vancomycin in patients failing vancomycin taper or pulse.[14] However, there has not been any evidence to support adding rifampin in the primary episode of CDI.[15]

Rifaximin may be used in combination or following vacomycin in patients failing vancomycin taper or pulse. It has a higher concentration in the gut lumen than rifampin; however, resistant isolates of *C. difficile* have been identified.[16,6]

Probiotics have not shown convincing evidence of their effect in the treatment or prevention of recurrence.[17]

IVIG is often considered in refractory cases. Its efficacy is uncertain and carries a high cost.[6,18]

Stool infusion therapy, also known as stool transplant, has low failure rates in small studies. Furthermore, it has only been studied in recurrent cases.[6,19] A randomized controlled study is underway, comparing vancomycin and fecal transplant for recurrent CDI in The Netherlands.[20]

Resins have shown limited efficacy and have the potential to bind metronidazole, as well as vancomycin. They have not been shown to be more effective than either metronidazole or vancomycin.[5]

Nitazoxanide is an antiparasitic drug and was shown in several small studies to be as effective as metronidazole.[21]

Monoclonal antibodies directed against *C. difficile* toxins reduced the recurrence of CDI when used in addition to antibiotics (7% vs. 25%); however, confirmatory studies are needed.[22]

C. difficile toxoid vaccine for recurrent CDI was tested in three patients and all were able to stop therapy with vancomycin.[23]

Resolution

- No need for repeat stool testing;
- Based on the clinical picture.

C. difficile toxins may persist in stool for a prolonged period of time. It is thus not recommended to perform repeat stool testing. Patients may be taken off contact isolation once their symptoms have resolved.

Prevention

- Carry out contact isolation of patients with CDI, and maintain this for the duration of diarrhea.

- Good hand-washing with soap and water. (Spores are highly resistant to alcohol.)
- Cohort CDI patients if single rooms are not available.[3]

Contact isolation and hand-washing with soap and water are recommended when, caring for any CDI patient.[24] Compliance with such techniques will decrease the rate of hospital-acquired *C. difficile*.[25] Decreasing or restricting antimicrobial prescribing practices may decrease the incidence of CDI as well.

References

1. Curry S. (2010) *Clostridium difficile*. *Clin Lab Med* **30**(1): 329–342. Review.
2. Bartlett JG and Gerding DN. (2008) Clinical recognition and diagnosis of *Clostridium difficile* infection. *Clin Infect Dis* **46**(Suppl 1): S12–S18.
3. Cohen SH, Gerding DN, Johnson S, *et al*. (2010) Clinical practice guidelines for *Clostridium difficile* infection in adults: 2010 update by the Society for Healthcare Epidemiology of America (SHEA) and the Infectious Diseases Society of America (IDSA). Society for Healthcare Epidemiology of America; Infectious Diseases Society of America. *Infect Control Hosp Epidemiol*. **31**(5): 431–455.
4. Shim JK, Johnson S, Samore MH, *et al*. (1998) Primary symptomless colonisation by *Clostridium difficile* and decreased risk of subsequent diarrhoea. *Lancet* **351**(9103): 633–636.
5. Mandell GL, Bennett JC, Dolin R, (eds.). (2009) *Mandell, Douglas, and Bennett's Principles and Practice of Infectious Disease*, Vol. 1, 7th ed. Elsevier, Philadelphia, PA.
6. McDonald LC, Killgore GE, Thompson A, *et al*. (2005) An epidemic, toxin gene-variant strain of *Clostridium difficile*. *N Engl J Med* **353**: 2433–2441.
7. Warny M, Pepin J, Fang A, *et al*. (2005) Toxin production by an emerging strain of *Clostridium difficile* associated with outbreaks of severe disease in North America and Europe. *Lancet* **366**: 1079–1084.

8. Kim JW, Lee KL, Jeong JB, *et al.* (2010) Proton pump inhibitors as a risk factor for recurrence of *Clostridium-difficile*–associated diarrhea. *World J Gastroenterol* **16**(28): 3573–3577.
9. Vaishnavi C. (2009) Established and potential risk factors for *Clostridum difficile* infection. *Indian J Med Microbiol* **27**: 289–300.
10. Musher DM, Musher, BL. (2004) Contagious acute gastrointestinal infections. *N Engl J Med* **351**: 2417.
11. Byrn JC, Maun DC, Gingold DS, *et al.* (2008) Predictors of mortality after colectomy for fulminant *Clostridium difficile colitis*. *Arch Surg* **143**(2): 150–154.
12. Zar FA, Bakkanagari SR, Moorthi KM, Davis MB. (2007) A comparison of vancomycin and metronidazole for the treatment of *Clostridium difficile*–associated diarrhea, stratified by disease severity. *Clin Infect Dis* **45**(3): 302–307. [Epub 2007, Jun. 19].
13. Salkind A. (2010) *Clostridium difficile*: An update for the primary care clinician. *South Med J.* **103**(9): 896–902.
14. Buggy BP, Fekety R, Silva J Jr. (1987) Therapy of relapsing *Clostridium difficile*–associated diarrhea and colitis with the combination of vancomycin and rifampin. *J Clin Gastroenterol* **9**: 155–159.
15. Lagrotteria D, Holmes S, Smieja M, *et al.* (2006) Prospective, randomized inpatient study of oral metronidazole versus oral metronidazole and rifampin for treatment of primary episode of *Clostridium difficile*–associated diarrhea. *Clin Infect Dis* **43**: 547–552.
16. O'Connor J, Galang M, Sambol SP, *et al.* (2008) Rifampin and rifaximin resistance in clinical isolates of *Clostridium difficile*. *Antimicrob Agents Chemother* **52**: 2813–2817.
17. Gerding DN, Muto CA, Owens RC Jr. (2008) Treatment of *Clostridium difficile* infection. *Clin Infect Dis* **46**(Suppl 1): S32–S42.
18. Abougergi MS, Broor A, Cui W, Jaar BG. (2010) Intravenous immunoglobulin for the treatment of severe *Clostridium difficile colitis*: An observational study and review of the literature. *J Hosp Med* **5**(1): E1–E9. Review.
19. Yoon SS, Brandt LJ. (2010) Treatment of refractory/recurrent *C. difficile*–associated disease by donated stool transplanted via

colonoscopy: A case series of 12 patients. *J Clin Gastroenterol* **44**(8): 562–566.

20. E van Nood, Speelman P, Kuijper E J, Keller J J. (2009) Struggling with recurrent *Clostridium difficile* infections: Is donor faeces the solution? *Euro Surveill* **14**(34).
21. Venuto C, Butler M, Ashley ED, Brown J. Alternative therapies for *Clostridium difficile* infections. *Pharmacotherapy* **30**(12): 1266–1278.
22. Lowy I, Molrine DC, Leav BA, *et al.* (2010) Treatment with monoclonal antibodies against *Clostridium difficile* toxins. *N Engl J Med* **362**: 197.
23. Sougioultzis S, Kyne L, Drudy D, *et al.* (2005) *Clostridium difficile* toxoid vaccine in recurrent *C. difficile*–associated diarrhea. *Gastroenterology* **128**: 764–770.
24. Vonberg RP, Kuijper EJ, Wilcox MH, *et al.* (2008) Infection control measures to limit the spread of *Clostridium difficile. Clin Microbiol Infect* **14**(Suppl 5): 2–20.
25. Boyce JM, Pittet D.(2002) Guideline for Hand Hygiene in Health-Care Settings. Recommendations of the Healthcare Infection Control Practices Advisory Committee and the HICPAC/SHEA/APIC/IDSA Hand Hygiene Task Force. Society for Healthcare Epidemiology of America/Association for Professionals in Infection Control/Infectious Diseases Society of America. *MMWR Recomm Rep* **51**: 1–45.
26. Riggs MM, Sethi AK, Zabarsky TF, *et al.* (2007) Asymptomatic carriers are a potential source for transmission of epidemic and nonepidemic *Clostridium difficile* strains among long-term care facility residents. *Clin Infect Dis* **45**: 992.

Chapter 60

Catheter-Associated Bloodstream Infections

*David P. Calfee**

Key Pearls

- In suspected central-line-associated bloodstream infections (CLABSIs), blood cultures should be obtained before the initiation of antimicrobial therapy and at least one blood sample should be drawn from a peripheral vein.
- A central venous catheter that is the suspected or confirmed source of bloodstream infection should be removed immediately if the patient is demonstrating evidence of severe illness (e.g. hypotension, organ failure).
- Empiric antimicrobial therapy of CLABSI should be directed toward the pathogens most likely to be causing the infection, including coagulase-negative Staphylococci, *S. aureus* (including MRSA), gram-negative bacilli and, in certain patients (such as those with femoral catheters and high-risk medical conditions), *Candida* species.
- When one is attempting to salvage a catheter implicated in an episode of CLABSI, antibiotic lock therapy may increase the likelihood of successful catheter salvage.

*Weill Cornell Medical College, New York, NY, USA.

- The key aspects of CLABSI prevention include hand hygiene, use of maximal sterile barriers during insertion, use of chlorhexidine for skin preparation prior to insertion and during subsequent exit site care, avoidance of the femoral vein site, aseptic technique during catheter use, application of an antiseptic to the catheter hub prior to accessing the lumen, and removal of the catheter as soon as it is no longer needed.

Introduction and Epidemiology

It has been estimated that over 90,000 catheter-associated bloodstream infections occur in US hospitals each year.[1] The reported incidence of CLABSI varies among different patient populations.[2] Compared to patients without CLABSI, patients who develop CLABSI have longer hospital stays, face an increased risk of death, and incur substantially greater hospital costs. In fact, CLABSIs have been estimated to cost the US healthcare system up to US$2.7 billion per year.[1]

These infections, though, are largely preventable. Thus, many hospitals have appropriately given increased attention to CLABSI and efforts to prevent these infections. In addition to preventive efforts at individual healthcare facilities, CLABSI prevention has received significant attention at a higher level. For instance, the Centers for Medicare and Medicaid Services (CMS) has designated CLABSI as a reasonably preventable hospital-acquired condition for which, as of October 2008, it will no longer reimburse hospitals for the costs associated with treatment. In 2010, the Joint Commission added prevention of CLABSI to its National Patient Safety Goals.

Although much of the study and discussion of CLABSI has focused on the intensive care unit (ICU) setting, this topic is quite relevant to patients outside the ICU as well. Although a lower percentage of patients outside the ICU have central venous catheters (CVCs), the absolute number of patients with central lines outside the ICU typically exceeds the number of ICU patients with CVCs.[3,4] For instance, a point prevalence study conducted in six major medical centers found that only 30% of patients with CVCs were in ICUs.[3] In addition, data from the US and other countries indicate that the rates of CLABSI in non-ICU areas are similar to or perhaps even higher than those in ICUs.[2,5,6]

Pathogenesis

Catheter-related infection is preceded by asymptomatic bacterial or fungal colonization or contamination of the catheter. There are a number of ways in which this device can become colonized. First, organisms can colonize the external surface of the catheter during insertion or after insertion due to migration of organisms from the skin at the catheter exit site along the external surface of the device. Catheters can also become colonized through the introduction of organisms into the catheter hub during access or other manipulation of the device, with subsequent colonization of the catheter's internal surface. Less frequent causes of catheter colonization include hematogenous spread of micro-organisms from a distant site of infection and administration of contaminated medications, blood products, or other infusates through the device. The production of biofilm, a complex polysaccharide secreted by many pathogens, plays an important role in the epidemiology of catheter-related infections by protecting micro-organisms from host defenses and antimicrobial agents.

Microbiology

Gram-positive organisms are the most common cause of CLABSI.[7,8] For example, coagulase-negative staphylococci, such as *S. epidermidis*, cause approximately one third of these infections and *S. aureus* is responsible for an additional 10%–20%. Data submitted to the CDC's National Healthcare Safety Network (NHSN) for the period 2006–2007 demonstrated that methicillin-resistant strains of *S. aureus* (MRSA) were responsible for approximately 57% of all *S. aureus* CLABSIs.[7]

Gram-negative organisms, such as *Enterobacter* species, *E. coli.*, *Klebsiella* species, and *P. aeruginosa*, and *Candida* species each account for approximately 5% of reported cases.

Diagnosis

The diagnosis of CLABSI should be considered in a patient with fever or others signs and symptoms of infection in whom another source of infection is not immediately apparent. Blood cultures remain the primary diagnostic modality for identification of catheter-associated bloodstream infections. Symptoms or physical exam abnormalities at the catheter exit site or along the catheter tract are uncommon in CLABSI and their absence should not dissuade the clinician from considering a catheter-related infection in patients with otherwise compatible signs and symptoms.

For epidemiologic and surveillance purposes, a CLABSI is defined by the CDC as a primary bloodstream infection [i.e. positive blood culture(s) in the absence of an identifiable source of bloodstream infection (e.g. pneumonia, surgical site infection, urinary tract infection)] in a patient with a central venous catheter in place at the time of or within 48 hr before the blood sample was obtained (Table 1).[9] These or similar definitions are also frequently used for clinical diagnosis and management. It should be noted that the CDC definitions identify bloodstream infections that are associated with, but not necessarily due to, a central venous catheter and are thus not entirely specific for catheter-related bloodstream infections.

In situations where it is felt necessary to determine if the catheter is the true source of bacteremia, additional testing may be useful (Table 1).[10] An example of such a situation may be a clinically stable patient with a tunneled central venous catheter in whom removal and replacement of the catheter would pose significant risk or difficulty. In these situations, the use of diagnostic techniques such as quantitative blood cultures or differential time to positivity may be useful for determining if contamination of the catheter lumen is the cause of the bloodstream infection. These techniques may be most appropriate for use in patients with long-term catheters. Catheter segment cultures can also provide evidence to determine if a catheter is the source of a bloodstream infection but this technique can be performed only if the catheter is removed.

Table 1. Diagnosis of Catheter-Associated and Catheter-Related Bloodstream Infections

	Criterion	Description
Epidemiologic definitions[9] (i.e. catheter-*associated* bloodstream infection)	Criterion 1	• The patient has a recognized pathogen cultured from one or more blood cultures. and • The organism cultured is not related to an infection at another site.
	Criterion 2	• The patient has at least one of the following signs or symptoms: ○ Fever (>38°C) ○ Chills ○ Hypotension and • The signs, symptoms, and positive laboratory results are not related to an infection at another site. and • A common skin contaminant [e.g. diphtheroids (*Corynebacterium* species), *Bacillus* species (other than *B. anthracis*), *Propionibacterium* species, coagulase-negative Staphylococci, *viridans* group Streptococci, *Aerococcus* species, *Micrococcus* species] is cultured from two or more blood cultures drawn on separate occasions.
	Criterion 3	• A patient ≤1 year of age has at least one of the following signs or symptoms ○ Fever (>38°C, rectal) ○ Hypothermia (<37°C, rectal) ○ Apnea ○ Bradycardia and • The signs, symptoms, and positive laboratory results are not related to an infection at another site.

(*Continued*)

Table 1. (*Continued*)

	Criterion	Description
		and • A common skin contaminant [e.g. Diphtheroids (*Corynebacterium* species), *Bacillus* species (other than *B. anthracis*) *Propionibacterium* species, coagulase-negative Staphylococci, *viridans* group Streptococci, *Aerococcus* species, *Micrococcus* species] is cultured from two or more blood cultures drawn on separate occasions.
"Definitive" clinical diagnosis[10] (i.e. catheter-related bloodstream infection)	Catheter segment culture method	The same organism is isolated from at least one percutaneous blood sample and from the catheter tip.
	Quantitative blood culture method	The same organism is isolated from paired blood samples drawn from a peripheral vein and the catheter hub, and the colony count of organisms grown from the sample aspirated through the catheter hub is at least three times greater than that grown from the sample obtained from the peripheral vein.
	Differential time to positivity method	The same organism is isolated from paired blood samples drawn from a peripheral vein and the catheter hub, and growth is detected in the catheter-aspirated sample more than 120 min before growth is detected in the sample obtained from the peripheral vein.

Table 2. Management of Catheter-Associated Bloodstream Infections

Intervention	Recommendations
Catheter removal	Catheter removal is recommended in the setting of: • Complicated infections (e.g. CLABSI complicated by septic thrombophlebitis, endocarditis, osteomyelitis, tunnel infection, port abscess); • CLABSI in most patients with temporary central venous catheters. Catheter retention may be attempted in the setting of uncomplicated CLABSI due to coagulase-negative *Staphylococcus* or *Enterococcus* in patients with long-term central venous catheters. Catheter retention may also be considered in individual cases of uncomplicated CLABSI due to coagulase-negative *Staphylococcus* in patients with temporary central venous catheters and CLABSI caused by gram-negative bacilli in patients with long-term central venous catheters. When catheter retention (also known as catheter salvage) is attempted: • Antibiotic lock therapy should be included as part of the treatment regimen (i.e. in addition to systemic antimicrobial therapy). • The catheter should be removed if the patient remains bacteremic, if clinical deterioration occurs, or if evidence of complicated infection is identified.
Antimicrobial therapy	Empiric antimicrobial therapy should directed toward the most likely causative organisms and anticipated antimicrobial susceptibility patterns as determined based on national, local, and patient-specific data. Definitive therapy should be based on the identification of the causative organism and the results of antimicrobial susceptibility testing. The duration of antimicrobial therapy should be determined on the basis of: • The presence of complications: ○ Osteomyelitis in adults is typically treated for 6–8 weeks, but individual cases may vary. ○ Septic thrombophlebitis and endocarditis are typically treated for 4–6 weeks, but individual cases may vary.

(*Continued*)

Table 2. (*Continued*)

Intervention	Recommendations
	○ Catheter tunnel infections and port abscess are generally treated for 7–10 days following device removal. • The causative organism: ○ Uncomplicated coagulase-negative staphylococcal infections may be treated for 5–7 days if the device is removed or 10–14 days if the device is left in place. ○ *S. aureus* infections should be treated for a minimum of 14 days but many experts recommend treatment for at least 4 weeks due to concerns about the presence of undetected endocarditis. ○ CLABSI due to *Candida* species should be treated with antifungal therapy for two weeks after the first negative blood culture. ○ Uncomplicated CLABSI caused by other organisms (e.g. gram-negative bacilli, enterococci) should be treated for 7–14 days. When catheter salvage is attempted, antibiotic lock therapy, in addition to systemic antimicrobial therapy, should be included in the treatment regimen.

Treatment

Recently updated treatment guidelines from the Infectious Diseases Society of America provide recommendations for selection of an empiric antibiotic regimen, duration of antimicrobial therapy, and catheter removal for confirmed and suspected CLABSI in patients with short-term and long-term catheters.[10] Empiric antibiotic therapy should be guided by knowledge of the common causes of CLABSI, local antibiotic susceptibility patterns, and patient-specific considerations such as underlying medical conditions, severity of illness, and results of prior microbiologic test results. The initial empiric antimicrobial regimen should be adjusted as appropriate based on culture results. The recommended duration of therapy is dependent upon the organism, the rapidity of clearance of bacteremia or fungemia, and the presence or absence of complications (Table 2).

In addition to antimicrobial therapy, catheter removal often plays a significant role in the management of CLABSI. When there is infection of the catheter tunnel or of a subcutaneous port, treatment is unlikely to be successful without removal of the device. In general, temporary, nontunneled catheters should be removed in the setting of CLABSI, although catheter salvage may be considered in some patients with infections due to coagulase-negative staphylococci. For long-term CVCs, such as tunneled catheters and implanted ports, catheter removal is recommended in many situations, but catheter salvage may be considered in some situations, particularly for uncomplicated infections due to coagulase-negative staphylococci or enterococci and in patients in whom catheter removal or replacement is associated with significant potential for complications or difficulty. Regardless of the type of catheter or the infecting organism, catheter removal is always recommended in the management of patients who are clinically unstable, have complicated infections (e.g. endocarditis or septic thrombophlebitis), or have persistently positive blood cultures.

When catheter salvage is attempted, the use of antibiotic lock therapy (ALT), in addition to systemic antimicrobial therapy, is recommended. ALT involves the instillation of a concentrated antibiotic solution into the catheter lumen, where it is allowed to dwell while the catheter is not in use. This prolonged exposure to a concentration of the antibiotic that often exceeds the minimum inhibitory concentration (MIC) of the infecting organism by more than 1000 times may increase the likelihood of eradicating organisms from the catheter lumen. The use of antiseptics, such as ethanol, has also been evaluated for use in catheter lock therapy but routine use of these agents is not recommended.

Prevention

Scientific research and clinical evidence suggest that many CLABSIs can be prevented through the use of relatively simple practices that reduce the risk of catheter contamination and subsequent bloodstream infection (Table 3). These evidence-based practices have been outlined in a number of guidelines and recommendations.[11,12] The Institute for Healthcare

Table 3. Strategies to Prevent Central Line-Associated Bloodstream Infections

	Strategy	Comments
Routine strategies	Educate healthcare workers involved in catheter insertion, use, and/or maintenance.	• Research has demonstrated that HCW education regarding proper catheter insertion and use of techniques can reduce the rate of infection. • Periodic re-education is recommended for all healthcare providers involved in insertion, use, and maintenance of vascular access devices. • Trainees performing catheter insertion should be directly supervised.
	Perform hand hygiene.	• Hand hygiene must be performed prior to catheter insertion and before catheter use or manipulation.
	Select the optimal site for catheter insertion (i.e. avoid the femoral vein site when possible).	• The subclavian vein site has been associated with the lowest risk of infectious complications, while the femoral site has been associated with the highest risk of infectious and thrombotic complications. • The risks of infectious and noninfectious complications associated with each potential site of insertion must be considered for each patient.
	Use maximal sterile barriers during device insertion.	• "Maximal sterile barriers" refers to the use of a sterile gown and gloves and nonsterile cap and mask by all persons involved in the insertion procedure and coverage of the patient with a full-body sterile drape during the procedure.

(*Continued*)

Table 3. *(Continued)*

	Strategy	Comments
	Apply a cutaneous antiseptic at the insertion site prior to insertion and at the time of all dressing changes.	• 2% chlorhexidine gluconate is the preferred antiseptic for patients older than 2 months of age. • Alternative antiseptics include tincture of iodine, povidone-iodine, and 70% alcohol.
	Keep the catheter insertion site covered with a sterile dressing at all times.	• Gauze dressings should be changed every other day. • Semipermeable, transparent dressings should be changed at least every 7 days. • Dressings should be changed immediately if they become loose, damp, or soiled.
	Disinfect the catheter hub prior to accessing the catheter.	• Disinfect the catheter hub with chlorhexidine, alcohol, or an iodophor using friction in order to reduce the risk of contamination of the catheter lumen.
	Remove catheters that are no longer necessary.	• Review the necessity of vascular access devices on a daily basis and remove devices that are no longer necessary. • Studies suggest that patients outside the ICU are more likely to have catheters that are not considered to meet criteria for necessity.[4]
Additional approaches*	Use a catheter dressing impregnated with chlorhexidine or other antiseptic compound.	• Use of a chlorhexidine-impregnated sponge dressing has been associated with reductions in CLABSI rates. Other types of chlorhexidine-containing dressings are also available now.

(Continued)

Table 3. (*Continued*)

Strategy	Comments
Use antiseptic- or antibiotic-coated catheters.	• Catheters coated with antibiotics (e.g. rifampin and minocycline) or antiseptics (e.g. chlorhexidine and silver sulfadiazine), in some studies, have demonstrated the potential to reduce the incidence of CLABSI.
Bathe intensive care unit patients with chlorhexidine on a daily basis.	• Studies performed in intensive care units[15] and long-term acute care facilities[16] have suggested that daily bathing with chlorhexidine may reduce the risk of CLABSI.

* If not already implemented in an institution, these approaches should be considered when routine strategies fail to adequately reduce the incidence of CLABSI in specific patients or patient populations, or throughout a hospital.

Improvement (IHI) has promoted a "central line bundle," five evidence-based practices to be implemented together in order to reduce the risk of CLABSI (http://www.ihi.org/IHI/Topics/CriticalCare/IntensiveCare/Changes/ImplementtheCentralLineBundle.htm).

The components of the central line bundle are:

- Hand hygiene
- Maximal barrier precautions during catheter insertion
- Chlorhexidine-based skin antisepsis
- Avoidance of the femoral vein site in adult patients
- Daily review of catheter necessity with removal of catheters as soon as they are no longer necessary

The use of a checklist to ensure that all critical infection prevention strategies are performed during catheter insertion has also been promoted as an effective preventive measure. In addition to optimizing practices related to catheter insertion and timely removal, appropriate catheter use and maintenance techniques, such as disinfecting the catheter hub before accessing it and keeping the insertion site covered with a sterile dressing, are also critical components of a CLABSI prevention program. There is substantial evidence that these practices are effective in preventing CLABSI in routine clinical practice.[13,14]

References

1. Scott R. (2009) The direct medical costs of healthcare-associated infections in US hospitals and the benefits of prevention. Centers for Disease Control and Prevention.
2. Edwards J, Peterson K, Mu Y, *et al.* (2009) National Healthcare Safety Network (NHSN) report: Data summary for 2006 through 2008, issued December 2009. *Am J Infect Control* **37**: 783–805.
3. Climo M, Diekema D, Warren D, *et al.* (2003) Prevalence of the use of central venous access devices within and outside of the intensive care unit: Results of a survey among hospitals in the prevention epicenter program of the Centers for Disease Control and Prevention. *Infect Control Hosp Epidemiol* **24**(12): 942–945.
4. Trick W, Vernon M, Welbel S. (2004) Unnecessary use of central venous catheters: The need to look outside the intensive care unit. *Infect Control Hosp Epidemiol* **25**(3): 266–268.
5. Marschall J, Leone C, Jones M, *et al.* (2007) Catheter-associated bloodstream infections in general medical patients outside the intensive care unit: A surveillance study. *Infect Control Hosp Epidemiol* **28**(8): 905–909.
6. Vonberg R, Behnke M, Geffers C, *et al.* (2006) Device-associated infection rates for non-intensive care unit patients. *Infect Control Hosp Epidemiol* **27**(4): 357–361.
7. Hidron AI, Edwards HR, Patel J, *et al.* (2008) NHSN annual update: Antimicrobial-resistant pathogens associated with healthcare-associated infections: Annual summary of data reported to the National Healthcare Safety Network at the Centers for Disease Control and Prevention, 2006–2007. *Infect Control Hosp Epidemiol* **29**: 996–1011.

8. Wisplinghoff H, Bischoff T, Tallent S. (2008) Nosocomial bloodstream infections in US hospitals: Analysis of 24,179 cases from a prospective nationwide surveillance study. *Clin Infect Dis* **39**: 309–317.
9. Horan T, Andrus M, Dudeck M. (2008) CDC/NHSN surveillance definition of healthcare–associated infection and criteria for specific types of infections in the acute care setting. *Am J Infect Control* **36**: 309–332.
10. Mermel L, Allon M, Bouza E, Craven D, *et al.* (2009) Clinical practice guidelines for the diagnosis and management of intravascular catheter-related infection: 2009 Update by the Infectious Diseases Society of America. *Clin Infect Dis* **49**(1): 1–45.
11. O'Grady N, Alexander M, Burn LA, *et al.* (2011) Guidelines for the prevention of intravascular catheter-related infections. *Clin Infect Dis* **52**(9): e162–193.
12. Marschall J, Mermel L, Classen D, *et al.* (2008) Strategies to prevent central line–associated bloodstream infections in acute care hospitals. *Infect Control Hosp Epidemiol* **29** (Suppl 1): S22–S30.
13. Berenholtz S, Pronovost P, Lipsett P, *et al.* (2004) Eliminating catheter-related bloodstream infections in the intensive care unit. *Crit Care Med* **32**(10): 2014–2020.
14. Pronovost P, Needham D, Berenholtz S, *et al.* (2006) An intervention to decrease catheter-related bloodstream infections in the ICU. *N Engl J Med* **355**(26): 2725–2732.
15. Bleasdale S, Trick W, Gonzalez I. (2007) Effectiveness of chlorhexidine bathing to reduce catheter-associated bloodstream infections in medical intensive care unit patients. *Arch Intern Med* **167**(19): 2073–2079.
16. Munoz-Price L, Hota B, Stemer A, Weinstein R. (2009) Prevention of bloodstream infections by use of daily chlorhexidine baths for patients at a long-term acute care hospital. *Infect Control Hosp Epidemiol* **30**(11): 1031–1035.

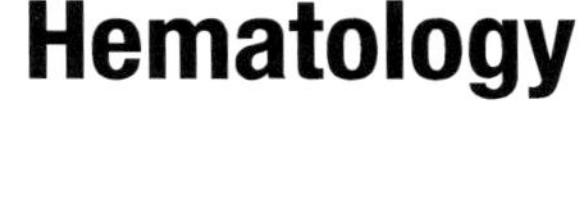

Hematology

Chapter 61

Anemia

Che-Kai Tsao and Louis Aledort**

Key Pearls

- The evaluation of anemia should always start with a comprehensive history and physical examination, and an accurate assessment of its acuity. The initial evaluation should include: CBC with evaluation of differentials, reticulocyte count, haptoglobin, lactate dehydrogenase, mean corpuscular value, electrolyte panel, and liver function testing.
- Autoimmune hemolytic anemia should always be differentiated from familial spherocytosis, as the two entities may appear similar on the peripheral smear. Family history and laboratory investigation (haptoglobin, LDH, direct Coombs test) should be carried out.
- When faced with multiple nutritional deficiencies (e.g. B12, folate, iron), gastrointestinal malabsorption should always be considered. An endoscopic procedure with tissue biopsy can be helpful in establishing the diagnosis.
- Hemoglobin electrophoresis will detect only beta thalessemia (elevated hemoglobin A2). Thus, alpha thalessemia should always be considered when a thorough investigation for microcytic anemia is nondiagnostic.
- Thrombotic thrombocytopenic purpura is often missed and can be rapidly fatal. Measurement of the ADAMST13 level is diagnostic, with an absolute deficiency usually less than 10% of normal activity. Treatment with plasmapheresis should always be initiated prior to definitive diagnosis.

*Mount Sinai School of Medicine, New York NY, USA.

Introduction

The evaluation of anemia is a complex process, necessitating a comprehensive understanding of the physiology of red blood cells (RBCs) and the processes of production and destruction. A systematic approach is essential, and it consists of a comprehensive history and physical exam, laboratory tests, and review of the peripheral blood smear.[1,2]

Anemia is defined by a decrease in circulating red blood cells in the body, as reflected by a reduction in hemoglobin (g/dL whole blood), hematocrit (% whole blood with intact RBCs), and/or RBCs (million cells/μL of blood).

Normal values can vary widely, depending on multiple factors (age, ethnicity, etc.).[3] Despite variability in the current literature, the World Health Organization defines anemia as Hg <14 in men and Hg <12 in women. An overview of the approach to anemia is presented in Fig. 1.

History

The first step is to quantify anemia-related symptoms (e.g. shortness of breath, fatigue) to determine the acuity of diagnostic workup and treatment.[4] Particularly in young women, pay close attention to patterns of menstruation, and characterize the bowel movement or stool appearance in the older population. Also, screen for symptoms relating to deficiencies in other blood lines (e.g. infection, bleeding). A comprehensive review of systems is particularly important, as specific symptoms can aid in focusing the workup.

- Medical history: many disease states can directly or indirectly cause anemia.
- Surgical history: various surgeries may contribute indirectly to anemia (bowel resection in nutritional deficiency).[5]
- Medications: can cause both increased destruction and decreased production of RBCs.
- Family history: familial hemoglobinopathies should be screened for.
- Social history: pay close attention to toxins and drug exposure.

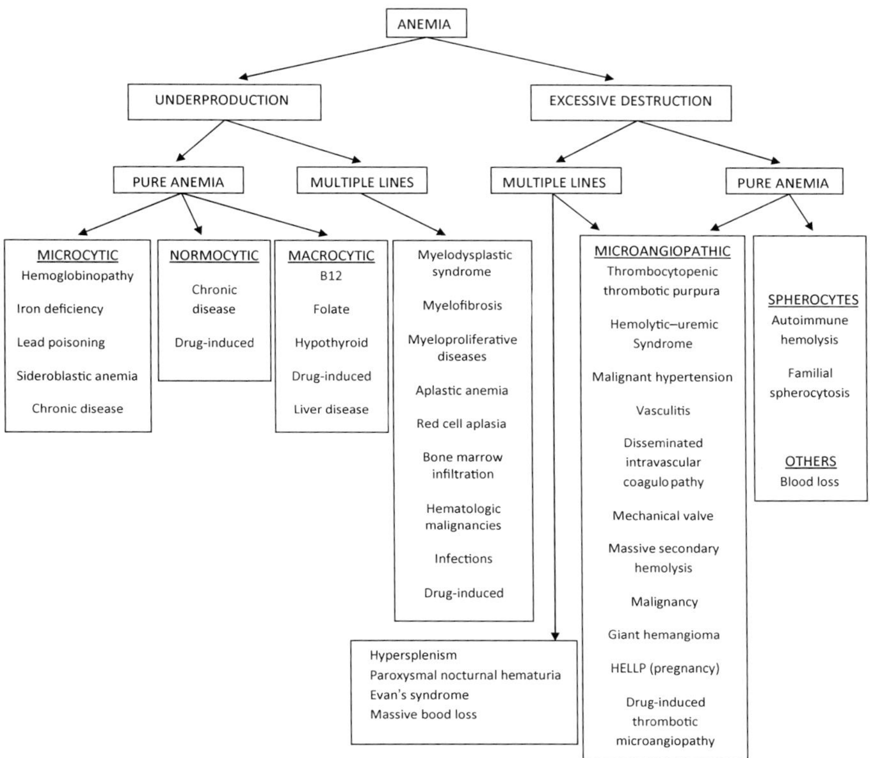

Fig. 1. Overview of anemia.

Physical Examination

A careful, comprehensive physical examination must be performed, as it can provide information on the severity and etiology of anemia. Careful attention should be paid to assessing for the presence of lymphadenopathy, the size of the liver or spleen, the neurological exam, and the underlying joint pathology.

Peripheral Smear

The smear should always be examined whenever possible, as it is often diagnostic.[6,7] An area where RBCs are close but not touching each other

Table 1. Laboratory Evaluation

Laboratory marker	Evaluation
Mean corpuscular volume (MCV)	Microcytic: MCV <80 Normocytic: MCV 80–100 Macrocytic:MCV >100
Mean corpuscular hemoglobin (MCH)	Low: iron deficiency anemia or thalessemia High: all forms of macrocytic anemia
Mean corpuscular hemoglobin concentration (MCHC)	High value = desiccation of RBC volume (e.g. spherocytosis, sickle cell anemia)
Reticulocyte count (% or absolute)	High: blood loss or RBC destructive process Low: abnormal bone marrow production
Lactate dehydrogenase (LDH)	High value may indicate destructive process vs. liver disease.
Haptoglobin	Low value indicates hemolysis vs. liver disease.
Bilirubin	High indirect bilirubin is consistent with hemolysis, while high direct bilirubin may indicate liver disease.
Serum creatinine	Renal insufficiency may contribute to low erythropoietin production.

should be found, and many fields should be examined prior to making a conclusion. RBC morphology should be examined first, and the size, shape, intracellular inclusions, abnormal cells, and cytoplasm to central pallor ratio should all be evaluated. White blood cell and platelet morphology should also be evaluated. Example findings from peripheral blood smears are shown in Fig. 2.

After the history, physical examination, examination of the peripheral blood smear, and laboratory evaluation, the anemia should be classified as being due to underproduction versus excessive destruction, and then to whether cells are microcytic, normocytic, or macrocytic.

Underproduction

Underproduction first needs to be classified as to whether only the red blood cell line is affected or multiple cell lines are affected. If only the red blood cell line is affected, the differential based on cell size is as follows:

Microcytic

- *Hemoglobinopathy*. Underlying structural hemoglobin abnormality can cause microcytic anemia, including sickle cell diseases and thalessemia. Hemoglobin electrophoresis can be diagnostic but alpha thalassemia cannot be diagnosed without genetic testing.

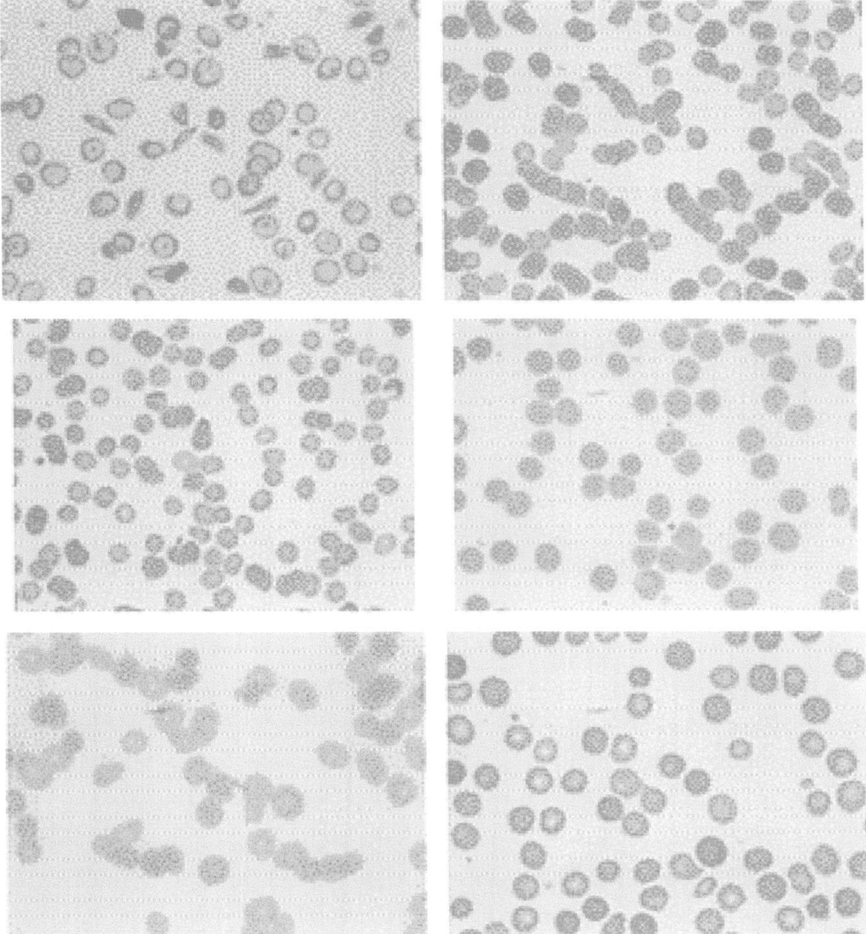

Fig. 2. Peripheral blood smear of various states of anemia: (1) sickle cell disease, (2) Rouleaux formation, (3) Burr cells, (4) teardrop cells, (5) sideroblastic anemia, (6) spherocytosis, (7) polychromasia, (8) schistocytes or "fragment cells," (9) target cells.

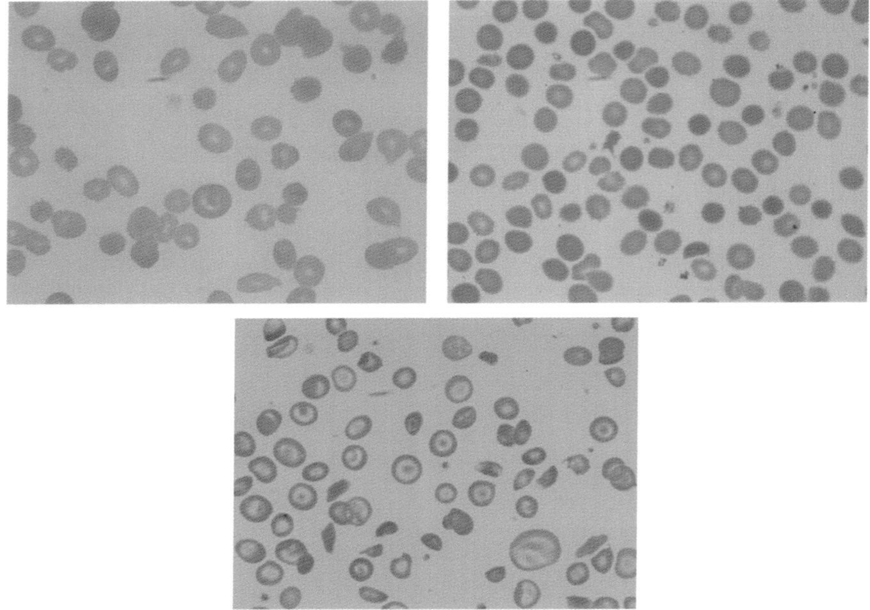

Fig. 2. (*Continued*)

- *Iron deficiency*. Diagnostic criteria include low serum ferritin (<15 mcg/L), and low serum iron, and high total iron binding capacity can be diagnostic, but often these tests can be unreliable (such as high ferritin in the inflammatory state). Bone marrow biopsy with iron stain is the gold standard for diagnosis. If the underlying etiology is unclear, one must rule out occult blood loss due to gastrointestinal or vaginal bleeding; consider screening colonoscopy and endoscopy, especially if the patient is above age 50. Note that a normal term pregnancy can deplete up to one third of the body's iron store.
- *Lead poisoning*. This is associated with multiple symptoms, including abdominal pain, headache, and neuropathy, and can lead to microcytic anemia, which often coexists with underlying iron deficiency. A peripheral smear can show basophilic stippling, although this is not a specific finding. Blood lead level should be ordered with clinical suspicion. Sideroblastic anemia can also be caused by lead toxicity.

- *Sideroblastic anemia.* This disease entity may be congenital (early onset), clonal with myelodysplastic syndrome (middle-aged/older), or acquired (drug-induced, lead poisoning, copper deficiency, alcoholism).
- *Anemia of chronic disease.* Many diseases can cause this entity, including vasculitis, rheumatoid disease, inflammatory disease, and chronic infections.

Normocytic

- *Anemia of chronic disease.* This entity can also present with normocytic anemia (see above section).
- *Drug-induced.* Many drugs can cause myelosuppression, resulting in drug-induced anemia. A careful history of the present illness should include a careful review of medications, especially recently added agents relative to the onset of anemia.

Macrocytic

- *Vitamin deficiency.* Folate and B_{12} deficiency both may cause megaloblastic anemia.[8] Note an elevated serum methylmalonic acid level and presence of neurologic deficit points to B_{12} deficiency. Also, folate deficiency may develop within weeks, whereas B_{12} deficiency can only develop after months of nonintake.
- *Hypothyroidism.* TSH screening should be performed, particularly when the patient is exhibiting signs of hypothyroidism (e.g. fatigue, weight gain.)
- *Drugs.* Several drugs, such as Zidovudine, can cause megaloblastic anemia.
- *Liver disease.* This can be either normocytic or macrocytic; consider screening for liver diseases, particularly with abnormal liver function testing.
- *Polychromasia due to blood loss or destruction.* Note that with an abundance of polychromatic cells, given that they are macrocytic, the MCV will often be elevated.

Underproduction with Multiple Cell Lines Affected

- *Myelodysplastic syndrome.* Often the patient may manifest with only anemia initially, and sequential decrease in other blood cell lines may follow. A review of the smear may show morphologically abnormal white blood cells (e.g. Peugher-huet). Bone marrow biopsy with cytogenetic evaluation is indicated but may initially not be diagnostic.
- *Myeloproliferative disease/myelofibrosis.* The patient may initially present with high hemoglobin (polycythemia vera) or a high platelet count (essential thrombocythemia), with development of anemia at a later time. Progression to pancytopenia with development of myelofibrosis (look for teardrop red cells on the peripheral smear) may follow, and secondary leukemia should be ruled out in this setting.
- *Aplastic anemia.* This entity may be idiopathic or iatrogenic (radiation, benzene, viral syndrome, etc.).
- *Red cell aplasia.* This can be caused by drugs or underlying disease (e.g. chronic lymphocytic leukemia).
- *Bone marrow infiltration.* Bone marrow infiltration by malignancies (e.g. breast cancer) or infectious agents (e.g. tuberculosis) will limit bone marrow production, resulting in pancytopenia.
- *Hematologic malignancy.* Leukemia, in both the acute and the chronic form, may affect any of the blood cell lines. A review of the peripheral smear and subsequent bone marrow biopsy with cytogenetic confirmation should be performed.
- *Multiple myeloma.* Quantitative immunoglobulin and electrophoresis of serum and urine to detect underlying monoclonal gammopathy can be used to screen patients with unexplained anemia. Unexplained protein gaps (serum protein minus albumin) and hypercalcemia may be suggestive. If a monoclonal paraprotein is discovered, proper staging with skeletal survey and bone marrow biopsy should be performed.
- *Infectious.* Human immunodeficiency virus, cytomegalovirus, Epstein–Barr virus, parvovirus B19, hepatitis B, and hepatitis C may

all cause pancytopenia. Patients at risk should be screened for these viral infections.

- *Drug-induced.* Refer to the "drug-induced" section above.

Excessive Destruction

Like in underproduction, one first needs to classify whether only the red blood cell line is affected or multiple cell lines are affected. In addition, clinicians should determine whether the peripheral blood smear demonstrates spherocytosis (presence of excessive spherocytes) or microangiopathy (presence of excessive schistocytosis). If only the red blood cell line is affected, the differential based on cell size is as follows:

Spherocytic

- *Hereditary spherocytosis.* Clinicians should always screen their patient for family and medical history of spherocytosis. High MCV and MCHC may be suggestive. When one is screening through the peripheral blood smear, it is important to screen multiple areas, as crowded areas where the red blood cells are overlapping may mimic its appearance.
- *Autoimmune hemolytic anemia.* This can be idiopathic or secondary to drugs and/or infections. In addition to anemia, a combination of high lactate dehydrogenase, high indirect bilirubin, and low haptoglobin is usually present. Diagnostic confirmation can be made with direct Coombs testing. If cold agglutinin disease is suspected, an indirect Coombs test can be confirmatory.

Nonspherocytic

- *Chronic blood loss.* Screening for gastrointestinal and uterine chronic blood loss should be considered for appropriate populations. Note that prior to depletion of the body's iron store, microcytosis may not be manifested.

Microangiopathic

- *Malignant hypertension.* With an abnormally high systolic blood pressure, the high shearing force on the red blood cells can cause fragmentation, resulting in formation of schistocytes.
- *Vasculitis.* In vasculitis, prominent vessel inflammation can result in red blood cell fragmentation. Low serum complement levels may be suggestive in the appropriate clinical setting.
- *Mechanical valve.* The presence of a metal mechanical valve, particularly in combination with malignant hypertension, can cause schistocytosis as red blood cells fragment upon encountering shearing force on the valve.
- *Massive secondary hemolysis.* Massive hemolysis can lead to microangiopathic disease, with schistocytosis as a predominant feature.
- *Malignancy.* Many cancers have been reported in the literature to cause microangiopathic anemia (e.g. gastric, ovarian, lung).
- *Giant hemangioma.* A large hemangioma (especially in the liver) can cause secondary microangiopathic disease, resulting in red blood cell fragmentation secondary to increased arterial blood flow.[9]

Excessive Destruction with Multiple Lines Affected

Microangiopathic

- *Thrombotic thrombocytopenic purpura.* TTP is one of the most-feared hematologic diseases, as it may be lethal without appropriate therapy. The underlying etiology can be idiopathic as well as acquired. A deficiency or inhibitor of ADAMST13 (a metalloproteinase enzyme cleaving vWF strands) results in excessive intravascular thrombosis and subsequent schistocytosis. This entity should always be ruled out first with unexplained and sudden onset schistocytosis. Urgent serum plasmapheresis should always be considered before definitive diagnosis. Measurement of the ADAMST13 level can be diagnostic; absolute deficiency is usually less than 10%, whereas

10%–40% is considered relative deficiency and other causes should also be entertained.

- *Drug-induced thrombotic microangiopathy*. Many pharmacologic agents have been associated with the development of this condition; cyclosporine, mitomycin-C, and ticlodipine are some examples that have been more commonly reported in the literature.
- *Hemolytic–uremic syndrome*. This disease entity is usually secondary to drugs or toxins (e.g. Shiga toxin). Patients will predominantly manifest renal failure and neurologic changes. The ADAMST13 level is above 10% and often can be normal.
- *Disseminated intravascular coagulopathy*. DIC is usually secondary to an underlying cause (e.g. retained fetus, sepsis), with activation of multiple coagulation factors resulting in consumptive coagulopathy. This results in worsening pancytopenia, coupled with elevated PT and PTT. An elevated *D*-dimer and low fibrinogen may be helpful in clinching the diagnosis. Schistocytosis is observed, but usually not abundant compared to TTP/HUS.
- *HELLP syndrome*. A life-threatening obstetric complication that is marked by hemolytic anemia, elevated liver enzymes, and a low platelet count. It occurs during the third trimester of pregnancy, often in a setting of known pre-eclampsia and prior to fulminant eclampsia. Delivery is the gold standard for treatment.

Non-microangiopathic

- *Hypersplenism*. This is often associated with existing liver disease, but may also occur with underlying hematologic, inflammatory, and infectious etiologies. Particularly in the setting of infection, increasing splenic sequestration or RBC destruction may manifest as worsening pancytopenia.
- *Evan's syndrome*. This is a rare disease characterized by simultaneous or sequential development of autoimmune hemolytic anemia,

idiopathic thrombocytopenia purpura, and/or autoimmune neutropenia without any identifiable underlying etiology.
- *Paroxysmal nocturnal hematura.* Patients will often present with a history of unprovoked thrombosis (e.g. Budd Chiari) and unexplained nocturnal hematuria. Diagnostic confirmation is made by flow cytometry of serum; CD55 and CD59 positivity coupled with the above history is diagnostic.
- *Acute blood loss.* In a surgical or trauma setting, large volume blood loss may cause rapid loss of all blood cell lines.

Management of Anemia

The management of anemia, while at first it may seem simplistic, can often be challenging when clinicians face numerous confounding factors. A stepwise approach should be established when one is considering the management of anemia.

The first step in management is to assess the acuity of the anemia. This is determined by the severity of symptomatic anemia, which should reflect the acuteness of symptom progression. Packed red blood cell should always be considered in this setting. The priority should be to ensure stability of the anemia, and further workup can ensue. Note that patients with underlying diseases (e.g. coronary heart disease, sickle cell anemias warrant differing levels of target transfusion goals.

An extensive workup as recommended above should be performed. Pay special attention to cases that may involve multiple etiologies (such as patients with CLL and concurrent autoimmune hemolytic anemia), requiring multimodality treatment.

The underlying etiology of the anemia should be treated:

- *Always correct the underlying etiology.* If the workup is nondiagnostic, hematologic consultation and bone marrow biopsy should be considered.

- *Nutritional deficiency*. Exploring the etiology of nutritional deficiency is particularly important, as specific nutritional malabsorption may warrant parenteral replacement.
- *Iatrogenic*. Stop the offending agent.
- *Anemia of chronic disease*. Consider transfusion as needed or using erythropoietin if the anemia cannot be corrected to target hematocrit.
- *Underlying hematologic disease*. Treatment of underlying disease may lead to correction of anemia.
- *Autoimmune hemolysis*. Consider starting prednisone at 1 mg/kg initially; second-line agents can be considered if there is inadequate effect with steroids.
- *Microangiopathic disease*. Prior to definitive diagnosis, plasma exchange should always be considered for underlying TTP. A through investigation of other causes should be made to rule out other causes, and proper treatment for appropriate etiologies should be performed without delay (e.g. fetal delivery in HELLP, supportive care or removal of the causative agent in HUS).

References

1. Hillman RS, Ault KA, (eds). (2001) Clinical approach to anemia. In *Hematology in Clinical Practice*. McGraw-Hill, New York, pp. 3, 29.
2. Tefferi A. (2003) Anemia in adults: A contemporary approach to diagnosis. *Mayo Clin Proc* **78**: 1274.
3. Beutler E, Waalen J. (2006) The definition of anemia: What is the lower limit of normal of the blood hemoglobin concentration? *Blood* **107**: 1747.
4. Gjorup T, Bugge PM, Hendriksen C, Jensen AM. (1986) A critical evaluation of the clinical diagnosis of anemia. *Am J Epidemiol* **124**: 657.
5. World Health Organization. (1968) *Nutritional Anaemias: Report of a WHO Scientific Group.*

6. Morris MW, Williams WJ, Nelson DA. (1995) Automated blood cell counting. In: Beutler E, Lichtman MA Coller BS, *et al.* (eds), *Williams' Hematology*, 5th ed. McGraw-Hill, New York, p. L3.
7. Williams WJ, Morris MW, Nelson DA. (1995) Examination of the blood. In: Beutler E, Lichtman MA, Coller BS, *et al.* (eds), *Williams' Hematology,* 5th ed. McGraw-Hill, New York, p. 8.
8. Davenport, J. (1996) Macrocytic anemia. *Am Fam Physician* **53**: 155.
9. Propp RP, Scharfman WB. (1966) Hemangioma–thrombocytopenia syndrome associated with microangiopathic hemolytic anemia. *Blood* **28**(5): 623–633.

Chapter 62

Thrombocytopenia

*Caroline Cromwell**

Key Pearls

- There is little risk of spontaneous bleeding unless the platelet count is <5000/μL.
- Prophylactic platelet transfusions are usually initiated at platelet counts <10,000/μL.
- Medications are often implicated in the hospitalized patient who develops thrombocytopenia.
- Immediately discontinue all heparin containing products if heparin-induced thrombocytopenia is suspected.
- Patients with a platelet count >50,000/μL are considered safe to participate in unrestricted activity if all other hemostatic parameters are normal.

Introduction

Approximately 5%–10% of all hospitalized patients will be found to have thrombocytopenia.[1] Thrombocytopenia is defined as a platelet count <150,000/μL, and it must be noted that 2.5% of the population will have a platelet count lower than this. For the purpose of this review, relevant thrombocytopenia will be defined as a platelet count <100,000/μL, since a count >100,000/μL is rarely associated with a significant

*Mount Sinai School of Medicine, New York, NY, USA.

bleeding risk. Patients with a platelet count >50,000/μL are usually asymptomatic, and patients with a platelet count of 25,000–50,000/μL may have bruising and petechiae. Based on studies of leukemic patients, there is little risk of spontaneous bleeding until the platelet count is < 5000–10,000/μL.[2]

Thrombocytopenia in the hospitalized patient must be evaluated to ascertain the risk of bleeding, to establish the underlying cause and determine treatment (if needed).

Causes of Thrombocytopenia

Table 1 lists the common causes of thrombocytopenia. Pseudothrombocytopenia is an easily diagnosed cause of thrombocytopenia, with review of the peripheral smear revealing platelet clumping. This can be easily ameliorated by the collection of blood in a heparinized tube. It should be suspected in the asymptomatic patient with a very low reported platelet count. Splenic sequestration of platelets due to liver disease or splenomegaly of any etiology is often seen in the hospital setting. Usually a platelet count of approximately 30,000–60,000/μL is found in such patients. If the platelet count is much lower than this, other causes for thrombocytopenia should be investigated. Dilutional thrombocytopenia is a rare cause of thrombocytopenia in patients who have received massive transfusions of plasma, blood, and intravenous fluids.

Other causes of thrombocytopenia can be divided into causes related to decreased production or increased destruction of platelets, or a combination of the two (Table 1).

Increased platelet destruction occurs frequently in the hospital setting, for a wide variety of reasons. DIC is often suspected, due to other marked abnormalities such as prolonged PT, PTT, and anemia, with a relatively obvious cause of the DIC identified, such as sepsis or malignancy. Immune causes of thrombocytopenia include ITP, and heparin-induced thrombocytopenia. ITP should be suspected in a patient with a normal white blood cell count and hemoglobin. A fall in the platelet count by

Table 1. Causes of Thrombocytopenia

Increased Destruction	Decreased Production
Idiopathic/immune thrombocytopenic purpura (ITP)	Primary bone marrow disorder — myeloproliferative or lymphoproliferative disorders
Disseminated intravascular coagulation-(DIC)	Infections
Splenomegaly	Medications
Thrombotic thrombocytopenic purpura (TTP)/hemolytic–uremic syndrome (HUS)	Chemotherapy
Antiphospholipid antibody syndrome	Radiation
Infections — bacterial, viral	Hepatitis
Medications	Drugs
Mechanical destruction — due to cardiopulmonary bypass, giant hemangiomata (Kasabach–Merritt syndrome)	B12/folate deficiency
Sepsis	Acute alcohol ingestion
Burns	Hypothyroidism
	Adrenal insufficiency

one-half, even if the platelet count remains in the normal range, should raise the suspicion of heparin induced thrombocytopenia. If HIT is suspected, all heparin should be discontinued.

Decreased production can occur in a number of settings: alcohol ingestion, vitamin deficiencies, and medications can all decrease megakaryopoiesis. Generally, these are associated with a decrease in other cell lines as well. Bacterial and viral infections, including HIV, can lead to direct bone marrow suppression, and megakaryocyte apoptosis. Particularly in the inpatient setting, when a patient may have just been initiated on a number of medications, these medications must also be assessed. The most important causes of thrombocytopenia to discover early are DIC, TTP, and HIT, as these can have the most rapid devastating consequences if left untreated. It is important to note that TTP is an infrequent but known side effect of clopidogrel therapy.

Evaluation of the Thrombocytopenic Patient

History: Detailed history-taking is key in the evaluation of thrombocytopenia. If bleeding has occurred, it is important to establish the onset and duration, so as to help elucidate the cause. Other key components of the history are:

(1) Recent infection, HIV risk factors.
(2) Drug history, particularly antibiotics, heparin, quinine, sulfa drugs. Recent initiation of new medications.
(3) Family history. This should include a detailed evaluation for familial bleeding disorders, history of thrombocytopenia or autoimmune disorders.
(4) History of prior thrombocytopenic episodes, history of anemia.
(5) Personal history of autoimmune disorder.
(6) Alcohol/drinking history.
(7) Diet/food history.

Physical Exam

A comprehensive physical exam is essential for the evaluation of any sign of bleeding. Patients with moderate thrombocytopenia are often asymptomatic. If bleeding occurs, it is usually mucocutaneous. The most common manifestations are petechiae, bruising ecchymoses, epistaxis, and gingival or gastrointestinal bleeding. Deep muscular bleeding and hemarthroses are more consistent with a coagulation disorder. Particularly in patients with platelet counts of 10,000/μL, careful neurologic assessment is warranted, due to the risk of intracranial hemorrhage. Stool guiac evaluation can be helpful. Abdominal assessment for splenomegaly is important as well. Of note is that, ITP is not associated with splenomegaly. Fever, adenopathy, or splenomegaly may suggest infection or malignancy.

Review of the Peripheral Smear

The peripheral smear should always be evaluated in a patient with thrombocytopenia. This review should include examination for platelet clumping, platelet size, presence of schistocytes, white blood cell abnormalities, and nucleated red blood cells. This can help guide the next diagnostic steps.

Laboratory Evaluation

Laboratory evaluation of thrombocytopenia can be wide-ranging and costly. Physicians must use clinical suspicion to determine which studies are appropriate for evaluation. Certain tests may take time to result and thus are used to confirm clinical suspicion. However, clinical judgment should dictate patient management. Laboratory testing may include:

- Repeat CBC
- Review peripheral smear
- CBC — in a heparinized tube
- PT, PTT
- D-dimer, fibrinogen degradation products
- Antiphospholipid antibody testing
- Platelet factor 4 assay and antiplatelet antibodies — for heparin-induced thrombocytopenia (HIT) antibodies
- Direct antiglobulin test
- Hepatitis screen
- Abdominal ultrasound — assess spleen size
- Bone marrow biopsy and aspiration
- Platelet function testing (if qualitative disorder is suspected)

Treatment of Thrombocytopenia

Cause specific treatment: If an underlying etiology is found for thrombocytopenia, one must proceed with appropriate treatment and supportive therapy as needed. For ITP, immunomodulatory therapy is usually initiated, with steroids and IVIG as first-line treatments. In the case of HIT, heparin must be stopped and alternative anticoagulation initiated with a direct thrombin inhibitor. In the case of DIC, while there is a role for supportive care with platelet, plasma, and red blood cell transfusion, treatment of the underlying cause is needed to correct the DIC. In the case of TTP, plasma exchange should be initiated. These treatments should proceed in consultation with a hematologist. B12 injections should be initiated in the case of B12 deficiency, and oral folate in the setting of folic acid deficiency.

Typically, anticoagulation and antiplatelet therapy are held for a platelet count <50,000/μL. However, in conditions of high thrombotic risk, anticoagulation can be considered on a case-by-case basis. Anticoagulation and antiplatelet therapy are generally considered safe at platelet counts >50,000/μL.

Platelet Transfusion Guidelines

Platelet transfusions are generally overutilized in patients with asymptomatic thrombocytopenia. In the case of TTP, HIT, and ITP, platelet transfusions are generally not advisable.

Consensus guidelines have established the prophylactic platelet transfusion trigger to be 10,000/μL.[3,4] The true efficacy of prophylactic platelet transfusion still remains to be determined.

Procedure specific target platelet counts

While there have been no randomized clinical trials regarding this, general guidelines have been set forth by consensus groups[5–8] (Table 2).

Table 2. Platelet Transfusion Guidelines

Routine dentistry	10,000/μL
Lumbar puncture, liver biopsy, endoscopy, bronchoscopy, central venous catheter insertion, tooth extraction	>50,000/μL
Neurosurgery/ophthalmic surgery	>100,000/μL

Complications of Platelet Transfusion

Risks associated with platelet transfusions include alloimmunization, transmission of infection, allergic reactions, and transfusion-related acute lung injury (TRALI). While the rates of these complications continue to improve, these risks should not be ignored.

Discharge Planning

Decisions for discharge must be made on a case-by-case basis. Patients with a platelet count >50,000/μL are considered safe to participate in unrestricted activity if all other hemostatic parameters are normal. Patients with moderate thrombocytopenia should avoid contact sports, but can otherwise participate in all activities. Patients with chronic ITP have young active platelets and often do not have any signs of bleeding even in the setting of severe thrombocytopenia. Discharge planning for those patients should occur in conjunction with the treating hematologist.[9]

References

1. Akca S, Haji-Michael P. (2002) Time course of platelet counts in critically ill Patients. *Crit Care Med* **30**: 753–756.
2. Gaydos LA, Freireich EJ. (1962) The quantitative relationship between platelet count and hemorrhage in patients with acute leukemia. *N Engl J Med* **266**: 905–909.
3. Rebulla P, Finazzi G. (1987) The threshold for prophylactic platelet transfusion in adults with acute myeloid leukemia. *N Engl J Med* **337**: 1870–1875
4. Slicheter S. (2007) Platelet transfusion therapy. *Hematol Oncol Clin* **21**: 697–729.
5. Tosetto A, Balduini CL, Cattaneo M. (2009) Management of bleeding and of invasive procedures in patients with platelet disorders and/or thrombocytopenia: Guidelines of the Italian Society for Haemostasis and Thrombosis (SISET). *Thromb Res* **124**(5): e13–e18.

6. Schiffer CA, Anderson KC. (2001) Platelet transfusion for patients with cancer: Clinical practice guidelines of the American Society of Clinical Oncology. *J Clin Oncl* **19**: 1519–1538.
7. Kelsey P. (2003) Guidelines for the use of platelet transfusions. *Br J Haematol* **122**: 10–23.
8. Marwaha N, Sharma RR. (2009) Concensus and controversies in platelet transfusion. *Tran Aph Sci* **41**: 127–133.
9. Lacy JV. (1977) Management of idiopathic thrombocytopenic purpura in the adult. **3**(3): 160–174.

Chapter 63

Venous Thromboembolism Prevention in Hospitalized Medical and Surgical Patients[§]

Charles E. Mahan,† and Alex C. Spyropoulos‡*

Key Pearls

- Venous thromboembolism (VTE) is a highly preventable disease in both the medical and the surgical patient if the appropriate type, dose and duration of prophylactic agent are used.
- Low molecular weight heparin (LMWH), unfractionated heparin (UFH), fondaparinux, warfarin, and mechanical methods are options to prevent VTE.
- Pharmacologic methods are more effective than mechanical methods.
- A combination of pharmacologic and mechanical is most efficacious.
- VTE prevention programs should be multifaceted, contain perpetual education, have active reminders, utilize clinical decision systems support, contain audit and feedback to providers, and monitor for appropriate and inappropriate use of thromboprophylaxis.

[*]New Mexico Heart Institute; Director, Department of Outcomes Research, 502 Elm Street NE; Albuquerque, New Mexcio, USA.
[†]University of New Mexico College of Pharmacy, Albuquerque, New Mexcio, USA.
[‡]University of Rochester Medical Center, Rochester, New York, USA
[§]We would like to dedicate this article to our loving wives, Dr. Stefanie Mahan and Dr. Jelena Sterio Spyropoulos, as well as to our families who have given us time and support to complete the work.

Epidemiology

Fatal pulmonary embolism (PE) remains the leading cause of preventable death in the hospitalized patient.[1] Despite available data for over 50 years on VTE prevention,[2] appropriate (type, dose, duration) prophylaxis remains suboptimal, with the current rates between 13% and 34%.[3–5] Approximately 25% and 75% of VTE-related deaths in the hospital occur in surgical and nonsurgical patient populations, respectively.[6] Longitudinal studies on both medical and surgical patients have revealed that VTE risk continues for 90 days or more following hospitalization, with a majority of VTEs occurring postdischarge.[7,8] Due to the poor performance of US hospitals, leading US quality entities have prioritized VTE prevention as a key quality measure to better protect patients.[9,10]

The rates of proximal deep vein thrombosis (DVT) and fatal PE are approximately 5% and 0.1%–1.2% in hospitalized medical patients[11–14] and 7%–23% and 0.9%–12.9% in hospitalized surgical patients,[15,16] respectively. The frequency of DVT in the absence of prophylaxis ranges from 10% to 60% in a wide range of patients.[1,14,15] (Table 1).

Risk Factors for Venous Thromboembolism and Risk Assessment Models

Upon hospital presentation, patients have both disease-specific (i.e. exposing) and patient-specific (i.e. predisposing) risk factors that are associated with increased VTE risk.[14] Existing data on individual risk factors have been derived from patient subgroups within placebo-controlled randomized trials or trials where no thromboprophylaxis was utilized. Many risk factors are well-established, and they are included in Tables 2 and 3.[1,14] These risk factors are used primarily in surgical patient groups. In the medical patient, a set of "probable" (significantly associated) and "possible" (not as rigorously studied) risk factors also exist, and they are listed in Table 3.[14]

VTE risk assessment models (RAMs) include "individualized" (one form for all patients based on individual VTE risk factors) or "group-based"

Table 1. Frequency of Deep Vein Thrombosis with Objective Diagnostic Testing in the Absence of Prophylaxis[1,15]

Condition/Patient Group	Risk of DVT
General medical patients	10%–26%
Myocardial infarction	17%–34%
Congestive heart failure	20%–40%
General surgery	15%–40%
Major gynecologic surgery	15%–40%
Major urologic surgery	15%–40%
Neurosurgery	15%–40%
Medical intensive care	25%–42%
Knee or hip arthroplasty, hip fracture surgery	40%–60%

Table 2. ACCPs Well-Established Risk Factors[1]

Surgery
Trauma (major trauma or lower-extremity injury)
Immobility, lower-extremity paresis
Cancer (active or occult)
Cancer therapy (hormonal, chemotherapy, angiogenesis inhibitors, radiotherapy)
Venous compression (tumor, hematoma, arterial abnormality)
Previous VTE
Increasing age
Pregnancy and postpartum period
Estrogen-containing oral contraceptives or hormone replacement therapy
Selective estrogen receptor modulators
Erythropoiesis-stimulating agents
Acute medical illness
Inflammatory bowel disease
Nephrotic syndrome
Myeloproliferative disorders
Paroxysmal nocturnal hemoglobinuria
Obesity
Central venous catheterization
Inherited or acquired thrombophilia

Adapted from Ref. 1.

Table 3. Risk Factors for VTE in Hospitalized Medical Patients[14]

High Risk (i.e. Well-Established)	Probable Risk
• History of DVT or PE	• High-dose estrogen therapy
• Family history of thrombosis	• Obesity (BMI >25)
• Acute infection	• Varicose veins
• Malignancy	• Heparin-induced thrombocytopenia (HIT)
• Age >75 years	• Congenital or acquired thrombophilia
• Congestive heart failure	• Antithrombin deficiency
• Stroke	• Positive lupus anticoagulant
• Myocardial infarction	• Antiphospholipid antibodies
• Prolonged immobility (≥4 days)	• Protein S deficiency
• Pregnancy or postpartum	• Protein C deficiency
• Acute or chronic lung disease	• Positive factor V Leiden
• Acute inflammatory disease	• Elevated anticardiolipin antibodies
• Inflammatory bowel disease	• Positive prothrombin gene mutation 20210A
• Shock	
Possible Risk	
• Paraproteinemia	
• Behcet's disease	
• Disorders of plasminogen and plasminogen activation	
• Nephrotic syndrome	
• Polycythemia	
• Paroxysmal nocturnal hemoglobinuria	
• Elevated serum homocysteine	
• Dysfibrinogenemia	
• Myeloproliferative disorders	
• Age ≥41 years	
• Sepsis (<1 month)	

(organized by diagnoses or clinical characteristics)[1,14] and scoring and computerized support may be used with either model.[1,17] Guidelines currently recommend a group-specific approach for simplicity.[1,15] Multiple RAMs are now available (e.g. Table 4),[17–19] including RAMs to calculate the risk for bleed in medical patients[20] (Table 5). Recent data suggest, however, that risk factors are not equally associated with thrombotic risk, and RAMs listing more risk factors have higher sensitivity.[17] Healthcare appears to be entering a new era, with RAMs being used to identify patients who are at higher risk for bleeding and VTE.[17]

Table 4. Risk Assessment Model: Risk Score Points Assigned to Each Independent VTE Risk Factor in Hospitalized Acutely Ill Medical Patients.

VTE Risk Factor	Points for the Risk Score
Previous VTE	3
Thrombophilia	2
Lower limb paralysis	2
Current cancer	2
Immobilization ≥7 days	1
ICU/CCU stay	1
Age >60 years	1

Abbreviations: ICU — intensive care unit; CCU — coronary care unit.
Scores: 0–1 = low risk; 2–3 = moderate risk; ≥4 = high risk. (Adapted from Ref. 18.)

Table 5. Medical Patients: Bleeding Risk Score Points Assigned to Each Independent Factor Identified with the Multiple Logistic Regression Model[20]

Bleeding Risk Factor in Medical Patients	Points
Moderate renal failure GFR 30–59 versus ≥60 mL/min/m^2	1
Male versus female	1
Age 40–84 versus <40	1.5
Current cancer	2
Rheumatic disease	2
Central venous catheter	2
Intensive care unit / coronary care unit	2.5
Severe renal failure GFR <30 versus ≥60 mL/min/m^2	2.5
Hepatic failure (international normalized ratio >1.5)	2.5
Age ≥85 versus <40	3.5
Platelet count $<50 \times 10^9$ cells/L	4
Bleeding in 3 months before admission	4
Active gastroduodenal ulcer	4.5

GFR = glomerular filtration rate.
Scores of 7 or greater are associated with an exponentially increased risk of major or clinically relevant nonmajor bleeding.
IMPROVE Bleed Risk Calculator available at:http://www.outcomes-umassmed.org/IMPROVE/bleeding_risk_score.cfm

Clinical Data — Primary Studies, Systematic Reviews, and Meta-Analyses

Hundreds of primary studies have been undertaken on medical and surgical patients over the last half-century.[1,15] While medical studies began emerging in the late 1970s and the 1980s, surgical studies began to appear in the 1960s. US quality entities have initiated surgical care VTE measures which have been mandated since 2007, while VTE measures for medical patients are an option for core measure reporting and will likely soon be mandated.

Medical Patients

Despite the many earlier studies, prevention in US medical patients was not widespread until after the placebo-controlled study with enoxaparin (MEDENOX) was published.[13] Compared to no thromboprophylaxis, anticoagulants have reduced the relative risk of DVT by 40%–80% while not significantly increasing bleeding.[1] Studies comparing LMWH and UFH have demonstrated that LMWH is as safe and effective as, if not more effective than, UFH, with one clear advantage being that LMWH causes less injection site hematomas than UFH.[1]

Meta-analyses, Cochrane reviews, and systematic reviews comparing LMWH to UFH in the medical patient have demonstrated that LMWH has either the same or improved major bleeding rates and injection site hematomas, and significantly lower rates (or strong trends) of VTE, proximal DVT, and fewer PE, than UFH.[21–24] The reviews have shown various effects on mortality, with some studies indicating a positive effect or trends,[25] and some no effect.[21,26] Additionally, several analyses on medical patients and one recent review[27] have concluded that TID (thrice daily) UFH is more effective than BID (twice daily) UFH, even if one takes into consideration the increased risk of major bleeding.[21,24,28,29] One niche of BID UFH may be in patients with severe renal failure, as LMWH can accumulate in patients with severely reduced renal function.

Surgical Patients

Guidelines have applicable recommendations for the medical, general-surgical, gynecologic, urologic, laparoscopic, bariatric, thoracic and coronary artery bypass, orthopedic, elective spine, isolated lower extremity, and neurosurgical populations.[1,15] A 2001 meta-analysis demonstrated a positive trend on mortality in surgical patients with LMWH.[30] In addition, higher doses of LMWH demonstrated a higher rate of major bleeding.[30] Overall, in this analysis, LMWH was deemed as safe and effective as UFH. In the surgical patient, heparin-induced thrombocytopenia (HIT) rates with UFH appear to be 3–10-fold higher compared to LMWH. In general, for the moderate-risk surgical population, LMWH is similar in safety and efficacy to UFH. However, for higher-risk surgical patients such as orthopedic patients or patients with multiple risk factors, LMWH appears better than UFH.

Overview of Guideline Recommendations

The American College of Chest Physicians (ACCP) guidelines on the prevention of VTE were published in June of 2008[1] and are the most widely cited guidelines. Table 6 includes current recommendations for VTE prevention in medical and surgical patients.[1] The key guideline points for surgical patients include:

- Warfarin may be used for the orthopedic population, with a target INR of 2.5.[1,15]
- Select mechanical methods may be used alone for total knee replacements (TKRs), gynecologic, urologic, laparoscopic, coronary artery bypass surgical groups, elective spine, and neurosurgery.[1,15]
- LMWH, fondaparinux, and TID UFH are typically options for moderate- and high-risk surgical patients with LMWH, and fondaparinux being preferred to TID UFH in high-risk, and BID UFH as an option in some moderate-risk, surgical groups.[1,15]
- Combination of intermittent pneumatic compression (IPC) and graduated compression stockings (GCSs) with anticoagulants typically provides a 60% further risk reduction in VTE events.[1,15,31]

Table 6. ACCP 8th Edition Levels of VTE Risk and Generally Recommended Thromboprophylaxis Strategies for Hospital Patients[1]

Levels of Risk	Approximate DVT Risk Without Thromboprophylaxis (%)*	Suggested Thromboprophylaxis Strategies
Low risk		
Minor surgery in mobile patients	<10	No specific thromboprophylaxis
Medical patients who are fully mobile		Early and "aggressive" ambulation
Moderate risk		
Most general, open gynecologic or urologic surgery patients	10–40	LMWH (at recommended doses), UFH BID or TID, fondaparinux
Medical patients, bed rest or sick		
Moderate VTE risk plus high bleeding risk		Mechanical thromboprophylaxis†
High risk		
Hip or knee arthroplasty, hip fracture surgery	40–80	LMWH (at recommended doses), fondaparinux, oral vitamin K antagonist (INR 2–3)
Major trauma, spinal cord injury		
High VTE risk plus high bleeding risk		Mechanical thromboprophylaxis†

* Based on objective diagnostic screening for asymptomatic DVT in patients not receiving VTE prophylaxis.

† Mechanical thromboprophylaxis includes intermittent pneumatic compression or venous foot pumps and/or graduated compression stockings. Clinicians should consider switching to anticoagulant thromboprophylaxis when high bleeding risk subsides.

Controversies in VTE Prevention

LMWH vs. UFH

In general, LMWH has demonstrated superior efficacy and safety compared to UFH in primary studies as well as meta-analyses and Cochrane reviews on both medical and surgical patient.[21,22,24,28,32] LMWH has also demonstrated improved efficacy trends in TKR over warfarin, and thus guidelines have given warfarin a lower grade recommendation.[15,16,32] Moreover, UFH has demonstrated increased major and minor bleeding,[21,33–36] increased HIT rates,[1] and requires BID or TID dosing compared to once daily dosing with LMWH.[27] In summary, LMWH should be considered superior to warfarin and UFH due to its efficacy and safety.

Extended Prophylaxis

While extended prophylaxis is well-established in certain surgical groups, such as in major abdominal, pelvic cancer, or major orthopedic surgery,[1,15] clinical trial data on medical patients support only up to 14 days of pharmacologic thromboprophylaxis.[11–13] Further studies are needed to evaluate if other surgical groups may benefit from extended prophylaxis and to determine the optimal duration for medical patients in light of a study favoring extended prophylaxis in patients over 75 years old, those with level 1 mobility (i.e. sedentary without bathroom privileges or on total bedrest), and women.[37]

Mechanical Prophylaxis

Another controversy surrounds the use of mechanical prophylaxis in the medical and the surgical patient. No studies of mechanical methods have shown a reduction in PE or death, and compliance with keeping the mechanical methods applied is low.[1] Currently, mechanical methods should only be utilized[1,15]:

- In at-risk medical patients who are actively bleeding or at high risk for bleeding;
- In surgical groups at high risk for bleeding as recommended by guidelines;
- As an adjunct to pharmacologic prophylaxis.

Systems should be put in place for optimal use of mechanical methods for hospitalized patients, to ensure that compliance is maximized.

Enhancing Hospital Systems to Increase Thromboprophylaxis and Decrease Hospital-Acquired Venous Thromboembolism

Approximately 50 VTE prevention studies have been published to date[17] and recent reviews of these studies[17,38] suggest that programs should be multifaceted; contain perpetual education; have active reminders; utilize clinical decision systems support; contain audit and feedback to providers — especially of those ignoring active reminders; and monitor for appropriate and inappropriate use of thromboprophylaxis.[17] VTE programs are most successful when they are multidisciplinary, with pharmacy-driven programs being favored in studies.[17]

References

1. Geerts WH, Bergqvist D, Pineo GF, *et al.* (2008) Prevention of venous thromboembolism: American College of Chest Physicians Evidence-Based Clinical Practice Guidelines (8th ed.), *Chest* **133**: S381–S453.
2. Sevitt S, Gallagher NG. (1959) Prevention of venous thrombosis and pulmonary embolism in injured patients: A trial of anticoagulant prophylaxis with phenindione in middle-aged and elderly patients with fractured necks of femur. *Lancet* **2**: 981–989.
3. Amin A, Spyropoulos AC, Dobesh P, *et al.* (2010) Are hospitals delivering appropriate VTE prevention? The venous thromboembolism study to assess the rate of thromboprophylaxis (VTE start). *J Thromb Thrombolysis* **29**: 326–339.
4. Amin A, Stemkowski S, Lin J, Yang G. (2007) Thromboprophylaxis rates in US medical centers: Success or failure? *J Thromb Haemost* **5**: 1610–1616.
5. Yu HT, Dylan ML, Lin J, Dubois RW. (2007) Hospitals' compliance with prophylaxis guidelines for venous thromboembolism, *Am J Health Syst Pharm* **64**: 69–76.

6. Geerts WH, Pineo GF, Heit JA, *et al*. (2004) Prevention of venous thromboembolism: The Seventh ACCP Conference on Antithrombotic and Thrombolytic Therapy, *Chest* **126**: S338–S400.
7. Spyropoulos AC, Hussein M, Lin J, Battleman D. (2009) Rates of symptomatic venous thromboembolism in US surgical patients: A retrospective administrative database study, *J Thromb Thrombolysis* **28**: 458–464.
8. Spencer F A, Lessard D, Emery C, *et al*. (2007) Venous thromboembolism in the outpatient setting, *Arch Intern Med* **167**: 1471–1475.
9. SCIP website.
10. NQF website.
11. Cohen AT, Davidson BL, Gallus AS, *et al*. (2006) Efficacy and safety of fondaparinux for the prevention of venous thromboembolism in older acute medical patients: Randomised placebo controlled trial, *BMJ* **332**: 325–329.
12. Leizorovicz A, Cohen AT, Turpie AG. *et al*. (2004) Randomized, placebo-controlled trial of dalteparin for the prevention of venous thromboembolism in acutely ill medical patients, *Circulation* **110**: 874–879.
13. Samama MM, Cohen AT, Darmon JY, *et al*.(1999) A comparison of enoxaparin with placebo for the prevention of venous thromboembolism in acutely ill medical patients. Prophylaxis in Medical Patients with Enoxaparin Study Group. *N Engl J Med* **341**: 793–800.
14. Spyropoulos AC. (2005) Emerging strategies in the prevention of venous thromboembolism in hospitalized medical patients, *Chest* **128**: 958–969.
15. Nicolaides AN, FJ, Kakkar AK, *et al*. (2006) International Consensus Statement, *Int Union Angiol* **25**: 101–161.
16. Mismetti P, Laporte S, Zufferey P, *et al*. (2004) Prevention of venous thromboembolism in orthopedic surgery with vitamin K antagonists: A meta-analysis, *J Thromb Haemost* **2**: 1058–1070.
17. Mahan CE and Spyropoulos AC. (2010) Venous thromboembolism prevention: A systematic review of methods to improve prophylaxis and decrease events in the hospitalized patient, *Hosp Pract (Minneap)* **38**: 97–108.

18. Spyropoulos AC, Anderson FA, Fitzgerald G, *et al.* (2009) Venous thromboembolism risk factors in acutely ill hospitalized medical patients: Findings from the IMPROVE registry, *J Thromb Haemost* **7**: Abstract OC-MO-052.
19. McCaffrey R, Bishop M, Adonis-Rizzo M, *et al.* (2007) Development and testing of a DVT risk assessment tool: Providing evidence of validity and reliability, *Worldviews Evid Based Nurs* **4**: 14–20.
20. Decousus H, Tapson VF, Bergmann JF, *et al.* (2010) Factors at admission associated with bleeding risk in medical patients: Findings from IMPROVE, *Chest*.
21. Wein L, Wein S, Haas SJ, *et al.* (2007) Pharmacological venous thromboembolism prophylaxis in hospitalized medical patients: A meta-analysis of randomized controlled trials, *Arch Intern Med* **167**: 1476–1486.
22. Mismetti P, Laporte-Simitsidis S, Tardy B, *et al.* (2000) Prevention of venous thromboembolism in internal medicine with unfractionated or low-molecular-weight heparins: A meta-analysis of randomised clinical trials, *Thromb Haemost* **83**: 14–19.
23. Alikhan R, Cohen AT. (2003) A safety analysis of thromboprophylaxis in acute medical illness, *Thromb Haemost* **89**: 590–591.
24. Shorr AF, Jackson WL, Sherner JH, *et al.* (2008) Differences between low-molecular-weight and unfractionated heparin for venous thromboembolism prevention following ischemic stroke: A metaanalysis, *Chest* **133**: 149–155.
25. Burleigh E, Wang C, Foster D, *et al.* (2006) Thromboprophylaxis in medically ill patients at risk for venous thromboembolism, *Am J Health Syst Pharm* **63**: S23–S29.
26. Dentali F, Douketis JD, Gianni M, *et al.* (2007) Meta-analysis: Anticoagulant prophylaxis to prevent symptomatic venous thromboembolism in hospitalized medical patients, *Ann Intern Med* **146**: 278–288.
27. Mahan CE, Pini M, Spyropoulos AC. (2010) Venous thromboembolism prophylaxis with unfractionated heparin in the hospitalized medical patient: The case for thrice daily over twice daily dosing, *Intern Emerg Med* **5**: 299–306.

28. Yalamanchili K, Sukhija R, Sinha N, *et al.* (2005) Efficacy of unfractionated heparin for thromboembolism prophylaxis in medical patients, *Am J Ther* **12**: 293–299.
29. King CS, Holley AB, Jackson JL, *et al.* (2007) Twice vs three times daily heparin dosing for thromboembolism prophylaxis in the general medical population: A metaanalysis, *Chest* **131**: 507–516.
30. Mismetti P, Laporte S, Darmon JY, *et al.* (2001) Meta-analysis of low molecular weight heparin in the prevention of venous thromboembolism in general surgery, *Br J Surg* **88**: 913–930.
31. Kakkos SK, Caprini JA, Geroulakos G, *et al.* (2008) Combined intermittent pneumatic leg compression and pharmacological prophylaxis for prevention of venous thromboembolism in high-risk patients, *Cochrane Database Syst Rev*, CD005258.
32. Howard AW and Aaron SD. (1998) Low molecular weight heparin decreases proximal and distal deep venous thrombosis following total knee arthroplasty: A meta-analysis of randomized trials, *Thromb Haemost* **79**: 902–906.
33. Harenberg J, Roebruck P, Heene DL. (1996) Subcutaneous low-molecular-weight heparin versus standard heparin and the prevention of thromboembolism in medical inpatients. The Heparin Study in Internal Medicine Group, *Haemostasis* **26**: 127–139.
34. Kleber FX, Witt C, Vogel G, *et al.* (2003) Randomized comparison of enoxaparin with unfractionated heparin for the prevention of venous thromboembolism in medical patients with heart failure or severe respiratory disease, *Am Heart J* **145**: 614–621.
35. Lechler E, Schramm W, Flosbach CW. (1996) The venous thrombotic risk in non-surgical patients: Epidemiological data and efficacy/safety profile of a low-molecular-weight heparin (enoxaparin). The Prime Study Group. *Haemostasis* **26** (Suppl 2): 49–56.
36. Bergmann JF, Neuhart E. (1996) A multicenter randomized double-blind study of enoxaparin compared with unfractionated heparin in the prevention of venous thromboembolic disease in elderly in-patients bedridden for an acute medical illness. The Enoxaparin in Medicine Study Group. *Thromb Haemost* **76**: 529–534.

37. Hull RD, Schellong SM, Tapson VF, *et al.* (2010) Extended-duration venous thromboembolism prophylaxis in acutely ill medical patients with recently reduced mobility: A randomized trial, *Ann Intern Med* **153**: 8–18.
38. Tooher R, Middleton P, Pham C, *et al.* (2005) A systematic review of strategies to improve prophylaxis for venous thromboembolism in hospitals, *Ann Surg* **241**: 397–415.

Chapter 64

Diagnosis and Treatment of Venous Thromboembolic Disease

Scott Kaatz and David G. Paje**

Key Pearls

- Newly admitted patients who are clinically unlikely to have VTE based on a validated clinical prediction rule and who have a negative *D*-dimer can be safely ruled out for VTE.
- Patients with hemodynamically unstable PE should be treated with systemic thrombolysis or pulmonary embolectomy.
- Patients with hemodynamically stable PE and who do not have significant clinical or cardiac risk factors may be candidates for outpatient treatment or early discharge.
- Parenteral anticoagulants and warfarin should be overlapped for a minimum of five days and parenteral agents should not be stopped until the INR has been above 2.0 for 24 hr.
- Patients with cancer-related VTE should be treated with LMWH for the first 3–6 months.

Introduction

Deep vein thrombosis (DVT) and pulmonary embolism (PE) are different clinical manifestations of venous thromboembolism (VTE), and cause

*Henry Ford Hospital, Wayne State University School of Medicine, Detroit, MI, USA.

substantial morbidity. Over 900,000 patients suffer either an initial or a recurrent VTE each year in the United States.[1] Many patients are admitted for VTE and up to one-third of cases occur while the patients are in the hospital, which makes VTE a common disease that a hospitalist must diagnose and treat.

Diagnosis

Clinical Prediction Rules

An essential prerequisite to the diagnosis of VTE is the estimation of the clinical probability of the disease. If the subsequent test result is discordant with the pretest clinical probability, the diagnosis has to be reconsidered. Clinical prediction rules offer a systematic approach to estimating the probability of disease. Several prediction rules have been developed for DVT and PE. The Wells model (Table 1) has been well validated in randomized diagnostic management trials.[2,3] However, it is important to note that the Wells clinical model was developed as an evaluation tool in the outpatient setting. Thus, it should only be used for patients who are newly admitted or who are in an observation unit. It has limited utility for patients who develop symptoms while already admitted to the hospital, particularly those who have undergone surgery.

If the clinical suspicion for VTE is high, anticoagulation should be initiated promptly while completing diagnostic testing.[4] If the clinical suspicion for VTE is low, then *D*-dimer testing is useful for ruling out VTE.

D-Dimer

D-dimer is a breakdown product of fibrin, and its serum level may be used as a marker for clotting activity. If the clinical probability is low based on prediction rules, VTE may be safely ruled out with a negative *D*-dimer test using a sensitive assay.[2,3] Patients who have a low-probability Wells score and a negative *D*-dimer result and who do not receive anticoagulation have

Table 1. Clinical Model for Predicting Pretest Probability for Pulmonary Embolism

Clinical Feature	Points
Clinical signs and symptoms of DVT (minimum of leg swelling and pain with palpation of the deep vein)	3
An alternative diagnosis is less likely than PE	3
Heart rate greater than 100	1.5
Immobilization or surgery in the previous 4 weeks	1.5
Previous DVT/PE	1.5
Hemoptysis	1
Malignancy (on treatment, treated in the last 6 months, or palliative)	1
Clinical Probability (3 Levels)	**Total**
Low	0–1
Intermediate	2–6
High	≥7
Clinical Probability (2 Levels)	
PE unlikely	0–4
PE likely	>4

DVT = deep vein thrombosis; PE = pulmonary embolism.

only a 1-in-200 risk of VTE being diagnosed within the following three months.[2,3] This simple and inexpensive diagnostic strategy can be applied to approximately one-third of all patients presenting with possible VTE. It is most useful in the emergency department or upon hospital admission when appropriate.

If the Wells score indicates that VTE is unlikely but the *D*-dimer is positive, an imaging modality such as compression ultrasonography (CUS) for DVT or a multidetector computed tomography angiogram (CTA) for PE should be performed. If the Wells score shows that VTE is likely, *D*-dimer testing is not necessary since a CUS or CTA is indicated to evaluate for VTE regardless of the *D*-dimer result. In patients with renal failure, a ventilation–perfusion scan is the preferred alternative to CTA; however, this test can only definitively rule in (high probability) or rule out (normal) PE in 16% of patients.[5] Magnetic resonance imaging is not effective in the diagnosis of PE.[6]

Management of Acute VTE

Parenteral Anticoagulants

Prompt initiation of anticoagulation is required in the acute treatment of VTE. As it takes approximately five days for warfarin to lower serum factor II (prothrombin) to a level that does not promote further clotting, a rapidly acting parenteral anticoagulant is required to provide immediate therapy. It is administered concurrently with warfarin for at least five days and continued until the international normalized ratio (INR) of the prothrombin time is ≥ 2.0 for 24 hr.[4] Options for rapidly acting anticoagulants include unfractionated heparin (UFH), subcutaneous low-molecular-weight heparin (LMWH) and fondaparinux (Table 2).

Cancer-related Thrombosis

Patients with VTE associated with cancer constitute a unique group for which warfarin treatment can be very challenging because of the many potential drug interactions, fluctuating platelet counts, procedures, and dietary changes from chemotherapy-induced nausea. LMWH has been shown to be superior to warfarin for this particular group in terms of more effective prevention of recurrence and a lower bleeding risk. Therefore, patients with cancer-related VTE should receive at least 3–6 months of full therapeutic dose LMWH instead of warfarin.[4]

Warfarin

Age, gender, comorbidities, medications and genetics all influence warfarin dosing. One study on warfarin initiation showed that a starting dose of 5 mg is superior to 10 mg; this trial included predominantly older hospitalized patients.[7] On the other hand, a different study on mostly younger patients in the ambulatory setting favored the 10 mg initial dose.[7] In general, a 5 mg starting dose is recommended for older hospitalized patients with comorbidities. The routine use of pharmacogenomic testing is not recommended[7] until trials show that there is value added to warfarin dosing.

Table 2. Anticoagulant Regimens for Initial Treatment of VTE

Unfractionated heparin (UFH)[a] — preferred if CrCl <30 mL/min

- ***Monitored intravenous*** — 80 U/kg or 5000 U IV bolus, followed by 18 U/kg/hr or 1300 U/hr continuous infusion; aPTT monitored every 6 hrs and adjusted to 1.5–2.5 times control (0.3 – 0.7 IU/mL factor Xa inhibition)
- ***Monitored weight-based subcutaneous*** — 250 U/kg or 17,500 U SC bid; aPTT monitored every 6 hrs and adjusted to 1.5 – 2.5 times control (0.3 – 0.7 IU/mL factor Xa inhibition)
- ***Fixed-dose weight-based subcutaneous*** — 333 U/kg SC once, then 250 U/kg SC bid

Low-molecular-weight heparin (LMWH)

- ***Enoxaparin*** 1 mg/kg SC bid or 1.5 mg/kg SC daily; if CrCl < 30 mL/min, reduce dose to 1 mg/kg SC daily or consider UFH as an alternative
- ***Dalteparin*** 100 IU/kg SC bid or 200 IU/kg SC daily; adjust if CrCl < 30 mL/min
- ***Tinzaparin*** 175 IU/kg SC daily; if CrCl < 30 mL/min, consider UFH as alternative

Fondaparinux[b] — contraindicated if CrCl < 30 mL/min

- BW < 50 kg: 5 mg SC daily
- BW 50–100 kg: 7.5 mg SC daily
- BW > 100 kg: 10 mg SC daily

Initiate VKA at 2.5 – 10 mg/day on the first treatment day and overlap with any of the above parenteral anticoagulants for at least 5 days until the INR is >2.0 for 24 hr.

[a]Monitor platelet count at baseline and every other day from day 4 to day 14 or until heparin is stopped.
[b]No routine platelet monitoring is necessary.
CrCl = creatinine clearance; IV = intravenous; SC = subcutaneous; aPTT = activated partial thromboplastin time; bid = twice daily; BW = body weight; VKA = vitamin K antagonist; INR = international normalized ratio.

Thrombolysis

DVT

The primary reason to use thrombolytics in patients with DVT is to prevent the long-term consequences of postthrombotic syndrome (PTS), which can occur in as much as 50% of patients. Two earlier studies on systemic thrombolysis involving a total of 101 patients, evaluated this outcome in randomized trials,[8] leading to a weak suggestion to consider thrombolysis in highly selected patients, such as those with iliofemoral or extensive proximal DVT.[4] A more recent open-label randomized controlled trial on 209 patinets with iliofemoral DVT showed than the rates of PTS were 56% with conventional anticoagulation treatment alone and 41% with additional catheter-directed thrombolysis (p = 0.047), but there was a small increase in the risk of bleeding.[9] The ATTRACT randomized trial, which should be completed in 2015, is designed to determine if thrombolysis can safely prevent PTS (ClinicalTrials.gov number NCT00790335).

PTS can also be prevented with the use of compression stockings that provide 30–40 mmHg at the ankle, and guidelines recommend their use for at least two years after a DVT.[4] However, the diagnosis of PTS is very subjective and the efficacy of compression stockings has never been evaluated in a blinded randomized trial.

PE

Patients with hemodynamically unstable PE have a mortality rate of 58%, compared to only 15% in patients without shock or sustained hypotension.[10] A systematic review showed a reduction in mortality and recurrent PE in thrombolysis trials that included patients with hemodynamic compromise, but not in trials that excluded these patients.[11] Systemic thrombolysis with a short-acting agent is indicated for patients with hemodynamically unstable PE. Thrombolysis should also be considered in select hemodynamically stable yet high-risk patients (see Fig. 1) who are at low risk of bleeding.[12]

Indicators of poor prognosis in PE include age greater than 75 years, cardiac disease, respiratory disease, cancer, immobility from neurologic disease, ventricular dysfunction on echocardiogram, right ventricular dilatation on CT scan, and elevated troponin or elevated B-type natriuretic peptide.[12] Based on these factors, patients with hemodynamically stable PE may be triaged to the intensive care unit, where thrombolysis can be administered rapidly if the patient deteriorates, or to a general medical ward for continued monitoring and initiation of anticoagulation. Alternatively, outpatient treatment or early discharge may be considered for patients at low risk (see Fig. 1).[12]

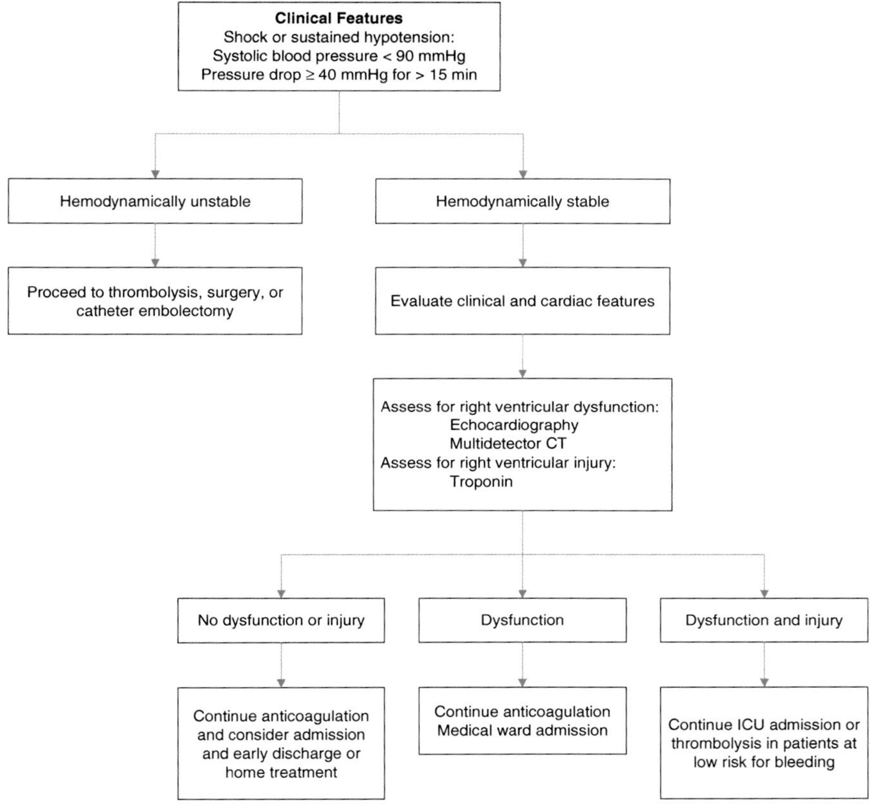

Fig. 1. Clinical management of confirmed acute pulmonary embolism. ICU denotes "intensive care unit." (Adapted from Ref. 12.)

IVC Filters

The routine use of inferior vena cava (IVC) filters for DVT or PE is not recommended. Their use is indicated when anticoagulation therapy is contraindicated, in which case anticoagulation should be started once the increased bleeding risk resolves.[4] In a randomized trial that compared conventional anticoagulation plus an IVC filter to conventional anticoagulation alone, the incidence of PE was reduced at 12 days and at 8 years after filter insertion. However, recurrent DVT increased, and there was no difference in total VTE recurrence at the end of 8 years of followup.[4]

Retrievable filters offer an option of removal if contraindications to anticoagulation therapy are transient, but their efficacy and safety compared to traditional permanent filters have not been adequately evaluated.[4]

Transitions of Care

Guidelines recommend treatment of DVT with LMWH in the outpatient setting whenever possible.[4] Many patients admitted for VTE to the hospital are candidates for early discharge. Important issues when transitioning a patient to postdischarge care that are part of the Joint Commission VTE core measure set include ensuring adequate overlap of warfarin with parenteral anticoagulants for at least five days and until the INR is stable, and providing appropriate patient education on warfarin that covers drug, disease and diet interactions.[7]

The duration of anticoagulation therapy is defined by the clinical scenario in which the index VTE event developed and this can be classified as provoked, cancer-related, idiopathic or recurrent. Provoked VTE, which includes those related to surgery or injury, has a low recurrence rate and requires only three months of treatment.[4] Cancer-related VTE should be treated with LMWH for the first 3–6 months and anticoagulation treatment should continue until the cancer has resolved.[4] Patients with idiopathic (unprovoked) VTE require a minimum of three months of treatment and should be considered for indefinite anticoagulation.[4] Long-term warfarin seems reasonable for patients with recurrent unprovoked VTE. Indefinite anticoagulation may not be necessary for patients with two or more episodes of VTE that were clearly provoked by surgery or injury.[4]

Summary

Clinical prediction rules combined with D-dimer testing provide an inexpensive and rapid way to rule out VTE for many patients presenting to the ED with acute symptoms. Parenteral anticoagulants should be started promptly while completing diagnostic testing if VTE is likely. Most patients with DVT may be treated in an outpatient setting and, if admitted, discharged early from the hospital. Patients with PE should be rapidly assessed for right ventricular strain or injury and then appropriately triaged for possible thrombolytic therapy. Inferior vena cava filters should be reserved for patients with absolute contraindications to anticoagulation. Prior to hospital discharge, warfarin and/or parenteral anticoagulant teaching is mandatory and adequate follow up for INR monitoring must be ensured.

References

1. Heit JA. (2008) The epidemiology of venous thromboembolism in the community. *Arterioscler Thromb Vasc Biol* **28**: 370–372.
2. Wells PS, Anderson DR, Rodger M, *et al.* (2003) Evaluation of *D*-dimer in the diagnosis of suspected deep-vein thrombosis. *N Engl J Med* **349**: 1227–1235.
3. van Belle A, Buller HR, Huisman MV, *et al.* (2006) Effectiveness of managing suspected pulmonary embolism using an algorithm combining clinical probability, *D*-dimer testing and computed tomography. *JAMA* **295**: 172–179.
4. Kearon C, Akl E, Comerota A, *et al.* (2012) Antithrombotic therapy for VTE disease: antithrombotic therapy and prevention of thrombosis, 9th ed: American College of Chest Physicians Evidence-Based Clinical Practice Guidelines. *Chest* **141**: e419S–e494S.
5. The PIOPED Investigators. (1990) Value of the ventilation/perfusion scan in acute pulmonary embolism. Results of the prospective investigation of pulmonary embolism diagnosis (PIOPED). *JAMA* **263**: 2753–2759.
6. Stein PD, Chenevert TL, Fowler SE, *et al.* (2010) Gadolinium-enhanced magnetic resonance angiography for pulmonary embolism: A multicenter prospective study (PIOPED III). *Ann Intern Med* **152**: 434–443, W142–143.7.
7. Ansell J, Hirsh J, Hylek E, *et al.* (2008) Pharmacology and management of the vitamin K antagonists: American College of Chest Physicians Evidence-Based Clinical Practice Guidelines (8th Edition). *Chest* **133**: 160S–198S.

8. Watson LI, Armon MP. (2004) Thrombolysis for acute deep vein thrombosis. *Cochrane Database Syst Rev* CD002783.
9. Enden T, Haig Y, Klow N, *et al*. (2012) Long-term outcomes after additional catheter-directed thrombolysis versus standard treatment for acute iliofemoral deep vein thrombosis (the CaVenT study): a randomised controlled trial. *Lancet* **379**: 31–38.
10. Goldhaber SZ, Visani L, De Rosa M. (1999) Acute pulmonary embolism: clinical outcomes in the International Cooperative Pulmonary Embolism Registry (ICOPER). *Lancet* **353**: 1386–1389.
11. Wan S, Quinlan DJ, Agnelli G, Eikelboom JW. (2004) Thrombolysis compared with heparin for the initial treatment of pulmonary embolism: A meta-analysis of the randomized controlled trials. *Circulation* **110**: 744–749.
12. Agnelli G, Becattini C. (2010) Acute pulmonary embolism. *N Engl J Med* **363**: 266–274.

Chapter 65

Inpatient Management of Sickle Cell Disease

Jeffrey Glassberg and Patricia Shi†*

Key Pearls

- Use hypotonic fluids when managing complications of SCD to decrease the concentration of intracellular hemoglobin S.
- Prompt achievement and maintenance of pain control is important for preventing progression of complications.
- Incentive spirometry during an acute pain episode, particularly with back or chest pain, may prevent acute chest syndrome.
- Supplemental oxygen in the absence of hypoxia may worsen anemia.
- Magnetic resonance imaging is far more sensitive than plain film radiographs for detection of early avascular necrosis (AVN).

Background

Sickle cell disease (SCD) is a group of genetic disorders in which two mutant copies of the β-globin gene are inherited. The substitution of valine for glutamic acid at codon six of the β-globin chain causes production of abnormal hemoglobin (HbS), which polymerizes when deoxygenated to form rigid chains that deform the red blood cell into its

*Mount Sinai School of Medicine, Department of Emergency Medicine, New York, NY, USA.
†Mount Sinai School of Medicine, Department of Medicine, New York, NY, USA.

Table 1. Common Hemoglobin Patterns of Sickle Cell-Related Genotypes

Genotype	% of Hb Type/Total Hb in a Typical Patient				
	HbS	HbA	HbF	HbC	HbA_2
HbAA (normal)	—	96	2	—	2
HbSA (trait)	40	55	2		3
HbSS (severe)	95	—	3	—	2
HbSC (moderate to severe)	48	—	3	47	2
$HbS\beta^0$ (severe)	93	—	2	—	5
$HbS\beta^+$ (moderate)	85	6	5	—	4
$HbS\beta^+$ (mild)	70	23	3	—	4

characteristic sickle shape. These rigid cells cause vaso-occlusion and hemolytic anemia, along with a complex state of inflammation, endothelial dysfunction, and abnormal cell adhesion.[1]

It is important to review a hemoglobin fractionation so as to determine the genotype of SCD (Table 1). In general, the SCD severity varies according to the genotype, with SS and $S\beta^0$ thalassemia being more severe with greater anemia than SC and $S\beta^+$ thalassemia, but there are many exceptions, and higher hematocrit is associated with more frequent pain episodes and avascular necrosis.[2]

Past medical history is important for assessing disease severity and risk of complications during admission. Frequency of acute pain episode hospitalizations, history of acute chest syndrome, renal insufficiency, pulmonary hypertension, and diastolic dysfunction are each associated with increased mortality.[2–4] Red cell units should be leukoreduced and at least phenotype-matched at Cc, Ee, and K red cell antigens, against which African-Americans are most likely to develop alloantibodies. The indications for simple or exchange transfusions are listed in Table 2. Transfusion to a hemoglobin above 10 mg/dL is not indicated, due to the risk of hyperviscosity. Sickle cell patients are at high risk of developing red cell alloantibodies and thus hemolytic transfusion reactions, which may be complicated by hyperhemolysis (where the patient's own red cells are also destroyed). Therefore an increase in hemolysis labs (indirect bilirubin, LDH, AST) or a drop in hemoglobin within two weeks of

Table 2. Indications for Red Cell Transfusion

Simple transfusion

- Transient red cell aplasia
- Symptomatic anemia
- Low and falling hemoglobin with inadequate reticulocytosis (except with hyperhemolysis)
- Hepatic or splenic sequestration
- Moderate-risk surgery

Consider exchange transfusion:

- Acute chest syndrome
- Fat embolism syndrome
- Acute multiorgan failure syndrome
- Stroke
- Retinal artery occlusion
- Priapism
- High-risk surgery

a red cell transfusion mandates a direct antiglobulin (Coomb's) test and repeat type and screen. Importantly, even though hyperhemolysis presents with severe anemia, often a negative direct antiglobulin test, and reticulocytopenia 7–10 days after a transfusion, it is best treated, if possible, by avoidance of further transfusion to avoid worsening the hemolysis. Instead, corticosteroids, IVIg, and erythropoietin are indicated.

Acute Pain Episodes

Acute pain episodes are the most common cause of hospital and ED admissions.[2] Patient assessment should include location, severity, and trigger stimuli such as concurrent infection, emotional or physical stress, dehydration, or asthma exacerbation.[5]

Vaso-occlusion can occur in any vascular bed, but particularly in the bone marrow due to its slow venous flow, and therefore pain in the back and extremity long bones is common.[6] Expeditious treatment may prevent possible progression to *acute multiorgan failure* or *fat embolism syndrome*, the majority of which present initially as simple acute pain

Table 3. Acute Pain Episode Guidelines

- Labs:
  - CBC, reticulocyte count
  - ALT, LDH, fractionated bilirubin if worsened icterus
  - Type and screen if Hb >1 gm/dL below baseline
  - Hypotonic fluids (e.g. D5$^1/_2$– $^1/_4$ NS with 20 mEq KC1/L at 1–1$^1/_2$ times maintenance. Reassess every 24 hrs
- Quickly achieve and maintain pain control with pain management consultation
- Adjuvant analgesic: acetaminophen ± muscle relaxant
- Laxatives: docusate and senna
- Deep venous thrombosis prophylaxis with low molecular weight or standard heparin
- Supplemental oxygen only if needed to keep O_2 saturation ≥92%
- Incentive spirometry, especially with chest or back pain
- Continue outpatient folate and hydroxyurea

episodes.[7, 8] Acute multiorgan failure typically presents with a rapid drop in Hb and platelets accompanied by fever, hypoxia, hepatic dysfunction, and renal insufficiency. Fat embolism syndrome, due to extensive bone marrow infarction and necrosis, typically presents with hypoxemia, non-focal encephalopathy, thrombocytopenia, and skin and mucosal petechiae.

Table 3 shows general management guidelines. Less recognized but important points are to use *hypotonic* fluids because of their beneficial effect on sickling,[9] DVT prophylaxis,[10] and incentive spirometry, especially if the patient is presenting with chest or back pain.[11] Isotonic fluids should be avoided unless the patient is hypovolemic. Supplemental oxygen has been associated with reticulocyte depression severe enough to require transfusion, and thus should be used only if needed to maintain the oxygen saturation > 92%.[12] Consultation with a hematologist is especially recommended with clinical deterioration or pain persisting for more than five days.

A history of pain medication use in the last 24 hours prior to hospital presentation is important. In patients with outpatient opioid prescriptions, emergent hospital presentation usually means that they have failed pain control with oral opioids. Intravenous (IV) opioids (typically morphine, hydromorphone, or fentanyl) should thus be given with the initial dose adjusted for outpatient opioid usage, pain reassessed *every 15–30 min,* and

IV opioids re-dosed until pain is relieved. Hydromorphone has several advantageous features, including its relatively low side effect profile and lack of active metabolites.[10] Pain usually improves after 2 to 3 doses of IV opioids if administered in rapid succession.

Maintenance of initial pain relief usually requires around-the-clock (ATC) dosing and not just on an as needed (PRN) basis, ideally in concert with a pain management team. Two options are listed in Table 4, along with tapering recommendations. Weaning should be withheld during the first 24 hrs of admission and commence early in the morning, not at night when pain tends to be worse.

Adjuvant acetaminophen and muscle relaxants are often helpful for opioid sparing effects. A small randomized trial in adults showed no benefit from ketoprofen,[13] and due to potential nephrotoxicity, treatment with nonsteroidal anti-inflammatory drugs is not recommended for more than 5 days. If transitioning to a long-acting oral opioid, start at least 1–2 days

Table 4. Around-the-Clock Options for Adults (>50 Kg)

Patient controlled analgesia (PCA) with hydromorphone (1 mg/mL)	Base initial dosing on at least the last 4 hr of opioid use. Strongly consider a basal rate, especially at night for sleep and in opioid-tolerant patients. Demand dose: 0.1–0.3 mg q8 mins
Long-acting opioid agonist (controlled-release morphine or oxycodone or transdermal fentanyl)	Base initial dosing on short-acting opioid requirements. Rescue doses equal 10%–15% of the total 24 hr dose or 50% of the 4 hr dose. Rescue opioid should be the same (in immediate release form) as the ATC opioid, available q1–2 hr prn.
Tapering opioids	Wean dose by 10%–20% every 8 hrs as tolerated to keep pain score <5. Once opioid doses 25%–30% of initial level, can switch to equianalgesic oral opioids and consider discharge.

before the date of anticipated discharge to adjust for the 3–4 doses required for steady-state levels.

Acute Chest Syndrome

Acute chest syndrome (ACS) is typically defined by a new infiltrate on chest X-ray, with respiratory symptoms, fever >38.5°C, or chest pain. Often ACS is not the presenting diagnosis, but develops during hospital admission, most frequently for an acute pain episode[14] or following anesthesia. Possible precipitants may be fat embolism from bone marrow infarction, pulmonary infarction, or pneumonia, with the most frequent organisms isolated being *Chlamydia pneumoniae* or *Mycoplasma pneumoniae*.

ACS accompanied by hypoxia with an oxygen saturation <90% or increasing respiratory distress is a strong indication for *red cell transfusion*. Exchange transfusion to achieve a HbA level > 70% is indicated with severe ACS, or where simple transfusion of two red cell units would increase the Hb > 10 gm/dL or Hct > 30%, which is contraindicated due to increased blood viscosity.

Additional important treatment includes optimal pain management, and especially *incentive spirometry* and *pain control* to prevent respiratory splinting. Patients should receive intravenous *antibiotics* with coverage for community-acquired and atypical pneumonia until fever is absent for at least 24 hrs, at which time the patient can be switched to oral antibiotics. *Bronchodilator therapy* is indicated for concurrent airway hyperreactivity.

Hepatobiliary and Splenic Complications

Although vaso-occlusion in the liver sinusoids can cause hepatic crisis and/or sequestration, patients may alternatively have *asymptomatic* hepatomegaly and marked hyperbilirubinemia, (including elevation of direct bilirubin), which often resolves spontaneously within weeks without intervention.[13]

Hepatic Crisis

Typical findings in hepatic crisis are right upper quadrant pain and tenderness, fever, and leukocytosis with variable increases in transaminases (typically >1–3 times ULN) and bilirubin, primarily conjugated. Coagulation parameters are normal. Supportive treatment (Table 2) usually normalizes manifestations in one week. Rarely, there is progression to hepatic ischemia and failure, termed "intrahepatic cholestasis," thus mandating exchange transfusion and repletion of coagulation factors, termed "intrahepatic cholestasis," with fresh frozen plasma, but high mortality remains.

Sequestration

In splenic or hepatic sequestration, vaso-occlusion causes sequestration of a large volume of blood in the affected organ with secondary pain and enlargement, hypotension, and hemoglobin reduction. Splenic sequestration is relatively uncommon in adults (compared to children) due to their larger blood volume, but may be seen in adults with SC or $S\beta^+$ thalassemia due to retained splenic function. In hepatic sequestration, which can occur with any sickle genotype, there are usually increases in liver enzymes, and bilirubinemia (often >20 mg/dL).

Treatment is supportive (Table 2) with simple transfusions for symptomatic anemia. Red cells should be transfused slowly, with reassessment after each unit, because with resolution, red cells re-entering the circulation may cause erythrocytosis, hyperviscosity, and hypervolemia, with possible intracerebral hemorrhage.

Biliary Colic and Cholecystitis

Many patients develop bilirubin gallstones early in life due to chronic hemolysis, but acute cholecystitis is relatively rare due to the small size and friability of bilirubin gallstones. Therefore, mild conjugated hyperbilirubinemia may be seen but without bile duct dilatation or increased alkaline phosphatase. However, any patient presenting with acutely elevated liver function tests requires a right upper quadrant ultrasound to rule out acute cholecystitis. If symptomatic, cholecystectomy should be done electively rather than during an acute obstruction.

Infections

Streptococcus pneumoniae infection in functionally asplenic adults is now relatively uncommon due to vaccination. *Bacteremia* is probably the most common infectious complication (Table 5), usually associated with indwelling central venous catheters but also with urinary tract infections, pneumonia, and infections of the biliary tract.[15] *Osteomyelitis* and *septic arthritis* can also be seen,[16] and orthopedics should be consulted for diagnostic aspiration of swollen joints. Infection of leg ulcers is usually local without underlying bone involvement.

Lastly, worsened anemia due to inadequate reticulocytosis (absolute reticulocyte count $<$50,000/uL) may be due to acute *Parvovirus B19 infection*, confirmed by IgM testing. Treatment is supportive with red cell transfusions, as patients should adequately clear the infection. A rare complication, however, is nephrotic syndrome.

Complications Requiring Immediate Subspecialty Evaluation

Stroke

Adults with SCD have an increased risk of stroke compared to racially matched controls,[17] with hemorrhagic as well as thrombotic strokes seen.

Table 5. Typical Organisms Isolated with Infections

Central venous catheter–associated bacteremia	Coag-negative Staphylococci > *Staphylococcus aureus* > gram-negative bacilli
Non-catheter-associated bacteremia	Gram-negative bacilli > gram-positive cocci > anaerobes
Osteomyelitis	*Salmonella*
Septic arthritis	*Staphylococcus aureus*, gram-negative bacilli

Management is the same as without SCD. Immediate neurologic/neurosurgical evaluation should be obtained. In addition, *exchange transfusion* to reduce the hemoglobin S level to < 30% may be indicated, especially in thrombotic strokes.

Priapism

Priapism is caused by vaso-occlusion in the corpora cavernosa. Physical exam reveals a hard penis with soft glans. If not rapidly treated, fibrosis and impotence may result. Treat with *hypotonic saline, analgesics,* and *encouragement to urinate* while awaiting immediate urologic consultation. If aspiration from the corporus cavernosa followed by irrigation with dilute epinephrine fails, exchange transfusion should be considered. Anecdotal association with neurologic events such as seizures or stroke (the ASPEN syndrome) is probably related to acute increases in blood viscosity, avoidable by targeting a post-procedure hematocrit close to the patient's baseline.

Eye Trauma

Direct eye trauma may cause bleeding into the anterior chamber, where sickle erythrocytes can occlude the trabecular channels, causing increased intraocular pressure and acute glaucoma. Immediate ophthalmologic consultation is required.

Special Topics

Pregnancy

Patients should not be discouraged from desired pregnancy, as maternal mortality is low despite increased risks of hypertension, pre-eclampsia, pain crises (especially 3rd trimester), and infections such as pyelonephritis. Preconception consultation with a maternal fetal medicine specialist is standard of care.[18] Overall fetal outcome is also good with >90% of infants having Apgar scores >7[19, 20] despite increased risks compared to race-matched controls of miscarriage or stillborn births, preterm delivery, and infants born with low birth weight or small for gestational age.

Hydroxyurea should be discontinued once pregnancy is confirmed due to its potential teratogenic effects. Referral to a high-risk obstetrician experienced in sickle cell disease is mandatory. Prophylactic transfusions generally are only considered with pre-eclampsia, symptomatic anemia, severely worsened sickle cell manifestations, or multiple gestations. Patients have an increased risk of C-section delivery, and postpartum early ambulation and prophylaxis with heparin is advised due to increased risk of venous thromboembolism in sickle cell disease.

Avascular Necrosis

Magnetic resonance imaging is far more sensitive than plain film radiographs for detection of early avascular necrosis (AVN). Symptomatic AVN is an indication for intervention, as 98% of hips will progress to femoral head collapse, the majority within five years of symptoms.[21] Even asymptomatic AVN has a risk of progression as high as 80%.[22] Symptoms of AVN are pain in the groin, thigh, or buttock with weight-bearing and motion, but often even at rest. Core decompression significantly prolongs hip survival when done at Steinberg stage I and II disease. Improvements in the care of sickle cell patients with total hip arthroplasty have led to a current short- and long-term orthopedic complication rate of approximately 10% compared to the 30%–50% historically reported.[23]

Perioperative Care to a Hb of 10 g/dL

Pre-op transfusion is recommended for surgeries requiring general anesthesia other than low-risk procedures such as dilation and curettage. Common surgical procedures requiring general anesthesia in adults are cholecystectomy for gallstones and orthopedic procedures such as core decompression and joint replacement. Even with preoperative transfusion,

Table 6. Perioperative Care Guidelines

- Hydration: A minimum of 8 hr preoperative hydration as well as postoperative hydration as tolerated
- Preoperative transfusion:
  - Only antigen-matched blood should be used;
  - With SS, Sβthal^0, or SC genotypes, simple transfusion is indicated for all but the lowest-risk procedures with a target Hb of 10 mg/dL;
  - For high-risk surgery (e.g. cardiothoracic, major abdominal, neurosurgical, prolonged anesthesia time), exchange transfusion may be indicated.
- Temperature: Keep patients warm perioperatively, as hypothermia will increase the risk of sickling.
- Oxygenation: Careful monitoring of oxygenation and oxygen saturation perioperatively, along with incentive spirometry postoperatively
- Pain control with patient controlled analgesia

up to 30% of patients still have postoperative complications, with the most common being acute painful episodes and acute chest syndrome.[24–26] Patients with poor cardiopulmonary status or undergoing high-risk surgeries (e.g. severe pulmonary hypertension, interstitial lung disease or myocardial dysfunction) should be considered for exchange rather than simple transfusion.

Acknowledgment

The authors thank Dr. Stelian Serban, (Director, Pain Service), and Jay Horton, (Clinical Program Manager, Palliative Care), for critical review of the opioid recommendations.

References

1. Conran N, Franco-Penteado CF, Costa FF. (2009) Newer aspects of the pathophysiology of sickle cell disease vaso-occlusion. *Hemoglobin* **33**: 1–16.

2. Platt OS, Thorington BD, Brambilla DJ, *et al.* (1991) Pain in sickle cell disease. Rates and risk factors. *N Engl J Med* **325**: 11–16.
3. Platt OS, Brambilla DJ, Rosse WF, *et al.* (1994) Mortality in sickle cell disease. Life expectancy and risk factors for early death. *N Engl J Med* **330**: 1639–1644.
4. Sachdev V, Machado RF, Shizukuda Y, *et al.* (2007) Diastolic dysfunction is an independent risk factor for death in patients with sickle cell disease. *J Am Coll Cardiol* **49**: 472–479.
5. Field JJ, DeBaun MR. (2009) Asthma and sickle cell disease: Two distinct diseases or part of the same process? *Hematology Am Soc Hematol Educ Program* 45–53.
6. McClish DK, Smith WR, Dahman BA, *et al.* (2009) Pain site frequency and location in sickle cell disease: The PiSCES project. *Pain* **145**: 246–251.
7. Hassell KL, Eckman JR, Lane PA. (1994) Acute multiorgan failure syndrome: A potentially catastrophic complication of severe sickle cell pain episodes. *Am J Med* **96**: 155–162.
8. Dang NC, Johnson C, Eslami-Farsani M, Haywood LJ. (2005) Bone marrow embolism in sickle cell disease: A review. *Am J Hematol* **79**: 61–67.
9. Guy RB, Gavrilis PK, Rothenberg SP. (1973) *In vitro* and *in vivo* effect of hypotonic saline on the sickling phenomenon. *Am J Med* Sci **266**: 267–277.
10. Austin H, Key NS, Benson JM, *et al.* (2007) Sickle cell trait and the risk of venous thromboembolism among blacks. *Blood* **110**: 908–912.
11. Bellet PS, Kalinyak KA, Shukla R, *et al.* (1995) Incentive spirometry to prevent acute pulmonary complications in sickle cell diseases. *N Engl J Med* **333**: 699–703.
12. Lane PK, Embury SH, Toy PT. (1988) Oxygen-induced marrow red cell hypoplasia leading to transfusion in sickle painful crisis. *Am J Hematol* **27**: 67–68.
13. Bartolucci P, El Murr T, Roudot-Thoraval F, *et al.* (2009) A randomized, controlled clinical trial of ketoprofen for sickle-cell disease vaso-occlusive crises in adults. *Blood* **114**: 3742–3747.

14. Vichinsky EP, Neumayr LD, Earles AN, *et al.* (2000) Causes and outcomes of the acute chest syndrome in sickle cell disease. National Acute Chest Syndrome Study Group. *N Engl J Med* **342**: 1855–1865.
15. Chulamokha L, Scholand SJ, Riggio JM, *et al.* (2006) Bloodstream infections in hospitalized adults with sickle cell disease: A retrospective analysis. *Am J Hematol* **81**: 723–728.
16. Hernigou P, Daltro G, Flouzat-Lachaniette CH, *et al.* (2010) Septic arthritis in adults with sickle cell disease often is associated with osteomyelitis or osteonecrosis. *Clin Orthop Relat Res* **468**: 1676–1681.
17. Strouse JJ, Jordan LC, Lanzkron S, Casella JF. (2009) The excess burden of stroke in hospitalized adults with sickle cell disease. *Am J Hematol* **84**: 548–552.
18. Barfield WD, Barradas DT, Manning SE, *et al.* Sickle cell disease and pregnancy outcomes: Women of African descent. *Am J Prev Med* **38**: S542–S549.
19. Smith JA, Espeland M, Bellevue R, *et al.* (1996) Pregnancy in sickle cell disease: Experience of the Cooperative Study of Sickle Cell Disease. *Obstet Gynecol* **87**: 199–204.
20. Barfield WD, Barradas DT, Manning SE, *et al.* (2010) Sickle cell disease and pregnancy outcomes: Women of African descent. *Am J Prev Med* **38**: S542–S549.
21. Hernigou P, Bachir D, Galacteros F. (2003) The natural history of symptomatic osteonecrosis in adults with sickle-cell disease. *J Bone Joint Surg Am* **85**A: 500–504.
22. Hernigou P, Habibi A, Bachir D, Galacteros F. (2006) The natural history of asymptomatic osteonecrosis of the femoral head in adults with sickle cell disease. *J Bone Joint Surg Am* **88**: 2565–2572.
23. Hernigou P, Zilber S, Filippini P, *et al.* (2008) Total THA in adult osteonecrosis related to sickle cell disease. *Clin Orthop Relat Res* **466**: 300–308.
24. Vichinsky EP, Haberkern CM, Neumayr L, *et al.* (1995) A comparison of conservative and aggressive transfusion regimens in the perioperative management of sickle cell disease. The Preoperative Transfusion in Sickle Cell Disease Study Group. *N Engl J Med* **333**: 206–213.

25. Koshy M, Weiner SJ, Miller ST, *et al.* (1995) Surgery and anesthesia in sickle cell disease. Cooperative Study of Sickle Cell Diseases. *Blood* **86**: 3676–3684.
26. Al-Mulhim AS, Al-Mulhim AA. (2009) Laparoscopic cholecystectomy in 427 adults with sickle cell disease: A single-center experience. *Surg Endosc* **23**: 1599–1602.

Chapter 66

Transfusion Medicine

*Patricia Shi**

Key Pearls

- Avoid unnecessary transfusions, so as to reduce the risk of transfusion-related morbidity and mortality.
- Premedication for transfusion is usually unnecessary in the absence of a transfusion reaction history and may mask early signs of a reaction.
- Blood bank physicians can assist with diagnosis and management of transfusion-related problems.
- The five most frequent causes of transfusion-related deaths are: transfusion-related acute lung injury, hemolytic transfusion reactions, transfusion-associated sepsis, and transfusion-associated circulatory overload.
- Understand the indications for special processing of cellular blood components.

Background

One of the most important functions of the blood bank is to prevent the occurrence of immune-mediated hemolytic transfusion reactions. Hemolytic transfusion reactions are caused by a mismatch of red cell antigens between the donor and the recipient. The ABO system is a group of carbohydrate antigens (A, B, O) defined by their terminal saccharide moiety. It is the most important blood group system in transfusion, because, unlike

*Department of Medicine, Mount Sinai School of Medicine, New York, NY, USA.

other red cell alloantibodies, antibodies to ABO antigens that are absent on one's own cells are spontaneously produced. These IgM antibodies are able to fix complement efficiently and cause acute intravascular hemolytic transfusion reactions. The Rh blood group system is next in importance, and encodes protein antigens, the most important of which is the D antigen, because it is highly immunogenic. Approximately 80% of D-negative individuals exposed to D develop anti-D alloantibody which can cause hemolytic transfusion reactions and hemolytic disease of the newborn.

A routine procedure in blood banking is to type donor blood products and recipients for the ABO and D antigens. "Forward" typing is performed to detect the presence of A, B, and D antigens on donor or recipient red cells using reagent anti-A, anti-B, and anti-D. "Reverse" typing is also performed to confirm the forward ABO type by detecting the presence of anti-A and anti-B in recipient serum only using commercially available reagent red cells.

Due to transfusion or pregnancy, recipients can develop red cell alloantibodies to other clinically relevant red cell antigens, most commonly in the Rh, Kell, Kidd, Duffy, and MNS systems. Therefore routine blood banking procedure also includes an antibody screen to detect such alloantibodies in the recipient's serum.

Finally, routine blood banking procedure also includes a crossmatch, where patient plasma is mixed with the actual selected donor unit. The crossmatch serves as a final confirmation of ABO incompatibility and can detect antibodies to low-incidence antigens that may be missed on the antibody screen.

Additional Compatibility Issues

Routine type, screen, and crossmatch take 45–60 minutes to complete, and if alloantibodies are detected, matching antigen-negative units for that patient may take over 24 hours. With severe transfusion emergencies, uncrossmatched, group O, Rh-negative red cells can be administered, but at the increased risk of non-ABO hemolytic transfusion reactions. If possible, the 15–20 min required for at least an ABO typing and crossmatch is recommended. Table 1 summarizes ABO compatibility between the patient

Table 1. Recipient Compatibility with Donor Blood Components

Patient ABO Group	Packed Red Blood Cells	Platelets*	Plasma
O	O	O	O > A > B > AB
A	A > O	A	A > AB
B	B > O	B	B > AB
AB	AB > A > B > O	AB	AB

*ABO matching of platelets is not required, but preferred to avoid potential hemolysis from passive transfer of ABO antibodies in plasma.

recipient and the blood product. Of note is that O patients can receive only O red cells but any ABO plasma, whereas AB patients can receive any ABO red cells but only AB plasma.

In addition to type and screen and crossmatch testing, other commonly ordered tests are:

(1) *Direct antigloblin test (direct Coombs test).* Commercial anti-IgG and anti-C3 are used to detect IgG and complement component C3d directly attached to red cells. This test is used to confirm a hemolytic transfusion reaction or autoimmune hemolytic anemia. A positive test may also be seen without any active hemolysis; for example, with hypergammaglobulinemia or after IVIG or WinRho®.

(2) *Platelet antibody screen.* Patient plasma is screened for the presence of antibodies, which may be produced due to previous transfusion or pregnancy, against platelet-specific and HLA antigens. This test should be ordered to confirm immune refractoriness to platelet transfusion. A positive test is defined by a corrected count increment <5000 (or, more roughly, a platelet count increase of <10,000/μL) within 1 hr of at least two ABO-compatible platelet transfusions. If the test is positive, the blood bank should obtain crossmatch-compatible platelets, or, in the case of only HLA antibodies, HLA-compatible or HLA-matched platelets.

Blood Components

In general, infusing any medications or solutions other than isotonic normal saline (0.9% USP), 5% albumin, or plasma through the same tubing with blood or components is contraindicated, due to potential life-threatening hemolysis or agglutination. The rate of infusion is guided by patient tolerance, but generally 100–300 mL/hr is recommended. Platelets can be transfused over 30 min if clinically tolerable. Any blood product must be infused within 4 hr of blood bank release, owing to the risk of bacterial growth. Descriptions and indications for commonly used blood products are listed in Table 2.[1–3]

The platelet transfusion threshold for prophylaxis is generally <10,000/μL, but might need to be ~20,000/μL with qualitative platelet dysfunction as in uremia, coagulopathy, severe uncorrected anemia, fever,

Table 2. Common Indications for Routine Blood Products

Blood Component	Indications	Average Product Volume (Dose)	Expected Increase
1 packed red blood cells (PRBCs) unit	Hb <7 g/dL* Hct <21%	300 mL 200 mL is red cells	Hb: 1 g/dL Hct: 3%
1 single donor platelet unit or 1 pool of whole-blood-derived platelets (4–6 units)	Prophylaxis: < 10,000/μL < 50,000/μL if invasive procedure or surgery or active bleeding < 100,000/μL neurosurgery	200–400 mL ~3 × 10^{11} platelets	30–50,000/μL
1 fresh frozen or thawed† plasma unit	INR > 1.5 prior to invasive procedure Bleeding coagulopathy	200 mL Coag. factors 1 U/ml Fibrinogen 2–4 mg/mL	10 mL/kg increases factor levels by ~25%
1 cryoprecipitate pool (usually 5 units)	Fibrinogen < 100 mg/dL with bleeding Factor XIII deficiency	15 mL FVIII ≥ 80 IU Fibrinogen 150 mg	~7 mg/dL increase in fibrinogen per unit

* Higher Hb[7–9] may be indicated with cardiopulmonary or cerebrovascular risk factors.

† Same coagulation factor content as fresh frozen except for reduced factors V and VIII.

uncontrolled hypertension, or acute pulmonary processes. Less commonly used blood products should be ordered with blood bank consultation, and include: *granulocyte* transfusions for neutropenia refractory to antibiotics, *Rh immune globulin* for Rh-negative recipients exposed to Rh-positive transfusions, and *recombinant factor VII* or *prothrombin complex concentrate* for coagulopathy.

Cellular blood components (red cell and platelet units) should be further processed for various indications, as outlined in Table 3.

Table 3. Indications for Further Processing of Cellular Blood Components

Processing	Indications	Examples of Indicated Recipients
Leukoreduction	• Prevention of febrile nonhemolytic reactions • Reduction in HLA alloimunization risk • Reduction in platelet refractoriness risk • Reduction in CMV transmission risk • Mortality reduction in cardiac surgery[4]	• History of recurrent febrile reactions • Potential and current transplant recipients • Platelet-transfusion-dependent • CMV-negative and immunosuppressed • Cardiac surgery patients
Irradiation	Elimination of transfusion-associated graft-versus-host disease risk	• Bone marrow transplant recipients • Hematologic malignancies • Treatment with nucleoside analog drugs • Congenital immunodeficiencies
Washing	Prevention of severe allergic or anaphylactic reactions	• IgA-deficient recipients • History of anaphylaxis or recurrent severe allergic reactions
Volume reduction	• Applicable mainly to platelet units • Reduction in circulatory overload risk	• Recipients with congestive heart failure, renal insufficiency; elderly

Table 4. Description and Management of Acute Transfusion Reactions by the Main Symptom

	Cause	Differentiating Signs/Symptoms	Management
Fever			
Acute hemolytic	Incompatible red cells or plasma	Hemoglobinemia and -uria	Confirm with repeat type and screen, direct antiglobulin test. Support blood pressure, renal function, DIC coagulopathy.
Septic	Bacterial contamination of platelets (usually gram-positive) or red cells (usually gram-negative)	Hypotension	Broad spectrum antibiotics pending gram stain and culture
Febrile	Donor unit cytokines or patient antileukocyte Abs	Hypertension	Demerol Prevention: acetaminophen or leukoreduction (Table 3)
Dyspnea			
Tranfusion-related acute lung injury	Donor antileukocyte Abs or lipids/cytokines in unit activate patient neutrophils	Within 6 hr of transfusion Fever Bilateral lung infiltrates Hypotension	Oxygen, pressors Steroids/diuretics not indicated Prevention: donor exclusion, leukoreduction[5]
Circulatory overload	Volume infused too much or too fast	Jugular venous distension Hypertension	Diuretics Prevention: volume reduction (Table 3)
Anaphylactoid	IgA deficiency with anti-IgA, hypersensitivity to donor allergens	Clear CXR Hypotension	Epinephrine, antihistamines, IV steroids
Hives			
Allergic	Hypersensitivity to donor allergens	Facial edema	Prevention: washing (Table 3) Antihistamine, steroids

Transfusion Reactions

Any adverse event due to a blood transfusion is regarded as a transfusion reaction.[1] Acute transfusion reactions generally occur during or within 4–6 hr of transfusion (Table 4). Despite routine antibody screening, an alloantibody may not be detected because of low titer or absence of its corresponding antigen on reagent red cells.

When an acute transfusion reaction occurs, the transfusion should be immediately stopped, a transfusion reaction report completed, posttransfusion samples collected, and the unit and attached tubing returned to the blood bank. Delayed transfusion reactions (Table 5) generally occur 1–2 weeks after transfusion, so recognition of transfusion as the cause is key.

Special Situations

Table 6 lists guidelines for management of special transfusion situations. Indications for red cell transfusion in hospitalized patients with sickle cell disease are discussed in a separate chapter. Platelet transfusions are generally ineffective in untreated idiopathic thrombocytopenic purpura and relatively

Table 5. Description and Management of Delayed Hemolytic Transfusion Reactions

	Cause	Major Signs/ Symptoms	Management
Delayed hemolytic	Anamnestic alloantibody to donor red cell antigens	Decreased hematocrit, elevated indirect bilirubin, usually 5–10 days posttransfusion	Supportive care. Confirm with type and screen and direct antiglobulin test.
Transfusion-associated graft-versus-host disease	Donor lymphocytes attack immuno-suppressed recipient	Fever, pancytopenia, skin rash, hepatitis, diarrhea	Supportive care. Consult hematology–oncology.
Posttransfusion purpura	Anamnestic allo/auto-antibody to donor platelets	Severe thrombocytopenia within 3 weeks of transfusion	Intravenous gammaglobulin/ steroids. Consult blood bank for alloantigen-negative platelets.

Table 6. Description and Management of Special Transfusion Situations

	Description	Important Clinical Points	How to Dose
Massive transfusion	Potential coagulopathy with ≥10 RBC unit bleed over 24 hr	Monitor for hypocalcemia due to citrate accumulation with liver dysfunction.	Monitor PT, aPTT, fibrinogen, platelets. 1 unit of FFP = 2 units of cryoprecipitate.
Emergent warfarin reversal	Fresh frozen plasma indicated only for serious bleeding[6]	For emergent reversal or volume issue, also consider prothrombin complex concentrate or recombinant factor VIIa.	Fresh frozen plasma: 10–15 cc/kg. Prothrombin complex concentrate: 25–50 IU/kg. Factor VIIa: consult hematology.
Reversal of platelet inhibitor drugs	Recommended only for bleeding and not prophylaxis[7]	Platelet inhibition irreversible with aspirin/ADP antagonists but not GPIIb/IIIa inhibitors.	Time platelet transfusion past half-life of active drug and last drug dose.
Platelet refractoriness	Confirm with platelet Ab screen after within 1 hr platelet count inadequate post-ABO-matched transfusions × 2	Possibilities are cross-matched, HLA-matched, or HLA-compatible units: consult with blood bank about best option.	Advance order needed for matched units. Leukoreduction to reduce further HLA alloimmunization.
Autoimmune hemolytic anemia	Indirect and direct antiglobulin tests to differentiate between warm and cold Abs	Test sample must be kept warm throughout transport to blood bank.	Transfuse slowly (~50 mL/hr) for first 15 min to observe for ↑ hemolysis due to undetected alloantibodies.
ABO-incompatible bone marrow transplants	• Hemolysis with minor incompatibility • Delayed red cell engraftment with major incompatibility	Blood must be ABO-compatible with both ABO types until recipient ABO type completely converts to donor and DAT is negative.	Blood bank should release dual ABO-compatible blood product as indicated by testing. Irradiation of all cellular blood products.

contraindicated in thrombotic thrombocytopenia purpura (TTP) and heparin-induced thrombocytopenia. If plasma exchange is not immediately available for TTP, simple transfusion of fresh frozen plasma (FFP) 15–30 mL/kg daily is indicated as a temporizing measure.

Therapeutic Apheresis Considerations

Table 7 lists important considerations in apheresis and more common category I (i.e. first-line therapy) indications for therapeutic apheresis.[8] Expeditious consultation with the blood bank to assess the need for

Table 7. Therapeutic Apheresis Guidelines

Preapheresis Arrangements	Important Clinical Points	Common Category I Indications
Arrange for catheter placement. Obtain patient weight; current CBC, PT, and aPTT; active type and screen; order for blood products from Blood Bank	• Withhold ACE inhibitors for 24 hr preapheresis, due to bradykinin inhibition. • Plasma exchange may ↓ platelet count, fibrinogen, immunoglobulins. • Dose crucial medications postapheresis if possible. • Citrate (not heparin) is used for anticoagulation and may cause hypocalcemia.	*Plasmapheresis*: TTP Ticlopidine/clopidogrel microangiopathy Various neurologic syndromes* Goodpasture's syndrome Wegener's granulomatosis Recurrent focal segmental glomerulosclerosis Cryoglobulinemia Hyperviscosity syndrome Wilson's disease Humoral kidney rejection *Red cell exchange*: Sickle cell disease indications High red cell parasitemia *Cytapheresis*: Leukostasis Erythrocytosis Thrombocytosis

*Guillain–Barre syndrome, chronic inflammatory demyelinating polyneuropathy, myasthenia gravis, paraproteinemic polyneuropathies.

central venous catheter placement is recommended, as delay in adequate venous access is often the main barrier to initiating treatment.

Acknowledgment

The author would like to thank Dr. Benjamin Greco, Medical Director at NYBC, for his careful review of the chapter.

References

1. *Circular of Information for the Use of Human Blood and Blood Components*, 2009 (accessed Oct. 10, 2010) at http://www.aabb.org/resources/bct/pages/ aabb_coi.aspx#blood.
2. Slichter SJ. (2007) Evidence-based platelet transfusion guidelines. *Hematol Am Soc Hematol Educ Program* **2007**: 172–178.
3. Roback JD, Caldwell S, Carson J, *et al.* (2010) Evidence-based practice guidelines for plasma transfusion. *Transfusion* **50**: 1227–1239.
4. Romano G, Mastroianni C, Bancone C, *et al.* (2010) Leukoreduction program for red blood cell transfusions in coronary surgery: Association with reduced acute kidney injury and in-hospital mortality. *J Thorac Cardiovasc Surg* **140**: 188–195.
5. Blumberg N, Heal JM, Gettings KF, *et al.* (2010) An association between decreased cardiopulmonary complications (transfusion-related acute lung injury and transfusion-associated circulatory overload) and implementation of universal leukoreduction of blood transfusions. *Transfusion.*
6. Ansell J, Hirsh J, Hylek E, *et al.* (2008) Pharmacology and management of the vitamin K antagonists: American College of Chest Physicians Evidence-Based Clinical Practice Guidelines (8th Edition). *Chest* **133**: S160–S198.
7. Lecompte T, Hardy JF. (2006) Antiplatelet agents and perioperative bleeding. *Can J Anaesth* **53**: S103–S112.
8. Szczepiorkowski ZM, Winters JL, Bandarenko N, *et al.* (2010) Guidelines on the use of therapeutic apheresis in clinical practice — evidence-based approach from the Apheresis Applications Committee of the American Society for Apheresis. *J Clin Apher* **25**: 83–177.

Rheumatology

Chapter 67

Acute Arthritis

Ruchi Jain[†] *and Peter D. Gorevic*[*]

Key Pearls

- The cause of acute arthritis can be determined in most instances by a detailed history and physical examination, laboratory testing, radiologic studies, and synovianalysis.
- Arthritis should be defined as to onset, pattern of development, aggravating factors, and number of joints involved: monoarticular (1 joint), oligoarticular (1–4 joints), or polyarticular (more than 4 joints).
- What is perceived as "arthritis" may originate from periarticular structures such as tendon sheaths, bursae, or muscles.
- Synovianalysis distinguishes between inflammatory and noninflammatory causes of acute arthritis, is the "gold standard" for the diagnosis of crystal arthropathy, and is critical to the proper workup of septic arthritis.
- Acute gout, pseudogout, and infection are the most common causes of acute attacks of monoarthritis in the hospitalized patient.

Introduction

Arthritis is a significant cause of acute and chronic disability in the inpatient setting. The hospitalist plays a central role in the initial evaluation of

*Mount Sinai Medical Center, New York, NY, USA.
†Montefiore Medical Center, Bronx, NY, USA.

such patients, and can orchestrate diagnostic workups and treatments in-hospital, as well as coordinate posthospitalization care. Osteoarthritis (OA) and crystal arthropathy are particularly prevalent among the geriatric inpatient population, and may significantly impact length-of-stay and convalescence. Acute arthritis is especially challenging in the critically ill patient who is immunosuppressed, has portals for infection, is receiving polypharmacy, and is susceptible to fastidious organisms.[1–3] The cause of acute arthritis can be determined by a detailed history and physical examination, appropriate laboratory testing, radiographic studies, and synovianalysis.

The Spectrum of Inpatient Rheumatology Consultations

Inpatient consultations for acute arthritis often vary with the hospital setting (e.g. community-based, referral, VA), geography, and demographics. Table 1 compares a recent (2009–2010) experience at Mount Sinai Medical Center in New York City with an earlier (1994–2003) report from the VA and University Hospitals affiliated with the University of Washington. In both series, 38% of consultations were for "arthritis," with the remainder being for systemic disease. Approximately 40% of consults were for acute

Table 1. Inpatient Consultations (University Hospitals)

Nature of Consults	University of Washington (1994–2003)	Mount Sinai Medical Center (2009–2010)
Total number of consults	1409	324
Arthritis	632 (38%)	122 (38%)
Monoarticular		49/122 (40%)
Oligoarticular		35/122 (29%)
Polyarticular		37/122 (30%)
Crystal arthropathy	197 (14%)	68/122 (56%)
Mechanical/osteoarthritis	111 (8%)	21/122 (17%)
Septic arthritis	70 (5%)	5/122 (4%)

Ref 7.

monoarticular arthritis at the New York City hospital, which reflected a higher (56% versus 14%) representation of acute monoarthritis and crystal arthropathy compared to the University of Washington hospitals. Longitudinal studies at the University of Washington showed a decreasing incidence of rheumatoid arthritis from 13% to 5% over the 10 year sampling, possibly reflecting improving therapies for this disease. Septic arthritis (4%–5%) and OA (8%–17%) accounted for a similar representation in both series.

Initial Approach

Patterns of Joint Disease

Acute arthritis causes pain, swelling, and loss of function. It should be defined as to *onset* (insidious, subacute, or chronic), *pattern of development* (symmetrical or asymmetrical, proximal or distal, single event or occurring in the setting of intermittent episodes), *aggravating factors* (recent surgery, change in medications, trauma), and *number of joints involved*: monoarticular (1 joint), oligoarticular (1–4 joints), or polyarticular (>4 joints). In the inpatient setting, the most important causes of monoarticular arthritis are infection and the crystal arthropathies (gout and pseudogout) (Table 2). Asymmetrical oligoarticular joint symptoms are seen in lyme disease, spondyloarthropathies, and crystal-induced arthritides. Polyarticular symptoms occur in established rheumatic disease, with the pattern of distribution being suggestive of specific diagnoses [e.g. distal interphalangeal and carpometacarpal involvement in OA, or proximal interphalangeal and metacarpophalangeal involvement in rheumatoid arthritis (RA)].

Mimics of Acute Arthritis

The predominating complaint may be pain, inflammation, or both, with the relative contribution of each varying considerably even among patients with established disease. "Arthritis" pain may be periarticular,

Table 2. Patterns of Acute Arthritis

Monoarticular	Oligoarticular	Polyarticular
Trauma (may be very rapid in onset)	Spondyloarthropathies: ankylosing spondylitis, psoriatic arthritis, colitic arthritis — all often with axial involvement)	RA. other connective tissue diseases
Noninflammatory: osteoarthritis	Migratory: rheumatic fever, sarcoidosis	Infections: gonococcus, hepatitis C
Infection (consider risk factors, pre-existent joint disease, age, systemic and local portals for infection)		Crystal arthropathy: gout, and pseudogout
Crystal-induced arthritis: calcium pyrophosphate crystals indicative of pseudogout may require a detailed search for joint fluid or for chondrocalcinosis; monosodium urate crystals are indicative of gout		
Onset of a systemic arthropathy: RA		

and may originate from tendon sheaths, bursae, or muscles. Even pain originating from such frequently "arthritic" joints as the knee may arise from causes other than synovitis, including dystrophic calcifications, bone spurs, collateral ligament instability, vascular compromise, and disuse.

Extraarticular Disease

Other system involvement may suggest specific forms of arthropathy. Systemic lupus erythematosus (SLE) may be associated with dermatologic manifestations, including alopecia, malar rash, photosensitivity, and Raynaud's. Ocular symptoms, including xerophthalmia and inflammatory eye disease, may suggest the need for ophthalmologic evaluations for

Sjogren's syndrome or uveitis; the latter may also be associated with seronegative spondyloarthropathies. Pleuritis, pericarditis, or hepatitis may prompt an evaluation for arthropathy secondary to an underlying connective tissue disease, or for arthropathy associated with autoimmune hepatitis, or chronic hepatitis B or C infection. Purpura, most commonly on the lower extremities around the malleoli, may indicate an underlying vasculitis. Small necrotic pustules over distal extremities with or without evident urethritis may suggest disseminated gonoccocal infection. Nail pitting and/or the presence of plaque may implicate psoriatic arthritis, and subcutaneous nodules may be part of RA or gout.

Laboratory Testing

The distinction between inflammatory and mechanical causes of arthritis may be found in the appearance of the joint, and confirmed by laboratory markers of inflammation, though both may be less apparent in the elderly and immunosuppressed patient. Inflammation may cause fever or an elevated platelet count. The erythrocyte sedimentation rate (ESR) may be affected by anemia or heart failure, and is best confirmed by specific acute-phase reactants (APRs), such as the C-reactive protein (CRP), which may go up by several hundred times in the course of acute infections or inflammatory disease.

Antinuclear antibodies (ANAs) and rheumatoid factor (RF) measure immune responses to a variety of nuclear antigens and immunoglobulin G, respectively. These autoantibodies have a significant baseline prevalence in the geriatric population. Both may be positive in nonconnective tissue disease states such as chronic viral (hepatitis C or HIV) infections, or liver disease. In addition, both antibodies may occur in rheumatic disorders other than SLE or RA.

Radiography

Radiographic studies provide information regarding the area of pain and swelling, and may yield objective evidence for joint pathology, including the presence of effusions. They can be followed serially for disease progression (such as joint destruction in a patient with a septic process). Radiographic evidence of degenerative joint disease (e.g. joint space narrowing, sclerotic changes, osteophytosis) in certain anatomic locations (e.g. lumbar spine, first metatarsal joint) increases in incidence with age, and may be subclinical or asymptomatic. CT imaging characterizes bone abnormalities, and MRI or ultrasound is useful for pathology involving ligaments, cartilage, tendons, and bursae. Lastly, nuclear scans (e.g. bone, indium) may have utility in the delineation of specific pathology (e.g. osteonecrosis) in bony structures around joints, or for infectious processes such as septic arthritis or osteomyelitis.

Synovianalysis

If the cause of acute arthritis remains unclear, arthrocentesis should be considered and synovianalysis performed. Referral to a rheumatologist may be requested to carry out this procedure, process material obtained for appropriate tests, and interpret direct examination of synovial fluid. Technically difficult arthrocenteses (e.g. hip, sacroiliac joints) may be directed by CT or ultrasound guidance. Arthrocentesis is relatively contraindicated if there is an overlying cellulitis or if the patient has coagulopathy.

Synovianalysis answers three important questions (Table 3):

- Is the fluid inflammatory or noninflammatory?
- Is it infected?
- Are there crystals?

The cell count, viscosity, and ability to form a mucin clot can be used to answer the first question.[4,5] The aspirate should be sent for gram stain and culture, with specific cultures or PCR techniques being relevant to anaerobes, fungus, AFB, GC, and Lyme disease if these infections are under consideration.[6] The rheumatologist is best able to examine joint fluid for crystals, consider the significance of unusual findings (e.g. hemarthrosis), and perform additional studies which may guide diagnostic testing and therapy.

Table 3. Synovial Fluid Analysis

Measure	Normal	Noninflammatory	Inflammatory	Septic
Clarity	Transparent	Transparent	Translucent/ cloudy	Opaque
Color	Clear	Yellow	Yellow	Yellow, brown, or green
White blood cells per microliter	<200	<2000	>2000	>50,000
Polymorphonuclear leukocytes (%)	<25%	<25%	50% or more	Usually 75% or more
Culture	Negative	Negative	Negative	Usually positive
Examples		OA, mechanical derangement	Crystal arthropathy, RA, seronegative arthritis	Bacterial infections (gonococcal vs. nongonococcal vs. fastidious organisms)

Monoarticular Acute Arthritis

Acute gout, pseudogout, and infection are the most common causes of attacks of monoarthritis.[8] Risk factors include trauma, surgery, renal insufficiency, diuretic use, and myocardial infarction.[9]

Gout/Pseudogout

Acute gout typically presents as a painful, erythematous, swollen great toe (i.e. podagra). The features of an acute monoarthritis that suggest gout include:

- Previous history of podagra
- Use of diuretics or other medications that may affect uric acid excretion (cyclosporine, low-dose aspirin)
- Presence of tophi in typical locations (e.g. helix of the ear, olecranon bursa)

In addition to the great toe, the ankle and knee are commonly involved. Fifteen percent of patients with acute gout may have normal or low uric acid levels during the acute attack, rising above the normal range only after resolution.[9] Acute pseudogout may be suggested by wrist/shoulder involvement, radiographic evidence of chondrocalcinosis, or associated metabolic disease (e.g. hypothyroidism, hyperparathyroidism, hypomagnesemia, hemochromatosis).[10] Gout and pseudogout can both present with polyarticular symptoms, particularly in chronic disease, and may be associated with fever.

Since crystal disease and infection can coexist, gram stain and culture should be a routine part of synovianalysis.[11] Gout is caused by monosodium urate crystals, which are needle-shaped, and *strongly* and negatively birefringent. By contrast, pseudogout is defined by calcium pyrophosphate dihydrate crystals, which are rhomboid-shaped, and *weakly* and positively birefringent.

For acute crystal arthropathy, nonsteroidal anti-inflammatory drugs (NSAIDs) can be employed. However, in the inpatient setting, concomitant medical conditions such as renal insufficiency, diabetes, or heart failure may militate against their use and create a need for appropriate precautions (e.g. cytoprotection, blood pressure control).[12] Colchicine is also effective for acute gout; however, it is limited by a low therapeutic index[13] and the side effect of diarrhea when the maximal effective dose is reached. Colchicine should be used with care in patients with renal insufficiency and known bone marrow suppression. Intra-articular steroids can be administered for acute monoarticular crystalline arthropathy, and systemic oral (or intravenous) formulations may be effective for polyarticular gout/pseudogout. Urate-lowering agents such as allopurinol should not be started during an acute flare, as attacks can be provoked by either a rise (such as with progressive renal insufficiency or with diuresis) or lowering of the uric acid level. However, if the patient is already on these agents, they may be continued.

Septic Arthritis

Infection must always be considered, particularly in the inpatient setting. Risk factors for septic arthritis include[14]:

- A history of RA or other pre-existing joint disease
- Joint prosthesis
- Intravenous drug abuse
- Diabetes
- Alcoholism

Eliciting urethritis or sexually transmitted disease is important when considering gonococcal arthritis.

Infection can be introduced into a joint through hematogenous spread or direct inoculation (e.g. trauma or iatrogenically).[6,14] The most common organism identified in the synovial fluid across all age and risk groups is *Staphylococcus aureus*, followed by other gram-positive bacteria, including streptococci. There has also been an increase in methicillin-resistant *S. aureus*, especially among intravenous drug abusers, individuals with orthopedic procedures, and the elderly.[6,14] The frequency of gram-negative organisms causing septic arthritis is also higher among the elderly, likely given comorbidities such as urinary tract infections and decubitus ulcers.

Arthrocentesis and examination of the synovial fluid are also critical in the diagnosis and the choice of antibiotic treatment. Repeated arthrocenteses may be required to remove existing inflammatory joint fluid and to prevent destructive changes.

Conclusion

The rheumatologist and the hospitalist can coordinate care in substantiating and expanding the initial impression of acute arthritis, and in the interpretation of diagnostic tests. Together, they can formulate treatment strategies for guiding the proper use of therapeutic agents such as NSAIDs, for administering local injection therapy, and for evaluating the patient for appropriate rehabilitation and long-term care to avoid permanent disability and maintain function.

References

1. Lillicrap MS, Bytne E, Speeds CA. (2003) Musculoskeletal assessment of general medical inpatients—joints still crying out for attention. *Rheumatology* **42**: 951–954.
2. Nguyen-Oghalal TY, Ottenbacher KJ, Granger CV, Goodswin JS. (2005) Impact of osteoarthritis on the rehabilitation of patients following a stroke. *Arth Rheum* **53**: 383–387.
3. Raj JM, Sudhakar S, Sems K, Carlson EW. (2002) Arthritis in the intensive care unit. *Crit Care Clin* **18**: 767–780.
4. Courtney P, Doherty M. (2009) Joint aspiration and injection and synovial fluid analysis. *Best Pract Res Clin Rheumatol* **23**: 161–192.
5. Pascual E, Doherty M. (2009) Aspiration of normal or asymptomatic pathological joints for diagnosis and research: Indications, technique and success rate. *Ann Rheum Dis* **68**: 3–7.
6. Margaretten ME, Kohlwes J, Moore D, Bent S. (2007) Does this adult patient have septic arthritis? JAMA **297**: 1478–1488.
7. Kent TA, Gardner GC. (2007) Evaluation of the activity of an academic rheumatology consult service over 10 years: Using Data to shape curriculum. *J Rheumatol* **34**: 563–566.
8. Siva C, Velazquez C, Mody A, Brasington R. (2003) Diagnosing acute monoarthritis in adults: A practical approach for the family physician. *Am Fam Physician* **268**: 83–90.
9. Schlesinger N, Norquist JM, Watson DJ. (2009) Serum urate during acute gout. *J Rheumatol* **36**: 1287–1289.
10. Zhang W, Doherty M, Bardin T, *et al.* (2011) European League Against Rheumatism recommendations for calcium pyrophosphate deposition. Part I: Terminology and diagnosis. *Ann Rheum Dis* (Jan 7).

11. Yu KH, Luo SF, Liou LB, *et al*. (2003) Concomitant septic and gouty arthritis — an analysis of 30 cases. *Rheumatology (Oxford)*. **42**: 1062–1066.
12. Kitchen J, Kane D. (2010) Nonsteroidal anti-inflammatory drug prescriptions in hospital inpatients: Are we assessing the risks? *Ir J Med Sci* **179**: 357–360.
13. Richette P, Bardin T. (2010) Colchicine for the treatment of gout. *Expert Opin Pharmacother* **11**: 2933–2938.
14. Mathews CJ, Weston VC, Jones A, *et al*. (2010) Bacterial septic arthritis in adults. *Lancet* **375**: 846–855.

Chapter 68

Inpatient Management of Rheumatoid Arthritis

*Yousaf Ali**

Key Pearls

- Rheumatoid arthritis (RA) affects the small joints of the hands and feet, and is commonly associated with systemic manifestations.
- Rheumatoid flare is usually polyarticular and infection needs to be excluded prior to starting immunosuppressive therapy.
- Patients with chronic RA are at risk for atlantoaxial instability and need to have flexion extension cervical spine radiographs prior to any surgery.
- Rheumatoid vasculitis can be life-threatening and requires pulse dose IV steroids and cytotoxic therapy.
- Patients on biologic therapy are at greater risk of severe infections including TB, and a high index of suspicion should be maintained even if the patient is afebrile.

Introduction

Rheumatoid arthritis (RA) is one of the most common autoimmune diseases, affecting approximately 1% of the adult population. It is characterized by a symmetric inflammatory arthritis of the small joints of the hands and feet in the setting of a positive rheumatoid factor (RF) or cyclic citrullinated peptide (CCP) antibody. The mortality of RA is increased

*Mount Sinai School of Medicine, New York, NY, USA.

Table 1

	Inpatient Interaction
Active RA	Infection
	RA Disease Flare
	Complication of Therapy
	Felty's Syndrome
	Rheumatoid Vasculitis
	Rheumatoid Lung
Inactive RA	Surgical Procedure

when compared to age-matched controls and despite aggressive intervention the disease can progress, resulting in deformity and extra-articular complications.

Although this condition is primarily managed in the outpatient setting, it is important to realize that there are many instances where the RA patient is admitted to the hospital and requires more intensive therapy.

The interaction between the hospitalist and the RA patient can be summarized as in Table 1.

Rheumatoid Flare

RA is prone to intermittent flare-ups, which require more aggressive intervention. In the outpatient setting this usually constitutes the addition of a course of corticosteroid or an increase in the dose of baseline prednisone. When a patient with RA complains of increasing joint pain, it is important to distinguish active RA from other causes of joint pain, such as osteoarthritis/bursitis or infection. An infectious arthritis can manifest as a mono- or polyarticular flare and usually associated with fever, leucocytosis and erythema over the joint. These findings may be completely absent, particularly in the older patient. If an infection is suspected arthrocentesis should be performed to confirm the presence of an organism.

If a patient with RA is admitted due to RA flare, this usually constitutes a polyarticular exacerbation that cannot be managed as an outpatient. Once infection has been excluded, the patient can usually be improved by increasing the prednisone dosage either by using a short burst of oral prednisone (40 mg prednisone daily) or by injecting intra-articular (IA) cortisone into the affected joint. Pulse intravenous Solu-Medrol at 1 g daily for three days is usually reserved for RA with severe disease such as systemic vasculitis.

Rheumatoid Vasculitis

With the advent of more aggressive management of RA, rheumatoid vasculitis has become quite a rare occurrence. Nevertheless, vasculitis needs to be recognized early, since if it is untreated the consequences can be severe. Manifestations of rheumatoid vasculitis can be localized or systemic. Local vasculitis is typified by nail fold infarcts, sensory neuropathy, leg ulceration and digital tip ulceration (see Fig. 1). Typically, this occurs in a patient with known RA who either has been lost to followup or has very aggressive RA. The patients are usually seropositive and have markedly elevated inflammatory markers. Since this occurs in patients with severe disease, the prognosis tends to be poor.[1]

Occasionally, vasculitis can result in systemic manifestations such as progressive mononeuritis multiplex, CNS or visceral infarcts. This should be considered as life-threatening and is an indication for intravenous high dose corticosteroids and rapidly acting immunosuppressive therapy such as

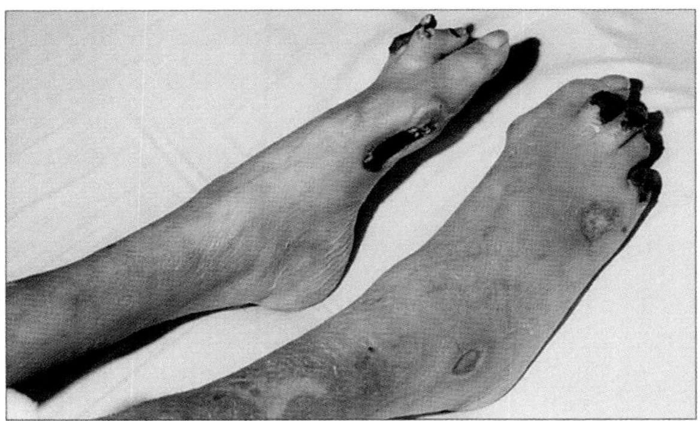

Fig. 1. Rheumatoid vasculitis with proximal ulceration and distal gangrene.

IV cyclophosphamide or intravenous anti-TNF agents such as infliximab. Generalized measures such as nicotine cessation, statin therapy and surgical debridement should also be part of the overall care of these patients.

Felty's Syndrome

Chronic neutropenia can occur in RA either with or without splenomegaly. When it is associated with splenic enlargement, it is termed "Felty's syndrome." Similar to vasculitis, this complication tends to occur in patients with chronic longstanding seropositive disease. The hospitalist may encounter these individuals as they are admitted for evaluation of neutropenia, suffer from infections or are undergoing therapeutic splenectomy. The patient may undergo bone marrow aspiration to determine the cause and this usually reveals a hypercellular or normal marrow. Since levels of proinflammatory cytokines are high in active RA, the bone marrow remains suppressed and normal hematopoiesis is inhibited. Treatment of this condition involves treating the underlying disease with immunosuppressive therapy. This is a difficult clinical decision, as additional immune modulating therapy can further potentiate the risk of infection. Splenectomy is sometimes required, although the neutropenia may persist. If the patient's WBC remains too low, a course of granulocyte colony-stimulating factor (GCSF) may be required, although it is important to note that this can occasionally result in an RA flare.

Cardiopulmonary Complications of RA

When a rheumatoid patient presents with dyspnea, the differential diagnosis is broad (Table 2).

Patients with RA do have accelerated atherosclerosis, which is most likely due to the underlying systemic inflammatory response and concomitant chronic corticosteroid usage. This milieu predisposes the patient to a higher risk of coronary artery disease (CAD),[2] and cardiac ischemia needs to be considered in a dyspneic patient. Some investigators have labeled accelerated CAD as an extra-articular manifestation of RA.[3]

Table 2. Dyspnea in a patient with RA

Cardiac	Pulmonary	Constitutional
Congestive Heart Failure	Cricoarytenoid Arthritis	Anemia
Myocarditis	Pleural Effusions	Infection
Pericardial Effusion	Rheumatoid Lung	
Aortitis	Bronchiolitis Obliterans Organizing Pneumonia	
Coronary Artery Disease	Pulmonary Fibrosis	
	Methotrexate Pneumonitis	
	Pneumonia	

Myocarditis and pericarditis are unusual clinical manifestations but are often seen in autopsy specimens of patients with longstanding RA. Coronary artery vasculitis has been described and also reflects underlying active systemic disease. The treatment of this includes aggressive pulse dose steroids and immunomodulatory therapy. Since the advent of coronary arteriography, this diagnosis has been easier to identify but should definitely be considered in the patient without traditional risk factors who presents with coronary ischemia.

Pleural effusions are commonly found in RA but are often incidental as opposed to symptomatic. This contrasts with SLE, in which serositis tends to be more problematic. The rheumatoid pleural effusion is exudative, with a low glucose count and is often associated with pericardial and interstitial lung disease.

Interstitial lung disease (ILD) occurs in about 5% of patients who have had RA for greater than 10 years and is associated with seropositivity, nicotine abuse and male sex (see Fig. 2). The presentation of ILD or rheumatoid lung is usually insidious and needs to be distinguished from methotrexate-induced alveolitis, which is more subacute and associated with cough, new pulmonary infiltrate and rapidly progressive pulmonary decompensation.[4] Treatment of RA-associated ILD is with high dose steroids and fortunately tends to be more responsive to immunosuppressive therapy compared to idiopathic ILD. In patients with progressive pulmonary symptoms a diagnosis of bronchiolitis obliterans with organizing

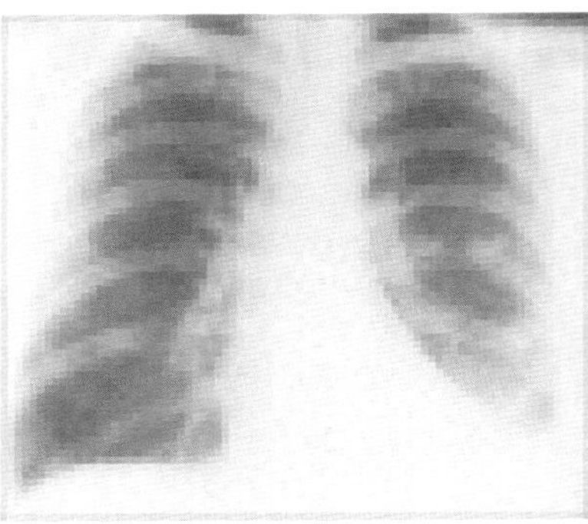

Fig. 2. ILD with pleural effusion and rheumatoid nodule.

pneumonia (BOOP) should be considered and referral for lung biopsy is advised.

Airway obstruction can occur in both the upper and lower airways, and may be due to cricoarytenoid arthritis or bronchiectasis. The symptoms of upper airway inflammation include dysphagia, hoarseness, pain with speech and globus pharyngeus. This can usually be diagnosed by direct visualization of the vocal cords and with the use of pulmonary function testing. Bronchiectasis is thought to occur in approximately 50% of cases with RA and may be due to recurrent pulmonary infections or genetic predisposition. Although treatment with corticosteroids will alleviate the inflammatory response, great care should be taken with biologic response modifiers (BRMs) given the risk of concomitant infection.[5]

Neurologic Impairment

A small subset of RA patients can develop a peripheral neuropathy, which is felt to be related to underlying vasculitis of the vasa nervorum supplying the nerves. This is usually seen in conjunction with rheumatoid vasculitis elsewhere but may occur as an isolated manifestation. This neuropathy usually manifests as a sensory neuropathy with parasthesias but mononeuritis multiplex can also occur in RA.

In patients with longstanding RA, erosions can occur at the atlantoaxial articulation of the cervical spine. This results in instability of the transverse ligament at C1 and subsequent myelopathy (see Fig. 3). Superior migration of the odontoid peg can also result in cord compression into the foramen magnum, resulting in hyperreflexia, positive Babinski sign and weakness. Surgical stabilization is required in these circumstances. If a patient with severe RA is undergoing surgery, the anesthetist should be made aware and preop flexion extension films should be obtained to assess the degree of C1/2 stability.

Fortunately, RA rarely involves the central nervous system, although angiitis has been reported. This usually presents with severe headache, fever and mental status changes. A brain biopsy is usually required to secure the diagnosis. Treatment is with high dose corticosteroids and cytotoxic agents.

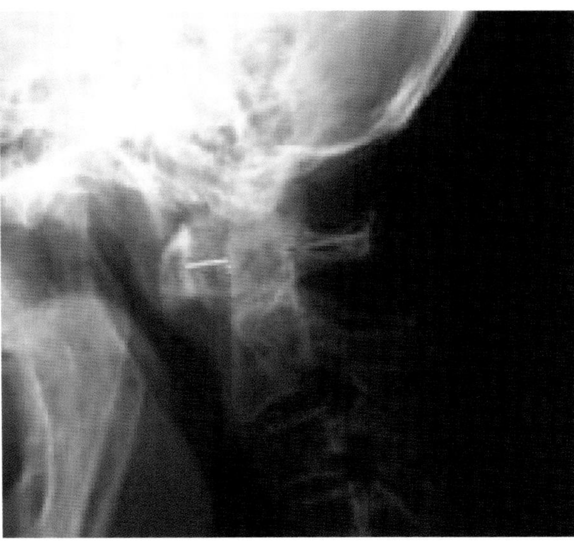

Fig. 3. Plain lateral radiograph of the normal cervical spine taken in extension, showing measurement of the anterior atlantodental interval (yellow line) and the posterior atlantodental interval (red line).

Use of Biologic Therapy in the Inpatient with RA

Tumor necrosis factor (TNF), interleukin (IL) 6, IL-1 and several other cytokines are recognized important mediators of inflammation. Over the past decade, bench-to-bedside research has allowed development of novel therapies to inhibit these molecules and has altered the disease process dramatically. In 1999, biologic therapy was approved by the FDA, and it has become part of the mainstream armamentarium. These drugs target the inflammatory cascade and are used in patients with active persistent RA who have failed conventional DMARD therapy. Examples of commonly used anti-TNF agents are etanercept, infliximab and adalimumab. Although these are agents highly effective at arresting disease activity, TNF is also important in maintaining host defense by destroying intracellular organisms such as mycobacteria and Listeria. It is now recognized that anti-TNF agents are associated with severe infections and reactivation of latent tuberculosis (TB). When a patient is admitted with a febrile illness on biologic therapy, the drug should be immediately discontinued and a high index of suspicion should be kept for an unusual infection or TB. Occasionally, fatal infections have occurred with these agents,[6] and early recognition is vital.

References

1. Turesson C, O'Fallon WM, Crowson CS, *et al.* (2002) Occurrence of extra-articular disease manifestations is associated with excess mortality in a population-based cohort of patients with rheumatoid arthritis. *J Rheumatol* **29**: 62–67.
2. Maradit-Kremers H, Nicola PJ, Crowson CS, *et al.* (2005) Cardiovascular death in rheumatoid arthritis: A population-based study. *Arthritis Rheum* **52**: 722–732.
3. Van Doornum S, McColl G, Wicks IP. (2002) Accelerated atherosclerosis: An extraarticular feature of rheumatoid arthritis? *Arthritis Rheum* **46**: 862–873.

4. Tanoue LT. (1998) Pulmonary manifestations of rheumatoid arthritis. *Clin Chest Med* **19**: 667–685.
5. Lieberman-Maran L, Orzano IM, Passero MA, Lally EV. (2006) Bronchiectasis in rheumatoid arthritis: report of four cases and a review of the literature — implications for management with biologic response modifiers. *Semin Arthritis Rheum* **35**(6): 379–387.
6. Moreland LW, Heck Jr LW, Koopman WJ. (1997) Biologic agents for treating rheumatoid arthritis. *Arthritis Rheum* **40**: 397–409.

Chapter 69

Systemic Lupus Erythematosus

Okey Justin Oparanaku and Leslie Dubin Kerr*

Key Pearls

- SLE and the drugs used for its treatment cause immunosuppression leading to a predisposition to infections. Thus infection/sepsis are the leading causes of hospitalization in SLE patients.
- Lupus nephritis is asymptomatic unless the initial presentation is uremia or nephrosis. Thus, a urinanalysis is mandatory in all hospitalized SLE patients.
- Fluctuations in laboratory test values are poor predictors of disease exacerbation in SLE. As such, laboratory tests directed at monitoring SLE autoantibodies are of limited utility in hospitalized SLE patients.
- Thrombotic events, including myocardial infraction, cerebrovascular accidents and pulmonary embolism are increased in SLE patients, so a high index of suspicion is needed to diagnose and treat these complications.
- Pulse IV steriods are not indicated as a global treatment of a lupus flare. Steroids should be given in the lowest possible doses needed to control disease activity and gradually tapered as soon as possible.

Introduction

In the study by Ward[11] using a state hospitalization registry to examine the association between a hospital's experience in treating patients with

*Mount Sinai School of Medicine, New York, NY, USA.

systemic lupus erythematosus (SLE) and in-hospital SLE mortality, it was observed that mortality was lower at hospitals in which there was more experience in caring for patients with SLE.

The association between a hospital's experience and in-hospital SLE mortality led to suggestions for several possible courses of action to improve the management of hospitalized SLE patients, including:

- Providing increased education to healthcare providers at hospitals with a large SLE population;
- Increasing the experience of providers at hospitals in which there is less experience;
- Developing regional centers.

Thus this chapter which highlights the management of SLE will add to other available resources in fulfilling the first strategy without belaboring the aspect of SLE diagnosis and continuity of care provided by community rheumatologists.

What is Systemic Lupus Erythematosus?

SLE is an autoimmune disease with multisystem involvement, characterized by the presence of autoantibodies directed against cellular antigens. The criteria for diagnosis were published by the American College of Rheumatology, revised in 1982 and updated in 1997 (see Table 1).

SLE is about 9–10 times more common in women, and has a nearly 9 times higher prevalence in those with African-American heritage.

Diagnostic Difficulties in SLE

SLE is a multisystem disease with an extensive differential diagnosis, whose manifestations vary with the type of tissue damage and degree of organ dysfunction. As such, SLE patients have different presentations and their management strategies therefore differ.

Table 1. The 1982/1997 American College of Rheumatology Revised Criteria for the Classification of Systemic Lupus Erythematosus

Cutaneous

1. Malar rash: fixed malar erythema, flat or raised.
2. Discoid rash: erythematous raised patches with keratic scaling and follicular plugging; atrophic scarring may occur.
3. Photosensitivity; skin rash as an usual reaction to sunlight; diagnosed by patient history or physician observation.
4. Oral ulcers; oral or nasopharyngeal ulcers, usually painless; observed by physician.

Systemic

5. Arthritis; nonerosive, involving two or more peripheral joints; characterized by tenderness, swelling, effusion.
6. Serositis; pleuritis (convincing history of pleuritic pain or rub heard by physician, or evidence of pleural effusion) or pericarditis (documented by electrocardiogram, rub or evidence of pericardial effusion).
7. Renal disorder; persistent proteinuria (>0.5 g/day or >3+) or cellular casts of any type.
8. Neurological disorder; seizure or psychosis in the absence of other causes.

Laboratory

9. Hematological disorder; hemolytic anemia or leucopenia (<4000 on two occasions), lymphopenia (<1500 on two occasions), or thrombocytopenia (<100,000 in the absence of an offending drug).
10. Immunological disorder; anti-ds DNA, or anti-Sm, or antiphospholipid antibodies (abnormal IgM or IgG anticardiolipin antibody, lupus anticoagulant or false-positive syphilis serology).
11. Antinuclear antibody in the absence of drugs known to be associated with the "drug-induced lupus syndrome.

For identifying patients in clinical studies, a patient is said to have SLE if any four or more of the 11 criteria are present either serially or simultaneously, during any interval of observation.

Fluctuations in laboratory test values are poor predictors of disease exacerbation in SLE. As such, laboratory tests directed at monitoring various autoantibodies seen in SLE are not very useful in hospitalized SLE patients.

Common Presentations of Hospitalized SLE Patients

Factors that lead to hospitalization have been found to differ from those that are associated with the usual morbidity in outpatient SLE management.

Infection and sepsis are the leading causes of hospitalization and this fact has been corroborated by many studies.

Infection/Fever

Zhou NJ *et al.*[13] reviewed the records of 1947 consecutive patients hospitalized for SLE. A total of 487 patients had fever, among whom 265 had fever from infection and 206 from SLE. Eight had both infections and active SLE. Four patients had fever caused by malignancies and four miscellaneous causes. The authors identified the most common sites of infection as the respiratory tract, urinary tract, skin and mucosa. Compared to patients with infection and fever, those with SLE fever were more likely to have lower serum complement C3 and a higher SLE disease activity index score. Risk factors for fever due to infection were the prior use of azathioprine for six or more months, leucocytosis in the absence of steroids and bandemia. SLE fever without infection is characterized by a low WBC (not explained by cytotoxics), normal or slightly increased CRP, low C3/C4 and increased dsDNA. Those with a SLE flare with fever as a part of it may require immune suppression, while those with fever due to infection will require anti-infective agents — antibacterial, antifungal or antiviral agents. However, SLE fever alone is not an indication for steroids or immunosuppression, as this can be treated with hydroxychloroquine or NSAIDs.

The workup of the febrile hospitalized lupus patient should be directed to the suspected source of infection, and the immunosuppressants stopped briefly during this period.

Renal Disease

Active lupus nephritis occurs in approximately 30% of patients with SLE and is still among the most important life-threatening complications of SLE.

Lupus nephritis is initially asymptomatic unless the initial presentation is uremia or nephrosis. Thus, it may be unrecognized unless a urinalysis is obtained revealing proteinuria, or an active sediment. Renal biopsy has led to the classification of the disease, which is now known by classes

Table 2. International Society of Nephrology and Renal Pathology Society (ISN/RPS) Classification of Lupus Nephritis (2004)

***Class* 1;** Minimal mesangial — normal glomeruli by light microscopy (LM), mesangial immune deposits by immunofluorescence.
***Class* 11:** Mesangial proliferative: mesangial hypercellularity or matrix expansion by LM with mesangial immune deposit.
***Class* 111:** Focal proliferative; focal, segmental, and/or global endo- and/or extracapillary involvement of <50% of glomeruli, with or without mesangial alteration.

111*(A)*: Purely active lesions.
111*(A/C)*: Active and chronic lesions.
111*(C)*: Chronic inactive with scarring.

***Class 1V*:** Diffuse proliferative — same as Class 111 but involving >50% of glomeruli.

1*V-S(A) or IV-G(A)*: Purely active, diffuse segmental or global proliferative.
1*V-S(A/C) or* 1*V-G(A/C)*: As above with active and chronic lesions.
1*V-S(C) or* 1*V-G(C)*: Inactive with scarring.

***Class V*:** Membranous — global or segmental subepithelial immune deposits with or without mesangial alteration.
***Class V1*:** Advanced sclerosing; >90% of glomeruli sclerosed with no activity.

1–6 (Table 2). There are no known clinical or laboratory markers with high reliability in predicting active renal disease in patients with SLE.

Therapy usually consists of high dose steroids (prednisone 1 mg/kg body weight or pulse steroid) tapered over time, and immunosuppressive regimens (mycophenolate mofetil, cyclophosphamide). This is often initiated in the hospital and continued as an outpatient treatment.

Pulmonary Disease

Lupus patients may be admitted for evaluation of pleuritic chest pain, cough and shortness of breath. The differential diagnosis includes serositis and pulmonary emboli, especially in those with antiphospholipid syndrome (APLS). Other causes are interstitial lung disease, pulmonary hypertension and pulmonary hemorrhage. Radiological investigation — chest X-ray, CT scan and CT angiography, and echocardiogram — is necessary for making the appropriate diagnosis.

The most severe (but rare) pulmonary manifestation of SLE is acute lupus pneumonitis. It is associated with acute shortness of breath, hemoptysis, fever and interstitial alveolar infiltrates. Infections, congestive heart failure and uremia must be excluded. The mortality is high despite treatment with high dose steroids and immunosuppressants.

Cardiovascular Disease

Chest pain is a common cause of hospitalization for SLE patients. Whenever a patient of the relevant age group and cardiovascular risk factors presents with chest pain, the workup should be geared toward excluding coronary artery disease and acute myocardial infarction. However, because most SLE patients are young women, an age group not typically associated with cardiovascular morbidity, they may be mistaken as a low risk group. It has been shown that SLE is an important independent risk factor for coronary artery disease and myocardial infarction.

Pericarditis is another cause of chest pain in SLE patients. The chest pain is substernal and may be associated with a friction rub. The echocardiogram may be normal or show a small pericardial effusion. Cardiac tamponade is very rare in SLE patients.

SLE can cause myocarditis in active systemic disease. Patients have a high CPK-MB and/or troponin with the new onset heart failure and arrhythmias without any evidence of myocardial infarction. Lupus myocarditis requires treatment with immunosuppressive agents.

Pulmonary hypertension in SLE patients may be secondary to ILD, vasculitis, or possibly due to microinfarction in APLS.

Neuropsychiatric Disease

Hospitalization of SLE patients for neuropsychiatric manifestations may pose serious challenges. This is because the symptoms are usually subtle, ranging from organic brain syndrome, manifesting as cognitive or behavioral problems, to psychosis which could still be difficult to differentiate from the frustration associated with chronic illness or steroid use.

Cognitive dysfunction in SLE could be due to atherosclerosis, infections, vasculitis, or the organic brain syndrome in lupus known as lupus cerebritis.

Other neurological complaints, such as headaches, seizures or a change in mental status, could be due to an array of factors such as infections, medications, hypertension, hemorrhage or vasculitis. Laboratory tests and imaging are often not helpful. Lumbar puncture is useful for ruling out infection.

CVA in SLE is multifactorial and the usual risk factors, such as hypertension, diabetes, atherosclerosis, coagulopathies and cardiac defects, must be ruled out. Workup for APLS and echocardiogram is mandatory. In rare cases of lupus cerebritis, immunosuppression is required to control inflammation. This consists of high dose steroids and/or cyclophosphamide. Confirmation of cerebritis might require MRI/MRA or brain biopsy which carries significant morbidity. APLS, structural brain lesions and infections must be excluded prior to the diagnosis of cerebritis.

Transverse myelitis is a rare and very serious complication of SLE, manifesting as rapidly ascending paralysis or weakness, loss of sensation and incontinence. It is an emergency arising from inflammation and/or infarction of the spinal cord, usually at T10. Diagnosis is by contrast MRI of the brain and spinal cord and lumbar puncture. Treatment consists of the use of pulse steroids, immunosuppressants and possibly plasmapheresis.

Musculoskeletal Disease

Arthritis and muscle pain are the most common presentations of SLE, and are occasionally severe enough to warrant hospitalization. Arthralgia is found in 80% of SLE patients, while arthritis in two or more joints is found in 50% of patients at some time in their disease. Polyarthritis is usually symmetrical, involving small joints of hands, wrists, and knees. It is the most common flare in SLE patients. An acute monoarthritis in an SLE patient, especially if the synovial fluid is inflammatory, is a septic arthritis until proven otherwise.

It is important to consider avascular necrosis (AVN) presenting as joint pain in SLE. Patients on chronic steroid therapy as well as SLE patients who have never been on steroids are at risk. AVN causes symptoms later in the course of the disease, and is monoarticular or oligoarticular rather than polyarticular. It usually affects the knees, hips and shoulders. MRI is diagnostic of AVN, and orthopedic evaluation might be necessary.

Skin manifestations in SLE include malar rash, photosensitive rash, subacute cutaneous lupus, discoid rash and painless mucus membrane lesions (oral, vaginal, nasal). They are seen in hospitalized patients as part of the SLE flare and are rarely by themselves the cause of admission. Cutaneous vasculitis in SLE usually affects small and medium-sized arterioles, and presents as palpable purpura with leucocytoclastic vasculitis on biopsy. Leucocytoclastic vasculitis in SLE usually responds to low dose steroids. More rarely, SLE patients may develop bullous lupus similar to pemphigus, which may be life-threatening, requiring high dose steroids and/or immunosuppressive medications.

Gastrointestinal Disease

Rarer reasons for hospitalization for SLE may be gastrointestinal problems. *Candida* esophagitis due to immunosuppression should be suspected in the SLE patient with dysphagia and/or abdominal pain. Abdominal pain may also be due to infection, peritonitis, gastroenteritis, appendicitis or vasculitis.

Mesenteric vasculitis and infarction is rare and insidious, leading to perforation, and is sometimes diagnosed only at laparotomy. It is seen in 1%–2% of lupus patients. APLS, which causes mesenteric ischemia should be a consideration and ruled out before high dose steroids or surgery.

Hematological Disease

Hematological manifestations — anemia, leucopenia, lymphopenia and thrombocytopenia — are seen in SLE patients. Autoimmune hemolytic anemia with a positive Coombs test, if severe, might require hospitalization for IV high dose steroids, IV immunoglobulin (IVIG) or immunosuppressive therapy.

Leucopenia often correlates with disease activity as well as asymptomatic thrombocytopenia. Thrombotic thrombocytopenic purpura (TTP) is a rare, severe complication of SLE, requiring admission. Like TTP without SLE, it is managed with plasmapheresis or rituximab in severe cases. Care should be taken to exclude cytopenias caused by medication used in the management of SLE.

Pharmacological Treatment of Hospitalized SLE Patients

The medications frequently used to treat patients with SLE and their common side effects are listed in Table 3.

Corticosteroids

Steroids are useful as an adjunctive short term treatment in lupus flares. They are used in forms such as hydrocortisone, prednisone, methylprednisolone and dexamethasone.

The general principle of steroid use is to give the lowest possible dose needed to control disease activity and withdraw by gradual tapering of the dose as soon as possible. If there is difficulty in withdrawal or anticipated difficulty, a steroid sparing agent is introduced. The aim is to eventually get the patient completely off steroids or to as low a dose as possible. SLE patients on steroids for three months or more should get calcium, vitamin D and bisphosphonates for bone health. Pulsed IV steroids are not indicated as a reflexive global treatment for a lupus flare.

Disease-Modifying Antirheumatic Drugs

Disease-modifying antirheumatic drugs (DMARDs) are used as steroid sparing agents as well as for immunosuppression of severe disease, and therefore their use increases the risk of infection. They should be

Table 3. Medication Uses and Side Effects

Medication	Uses	Side Effects		Special Considerations
Hydroxychloroquine	Discoid lupus, systemic lupus	Occasional rash, ocular defect	Ophthalmological monitoring	Response takes 8–12 wks. Do not discontinue on admission. No report of teratogenicity.
Azathioprine	Nephritis, serositis, myocarditis, cytopenias, vasculitis	Bone marrow suppression, nausea, vomiting, diarrhea, rash, liver toxicity	Baseline thiopurine methyltransferase, CBC, LFT repeat CBC after 1 wk	Response takes 2–4 mths. Converted to 6-MP (active)
Methotrexate	Arthritis	Oral sores, liver toxicity, acute pneumonitis, infection risks, BM suppression, teratogenic, lymphoma	LFT, CBC, CXR	4–8 wks for response. Folic acid and folinic acid reduce risks.
Mycophenolate mofitil/ mycophenolic acid	Nephritis, vasculitis, myocarditis, cytopenias	Nausea, vomiting, diarrhea, drug fever, infection risk, BM suppression, teratogenic	CBC, LFT, renal function	No impact on future fertility.
Rituximab	Refractory disease (off label)	Fatal infusion reaction, infections, BM suppression, pneumonitis, headaches, parasthesia	LFT, creatinine, CBC	4–8 wks for response.

discontinued if patients are hospitalized and there is a concern about infection and/or malignancy (except for hydroxychloroquine).

References

1. Ansell SM, Bedhesi S, Ruff B, *et al.* (1996) Study of critically ill patients with systemic lupus erythematosus. *Crit Care Med* **24**: 981–986.
2. Bosch X, Guilabert A, Pallares L, Cerveral R, *et al.* (2006) Infections in systemic lupus erythematosus: A prospective and controlled study of 110 patients. *Lupus.* **15**(9): 584–589.
3. Cervera R, Khamashta MA, Font J, *et al.* (1999) Morbidity and mortality in systemic lupus erythematosus during a 5-year period: A multicenter prospective study of 1000 patients. European Working Party on Systemic Lupus Erythematosus. *Medicine (Baltimore)* **78**: 167–175.
4. Hochberg MC. (1997) Updating the American College of Rheumatology revised criteria for the classification of systemic lupus erythematosus. *Arthritis Rheum* **40**: 1725.
5. Lash AA, Lusk B. (2004) Systemic lupus erythematosus in the intensive care unit. *Critical Care Nurse* **24**(2): 56–65.
6. Noel V, Lortholary O, Cassassus P, *et al.* (2001) Risk factors and prognostic influence of infection in a single cohort of 87 adults with systemic lupus erythematosus. *Ann Rheum Dis* **60**: 1141–1144.
7. Petri M, Genovese M, Engle E, Hochberg M. (1991) Definition, incidence and clinical description of flare in systemic lupus erythematosus: A prospective cohort study. *Arthritis Rheum* **34**: 937–944.
8. Thong BY, Tai DY, Goh SK, Johan A. (2001) An audit of patients with rheumatic disease requiring medical intensive care. *Ann Acad Med Singapore* **30**: 254–259.
9. Wallace DJ. (2008) Lupus. In: *The essential Clinician's Guide*. Oxford American Rheumatology Library, pp. 21–90.
10. Ward MM. (1999) Hospital experience and mortality in patients with systemic lupus erythematosus. *Arthritis Rheum* **42**(5): 891–898.

11. Ward MM. (2000) Hospital experience and expected mortality in patients with systemic lupus erythematosus: A hospital level analysis. *J Rheumatol* **9**: 2146–51.
12. Weening JJ, D'Agati VD, Schwartz MM, *et al*. (2004) The classification of glomerulonephritis in systemic lupus erythematosus revisited. *J Am Soc Nephrol.* **15**: 241–250.
13. Zhou WJ, Yang CD. (2009) The causes and clinical significance of fever in systemic lupus erythematosus: A retrospective study of 487 hospitalized patients. *Lupus* **18**(9): 807–812.

Oncology for the Hospitalist

Chapter 70

Malignancy Workup

*Tony Philip**

Key Pearls

- Thorough and accurate capturing of the patient's medical, surgical, social and family history remains essential.
- Tissue is the issue. Pathology is critical in providing a prognosis, diagnosis, and treatment plan for patients with malignancies.
- lnpatient management should be reserved for patients needing transfusion support or prolonged chemotherapy and for patients lacking the appropriate follow up to ensure timely diagnosis and treatment. The vast majority of oncology is practiced in the outpatient setting.
- The likelihood of lymphadenopathy being malignant increases with age and/or significant history of alcohol and tobacco use.
- Serum tumor markers are not a substitute for tissue diagnosis. The rare situations where tumor markers are diagnostic is AFP for hepatocellular carcinoma and beta-HCG or AFP in germ cell tumors.

Introduction

Patients presenting to the hospital with symptoms from a previously unknown malignant process are more likely to be at an advanced stage. A multi-disciplinary approach in caring for a patient with suspected

*Hofstra North Shore-Long Island Jewish Hospital System, Lake Success, NY, USA.

malignancy is of utmost importance. Having an experienced and trusted team of pathologists, radiologists, surgeons, and medical oncologists makes life easier. While working on a diagnosis, patients may need symptom management, i.e. pain, bleeding, dyspnea, or dysphagia.

Adrenal Mass

Unilateral adrenal masses are common and categorized as either functional (hormonesecreting) or silent, and as either benign or malignant. The majority are benign, nonfunctioning adenomas that are discovered incidentally on abdominal imaging done for other reasons. Functional tumors secrete hormones causing Cushing's syndrome, primary aldosteronism, or hypertension. Adrenocortical carcinomas are rare, aggressive tumors. Adrenal adenomas are less than 4 cm in diameter, while adrenocortical carcinomas are typically larger than 4 cm. The rich lipid nature of cortical adenomas helps to distinguish these benign tumors from carcinoma on CT imaging.

Pancreatic Mass

Pancreatic head masses typically present with painless jaundice from a pancreatic head mass causing biliary obstruction. However, the more common presentation is vague, nonspecific abdominal symptoms from metastatic disease to liver and local lymph nodes. Pancreatic masses are deemed unresectable if there is presence of metastatic disease, direct involvement of the superior mesenteric artery, inferior vena cava, aorta, celiac axis, or hepatic artery. Pancreatic tail masses that encase the splenic vein are not necessarily unresectable; if the tumor is otherwise potentially resectable, distal pancreatectomy and splenectomy can be considered. If there is no clear metastatic disease, the patient should be evaluated by an experienced surgeon to see if resection is feasible.

Colorectal Mass

A male or a post-menopausal female with iron deficiency anemia should undergo a colonoscopy to evaluate for colon cancer. Remember that iron deficiency is not a diagnosis but rather a symptom of another process causing blood loss or malabsorption. Other potential presenting symptoms can be abdominal pain, change in stool caliber, diarrhea, vomiting or obstruction. CT imaging of the chest, abdomen and pelvis should be performed to rule out metastatic disease. Colon cancer typically metastasizes to the lymph nodes and liver before going to the lung; however, rectal cancer due to its dual blood supply, can metastasize to the lung without involving the liver. If the disease is limited to the colon and/or local lymph nodes, then the patient should be referred for a curative resection. In the metastatic setting, the case should be discussed amongst a multidisciplinary team on the role of chemotherapy and surgery in the palliative setting.

Head and Neck Mass

A lymph node is more likely to be malignant in an older patient with a history of smoking and alcohol. However, with the emergence of HPV-associated head and neck cancers, there are an increasing number of cases in nondrinkers and nonsmokers. HPV related head/neck cancers have a better prognosis. The physical exam findings that raise suspicion for malignancy are nodes that are firm, fixed, and rapidly growing. In an adult with a suspicious neck mass, the mass should be evaluated by an otolaryngologist. An otololaryngologist can perform a fine needle aspiration (FNA) for histologic diagnosis and, if there is malignancy, can perform endoscopy looking for the primary site. CT scans of the neck and chest should be performed for staging. A PET scan is particularly useful in identifying a primary site and staging the disease.

If there is suspicion for lymphoma (i.e. rapid growth, multiple nodes, younger patient, or B symptoms), a core biopsy or excisional biopsy should be performed rather than FNA, because lymphoma cannot be as accurately diagnosed because FNA as it does not allow the pathologist to assess the lymph node architecture.

Anterior Mediastinum

Masses in the anterior compartment are more likely to be malignant than those found in the other compartments of the mediastinum. The differential diagnosis for anterior mediastinal tumors includes:

- Thymoma/thymic carcinoma
- Lymphoma (primary mediastinal vs. systemic lymphoma)
- Germ cell tumor (malignant teratoma vs. seminoma vs non-seminoma)
- Substernal thyroid tissue/goiter

Thymoma is the most common neoplasm of the anterior mediastinum. The presence of myasthenia gravis, pure red cell aplasia, or other paraneoplastic syndromes in a patient with an anterior mediastinal mass is highly suggestive of thymoma. Definitive diagnosis still requires surgical excision or biopsy. The patient should also be evaluated by a thoracic surgeon for resection. The primary treatment modality is surgery for invasive and non-invasive thymomas. Tumors that are deemed unresectable or metastatic can be treated with radiation or chemotherapy but outcomes are poorer.

Germ cell tumors are more common in young adults and men. They can be subdivided into benign teratomas, seminomas, and malignant teratomas/nonseminomatous germ cell tumors. Radiologically, seminomas are typically bulky, lobulated, and homogeneous, and rarely locally invasive. Nonseminomas, however, are large and irregularly shaped, with areas of necrosis or hemorrhage. The use of serum alpha-fetoprotein (AFP) and beta-HCG is important diagnostically. The presence of an elevated AFP along with a mediastinal mass would be sufficient for diagnosing nonseminoma. Nonseminomas have a poorer prognosis than pure seminomas.

Substernal goiter can be easily diagnosed on CT scans of the chest and neck. The primary treatment modality is surgical excision if symptomatic and also to reduce the risk of malignant transformation.

The diagnosis of Hodgkin's lymphoma (HL) or non-Hodgkin's lymphoma (NHL) in the mediastinum requires histopathologic examination, and therefore a larger biopsy piece, i.e. core biopsy, is needed rather than FNA. The distinction of HL vs. NHL dictates prognosis and chemotherapeutic options. It is also important to elicit history regarding the presence of B symptoms (fever, weight loss, and night sweats).

Lung Mass/Nodule

A lung nodule is typically identified when a patient presents with symptoms of metastatic disease (i.e. seizure from brain metastasis, local invasion of the chest wall or recurrent laryngeal nerve, and malignant pleural effusion). Occasionally, it is an incidental finding in a patient who may have chest X-ray or CT Chest for other reasons. The next step should be staging with CT Chest/Abdomen/Pelvis, MRI brain, PET/CT (if available) and bone scan. A biopsy should be performed to determine histology (small-cell vs. non-small-cell vs. metastatic disease). There is growing evidence that the specific histology of non-small-cell lung cancer is important for prognosis and treatment (i.e. squamous cell carcinoma or adenocarcinoma). Every effort should be made to obtain adequate tissue for necessary molecular studies.

After initial staging has been completed, the patient should be evaluated for resection by a thoracic surgeon if there is no evidence of metastatic disease or contralateral hilar lymphadenopathy. If there is metastatic disease or unresectable disease, then the patient may benefit from palliative chemotherapy, which has been shown to be better than the best supportive care.

A patient who presents with seizure from a solitary brain metastasis should be evaluated by a neurosurgeon for resection. Radiation oncology should also evaluate the patient for radiation therapy if the brain lesion is unresectable or for adjuvant therapy after surgery.

Renal Mass

A kidney mass can be detected as an incidental finding or during work up for hematuria. It is one of the few malignancies that can be reliably diagnosed via CT scans using the Bozniak criteria, which take into account fluid density with the presence and complexity of septa. The classic triad of renal cell carcinoma (RCC) is flank pain, hematuria, and palpable abdominal mass, which rarely occurs and is strongly suggestive of locally advanced disease. RCC comprises (80%–85%) primary renal neoplasms followed by transitional cell carcinoma. Bilateral RCC should raise suspicion of inherited conditions such as von Hippel–Lindau disease and tuberous sclerosis. Other risk factors include smoking, family history, and chemical exposure, i.e. thorotrast. Associated paraneoplastic syndromes include hypercalcemia, erythrocytosis, thrombocytosis, and Stauffer's syndrome (hepatic dysfunction in the absence of liver metastases).

Surgery is the primary treatment for curative intent in the majority of patients without metastatic RCC and is therefore the preferred recommendation for patients with stage I, II, and III disease. An RCC becomes T4 when it invades beyond Gerota's fascia, including contiguous extension into the ipsilateral adrenal gland, and therefore a T3c which grossly extends into the vena cava above the diaphragm or invades the wall of the vena cava could still be resectable with curative intent. Therefore, evaluation by an experienced urologist should be obtained.

Liver Mass

In a patient with a solitary liver lesion, an experienced radiologist can tell on CT and/or MRI if the lesion has features that raise suspicion of malignancy vs. benign etiology (i.e. focal nodule hyperplasia, hemangiomas, or cysts). Radiologic studies can rule out an extrahepatic primary such as gastrointestinal malignancies, lung cancer, breast cancer, or melanoma (specifically, ocular melanoma).

In a cirrhotic patient with a liver mass, the diagnosis is hepatocellular carcinoma until proven otherwise, especially if the serum AFP is elevated. Risk factors include viral hepatitis, hemochromatosis, and alcohol abuse.

Brain Mass

A patient who presents with a symptomatic isolated brain lesion should be evaluated for evidence of a primary lesion (for example, melanoma, lung, renal or breast cancer).

An experienced neuroradiologist can reliably tell you if the lesion is a meningioma vs. glioblastoma multiforme vs. metastatic lesion. If a primary site is not identified, the patient may need to go for biopsy/resection to determine the histology.

Patients who present with symptomatic brain lesions should be placed on high dose dexamethasone to reduce vasogenic edema and antiepileptics.

References

1. Winer-Muram HT. (2006) The solitary pulmonary nodule. *Radiology* **239**: 35–46.
2. Ost D, Fein D. (2000) Evaluation and management of the solitary pulmonary nodule. *Am J Respir Crit Care Med* **162**: 782–787.
3. Schwetschenau E, Kelley DL. (2002) The adult neck mass. *Am Fam Physician* **66**(5): 831–839.
4. Davis RD Jr, Oldham HN Jr, Sabiston DC Jr. (1987) Primary cysts and neoplasms of the mediastinum: Recent changes in clinical presentation, methods of diagnosis, management, and results. *Ann Thorac Surg* **44**(3): 229–37.
5. Duwe BV. (2005) Tumors of the mediastinum. *Chest* **128**(4): 2893–2909.
6. Atlains MB. Clinical manifestations, evaluation and staging of renal cell carcinoma. In: *UpToDate*, Baslow DS (ed).

Chapter 71

Chemotherapy and Associated Symptoms

Sonia M. Seng, Che-Kai Tsao[†] and William K. Oh[†]*

Key Pearls

- Doxorubicin-induced cardiomyopathy is dose-dependent. Around 6% of patients who receive a cumulative dose of over 550 mg/m^2 will experience chronic cardiomyopathy. Patients who have a pre-existing history of heart disease, are >70 years of age, receive concurrent chemotherapy or biotherapy, or have a history of radiation to the mediastinum are at greater risk. The cardioprotective benefit of the EDTA-like chelator dexrazoxane remains controversial.
- Up to 30% of patients receiving oxaliplatin experience an acute, reversible peripheral neuropathy manifested by jaw pain, difficulty in swallowing, shortness of breath, and oral parasthesias when exposed to the cold. Severe pharyngolaryngeal dysesthesia occurs in only 1%–2% of patients and may be avoided by increasing the infusion time or avoiding exposure to the cold.
- 10% of the US population harbor a genetic polymorphism in UDP-glucuronosyl transferase 1A, an enzyme that metabolizes irinotecan. Patients with this UGT1A1*28 polymorphism are seven times more likely to suffer severe diarrhea and myelosuppression when exposed to irinotecan.

*Southcoast Centers for Cancer Care, Fall River, MA, USA.
[†]Mount Sinai School of Medicine, New York, NY, USA.

- Chemotherapy-induced emesis can be classified as immediate (within hours), delayed (hours to days), or anticipatory (prior to infusion). Administration of prophylactic oral aprepitant, dexamethasone, and ondansetron for three days, starting on the first day of chemotherapy, is effective in preventing delayed emesis in highly emetogetic chemotherapy regimens.
- The exacerbation of cancer-related fatigue is one of the most common side effects of systemic chemotherapy. Methylphenidate improves opioid-induced sedation, depression, and cancer-related fatigue in randomized clinical trials. Patients with severe fatigue or advanced disease are more likely to benefit.

Cancer is the second leading cause of death in the United States. Chemotherapy, biotherapy, and immunotherapy are utilized with various goals, including cure, improvement in overall survival or progression-free survival, decrease in recurrence rates, tumor debulking and organ preservation, and palliation. Toxicity is dependent on multiple factors, including the drug, dose, schedule, route of administration, and combination with other drugs or therapies. An individual's genetics, bone marrow and organ reserve, and functional status may influence drug absorption, metabolism, and efficacy. Also, several genetic polymorphisms have been found to impact chemotherapy metabolism and toxicity. Monoclonal antibodies and small molecule tyrosine kinases that target specific receptors and genes expressed in cancer tissue have revolutionized oncology by enabling physicians to identify patients who are more likely to derive benefit from specific treatments. The administration of chemotherapy and biotherapy and the management of their associated side effects require an interdisciplinary approach between internists, radiologists, surgeons, pharmacists, and the oncologic team.

Chemotherapy-associated Complications

1. **Nausea/Emesis**: Prior to chemotherapy administration, assess the risk of emesis:
   - Immediate — within 24 hours after chemotherapy administration
   - Delayed — greater than 24 hours to days

Table 1. Chemotherapy and Associated Adverse Effects

Drug	Approved Use (Unlabeled Use)	Adverse Side Effects
Alkylating Agents: *Crosslink DNA and interfere with DNA synthesis. Not cell-cycle-specific.* All alkylating agents may cause secondary malignancies and infertility.		
Alkyl sulfonates		
Busulfan	Chronic myelogenous leukemia (CML), Hematopoeitic stem cell transplant (HSCT)	Marrow suppression, hyperpigmentation, hemorrhagic cystitis, seizures with high doses; pulmonary fibrosis, adrenal insufficiency, and veno-occlusive disease are rare.
Azridines		
Thiotepa	Hodgkin's disease, breast, ovarian, superficial bladder, malignant effusions (HSCT)	Myelosuppression, alopecia, rash, nausea/vomiting, central nervous system (CNS) toxicity with high doses.
Mitomycin	Pancreatic and gastric cancer (a variety of solid malignancies)	Myelosuppression, nausea/vomiting, hemolytic uremic syndrome, peripheral neuropathy, nephrotoxicity.
Nitrogen mustards:		
Melphalan	Multiple myeloma and ovarian cancer (CML and endometrial cancers)	Myelosuppression, hyperuricemia renal toxicity, hypersensitivity reactions, cholestasis cardiac toxicity is rare.
Chlorambucil	Chronic lymphocytic leukemia (CLL); also Hodgkin's and Non-Hodgkin's lymphoma (NHL)	Myelosuppression, skin reactions, neuropathies, seizures with high doses, rare pulmonary fibrosis and hepatic toxicity.
Cyclophosphamide	Leukemia, lymphoma, solid malignancies	Myelosuppression, immune suppression, nausea/vomiting, alopecia, hemorrhagic cystitis; cardiomyopathy, veno-occlusive disease (VOD), skin reactions/Stevens–Johnson syndrome, pulmonary toxicity and syndrome of inappropriate antidiuretic hormone secretion (SIADH) are rare.

(*Continued*)

Table 1. *(Continued)*

Drug	Approved Use (Unlabeled Use)	Adverse Side Effects
Ifosphamide	Testicular cancer, non-Federal and Drug Administration (FDA) uses acute lymphoblastic leukemia (ALL), a variety of solid tumors, lymphoma, multiple myeloma	Myelosuppression, alopecia, nausea/vomiting, hemorrhagic cystitis, metabolic acidosis, renal toxicity, CNS toxicity with high doses and associated with higher doses.
Bendamustine (Treanda)	CLL, NHL	Myelosuppression, infection, fever, nausea/vomiting, diarrhea, headache, infusion reactions, hyperbilirubinemia.
Nitrosureas		
Carmustine (BCNU)	CNS tumors and lymphomas	Bone marrow suppression, nausea/vomiting, phlebitis; liver, renal, pulmonary toxicity, and VOD with high doses.
Triazenes		
Dacarbazine	Hodgkin's disease and melanoma (sarcomas)	Nausea/vomiting, myelosuppression, flu–like illness, facial flushing, hypotension, polyneuropathy; hepatic necrosis reported.
Temozolomide	Anaplastic astrocytoma, glioblastoma multiforme	Myelosuppression, nausea/vomiting, seizure, headache, constipation, opportunistic infections/pneumocystis pneumonia.
Platinum Analogs		
Cisplatin	Bladder, testicular, ovarian cancer(multiple solid epithelial malignancies, HSCT)	Renal toxicity, ototoxicity, myelosuppression, nausea/vomiting, alopecia, peripheral neuropathy, metabolic disorders, anaphylaxis, pulmonary toxicity rare in high doses. Second and third generation platinum analogs have less renal insufficiency and more myelosuppression than cisplatin.

(Continued)

Table 1. *(Continued)*

Drug	**Approved Use (Unlabeled Use)**	**Adverse Side Effects**
Carboplatin	Ovarian cancer (a variety of solid malignancies, HSCT)	Myelosuppresion, nausea/vomiting, renal toxicity, hepatic toxicity, autonomic dysfunction, allergic reactions. Often substitutes for cisplatin in patients with renal toxicity.
Oxaliplatin	Colorectal cancer (multiple solid malignancies)	Nausea/vomiting, diarrhea, marrow suppression, dysesthesia, peripheral neuropathy, laryngospasm (cold-induced), hepatic toxicity, dyspnea, anaphylaxis rare.
Antimetabolites: Inhibit *dihydrofolate reductase* or *thymidilate synthase,* critical in folate metabolism and DNA/RNA synthesis.		
Folate antagonists		
Methotrexate	Leukemia, NHL, sarcoma, solid malignancies, neoplastic meningitis	Myelosuppression, nausea/vomiting, mucositis, diarrhea, renal and hepatic toxicity, CNS toxicity and seizures with high doses, pneumonitis rare with chronic low oral dose. Methotrexate accumulates in effusions.
Pemetrexed	Mesothelioma, nonsquamous non small cell lung cancer (NSCLC)	Myelosuppression, stomatitis/pharyngitis, anorexia, nausea/vomiting, rash, gastrointestinal (GI) toxicity. Toxicity ameliorated with B12 and folate supplementation.
***Purine analogs*:**		
6-mercaptopurine (6MP)	ALL	Myelosuppression, hyperuricemia with tumor lysis syndrome, nausea/vomiting, diarrhea, rare hepatotoxicity.

(Continued)

Table 1. *(Continued)*

Drug	Approved Use (Unlabeled Use)	Adverse Side Effects
Fludarabine	B-cell CLL, acute myleogenous leukemia (AML), NHL, mycosis fungoides	Myelosuppression, asthenia, pulmonary toxicity, immune suppression and opportunistic infections, nausea/vomiting, neurotoxicity progressive multifocal leukoencephalopathy (PML); transfusion-associated graft-versus-host disease (GVHD) and autoimmune hemolytic anemia or idiopathic thrombocytopenia purpura (ITP) rare.
Cladribine	Hairy cell leukemia (CLL, CML)	Myelosuppression, nausea, rash, CD4/CD8 suppression and opportunistic infections.
Clofarabine	Relapsed/refractory ALL (AML, myelodysplatic syndrome (MDS))	Myelosuppression, nausea/vomiting, tachycardia, hypotension, capillary leak syndrome, tumor lysis syndrome, liver and renal toxicity, hand–foot syndrome.
Hydroxyurea	CML, melanoma, ovarian cancer, head and neck cancer myeloproliferative disorders (MPD)	Myelosuppression, GI toxicity, rash, hyperpigmentation with extended therapy.
***Pyrimidine analogs*:**		
Fluorouracil (5FU)	Colorectal, breast, gastric, pancreatic, basal cell cancer (multiple solid malignancies)	Myelosuppresion, diarrhea, and mucositis are dose-limiting toxicities; also nausea/vomiting and hand–foot syndrome with high doses or continuous infusion, rare cerebellar syndrome, cardiac toxicity, and hypersensitivity reactions. 5FU is a radiosensitizer. Patients with dihydropyrimidine dehydrogenase (DPD) deficiency have severe toxicity.
Capecitabine (Xeloda) Oral prodrug of 5FU	Breast and colon cancer (GI malignancies)	Diarrhea, mucositis, hand–foot syndrome, hyperbilirubinemia. Less myelosuppression and nausea/vomiting than 5-FU. Used as a radiosensitizer. Patients with DPD deficiency have severe toxicity.

(Continued)

Table 1. *(Continued)*

Drug	Approved Use (Unlabeled Use)	Adverse Side Effects
Cytarabine	AML, ALL, CML in blast phase, CNS leukemia (lymphomas)	Dose-dependent marrow suppression, liver, GI (nausea, vomiting, diarrhea) and CNS toxicity/cerebellar toxicity. Acute pancreatitis is seen with continuous infusions. High dose Cytarabine is associated with conjunctivitis, hand–foot syndrome, mucositis. Intrathecal form associated with arachnoiditis and demyelinating leukencephalopathy when combined with other CNS-directed therapies.
Gemcitabine	Pancreatic, lung, breast, and ovarian, bladder cancers (NHL and other solid malignancies)	Edema, myelosuppression, nausea/vomitting, alopecia, rash, flulike syndrome, hepatic and renal toxicity, hematuria, proteinuria, hemolytic uremic syndrome (HUS) rare.
Topoisomerase Inhibitors: *Naturally occurring plant alkaloids that inhibit enzymes involved in cleaving and ligating DNA strands required for replication.*		
***Camptothecins*:**		
Irinotecan	Colorectal cancer; also lung cancer, leukemia, NHL, brain cancer, gastric cancer, and other solid malignancies	Diarrhea, myelosuppression, cholinergic toxicity, fever, alopecia, hyperbilirubinemia, interstitial lung disease rare. 10% of North Americans are homozygous for UGT1A1, the enzyme that converts irinotecan to its active metabolite. Patients with UGT1A1 genetic polymorphisms, Gilbert's, and Crigler–Najjar syndrome are more susceptible to severe diarrhea and myelosuppression.

(Continued)

Table 1. *(Continued)*

Drug	Approved Use (Unlabeled Use)	Adverse Side Effects
Topotecan	Ovarian, small cell lung cancer (SCLC), cervical cancer	Myelosuppression, nausea/vomiting, mucositis, diarrhea, alopecia, transaminitis.
***Anthracyclines*:**		
Doxorubicin	Leukemia, lymphoma, multiple myeloma, sarcoma, multiple solid malignancies including breast, ovarian, bladder, small cell lung, and gastric cancer	Acute and delayed cardiotoxicity (arrhythmia, tachycardia, congestive heart failure (CHF)), myelosuppression, nausea/vomiting, alopecia, mucositis, potent vesicant. Also radiation recall syndrome and secondary leukemias/MDS. Liposomal form associated with hand–foot syndrome and infusion reactions. Urine reddens after drug administration. Increased incidence of CHF with cumulative doses >300 mg/m^2.
Epirubicin	Breast cancer; also cervical, esophageal, gastric cancer and sarcomas	Myelosuppression, vesicant, diarrhea, stomatitis, amenorrhea, radiation recall syndrome. Dose-dependent cardiac toxicity; lifetime dose should not exceed 900 mg/m^2. Less cardiac toxicity, alopecia, and nausea than with doxorubicin. Urine turns red–orange after drug administration.
Daunorubicin	ALL, AML, NHL, Ewing's sarcoma	Myelosuppression, nausea/vomiting, diarrhea, alopecia, hepatic toxicity, vesicant, phlebitis. Dose-dependent cardiac toxicity; lifetime dose should not exceed 550 mg/m^2. Urine reddens after drug administration.
Idarubicin	AML (ALL)	Myelosuppression, nausea/vomiting, diarrhea, alopecia, cardiac toxicity (1%–5%), hepatic and renal toxicity, vesicant.

(Continued)

Table 1. *(Continued)*

Drug	Approved Use (Unlabeled Use)	Adverse Side Effects
***Anthracene-diones*:**		
Mitoxantrone	AML, prostate cancer	Myelosuppression, nausea, mucositis, alopecia, menstrual disorder/amenorrhea, liver toxicity; cardiotoxic at doses >160 mg/m^2. Urine turns green/blue after administration.
***Epipodophyllo-toxins*:**		
Etoposide	SCLC, testicular cancer; also multiple hematologic and oncologic malignancies	Myelosuppression, alopecia, nausea/vomiting, mucositis, fever, hepatic toxicity, leukemia and anaphylaxis-like reactions rare; hypotension with rapid infusions.
Antimicrotubule Agents: *Increase formation and stabilization of microtubules, leading to mitotic arrest and cell death.*		
***Taxanes*:**		
Paclitaxel	Kaposi's sarcoma, breast, ovarian cancer, and NSCLC (lymphoma and other solid cancers)	Neutropenia, thrombocytopenia, alopecia, nausea, hypersensitivity reactions, sensory neuropathies, myalgias, arthralgias, transient bradycardia, optic nerve disturbances.
Docetaxel	Breast, prostate, gastric, head and neck, and NSCLC (ovarian cancer)	Neutropenia, nausea/vomiting, mucositis, alopecia, rash, nail damage, stomatitis, hypersensitivity reactions, capillary leak syndrome, hand–foot syndrome, rash, peripheral neuropathy less common than with paclitaxel, diarrhea, transaminitis.
Cabazitaxel	Prostate cancer	Myelosuppression, nausea/vomiting, hypersensitivity reactions, diarrhea, constipation, asthenia, abdominal pain, hematuria, nephrotoxicity.

(Continued)

Table 1. *(Continued)*

Drug	Approved Use (Unlabeled Use)	Adverse Side Effects
***Vinca alkaloids*:**		
Vincristine	Acute leukemia, lymphoma mycosis fungoides, rhabdomyosarcoma	Peripheral neurotoxicity (bilateral peripheral motor–sensory autonomic polyneuropathy), myelosuppression, nausea/vomiting. Toxic autonomic neurotoxicity manifests as constipation, paralytic ileus, urinary retention, hypotension. Patients with antecedent neurologic disorders are more prone to neurotoxicity; vesicant.
Vinblastine	Testicular cancer, breast cancer, NHL, Kaposi's sarcoma, Hodgkin's disease, mycosis fungoides, choriocarcinoma	Myelosuppression, hypertension (HTN), neurotoxicity, constipation, jaw pain, mucositis, nausea/vomiting, vesicant.
Vinorelbine	NSCLC; also breast, cervical, lung, and ovarian cancers, lymphomas	Myelosuppression, nausea/vomiting, alopecia, diarrhea, rare pancreatitis, vesicant.
***Epothilones*:**		
Ixabepilone	Breast cancer	Peripheral neuropathy, myelosuppression, hypersensitivity reactions, alopecia, hand–foot syndrome, nausea/vomiting, stomatitis.
Histone Deacetylase Inhibitors/Demethylating Agents		
Vorinostat (Zolinza)	Cutaneous T-cell lymphoma	Thrombocytopenia, anemia, diarrhea, fatigue, nausea, anorexia, dysgeusia, hyperglycemia, transient renal insufficiency, proteinuria; <5% thromboembolic events.
Azacytidine (Vidaza)	Myelodysplatic syndrome (AML)	Myelosuppression, infections, renal and hepatotoxicity, nausea/vomiting, fever, diarrhea, constipation, ecchymosis, weakness, arthralgias, hypokalemia, injection site erythema.

Table 2. Targeted Therapies and Their Associated Side Effects

Drug (Trade Name)	Target	Approved Indications (Unlabeled Use)	Major Adverse Side Effects
Monoclonal Antibodies			
Bevacizumab (Avastin)	VEGF-A	Metastatic colorectal cancer, nonsquamous NSCLC, second line glioblastoma (GBM), metastatic breast cancer	Black box warning for gastrointestinal perforation, hemorrhage, wound healing; infusion reaction, hypertension, proteinuria, exfoliative dermatitis.
Cetuximab (Erbitux)	EGFR	Head and neck cancer, metastatic colorectal cancer	Dermatologic reactions, headache, diarrhea, infection, infusion reactions, electrolyte abnormalities, hypomagnesia; rare cardiopulmonary arrest (2%).
Panitumumab (Vectibix)	EGFR	Metastatic colorectal cancer	Skin toxicities (acneiform dermatitis, exfoliation, rash), photosensitivity, paronychia, hypomagnesemia, fatigue, abdominal pain, nausea, diarrhea, constipation; infusion reactions (4%).
Transtuzumab (Herceptin)	HER-2	Breast cancer	Infections, neutropenia, anemia, myalgia, dyspnea, rash, headache, diarrhea, nausea, fever, cough, infusion reactions, cardiac toxicity, CHF.

(*Continued*)

Table 2. *(Continued)*

Drug (Trade Name)	Target	Approved Indications (Unlabeled Use)	Major Adverse Side Effects
Euclizimab (Soliris)	Complement protein C5; inhibits MAC and complement-mediated intravascular hemolysis	Paroxysmal nocturnal hemoglobinuria (PNH)	Headache, nasopharyngitis, nausea, back pain, fatigue, cough; increases risk for serious meningococcal infections; meningococcal vaccine or booster required prior to treatment.
Rituximab (Rituxan)	Anti-CD20	NHL, CLL, rheumatoid arthritis (RA); also ITP, chronic GVHD	Severe, even fatal infusion reactions (80% with first exposure), fever, lymphopenia, neutropenia, tumor lysis syndrome, infections, mucocutaneous reactions, renal toxicity hepatitis B reactivation, PML, arrhythmias, bowel obstruction or perforation, reported autoimmune events.
Alemtuzuma (Campath)	CD52	B-CLL	Myelosuppression, infections, infusion reactions, fever, nausea, diarrhea, insomnia, HTN, edema, arrhythmia; injection site reaction with subcutaneous administration.
Tyrosine Kinase Inhibitors			
Erlotinib (Tarceva)	EGFR	Advanced NSCLC and pancreatic cancer	Rash, diarrhea, fatigue, anorexia, stomatitis, hyperbilirubinemia, infection, dyspnea, conjunctivitis; rare MI, cerebral vascular accident (CVA), corneal ulceration.

(Continued)

Table 2. *(Continued)*

Drug (Trade Name)	Target	Approved Indications (Unlabeled Use)	Major Adverse Side Effects
Gefitinib (Iressa)	EGFR	NSCLC	Diarrhea, rash, acne, nausea/vomiting, <1% interstitial lung disease (ILD) and hemorrhage.
Imatinib (Gleevac)	Bcr-Abl (Ph+), platelet-derived growth factor (PDGF), c-kit (CD117), stem-cell-derived factor	Ph+ CML, Ph+ ALL, MDS/MP, systemic mastocytosis, hypereosinophilic syndrome, gastrointestinal stromal tumor (GIST), dermato-fibrosarcoma	Myelosuppression, edema, nausea, vomiting, muscle cramps, myalgias, diarrhea, rash, fatigue, abdominal pain, hepatoxicity, severe hemorrhage; rare CHF, GI perforation.
Dasatinib (Sprycel)	Bcr-Abl, Src, c-kit, EPHA2, PDGFRβ	Imatinib-resistant CML and imatinib-resistant Ph+ ALL	Myelosuppression, hemorrhage (associated with thrombocytopenia), fluid retention, QT prolongation, diarrhea, rash, dyspnea; teratogenic.
Nilotinib (Tasigna)	Bcr-Abl, c-kit, PDGFR	Imatinib-resistant CML and imatinib-resistant CML in chronic phase	Black box warning for QTC prolongation, myelosuppression, liver toxicity, rash, nausea/vomiting, abdominal pain, urinary tract infection, electrolyte derangements, sudden death; contains lactulose.
Lapatinib (Tykerb)	EGFR, HER2	Metastatic breast cancer	Diarrhea, hand–foot syndrome, nausea/vomiting, stomatitis, rash, fatigue; myelosuppression, hepatotoxicity, decreased left ventricular ejection fraction (LVEF) (2%–5%), QT prolongation, ILD.

(Continued)

Table 2. (*Continued*)

Drug (Trade Name)	Target	Approved Indications (Unlabeled Use)	Major Adverse Side Effects
Sunitinib (Sutent)	VEGFR1–3, c-kit, PDGFR, CSF-1, Flt-3, RET	Imatinib-resistant GIST, renal cancer	Myelosuppression, fatigue, fever, diarrhea, nausea, mucositis/stomatitis, vomiting, dyspepsia, abdominal pain, constipation, HTN, peripheral edema, rash, hand–foot syndrome, skin discoloration, hair color changes, dysguesia, headache, arthralgia, dyspnea, anorexia, bleeding. Hepatotoxicity, decreased LVEF/CHF (11%–27%), hemorrhage, hypothyroidism, renal toxicity.
Sorafenib (Nexavar)	VEGFR2–3,c-kit, PDGFR, Raf, Flt-3, RET, FGFR-1	Hepatocellular carcinoma, renal cancer	Fatigue, weight loss, rash, hand/foot skin reaction, alopecia, diarrhea, anorexia, nausea, abdominal pain, HTN; hypophosphatemia, myelosuppression, elevated lipase; rarely cardiac ischemia (2.7%), GI perforation (<1%).
Pazopanib (Votrient)	VEGFR, PDGFR, FGFR, GIST c-kit, leukocyte-specific protein, transmembrane glycoprotein receptor	Renal cell cancer GIST	Diarrhea, hypertension, hair depigmentation, nausea, anorexia, vomiting, hepatotoxicity, hypothyroidism, QT prolongation (<2%), severe hemorrhage (92%), arterial thrombotic events (2%).

(*Continued*)

Table 2. *(Continued)*

Drug (Trade Name)	Target	Approved Indications (Unlabeled Use)	Major Adverse Side Effects
Everolimus (Affinitor)	mTOR, VEGF, hypoxia-inducible factor 1 (HIF-1)	Advanced renal cell carcinoma (after first-line tyrosine kinase)	Stomatitis, infections, asthenia, fatigue, cough, diarrhea, noninfectious pneumonitis, myelosuppression, hyperglycemia, hypertriglyceridemia, renal toxicity, myelosuppression, immunosuppression, infections including fungal and hepatitis B reactivation.
Temsirolimus (Torisel)	mTOR, VEGF, hypoxia-inducible factor 1 and 2 al pha (HIF-1 and-2 alpha)	Advanced renal cell carcinoma (poor risk)	Rash, asthenia, pyrexia, mucositis, nausea, anorexia, diarrhea, anemia, lymphopenia, thrombocytopenia, hyperglycemia, hyperlipidemia, renal and liver toxicity; <10% hypersensitivity reactions, HTN, ILD, PNA, bowel perforation.
Immune Modulating Drugs and Immunotherapy			
Thalidomide	Immunomodulator and inhibitor of angiogenesis and TNF-alpha	Multiple myeloma	Leukopenia, edema, constipation, hypocalcemia, CNS toxicity, hypersensitivity reactions, serious dermatologic reactions, peripheral neuropathy, severe birth defects, thromboembolic events.

(Continued)

Table 2. (*Continued*)

Drug (Trade Name)	Target	Approved Indications (Unlabeled Use)	Major Adverse Side Effects
Lenalidomide (Revlimid)	Immunomodulator, inhibitor of angiogenesis and TNF-alpha	Multiple myeloma and mylodysplastic syndrome with 5q- syndrome (CLL, NHL)	Thrombocytopenia, myelosuppression, peripheral edema, constipation, peripheral neuropathy, serious bullous dermatologic reactions, thromboembolic events <5%, severe birth defects, arrhythmia <5%.
Bortezomib (Velcade)	26S proteosome inhibitor blocks intracellular protein degradation	Multiple myeloma, mantle cell lymphoma	Diarrhea, nausea, constipation, peripheral neuropathy, pyrexia, thrombocytopenia, neutropenia, hepatic toxicity, hypotension, varicella reactivation.
Sipuleulcel- T (Provenge)	Autologous cellular immunetherapy against prostate-specific membrane antigen	Metastatic castration-resistant prostate cancer	Infusion reactions, chills, fatigue, fever, back pain, nausea, joint ache, headache.
Interferon (INF) alpha 2B	Immunomodulator enhances macrophage and lymphocyte activity	Melanoma, Kaposi's sarcoma, hairy cell leukemia, mantle cell lymphoma (renal cell carcinoma)	Influenza-like symptoms, nausea/vomiting, infections, hepatotoxicity, autoimmune disorders.
Interleukin-2	Immunomodulator enhances lymphocyte and natural killer cell activity, induces INF gamma	Melanoma, renal cell carcinoma	Hypotension, nausea/vomiting, stomatitis, influenza-like illness, cardiac arrhythmias, pulmonary edema, metabolic acidosis, neurotoxicity, capillary leak syndrome, sepsis.

Table 3. Management of Chemotherapy-associated Nausea/Vomiting

	Prophylaxis	**Treatment of Breakthrough Vomiting**
Minimal risk (<10%)	No prophylaxis is recommended.	*Add one class of medications at one time:* *Antiphychotic* Halperidol (1–2 mg po q4–6 hr)
Low risk (10%–30%)	Steroid or prochlorperazine or metoclopramide (consider PPI or H2 antagonist).	*Benzodiazepine* Lorazepam (0.5–2 mg po q4–6 hr) *Cannabinoid* Dronabinoid (5–10 mg po q3–6 hr)
Moderate risk (30%–90%)	Serotonin antagonist, steroid (consider PPI or H2 antagonist).	*Dopamine receptor antagonist* Metoclopromide (10–40 mg po/iv q4–6 hr) *Phenothiazine* Prochlorperazine (10 mg po/iv q4–6 hr)
High risk (>90%)	Neurokinin inhibitor, serotonin antagonist, steroid (consider PPI or H2 antagonist).	*Serotonin antagonist* Odansetron (8 mg iv q8–24 hr) *Steroid* Dexamethasone (12 mg po/iv q12–24 hr)

- Anticipatory — prior to infusion
  — Use benzodiazepine (lorazepam 0.5–2 mg po prior to infusion)

2. **Neurologic complications:** From direct effect to CNS or indirect effect by drug metabolites. The first step is to stop causative chemotherapy, particularly if severe, since the deficit may be irreversible. Neuropathy may be partially treated with pregabalin, gabapentin, or vitamin B6.
3. **Enterotoxicity**

- Diarrhea: direct intestinal mucosal damage, resulting in increasing small bowel fluid secretion greater than colonic reabsorption capacity, causing significant diarrhea.
- Constipation: slowing of bowel motility.
- Colitis: may take several forms in setting of chemotherapy use.
- Intestinal perforation: see Table 5.
- Other antidiarrheal agents: anticholinergic agent, tincture of opium, budesonide, cholestyramine, and absorbants.

Table 4. Management of Neurologic Complications

Neurologic Complication	Symptoms and Signs	Features/Treatment
Acute encephalopathy	Confusion, somnolence	Supportive care (usually resolves spontaneously without long term sequela)
Headache	Headache may be frontal or generalized	Opioid, Tylenol, or NSAID as needed
Aseptic meningitis	Headache, nausea, vomiting, nuchal rigidity	May be prevented with steroids; treatment is supportive with pain medications
Leukoencephalopathy	Progressive dementia, hemiparesis, ataxia, seizure	Irreversible effects; CT or MRI of head may be diagnostic; associated with concurrent methotrexate and whole brain radiation
Neuropathy	Motor	Proximal muscle weakness more common
	Cranial	Ototoxicity (tinnitus), extraocular palsy
	Sensory	Parasthesia, atypical arthralgia and myalgia
	Autonomic	Rare but reported with multiple agents

Table 5. Management of Chemotherapy-associated Enterotoxicity

Enterotoxicity	Severity	Features/Management
Diarrhea	Mild	Avoid lactose products, eat small and frequent meals, adequate hydration, and consider loperamide as needed.
	Moderate	Hold cytotoxic chemotherapy, start loperamide 2 mg orally every 2 hr, and consider adding oral antibiotics for infectious diarrhea.
	Severe	Hold chemotherapy, add IV hydration, IV antibiotics, bowel rest, continue loperamide, and consider octreotide (150 mcg/kg subcutaneously tid).

(*Continued*)

Table 5. (*Continued*)

Enterotoxicity	Severity	Features/Management
	Infectious	Hold antimotility agents (e.g. loperamide) with suspicion of severe infectious diarrhea, particularly *Clostridium difficile* colitis. Stool sample should be sent to rule out *C diff. E. coli. Campylobacter*, and other infectious agents).
Colitis	Neutropenic enterocolitis	Severe infectious colitis is associated with acute leukemia during induction therapy. It is caused by a combination of mucosal injury, severe neutropenia, and invasion by micro-organisms. It is associated with high mortality. Early recognition and appropriate medical management reduce mortality. Colitis is treated with broad spectrum antimicrobial therapy (bacterial, viral, and fungal coverage), bowel rest, and consider adding granulocyte colony stimulating factor (G-CSF).
	Ischemic colitis	Associated with several chemotherapeutic agents. Supportive care, bowel rest, and possible surgical resection.
	Clostridium difficile colitis	Commonly seen in the setting of prophylactic antibiotic use. The treatment of choice is oral metronidazole; but IV metronidazole, oral vancomycin, and intravenous immunoglobulin (IVIG) can be considered in the setting of resistant disease. A colectomy is associated with high mortality.
	Infectious	Consider bacterial (e.g. resistant gram negatives/anaerobes), viral (e.g. cytomegalovirus (CMV)), and fungal (e.g. invasive aspergillosis) coverage.
Bowel perforation	Any	Antiangiogenic agents. Induction chemotherapy for gastrointestinal malignancy, particularly with lymphoma.

(*Continued*)

4. **Infection:** As chemotherapy or underlying malignancy induces impaired immune function, consideration of prophylaxis and treatment of infection is imperative in this population.

	Prophylaxis	**Investigation/Treatment**
Low risk: neutropenia <7 days Solid tumor	None	1. History of present illness 2. Physical examination 3. Laboratory/radiographic testing
Intermediate risk: Lymphoma Myeloma Autologous stem cell tx Neutropenia 7–10 days	Bacterial: fluoroquinolone Viral: acyclovir Fungal: fluconazole	4. Broad spectrum antibiotic, with broadening of antiviral and antifungal coverage as needed: a. Bacteria: resistant gram-negative bacteria, MRSA; b. Viral/fungal: start with first line prophylaxis; if suspicion of specific causative disease, can have broad coverage.
High Risk: Acute leukemia Allogeneic stem cell tx Neutropenia >10 days	Bacterial: fluoroquinolone Viral: acyclovir, famciclovir, valacyclovir Fungal: fluconazole, micafungin, posoconazole	5. Serologic testing (e.g. CMV, galactomannan) may be helpful 6. Body fluid (sputum, nasal swab) 7. Tissue biopsy (lung, GI tract)
PCP: High dose steroid Allogeneic stem cell tx Alemtuzumab use	First line: sulfamethoxazole, trimethoprim Second line: dapsone, pentamidine, atavaquone	
CMV: Allogeneic stem cell tx	Use ganciclovir (oral) or valganciclovir/foscarnet (IV)	

Table 6. Other Chemotherapy-Associated Complications

Complication	Approach/Signs/Symptoms	Treatment/Adverse Effects
Pain		
Chemotherapy-associated pain is mostly neuropathic in nature. Most pains resolve spontaneously over time; some may become chronic. Supportive care with pain medication can be employed. G-CSF can cause atypical bone, joint, muscle pain.	History of present illness and physical examination are most helpful. Pain is persistent in nature; in most cases, intensity and duration of pain are correlated with cumulative dosage of chemotherapy.	Refer to pain control. Mild: nonopioid as needed. Moderate: opioid therapy, stop chemotherapy. Severe: opioid therapy, stop chemotherapy, and consider alternative agents (e.g. gabapentin for neuropathic pain).
Myelosuppression Management based on: 1. Current disease (MDS and myeloid malignancies vs. others) 2. Chemotherapy regimen 3. Patient risk factors (age, comorbidities, etc.) — Assess need for granulocyte-colony-stimulating factor.	*Febrile neutropenia* • Continue filgrastim or sargromostim if already on therapy. • Already received pegfilgrastim, no additional growth factor is required. • G-CSF can be considered when patient is at risk for poor clinical infectious outcome (age >65, sepsis, neutropenia expected >10 days, fungal infection, pneumonia, or ANC <100).	*Adverse effects of G-CSF* • Bone pain, arthralgia, or myalgia is commonly observed but gradually resolves over days to weeks. • Opioid or NSAID can be used as needed for pain control.

(*Continued*)

Table 6. (*Continued*)

Complication	Approach/Signs/Symptoms	Treatment/Adverse Effects
Fatigue • Persistent sense of physical and emotional exhaustion relating to cancer treatment • Interfering with daily functioning	• Thorough history of present illness and physical examination to identify severity of fatigue. • Rule out other causes: anemia, malnutrition, insomnia, medication side effects, substance abuse, medical comorbidities.	*Nonpharmacologic* • Activity enhancement (e.g. exercise program, physical therapy) • Psychosocial intervention (e.g. behavioral therapy) • Cognitive-behavioral therapy • Nutrition optimization *Pharmacologic intervention* • Stimulants (e.g. methylphenidate, modafinil) • Sleeping medication (e.g. mirtazapine, zolpidem) • Correction of anemia (e.g. blood transfusion, erythropoietin growth factors)
Cutaneous manifestation Skin	*Common reactions* Infusion reactions: 1. Type 1 (IgE-mediated) — urticaria, pruritus 2. Type 3 (immune complex) — Erythema multiforme/vasculitis 3. Type 4 (T-cell mediated) — skin rash	*Reactions (other)* Pigmentation: 1. Localized 2. Diffuse
Hair	Alopecia (usually reversible)	Pigmentation (temporary)
Nail	Onycholysis	Nail color change (temporary)

(*Continued*)

Table 6. (*Continued*)

Complication	Approach/Signs/Symptoms	Treatment/Adverse Effects
Cardiotoxicity		
Most commonly associated with anthracyclines	*Acute toxicity* (during or immediately after infusion; all agents)	*Cumulative toxicity* (months to years after infusion) (anthracycline use)
Other agents:	Arrhythmia	Ventricular dysfunction
Vinca-alkaloids		Management with beta-blocker and angiotensin-converting enzyme inhibitors has improved morbidity and mortality.
5-FU		
Monoclonal antibodies	Ventricular dysfunction	
Alkylating agents		
Tyrosine kinase inhibitors	Pericarditis–myocarditis	
Risk factors		
Cumulative dose	Often reversible.	Surveillance with echocardiograms or multigated blood pool imaging is necessary when employing anthracyclines and trastuzumab-containing regimens.
Age		
Concurrent chemotherapy	Use of valsartan may decrease incidence of acute toxicity.	
Concurrent radiation		

References

1. Ando Y, Saka H, Ando M, *et al.* (2000) Polymorphisms of UDP-glucuronosyltransferase gene and irinotecan toxicity: A pharmacogenetic analysis. *Cancer Res* **60**(24): 6921–6926.
2. Bruera E, Yennurajalingam. S (2010) Challenge of managing cancer-related fatigue. *J Clin Oncol* **28**(23): 3671–3672.
3. Chu E, DeVita VT. (2008) *Physician's Cancer Chemotherapy Drug Manual 2008.* Jones and Barlett, Sudbury, Massachusetts.
4. DeVita VT, Lawrence T, Rosenberg SA. (2008) *Cancer: Principles & Practice of Oncology*, 8th ed. Lippincott Williams & Wilkins, Philadelphia, Pennsylvania.
5. Holland J, Emil Frei III. (2010) *Cancer Medicine*, 8th ed. People's Medical Publishing House, Shelton, Connecticut.
6. Singal PK, Iliskovic N. (1998) Doxorubicin-induced cardiomyopathy. *N Engl J Med.* **339**(13): 900–905.
7. *Micromedex® Healthcare Series.* Version 2.0. Thomson Healthcare, Greenwood Village, CO.
8. National Comprehensive Cancer Network Guidelines for Supportive Care. V.1.2010 © National Comprehensive Cancer Network, Inc. (2010).
9. http://www.accessdata.fda.gov/scripts/cder/drugsatfda; last accessed Sep 21, 2010.

Chapter 72

Oncologic Emergencies

*Noa Biran, Keren Osman**

Key Pearls

- Superior vena cava (SVC) syndrome, most commonly occurring with lung cancer, can present with stridor, hemoptysis, or facial swelling and should be managed with chemotherapy or radiotherapy depending on the primary tumor.
- Spinal cord compression should be suspected in patients with severe back pain, lower extremity weakness and/or loss of bowel/bladder function. Treat immediately with dexamethasone 10–16 mg IV followed by 4–6 mg every 4 hours.
- Hyperleukocytosis, defined by a WBC >75,000 or a rapid rise, is most commonly seen in M4 or M5 AML. Watch for neurologic, pulmonary, ophthalmologic, and cardiovascular symptoms and treat with hydration and leukapharesis.
- Hypercalcemia of malignancy may present with constipation, lethargy, abdominal pain, or polyuria. Treat with bisphosphanates, IV fluids and calcitonin.
- A temperature >38.5°C in the context of absolute neutrophil count (ANC) <500 defines neutropenic fever. The patient should be pancultured and started on empiric broad-spectrum antibiotics. Overall mortality rate is 5%.

*Mount Sinai School of Medicine, New York, NY, USA.

An oncologic emergency is an acute, potentially life-threatening event related to a patient's cancer or its treatment. The presentation may be insidious and take months to develop or can develop over hours. The goal is to prevent, assess, diagnose, and treat the condition before it rapidly results in permanent morbidity or mortality. Oncologic emergencies arise from the ability of cancers to spread, from the abnormal production of cellular products, or from the effects of antineoplastic agents that can result in metabolic derangements or multi-organ failure. Some oncologic emergencies may arise in patients with previously unrecognized malignancies. Once an oncologic emergency is suspected, aggressive, prompt management is critical in preventing devastating outcomes such as paralysis or death. Physicians need to be familiar with these oncologic emergencies as immediate treatment is often necessary prior to consultation with the hematologist-oncologist.

Superior Vena Cava Syndrome

Epidemiology. SVC syndrome is most common in (1) Lung cancer (2–4% of all lung cancer, and as high as 10% in small-cell lung cancer); (2) Non-Hodgkins lymphoma; (3) Large B-cell lymphoma (highest in primary mediastinal large B-cell lymphoma with sclerosis).[1]

Physiology and Anatomy. Compression of the SVC is due to extrinsic masses in the middle or anterior mediastinum, right paratracheal or precarinal lymph nodes and tumors extending from the right upper lobe bronchus. Severity depends on rapidity of onset of obstruction as collaterals take several weeks to dilate sufficiently to accommodate diverted blood flow from SVC.[2]

Presentation. Most common presentation includes facial or neck swelling (82%), arm swelling (68%), dyspnea (66%), cough (50%), and dilated chest veins (38%).[1] Also reported are orthopnea, chest pain, dysphagia, hoarseness, headache, confusion, dizziness and syncope.

Red flags. Stridor indicates laryngeal edema. Confusion, obtundation or other evidence of respiratory and neurologic compromise are associated with fatal outcomes. Monitor for hemoptysis or thrombosis related to extrinsic compression of major airway.

Management. Depending on the tumor type, chemotherapy, radiation therapy, or endovascular stent placement may be indicated.

Spinal Cord Compression

Definition/Epidemiology. Spinal cord compression is due to neoplastic epidural invasion of the space between the vertebrae and spinal cord, often cauda equina compression. Usually, spinal cord compression is from bone metastases and 60% go to the thoracic spine. This neurologic complication occurs in approximately 1 in 12,700 cancer patients each year. Although all tumors have potential to cause malignant spinal cord compression, prostate, breast and lung each account for 15% to 20% of the cases, while non-Hodgkins lymphoma, renal cell carcinoma, and multiple myeloma each cause 5% to 10% of cases.[3]

Diagnosis. Severe local back pain is the first symptom in 85% to 95% of cases and usually precedes other symptoms. Motor loss and weakness are present in 60% to 85%, with hyperreflexia and extensor plantar response below the level of lesion.[3] Spinal sensory levels are typically one to five levels below the level of cord compression. Look for loss of bowel and bladder function. Imaging includes CT or MRI.

Treatment. Pain can be controlled with opiates and corticosteroids. High dose corticosteroids constitute the first-line treatment in most patients, as they reduce vasogenic edema and inflammation, and have been shown to preserve or improve neurologic function. Dexamethasone is typically given at 10 to 16 mg IV bolus, followed by 4 to 6 mg every 4 hours. The most important prognostic indicator for ambulatory outcome is pretreatment motor function. Immediate initiation of therapy is critical. Radiation therapy plays an important role, especially in the case of radiosensitive tumors such as myeloma and NHL. Decompressive radical surgery may improve outcomes and should be considered.

Hematologic Emergencies

Hyperleukocytosis

Definition/Epidemiology. Hyperleukocytosis is defined by a WBC >75–100,000 or a rapid rise. It is most commonly seen in AML (M4 or M5), acute promyelocytic leukemia, and 11q23 deletions. In CML, there is concern if WBC >250,000. Leukostasis in small vessels results in poorly deformable WBC with high oxygen consumption and local hypoxemia. The clinical presentation varies widely and can affect multiple organ systems (Table 1).

Management. Hydration, chemotherapy, leukapheresis, hydroxyurea and allopurinol are used in management. Avoid transfusions as this may increase whole blood viscosity.

Leukapheresis, requiring a central catheter, enables rapid removal of circulating blasts and may lead to recruitment of marginated leukemic cells into intravascular space. Administration of plasma and electrolytes may reduce the risk of hemorrhage and tumor lysis. Initially, it may worsen thrombocytopenia, but this should not delay initiation of specific treatment.

Tumor Lysis Syndrome

Definition and mechanism. Tumor lysis syndrome (TLS) is the combination of metabolic derangements resulting from rapid destruction of malignant cells and abrupt release of intracellular ions, nucleic acids and their metabolites into the extracellular space. Monitor for hyperuricemia, hyperkalemia, hyperphosphatemia, and hypocalcemia secondary to calcium phosphate precipitation. Precipitation of uric acid crystals can occur in many organs including the kidneys (causing renal failure), the

Table 1. Clinical Presentation of Hyperleukocytosis

Neurologic	Dizziness, tinnitus, headache, confusion, delirium, stupor, coma
Pulmonary	Dyspnea, hypoxemia, interstitial/alveolar infiltrates
Ophthalmologic	Diplopia, papilledema, retinal bleed
Cardiovascular	NSTEMI/STEMI, bowel infarction, renal vein thrombosis
Miscellaneous	DIC in 30–50%, hypoglycemia, pseudohyperkalemia

cardiac conduction system (causing arrhythmias), and the joint spaces (causing an acute gouty flare).[4]

Epidemiology. TLS occurs in highly proliferative tumors, most commonly Burkitt's lymphoma, lymphoblastic lymphoma, and mantle cell lymphoma of blastic variant.

Risk factors include renal insufficiency, hyperuricemia, highly chemosensitive malignancies, rapidly growing or large tumor burden, and intravascular volume depletion.

Diagnosis: Clinical diagnosis can be made if Cr ≥ 1.5 times of the upper limit of normal, cardiac arrhythmia/sudden death, or seizure. Other symptoms include nausea, vomiting, lethargy, seizures, edema, CHF, muscle cramps, tetany.

The CAIRO-BISHOP classification system is used to make the diagnosis of TLS.[4] Two or more of the following lab changes are needed, and must occur between 3–7 days of receiving cytotoxic therapy.

Uric acid ≥ 8 mg/dL
K ≥ 6 mEq/L
Phos ≥ 6.5 mg/dL
Ca ≤ 7 mg/dL

(Or, a 25% decrease from baseline.)

Treatment and Prevention. Adequate hydration is most important. Allopurinol is used more commonly for prevention of tumor lysis, while rasburicase is used for the treatment (Table 2).

Hypercalcemia of Malignancy

Incidence and Mechanism. Malignant hypercalcemia may occur in up to 30% of all cancer patients at some time in their disease course.[3] It is mediated by PTHrP, PTH oversecretion, overproduction of vitamin D, or direct osteolytic effect of tumor on bone. Tumors most commonly associated with PTHrP production are of squamous histology and usually arise from the lung, esophagus, head and neck and cervix. Ovarian, endometrial and renal carcinoma may also produce hypercalcemia.

Table 2. Comparison of Two Drugs Used in Prevention and Treatment of Tumor Lysis Syndrome

Drug	Mechanism	Use	Dose	Adverse Events
Allopurinol	Inhibits xanthine oxidase decreasing uric acid production	Moderate-risk situations 2–3 days prior to starting chemotherapy	100mg/m² every 8 hr po or 200–400 mg/m²/d in 1–3 divided doses IV	Renal failure; reduce dose in renal insufficiency
Rasburicase	Recombinant form of the enzyme urate oxidase leading to degradation of uric acid into water soluble allantoin	High risk cases	0.05 0 0.2 mg/kg IV over 30 min. Monitor uric acid levels	Contraindicated in G6PD deficiency

Symptoms. The clinical presentation is nonspecific. Symptoms include constipation, lethargy, abdominal pain, and polyuria. ECG may show shortened QT interval and arrhythmias. The rate of rise influences the appearance of neurologic symptoms. Without correction, acute renal failure, seizures, coma and death may occur. Immobilization and dehydration worsen outcomes.

Diagnosis. Obtain an ionized calcium level.

Management. Remove exogenous calcium including parenteral feeds and medications (lithium, thiazides, vitamin D). Increase mobility. Hydrate with normal saline as it acts as a calciuretic. Lasix can be used after rehydration. Hemodialysis is reserved for patients with a high risk for cardiovascular and renal failure.

The following treatments result in inhibition of bone resorption to decrease total body calcium[3]:

— Bisphosphonates (pamidronate, zoledronic acid): response takes 2–4 days, adjust for renal insufficiency

— Calcitonin: response takes 12–24 hours; tachyphylaxis occurs quickly
— Corticosteroids: 1mg/kg; role usually limited to lymphomas

Neutropenic Fever

Definition. Neutropenic fever is defined by temperature >38.5°C, lasting >1 hr in the context of absolute neutrophil count (ANC) $< 0.5 \times 10^9$/l. Overall mortality rates are 5% in patients with solid tumors (1% in low-risk patients) and as high as 11% in some hematological malignancies.[5]

Initial Assessment. Symptoms or signs may suggest a source of infection but often there are no symptoms, especially in patients on corticosteroids. Culture blood from peripheral veins and from any indwelling venous catheters. Sputum, urine and skin samples should also be sent before prompt institution of empiric broad-spectrum antimicrobial therapy.

Outcome Risk Assessment. The Multinational Association for Supportive Care in Cancer (MASCC) index allows rapid risk assessment.[6] The MASCC is based on several clinical parameters (Table 3).

Management. Prompt administration of empiric broad-spectrum antibiotics is critical. Supportive care in the form of IV fluids, oxygen, and clinical stabilization should be provided until the patient is afebrile and stable for at least 24 hr and the neutrophil count is $\geq 1.0 \times 10^9$/l. If the patient is febrile at 48 hr, continue empiric coverage. If the patient is clinically unstable at 48 hr, seek prompt advice from an infectious diseases specialist. If pyrexia lasts >4 days, initiate antifungal therapy.[6]

Table 3. The MASCC scoring index

Burden of illness; no or mild symptoms	5
No hypotension	5
No chronic obstructive pulmonary disease	4
Solid tumor or no previous fungal infection	4
No dehydration	3
Burden of illness; moderate symptoms	3
Outpatient status (at onset of fever)	3
Age <20	2

Low risk cases requires score ≥ 21.

Low Risk Patients. A low risk patient must score ≥ 21 on the MASCC scoring index, and must also be hemodynamically stable, without acute leukemia, end-organ damage, pneumonia, and does not have an indwelling catheter. Oral quinolones with amoxicillin plus clavulinic-acid can be used.[6]

Choice of Empiric IV Antimicrobials: Use local bacterial resistance patterns to determine first choice empiric IV therapy. The Infectious Disease Society of America (IDSA) 2002 Guidelines recommend[7]:

Two drugs without vancomycin:

- Aminoglycoside plus antipseudomonal penicillin
- Aminoglycoside plus antipsuedomonal cephalosporin (cefepime or ceftazidime)
- Aminoglycoside plus carbapenem (imipenem-cilastatin or meropenem)

Vancomycin plus 1 or 2 antibiotics if any of the following criteria are met: clinically suspected catheter-related infections, known colonization with penicillin- and cephalosporin-resistant pneumococci or methicillin-resistant *S. aureus*; positive results of blood culture for gram-positive bacteria, hypotension or other evidence of instability. Regimens are:

- vancomycin plus cefepime or ceftazidime +/– aminoglycoside
- vancomycin plus carbapenem +/– aminoglycoside
- vancomycin plus antipseudomonal penicillin plus an aminoglycoside.

Alternative therapy may be indicated in specific situations (Table 4).

Table 4. Choice of Antibiotics and Workup of Various Clinical Conditions

Clinical Situation	Empiric Coverage	Labs/Studies
Central catheter	Vancomycin	
Cellulitis	Vancomycin	
Candidiasis	Fluconazole	
Diarrhea	Metronidazole	C. diff
Vesicular lesions	Acyclovir/ganciclovir	CMV
Lung infiltrates	Fungal coverage/bactrim	CT chest, BAL for PCP
Suspected meningitis/ encephalitis	Ceftazidime or meropenem plus ampicillin, acyclovir	Lumbar puncture

References

1. Qint LE. (2009) Thoracic complications and emergencies in oncologic patients. *Cancer Imaging* **2**:9A:S75–82.
2. Rice TW, Rodriguez RM, Light RW. (2006) The superior vena cava syndrome: Clinical characteristics and evolving etiology. *Medicine* (Baltimore) **85**(1): 37–42.
3. Behl D, Hendrickson AQ, *et al*. (2010) Oncologic emergencies. *Crit Care Clin* **26**: 181–205.
4. Cairo MS, *et al*. (2010). Recommendations for the evaluation of risk and prophylaxis of tumour lysis syndrome (TLS) in adults and children with malignant diseases: An expert TLS panel consensus. *Br J Haematol* **149**(4): 578–86.
5. NCCN Practice Guidelines in Oncology: Prevention and Treatment of Cancer Related Infections. 2009.
6. Marti FM, Cullen MH, *et al*. (2009) Management of febrile neutropenia: ESMO Guidelines Working Group. *Ann Oncol* **20**(4): 166–169.
7. Hughes WT, *et al*. (2002). 2002 Guidelines of the Use of Antimicrobial Agents in Neutropenic Patients with Cancer. *Clin. Infect. Dis.* **34**: 732–51.

Transplant Medicine

Chapter 73

Transplantation Medicine for the Hospitalist

Sakshi Dua and Maria L. Padilla**

Key Pearls

- Rigorous pre-transplantation screening is performed to ensure successful outcomes after organ transplantation.
- There exist organ-specific and center-specific contraindications to organ transplantation.
- Maintenance immunosuppression usually involves the use of calcineurin inhibitors, cell cycle inhibitors, and steroids.
- Post-transplantation rejection can be acute or chronic and both have distinct pathophysiologic mechanisms.
- Post-transplantation infectious complications are determined by the duration since transplantation and the anti-microbiol prophylaxis used.

Introduction

Organ transplantation is an established treatment option for patients with a wide variety of end stage diseases. It is essential for hospitalists to familiarize themselves with the field of transplantation medicine, since an encounter with a transplant candidate or recipient is inevitable.

*Mount Sinai Medical Center, New York, NY, USA.

United Network for Organ Sharing (UNOS) and Organ Allocation

Transplantation uses allografts from living-related, living-unrelated, or deceased donors. Deceased donor organs can be recovered from heart-beating or "brain-dead" donors and non-heart-beating or "cardiac death" donors.

UNOS is a national, private, nonprofit organization that develops policies and guidelines, maintains data on wait lists, runs organ matches, and records all transplants.

In the US and Puerto Rico, 58 organ procurement organizations (OPOs) coordinate organ procurement in designated service areas.

Allocation of organs depends on disease severity for some organs (liver and heart) and on disease severity plus the time spent on the wait list for others (lung, kidney, and bowel). Hospitalists are in a unique position to identify potential donors and should contact their hospital's designated representative at or near the time of a patient's death. The representative then contacts the local OPO and provides confidential information to determine if the patient is a potential donor.

Pretransplantation Screening

Due to the scarcity of donor organs, potential organ transplant recipients are thoroughly screened for medical and nonmedical factors to improve the likelihood of success given the risk and expense of transplantation.

Tissue Compatibility

Both the donor and the recipient are universally tested for ABO antigens to ensure blood type compatibility and prevent hyperacute rejection. Recipients are also tested for presensitization to donor antigens by checking panel reactive antibodies (PRAs) against human leukocyte antigen (HLA). HLA tissue typing is most important for hematopoietic stem cell and kidney transplantation. However, due to time constraints, it is not typically performed prior to heart, lung, liver, and pancreas transplantation.

Infection

To diminish the risk of donor-transmitted infections and reactivation of latent infection in recipients, several tests are performed pretransplantation. These include serologic tests for cytomegalovirus (CMV), Epstein–Barr virus (EBV), herpes simplex virus (HSV), varicella-zoster virus (VZV), hepatitis B and C virus, human immunodeficiency virus (HIV), and the tuberculin skin test (TST).

Financial and Psychosocial

Given the expense and emotional burden of going through organ transplantation, candidates undergo consultations with financial coordinators and social workers for psychosocial screening.

Contraindications to Transplantation

Although these are very center- and organ-specific (such as age eligibility), there are certain contraindications, such as:

- ABO incompatibility
- Active uncontrolled infection or sepsis
- Cancer (except for certain neuroendocrine, skin, and brain tumors or hepatocellular cancer confined to the liver)
- Presence of advanced AIDS if the patient is HIV-positive

Relative contraindications include psychosocial morbidities such as substance addiction, known nonadherence to followup visits and medications, and active psychiatric problems. Extremes of body weight, poor functional status, and HIV status are considered contraindications on an individual basis.

Maintenance Immunosuppressive Agents

These can be divided into the following categories:

- Calcineurin inhibitors (CNIs) such as tacrolimus (Tac) and cyclosporine A (CsA)
- Antimetabolites such as mycophenolate mofetil (MMF) and azathioprine (AZA)
- Mammalian target of rapamycin (mTOR) inhibitors such as sirolimus (SRL)
- Corticosteroids

Calcineurin inhibitors

Drug Interactions

CNIs are metabolized in the liver by the cytochrome p450 family. Common drugs that cause an increase in Tac or CsA levels include cytochrome p450 inhibitors such as:

- Diclofenac, doxycycline, imatinib, isoniazid, propofol, protease inhibitors, quinidine, telithromycin
- Calcium channel blockers: diltiazem, verapamil, nicardipine
- Macrolides: clarithromycin, erythromycin
- Azole antifungals, especially voriconazole, for which the Tac dose must be decreased by 66%
- Metoclopramide

Common drugs that cause a decrease in Tac or CsA levels include cytochrome p450 inducers such as:

- Nafcillin, nevirapine
- Anticonvulsants: carbamazepine, phenobarbital, phenytoin, primidone
- Rifamycins: rifabutin, rifampin
- St John's wort

Other interactions worth mentioning are:

- Synergistic nephrotoxic effects with ganciclovir.
- Increased risk of hemolytic uremic syndrome (HUS) or thrombotic thrombocytopenic purpura (TTP) with SRL.
- Hyperkalemia when used in conjunction with K^+ sparing diuretics or angiotensin-converting enzyme inhibitors (ACEIs).
- Synergistic nephrotoxicity in conjunction with gentamicin, tobramycin, vancomycin, bactrim, and NSAIDs.
- Synergistic neurotoxicity can be seen with CsA and imipenem (seizures)
- H-2 blockers and allopurinol both increase CsA levels/toxicity.

Side Effects

- Nephrotoxicity: This may range from mild renal dysfunction to end stage renal disease requiring hemodialysis. This nephrotoxicity is often dose dependent, but may also be idiosyncratic. Renal dysfunction may be reversible if the drug is stopped early. Both acute and chronic renal insufficiency can be seen.
- Hypertension (HTN)
- Dyslipidemia
- Electrolyte disturbances such as hypokalemia and hypomagnesemia
- HUS
- Neurologic complications, including seizures, tremors, and headaches
- Post-transplantation diabetes (specific to Tac)
- Hirsutism and gingival hyperplasia (specific to CsA)

Antimetabolites

Mycophenolate Mofetil

Drug interactions

- Valganciclovir: The two increase each other's effects, and hence concurrent use can worsen myelosuppression.

- Metronidazole: Their use is not recommended together.
- Flouroquinolones: Use with norfloxacin is not recommended.
- Rifamycins: Not recommended together.
- Magnesium salts: Separate by 2 hr.
- CsA interferes with its enterohepatic circulation; the usual dose of MMF when used in conjunction with CsA should be 1500 mg BID.

Side effects

- GI distress is the most notable side effect, with manifestations such as nausea, vomiting, and diarrhea.
- Leucopenia, anemia, and general bone marrow suppression.

Azathioprine

Drug Interactions

- Allopurinol: Potentially fatal toxicity from pancytopenia. If coadministration cannot be avoided, then AZA should be administered at 20%–30% of the normal dose.
- Bactrim: Concurrent use may lead to exaggerated leucopenia.
- ACEI: Concurrent use can induce anemia and severe leucopenia.
- Warfarin: AZA may interfere with anticoagulant effect.

Side Effects

- Dose-dependent myelosuppression resulting in thrombocytopenia, leucopenia, and macrocytic anemia
- Hepatotoxicity and hepatic veno-occlusive disease
- Nausea, vomiting, diarrhea, and pancreatitis
- Skin rashes and alopecia
- Interstitial pneumonitis

Mammalian Target of Rapamycin (mTOR) Inhibitors

Sirolimus

Drug interactions

Sirolimus is also metabolized by the cytochrome p450 family of enzymes and is subject to the same drug interactions as CNI. Its use with voriconazole is not approved, since it causes an 11-fold increase in area under curve (AUC) of SRL.

Side effects

SRL does not independently cause renal insufficiency, but can potentiate CNI-induced nephrotoxicity by both increasing the levels and potentiating the mechanisms of nephropathy.

- Dyslipidemia
- Hypertension
- Myelosuppression (especially thrombocytopenia)
- Thrombotic microangiopathy
- Lymphocoeles and pleural/pericardial effusions
- Pulmonary toxicity ranging from interstitial pneumonitis to organizing pneumonia, lymphocytic alveolitis, alveolar hemorrhage, and pulmonary vasculitis
- Poor wound healing and anastomotic site complications including fatal airway dehiscence in the perioperative period due to antifibroproliferative effect

Post-transplantation Complications

Rejection

Hyperacute Rejection

Hyperacute rejection occurs within 48 hr of transplantation and is caused by pre-existing complement-fixing antibodies to graft antigens (presensitization). It is rare, due to pre-transplantation screening. It is characterized by small vessel thrombosis and graft infarction. No treatment is effective other than graft removal.

Accelerated rejection occurs 3–5 days after transplantation and is caused by pre-existing non-complement-fixing antibodies to graft antigens. It is also rare and is characterized by cellular infiltrate with or without vascular changes. Treatment is with high dose steroids or antilymphocyte preparations. Plasmapharesis can clear circulating antibodies rapidly.

Acute Rejection

This is caused by a T-cell mediated delayed hypersensitivity reaction to allograft histocompatibility antigens. It is characterized by a mononuclear infiltrate with varying degrees of edema, hemorrhage, and necrosis. Vascular endothelium is the primary target. Treatment includes high dose steroids, antilymphocyte preparations, or both. After the resolution of acute rejection, the severely damaged parts of the graft heal by fibrosis, whereas the rest of the graft functions normally. Mortality is low and the graft can survive for long periods thereafter.

Chronic Rejection

This leads to graft dysfunction occurring months to years after transplantation. Causes are varied, including early acute rejection episodes, periprocedural ischemia, graft reperfusion injury, and infections such as CMV. The histopathology is organ-specific, with this being an airway-based lesion in lung transplant recipients (obliterative bronchiolitis) and a vessel based lesion in others (transplantation atherosclerosis). Regardless, it is characterized by extracellular matrix deposition, intimal and smooth muscle proliferation, and fibrotic obliteration of structures.

Chronic rejection usually progresses insidiously despite immunosuppression, and no effective treatment exists.

Infections

The increased susceptibility of the immunosuppressed organ transplant recipient broadens the possible spectrum of infecting micro-organisms. Preventive antimicrobial strategies have reduced the incidence and altered the timing of infections from different microbes after transplantation. The sequence with which different organisms appear in the posttransplantation course is dependent on the time since transplantation.

- The first month after transplantation is influenced by the infectious risks posed by surgery and the intensive care unit. Nosocomial bacterial pathogens predominate in this period.
- The second-to-sixth month after transplantation is a period of sustained intense immunosuppression characterized by emergence of opportunistic infections.
- Beyond six months most patients with stable graft function have slightly lowered immunosuppression. This period is characterized by community-acquired pathogens. During periods of enhanced immunosuppression for episodes of acute rejection or for the treatment of chronic rejection, opportunistic infections can be anticipated and appropriate precautions taken.

Conclusion

As the overall expected survival of patients who have undergone transplantation has improved, and as more patients live longer, infectious and medical complications that arise as a consequence of immunosuppressive therapy are seen more frequently.

References

1. www.unos.org
2. Bhorade SM, Stern E. (2009) Immunosuppression for lung transplantation. *Proc Am Thorac Soc* **6**(1): 47–53.

3. Kotloff RM, Ahya VN, Crawford SW. (2004) Pulmonary complications of solid organ and hematopoietic stem cell transplantation. *Am J Respir Crit Care Med* **170**(1): 22–48.
4. Remund KF, Best M, Egan JJ. (2009) Infections relevant to lung transplantation. *Proc Am Thorac Soc* **6**(1): 94–100.
5. Lyu DM, Zamora MR. (2009) Medical complications of lung transplantation. *Proc Am Thorac Soc* **6**(1): 101–107.

Neurology

Chapter 74

Concepts of and Approach to Delirium

*Alan Briones**

Key Pearls

- Delirium is a syndrome of an acute change in attention and cognition most commonly seen among hospitalized vulnerable elderly patients.
- Delirium has been associated with increased morbidity, mortality, healthcare costs, and hospital length of stay.
- Delirium is usually caused by multiple inciting factors, many of which are preventable.
- Prompt recognition, screening and prevention are the first steps in the approach to delirium.
- Haloperidol is the drug of choice for the treatment of delirium with severe agitation.

Definition and Diagnostic Criteria

Delirium is an acute state of confusion diagnosed clinically by the following key features as defined by the American Psychiatric Association's *Diagnostic and Statistical Manual of Mental Disorders*, 4th Edition (DSM-IV)[1]:

- Disturbance of consciousness (i.e. clouding — reduced clarity of awareness of the environment), with reduced ability to focus, sustain, or shift attention;

*Mount Sinai School of Medicine, New York, NY, USA.

- Change in cognition (e.g. memory impairment, disorientation, language deficits and perceptual disturbance) that is not better accounted for by a pre-existing, established, or evolving dementia;
- Development over a short period of time (usually hours to days), and disturbance tends to fluctuate during the course of the day;
- There is evidence from the history, physical examination, or laboratory findings that the disturbance is caused by the direct physiological consequences of a general medical condition.

Additional features of delirium include psychomotor hyperactivity (i.e. agitation or vigilance) or hypoactivity (i.e. lethargy or decreased motor activity), altered sleep-wake cycle, and emotional disturbances (i.e. fear, paranoia, anxiety, depression, anger, apathy or euphoria).[1]

Concepts of Delirium

Context

Delirium, an acute alteration of attention and cognition, is a common clinical syndrome among older hospitalized patients. The hospitalist is regularly faced with the challenge of preventing, recognizing, diagnosing, and treating delirium to reduce the risk of mortality and morbidity, and decrease both healthcare costs and hospital length of stay (LOS). The hospital prevalence of delirium ranges from 14%–24% and the incidence during hospitalization form 6%–56%.[2]

More recent studies estimate the rates of occurrence to be 7%–10% of older patients in the emergency department[3] and 40.9 % in the acute geriatric unit,[4] and 48%–70% in the intensive care unit[5,6]. A meta-analysis reported an incidence of postoperative delirium that ranged from 4%–53% after hip surgery.[7]

Mortality/Morbidity

Delirium has been associated with both inpatient and postdischarge mortality. An observational study estimated a 12-month mortality rate of

63.3%.[8] In addition, a meta-analysis showed evidence that delirium is associated with an increased risk of death, institutionalization, and dementia, independent of age, sex, comorbid illness, illness severity, or baseline dementia.[9]

Healthcare Costs

The average cost per day survived among delirious patients is approximately 2.5 times more than for patients without delirium. The total one-year healthcare cost associated with delirium ranges from US$16,303 to US$64,421 per patient, or US$38 billion to US$152 billion nationally each year.[10]

Hospital LOS

Patients with delirium stay 3.3 days longer in the hospital compared to controls,[11] and incidental delirium was associated with an excess stay of 7.78 days.[12] In the intensive care unit (ICU), delirium was found to be the strongest independent predictor of hospital LOS.[13]

Pathophysiology, Risk Factors, and Causes

Although it is poorly understood, there are several theories proposed to explain the pathogenesis of delirium:

- *Cholinergic deficiency*. Anticholinergic drugs can cause delirium; however, recent evidence has shown that neither cholinesterase inhibitors nor procholinergic drugs are effective in preventing delirium.[14]
- *Dopaminergic excess*. Dopaminergic medications can trigger delirium, and dopamine antagonists (antipsychotic drugs) can effectively manage symptoms.
- *Inflammatory theory*. Cytokines interleukin-6 and interleukin-8 have been associated with delirious patients.[15]
- *Dysregulation of the sympathetic nervous system and the hypothalamic-pituitary-adrenal axis*. Illness or trauma causes high, sustained cortisol levels among delirious patients.

- *Disruption of the sleep–wake cycle.* An increase or decrease in melatonin secretion has been found among postoperative delirious patients.[16]

Table 1. Risk Factors for Delirium

Dementia/cognitive impairment
History of delirium
Elderly (age >65 years)
Sensory impairment and poor functional status *
Polypharmacy
Comorbid illness †

*Immobility, functional dependence, and falls
†Chronic medical (kidney/liver failure, stroke, etc.), severe, and terminal illnesses

Risk factors that predispose patients to delirium are summarized in Table 1. Delirium is usually precipitated by various harmful insults (Table 2) that will tip over the susceptible patient into an acute confusional state. Dementia is the single most important and leading risk factor for delirium. Delirium may persist over time and can last from months to years, and so may be difficult to differentiate from dementia.[1]

Approach to Delirium

Early detection, screening, and prevention are the most important steps in the approach to delirium. However, some studies have shown that systematic monitoring for early detection of delirium did not have better outcomes than routine care for admitted older patients.[17] Fig. 1 depicts a systematic approach to delirium by the hospitalist. The Confusion Assessment Method (CAM) (Table 3) is a validated screening tool most frequently used among hospitalized patients to promptly recognize the presence of delirium.

Management

It is imperative that the underlying cause of the delirium and other compounding variables or concurrent illnesses be treated and addressed.

Table 2. Common Causes of Delirium

Drugs
Anticholinergics
Narcotics
Sedative–hypnotics
Alcohol
Drug withdrawal
Polypharmacy
Surgery and anesthesia
Orthopedic and cardiac surgery
Noncardiac surgery
Postoperative pain
Medical and neurologic disorders
Infections (including CNS)
Stroke
Systemic organ failure
Dehydration
Hyperthermia/hypothermia
Head injury/trauma
Respiratory failure
Toxic/metabolic abnormalities
Hyperglycemia/hypoglycemia
Electrolyte derangement
Endocrine disturbance
Inborn errors of metabolism
Nutritional deficiencies
Environmental
Hospitalization and ICU
Physical restraints
Urinary catheters
Sleep deprivation and emotional stress

Nonpharmacologic care of the delirious patient should be an interdisciplinary approach. The goal is to provide supportive care and avoid complications.

- Airway protection
- Nutritional support

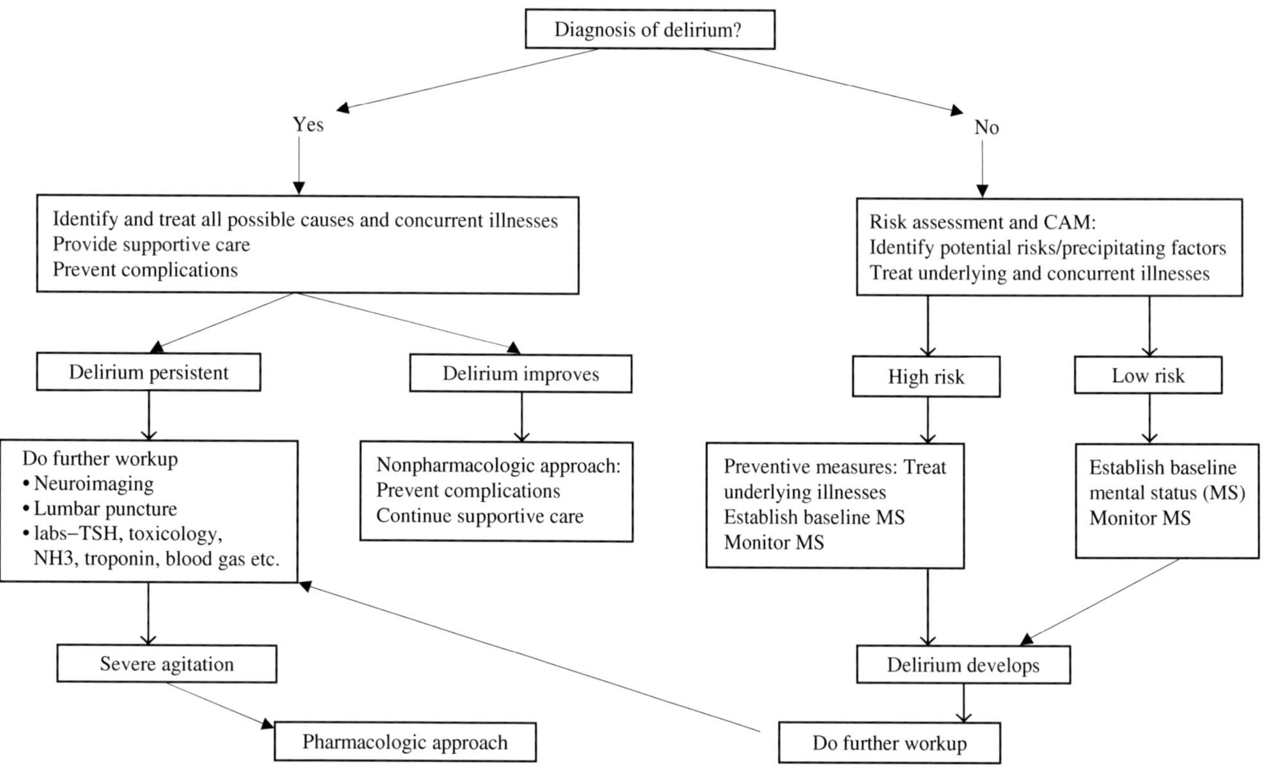

Fig. 1. An approach to delirium.

Table 3. Confusion Assessment Method (CAM) Diagnostic Algorithm*

Criteria	Assessment
1. Acute onset	Is there evidence of an acute change in mental status from the patient's baseline?
2. Fluctuating course	Did the abnormal behavior fluctuate during the day; tend to come and go or increase or decrease in severity?
3. Inattention	Did the patient have difficulty focusing attention, being easily distractible or having difficulty keeping track of what was being said?
4. Disorganized thinking	Was the patient's thinking disorganized or incoherent, such as rambling or irrelevant conversation, unclear or illogical flow of ideas, or unpredictable switching from subject to subject?
5. Altered level of consciousness	Shown by any answer other than "alert" to the following: Overall, how would you rate this patient's consciousness? Normal = alert Hyperalert = vigilant Drowsy, easily aroused = lethargic Difficult to arouse = stupor Unarousable = coma

Delirium diagnosis requires the presence of criteria 1 and 2 plus either 3 or 4.
*Inouye SK *et al.* (1990) Clarifying confusion: the CAM. *Ann Intern Med* **113**: 941–948.

- Skin care
- Medication review and reconciliation
- Mobility maintenance
- Venous thromboembolism prophylaxis
- Reorientation strategies
- Sleep–wake cycle restoration
- Avoidance of physical restraints and bladder catheters
- Use of sitters
- Use of relaxation techniques for agitation

Pharmacologic intervention is usually reserved for patients with severe symptoms of agitation that may disrupt medical therapy or compromise the safety of patients and others. Haloperidol is the mainstay treatment for severe agitation.

- Haloperidol 0.5 mg–1 mg (oral or intramuscularly) twice daily, with breakthrough doses every 4–6 hr as needed.[2]
- Risperidone 0.5 mg twice daily; olanzapine 2.5–5 mg once daily; quetiapine 25 mg twice daily.[2]

Extrapyramidal side effects are most commonly observed in patients treated with high dose haloperidol (>4.5 mg/day) but can be seen with low dose haloperidol and the atypical antipsychotics. Benzodiazepines should be avoided, as these agents can worsen confusion and agitation.

Reference

1. American Psychiatric Association. (1994) *Diagnostic and Statistical Manual of Mental Disorders*, 4th ed. APA Press, Washington, DC.
2. Inouye SK. (2006) Delirium in older persons. *N Engl J Med* **354**: 1157–1165.
3. Han JH, Wilson H, Ely EW. (2010) Delirium in the older emergency department patient: A quiet epidemic. *Emerg Med Clin North Am* **28**: 611–631.
4. Naughton BJ, Saltzman S, Ramadan F, *et al*. (2005) A multifactorial intervention to reduce prevalence of delirium and shorten hospital length of stay. *J Am Geriatr Soc* **53**: 18–23.
5. Thomason JW, Shintani A, Peterson JF, *et al*. (2005) Intensive care unit delirium is an independent predictor of longer hospital stay: A prospective analysis of 261 non-ventilated patients. *Crit Care* **9**: R375–R381.
6. McNicoll L, Pisani MA, Zhang Y, *et al*. (2003) Delirium in the intensive care unit: Occurrence and clinical course in older patients. *J Am Geriatr Soc* **51**: 591–598.
7. Bruce AJ, Ritchie CW, Blizard R, *et al*. (2007) The incidence of delirium associated with orthopedic surgery: A meta-analytic review. *Int Psychogeriatr* **19**: 197–214.

8. McCusher J, Cole M, Abrahamowicz M, *et al.* (2002) Delirium predicts 12-month mortality. *Arch Intern Med* **162**: 457–463.
9. Witlox J, Eurelings LS, Jonghe JF, *et al.* (2010) Delirium in elderly patients and risk of post-discharge mortality, institutionalization and dementia. *JAMA* **304**: 443–451.
10. Leslie DL, Marcantonio ER, Zhang Y, *et al.* (2008) One year healthcare costs associated with delirium in the elderly population. *Arch Intern Med* **168**: 27–32.
11. Boustani M, Baker MS, Campbell N, *et al.* (2010) Impact and recognition of cognitive impairment among hospitalized elders. *J Hosp Med* **5**: 69–75.
12. McCusker J, Cole MG, Dendukuri N, *et al.* (2003) Does delirium increase hospital stay? *J Am Geriatr Soc* **51**: 1539–1546.
13. Ely EW, Gautam S, Margolin R, *et al.* (2001) The impact of delirium in the intensive care unit on hospital length of stay. *Intensive Care Med* **27**: 1892–1900.
14. Campbell N, Boustani MA, Ayub A, *et al.* (2009) Pharmacological management of delirium in hospitalized adults: A systemic evidence review. *J Gen Intern Med* **24**: 848–853.
15. Van Munster BC, Korevaar JC, Zwindermann AH, *et al.* (2008) Time course of cytokines during delirium in elderly patients with hip fractures. *J Am Geriatr Soc* **56**: 1704–1709.
16. Shigeta H, Yaui A, Nimura Y, *et al.* (2001) Postoperative delirium and melatonin levels in elderly patients. *Am J Surg* **182**: 449–454.
17. Cole MG, McCusker J, Bellavance F, *et al.* (2003) Systematic detection and multidisciplinary care of delirium in older medical inpatients: A randomized trial. *CMAJ* **167**: 753–759.

Chapter 75

Acute Stroke and TIA

Qingliang T. Wang and Stanley Tuhrim**

Key Pearls

- Hypertension, smoking and diabetes together account for more than 50% of population attributable risk for ischemic stroke.
- Atrial fibrillation remains an important risk factor for embolic stroke and TIA. Patients with atrial fibrillation should be risk-stratified and managed for stroke risk reduction based on the CHADS2 scoring system.
- The clinical evaluation and management of acute ischemic stroke and of TIA are similar and time-sensitive, often requiring multidisciplinary collaboration and multimodality assessment and intervention. The ABCD2 scoring system is useful for assessing patients' recurrent stroke risk after a TIA or minor stroke.
- IV tPA remains the only FDA-approved treatment for acute ischemic stroke within 3 hr of the symptom onset, although it may also be effective in a select patient population for up to 4.5 hr after the symptom onset.
- The optimal parameters for blood pressure management in acute ischemic and hemorrhagic strokes, as well as the selection of particular antiplatelet and antihypertensive agents for primary and secondary stroke prevention, remain controversial.

*Mount Sinai Hospital, New York, NY, USA.

Definition, Epidemiology and Impacts of Acute Stroke and TIA

Stroke is the constellation of neurological symptoms caused by reduction or cessation of cerebral blood flow or extravasation of blood into the cerebral parenchyma and/or ventricular/subarachnoid space. Historically, symptoms lasting less than 24 hr have been defined as transient ischemic attacks (TIAs) However, recently developed advanced neuroimaging techniques and animal studies have demonstrated that cerebral ischemia of only a few minutes can cause infarction and irreversible neuronal injury and death.[1,2] Clinically, physicians often rely on magnetic resonance diffusion weighted imaging (MR-DWI) to differentiate infarction from TIA. However, the distinction is of limited clinical significance, because the clinical evaluation and management of TIA and of acute ischemic stroke are essentially the same. The management of intracerebral hemorrhage (10%–15% of all strokes) is distinct from that of ischemic stroke and TIA.

Stroke, the third leading cause of death and the first leading cause of disability in the United States, has been estimated to cost more than US$74 billion annually in the country in both direct healthcare cost and lost productivity.[3] The annual incidence of stroke in the US is about 790,000, of which about 130,000 are fatal.[3] African Americans have a significantly higher incidence rate and mortality from stroke than non-Hispanic whites and Asians.[3]

Although many nonmodifiable factors contribute significantly to stroke risk (Table 1), hypertension, diabetes, and smoking account for more than 50% of the population attributable risk for stroke.[4]

Approximately 20% of the strokes that occur in the US each year are recurrent strokes. The risk of recurrent stroke is highest within the first 30 days after the initial event (TIA or stroke) and remains elevated compared to healthy controls (Table 2). The ABCD2 scoring system has been shown to be useful for assessing recurrent stroke risk after a TIA or minor stroke[5]:

- Age >60 (score of 1)
- Blood pressure >140/90 at presentation (score of 1)

Table 1. Stroke Risk Factors

Nonmodifiable Risk Factors	Modifiable Risk Factors	Risk Reduction Measures
Age	Hypertension	Low-salt diet and medications
Gender	Diabetes	Diet, medications
Low weight at birth	Smoking	Smoking cessation
Race (black/white)	Hyperlipidemia	Diet, medications
Childhood nutritional status	Atrial fibrillation	Warfarin or ASA +/– clopidogrel
Sickle cell disease	Carotid/intracranial artery stenosis	Stenting +/– angioplasty or oral medications
Factor V Leiden	Cardiac causes	ASA + clopidogrel or PCI
Protein C deficiency	Migraine with aura	Antiplatelet agents; avoid triptans
Protein S deficiency	Physical inactivity	Physical exercise
Thrombophilia	Diet	Diet control and weight loss
Antithrombin mutation	Obesity (waist-to-hip ratio)	Diet, exercise, surgery
MTHFR mutation	Antiphospholipid syndrome (APLS)	ASA, warfarin, or heparin +/– immunomodulators
Homocysteinemia	Patent foraman ovale (PFO)	Antiplatelet agents vs. surgical closure
CADISIL	Hormone replacement therapy	Avoid HRT if possible
Moyamoya disease	Obstructive sleep apnea (OSA)	C-PAP, B-PAP, or surgical corrections

Table 2. Recurrent Stroke Risk After the Initial Event

	Percentage of Patients with Recurrent Stroke	
Time After Initial TIA/Stroke	**Initial Event TIA**	**Initial Event Stroke**
30 days	4%–8%	3%–10%
1 year	12%–13%	10%–14%
5 years	24%–29%	25%–40%

Data from Giles MF, Rothwell PM, *Lancet Neurol* **6**: 1063–1072 (2007) and Lovett, JK *et al.*, *Neurology* **62**: 569–573 (2004).

- Clinical symptoms of focal weakness or dysarthria (score of 2 if either present)
- Duration of symptoms >1 hr (score of 2 if >1 hr, 1 if >10 min but < 1 hr, 0 if <10 min)
- Diabetes mellitus (score of 1)

It is reasonable to hospitalize and work up patients with ABCD2 scores of 4–7 after a TIA or minor stroke.

Clinical Symptoms and Etiologies of Acute Stroke and TIA

Cerebral blood flow is proportionally related to cerebral perfusion pressure (CPP), which is the difference between systemic blood pressure (mean arterial pressure — MAP) and intracranial pressure (ICP). When CBF drops below 20 mL/100 mg brain tissue per minute (far below the normal range of 50–100 mL/100 mg per minute), neuronal dysfunction and irreversible neuronal damage/death occur, causing neurological symptoms. The constellation of stroke symptoms is largely determined by the vascular territory and the area of the brain involved (Table 3).

Table 3. Stroke Symptoms Based on Vascular Territories

Vascular Territories	Anatomic Structures	Clinical Symptoms
MCA	Lat. frontal lobe	(C) Weakness — arm, lower face > leg
	Operculum	(C) Sensory loss
	Sup. and lat. inf. temporal lobe	(C) Lateral gaze weakness, and
	Parietal lobe	(C) Homonomous hemianopsia
	Basal ganglia	(I) Gaze preference
	Anterior 2/3 of posterior limb of internal capsule	Aphasia (D)
		Hemineglect (ND)
		Constructional apraxia (ND)
		(C) Extrapyramidal signs
		Dysarthria
		Dysphagia (pseudobulbar)

(*Continued*)

Table 3. (*Continued*)

Vascular Territories	Anatomic Structures	Clinical Symptoms
ACA	Anterior 2/3 of medial frontal lobes Convexity Medial basal ganglia Corpus callosum genu Anterior limb of internal capsule	(C) Leg > arm weakness (C) Extrapyramidal signs (alien hand) (C) Neglect — motor (D) and sensory (ND) (C) Urinary incontinence Akinetc mutism or abulia Mood disturbance (depression or disinhibition) Gait apraxia Dysarthria
PCA	Midbrain Thalami Posterior 1/3 of posterior limb of internal capsule Optic tract Choroid plexus of third/lat. ventricles Posterior commissure Cerebral peduncles Splenum and posterior 1/3 of corpus callosum Posterior 1/3 of medial hemispheres Occipital lobe Inf. medial temporal lobe	Visual disturbances [(C) homologous hemianopsia, visual agnosia, palinopsia, macro-/micropsia, achromatopsia, Balint/Anton syndrome] Optic ataxia Asimultagnosia Prososagnosia Alexia/dyslexia (with/without agraphia) (C) Sensory loss (C) Weakness Altered consciousness and memory Dysarthria
ICA	MCA+ACA territory structures and eye (ophthalmic artery)	MCA + ACA symptoms and visual changes — visual field cut or acuity deficits
VA	Medulla Pontomedullary junction Lower pons Inf. lat. cerebellum	(I) Facial dysesthesia Dysarthria/hoarseness Horner's syndrome Lat. Medullary (Wallenberg) syndrome Nystagmus

(*Continued*)

Table 3. (*Continued*)

Vascular Territories	Anatomic Structures	Clinical Symptoms
		Dysphagia Ataxia Vertigo Nausea/vomiting (I) Loss of taste (I) Hearing loss (C) Weakness (C) Sensory changes
BA	Central pons, Midbrain	Loss of consciousness Papillary disturbance Dysarthria Dysphagia (bulbar dysfunctions) Asymmetric quadraperesis Occulomotor dysfunction Ataxia Nystagmus Locked-in syndrome Top of basilar syndrome
SCA	Sup. med. cerebellum	Dysarthria Ataxia Dysdiadochokinesia Vertigo Nystagmus Diplopia Nausea/vomiting Trunkal and apendicular ataxia (I) Weakness
AICA	Sup. lat. cerebellum Mid- and caudal lat. pons Middle cerebellar peduncle Pyramid	Ataxia Dysarthria (I) Hearing loss, tinnitus (I) Facial weakness (I) Limb weakness (I) Facial numbness (C) Sensory loss of body Vertigo Nystagmus Nausea/vomiting

(*Continued*)

Table 3. *(Continued)*

Vascular Territories	Anatomic Structures	Clinical Symptoms
		Dysphagia (I) Lateral gaze palsy
PICA	Inf. and lat. cerebellum Lat. medulla	Dysarthria Dysphagia Nausea/vomiting Vertigo Nystagmus Ataxia (I) Weakness Lat. medullary (Wallenberg) syndrome

C: contralateral; I: ipsilateral; B: bilateral; D: dominant hemisphere; ND: nondominant hemisphere; lat. lateral; sup. superior; inf. inferior.

The clinical and imaging characteristics, diagnostic modalities, and treatment options vary, depending on the stroke etiology (Table 4). Atrial fibrillation remains an important risk factor for cardioembolic strokes and will be discussed separately in a different chapter.

Diagnostic Approaches to Acute Stroke and TIA

Diagnosis of acute stroke involves an urgent evaluation of the patient's clinical history, general medical condition, and neurological status by emergency room physicians and experienced stroke neurologists with the assistance of neuroimaging studies, because it is often impossible to distinguish ischemic from hemorrhagic strokes solely based on clinical information.[8] Carotid and transcranial Dopplers (CD/TCD) are valuable noninvasive tools for evaluating carotid and intracranial artery stenosis. Transthoracic and transesophageal echocardiograms (TTE and TEE) are useful modalities for assessing embolic sources from the heart and great vessels. The cerebral angiogram remains the gold standard for evaluating both intracranial and extracranial vasculopathies, such as atherosclerosis/stenosis, dissection, aneursysm, AVM, and vasculitis.

Table 4. Etiologies of Stroke

Stroke Etiologies	Characteristics	Diagnostic Modalities	Treatment
Lacunar infarcts (<1.5 cm diameter)	Single, subcortical, basal ganglia, thalamocapsular or brain stem	CTH, MRI/ MRA, CD, TTE, and stroke labs	ASA or clopidogrel or aggrenox, with statin and antihypertensives and antidiabetics
Cardiac/artery–artery embolic infarcts	Multiple (or single if A–A) vascular territories, cortical	CTH, MRI/A, CD, TEE, and stroke labs	Warfarin (INR 2.0–3.0) if afib, or low EF (<30%) heparin if intracardiac thrombus
Hemodynamic failure	Border zone between MCA/ PCA, ACA / MCA, "beads on a string"	CTH, MRI/A, CD, CTA, TTE, and stroke labs	CEA or stenting if carotid stenosis >70% and symptomatic; otherwise, medical management with ASA, clopidogrel, or both
Air/tumor/ infectious emboli	Rare, multifocal	CTH, MRI/A, CD, TEE, and stroke labs	Air-hyperbaric O_2 chamber Tumor — chemo/radiation Infection — antibiotics
Venous sinus thrombosis	Venous infarctions, often with 2nd hemorrhage disorders	CTH, MRI/A, MRV, TTE, and stroke labs	Anticoagulation with heparin, then warfarin × 3–6 months
Vasculopathies	Multifocal, often associated with other autoimmnue disorders	CTA, MRA, CD, MRI cerebral angiogram	Target underline etiologies, often requires immune modulators

(*Continued*)

Table 4. (*Continued*)

Stroke Etiologies	Characteristics	Diagnostic Modalities	Treatment
Dissections	Trauma or congenital (Marfan's syndrome, fibromuscular dysplasia)	CTA/MRA, MRI, CD	Heparin, ASA, or stenting
Mechanical	Vascular occlusion from mass effect, herniation, etc.	CTH/CTA, MRI/A	Target underline etiologies Steroids and osmotic therapy may be helpful

CTA: CT angiography; CD: carotid Doppler; CEA: carotid endarterectomy.

Laboratory studies, such as a lipid panel, hemoglobin A1C, homocysteine, and urine toxicology testing, are also helpful in further stratifying patients' risk factors and identifying possible stroke etiologies. Patients under age 50 with stroke of otherwise undetermined etiology should be screened for hypercoagulable states such as cancer, systemic lupus erythematosus, granulomatous disease, factor V Leiden, protein C and protein S deficiencies, prothrombin G20210A and MTHFR (methyltetrahydrofolate reductase) mutations, and antiphospholipid antibody syndrome, MELAS (mitochondrial myopathy, encephalopathy, lactic acidosis, and stroke) syndrome and Fabry's disease. These conditions are rarely significant causes in elderly stroke patients.

Treatment Options for Acute Stroke and TIA

Since the landmark 1995 NINDS-sponsored IV tPA trial demonstrated a statistically significant favorable outcome in patients treated with IV tPA, management of acute stroke has become a time-sensitive emergency that requires coordination of multidisciplinary specialties, including EMS, emergency department, neurology, neuroradiology, neurointerventionalists, and pharmacy, in order to deliver appropriate and effective therapy in the shortest possible time frame.[9,10]

The IV tPA dose is 0.9 mg/kg, divided into a 10% bolus and a remaining 90% infusion within 1 hr, and should be administered within 3 hr of the symptom onset. The detailed inclusion and exclusion criteria of IV tPA treatment are listed in the most recent AHA/ASA guidelines.[8] Recently, the European-sponsored ECASS-III trial demonstrated persistent benefit of IV tPA treatment up to 4.5 hr from the symptom onset in a select population of ischemic stroke patients.[11,12]

Although rapidly improving stroke symptoms are a relative contraindication for administering IV tPA, consideration of tPA administration should still be given to those with significant residual neurological deficits, especially those with fluctuating symptoms. The neurological status of patients treated with tPA should be frequently reassessed to evaluate for secondary intracranial hemorrhage and the efficacy of tPA treatment. CT or MR angiography may be carried out for assessment of patency of vessels. In select centers that have the capacity to do so, intra-arterial administration of tPA and mechanical retrieval of thrombus (by MERCI, or Penumbra devices) within 6–8 hr of the time of the symptom onset may be considered as the next step in acute intervention.[8]

Antiplatelet agents such as aspirin (81 mg or 325 mg) and/or clopidogrel, and a statin should be given to those with ischemic stroke or TIA who are not candidates for IV tPA or endovascular interventions, mainly as secondary prevention measures to reduce recurrent stroke risks.

Blood pressure management in acute ischemic stroke remains a controversial issue. If IV tPA is administered, the blood pressure must be maintained below 185/110, with a goal of <180/105 for 24 hr post–tPA administration. However, in the absence of thrombolytic therapy, current AHA/ASA guidelines indicate that the blood pressure should not be lowered unless the patient's systolic blood pressure is >220 and diastolic blood pressure >110 during the first 24 hr after the stroke onset. If needed, a blood pressure reduction of 15% within the first 24 hr is reasonable. Patients with a prior history of hypertension should resume antihypertensive medications about 24 hr poststroke, often with a reduced dosage to keep blood pressure >140/90 for the next 72 hr. No data are available to guide the selection of particular antihypertensive medications.[8]

Table 5. National Institute of Health and Clinical Excellence (NICE) Criteria for Consideration of Decompressive Hemicraniectomy for Large Territory Stroke

Age	≤60
Clinical severity	Clinical deficits suggest MCA infarction with NIHSS >15.
Level of consciousness	Decreasing LOC with increase of score of 1 or more on Ia of NIHSS.
CT	>50% MCA territory infarct with/without ipsilateral ACA/PCA infarct.
MRI	>145 cm^3 of infarction on MR-DWI.

LOC: level of consciousness; MR-DWI: magnetic resonance diffusion-weighted imaging. Data are from Ref.[13]

Surgery for Acute Ischemic Stroke

Large volume hemispheric ischemic infarctions with mass effect and signs and/ or symptoms of imminent herniation, such as that in malignant MCA syndrome, stroke due to distal internal carotid artery occlusion, or cerebellar hemispheric infarctions, often necessitate decompressive hemicraniectomy/suboccipital craniectomy. However, improvement of both mortality and functional outcome has only been demonstrated in a select patient population within the first 48 hr of the stroke onset.[13] The National Institute of Health and Clinical Excellence (NICE) has issued guidelines for decompressive hemicraniectomy in large volume strokes (Table 5).

Management of Hemorrhagic Stroke

The common causes of intracerebral hemorrhage are listed in Table 6. The most common etiology of intracerebral hemorrhage is uncontrolled hypertension. Therefore, blood pressure control is again at the forefront of both primary and second prevention. The ideal systemic blood pressure in acute hemorrhagic stroke is unclear, although current AHA/ASA guidelines recommend keeping the systolic blood pressure at ≤180 mmHg and/or the mean arterial pressure (MAP) at ≤130 mmHg. A large-scale randomized trial (INTERACT II) is underway to address the issue of

Table 6. Common Causes of Hemorrhagic Strokes

Causes of Hemorrhage	Pathophysiology	Typical Locations	Other Characteristics
Hypertension	Lipohyalinosis, rupture of Charcot–Boucherd microaneurysms, fibroid necrosis of small arteries	Putamen, thalamus, pons, cerebellum	Most common cause
Coagulopathy	Anticoagulant use, clotting disorders, liver and renal diseases	Commonly multifocal; cerebellar vermis common	Prolonged ICH expansion and worsened outcome
Amyloid angiopathy	B-amyloid deposition in small- and medium-sized arteries	Lobar location, multicompartmental bleeds	Annual recurrent rate up to 10%, MR gradient echo — choice of study, associated with dementia
AVM	Direct shunting/ fistula of arteries to veins, leading to vascular malformation	Can be cortical or deep	Younger age, 2%–4% annual rate initial hemorrhage, 6%–18% recurrent annual rate
Aneurysm	Pathological dilation of arterial wall due to loss of integrity of internal elastic lamina	Typically at bifurcations, A-Com 30%, P-Com 25%, MCA 20%, ICA 8%. other 7%, multiple 20%–30%	Hemorrhage risks dependent on size, configuration, number of aneurysm, and prior history of hemorrhage
Cavernous angioma	Developmental large capillary anomaly without intervening neural tissue	Can be cortical or deep	Popcorn appearance on MR gradient echo with 0.25%–1.1%

(Continued)

Table 6. (*Continued*)

Causes of Hemorrhage	Pathophysiology	Typical Locations	Other Characteristics
			initial annual bleeding risk, 4.5% recurrent rate for anterior circulation, 2%–3% initial rate and 17%–21% recurrent rate for posterior circulation
Dural sinus thrombosis	Hypercoaguable, dehydrated, or inflammatory state causing thrombosis of venous sinuses	Most common superficial cerebral sinuses (superior sagittal, transverse, sigmoid, straight sinuses)	Can cause venous infarction and secondary hemorrhage; treat with anticoagulation even in the presence of hemorrhage
Vasculopathy	Congenital, autoimmune, infectious, or trauma	Typically involving small- and medium-sized arteries and multifocal, except for traumatic dissections	Usually preceded by periods of headache, cognitive decline, psychiatric symptoms, and recurrent strokes
Neoplasm	Primary CNS or metastatic tumor	Can occur anywhere; single or multifocal	Primary — GBM, oligo-dendroglioma, pituitary adenoma; Metastasis — lung, renal melanoma, thyroid, choriocarcinoma

(*Continued*)

Table 6. *(Continued)*

Causes of Hemorrhage	Pathophysiology	Typical Locations	Other Characteristics
Illicit drugs	Sympathomimetic effects from drugs such as cocaine, methamphetamine	Similar to hypertensive bleed	β-blocker is relatively contraindicated to avoid unopposed α-effect and sympathetic surge
Hemorrhagic conversion of ischemic infarction	Repurfusion injury or petechial hemorrhage	Within infarcted vascular territory	Common with large embolic infarcts or patients with coagulopathy
Trauma	Direct impact on parenchyma or rupture of blood vessels	Dependent on nature of injury, can be multifocal	Associated with skull fracture, SDH, ICH, IVH, or contusion

optimal blood pressure management in the acute phase of intracerebral hemorrhage.[14]

Nonsurgical therapeutic modalities for acute hemorrhagic strokes include:

- Osmotic therapy (with mannitol or hypertonic saline)
- Antiepileptic drugs (AEDs)
- Fever and infection control
- Reversing coagulopathies
- Intracranial pressure (ICP) monitoring
- Continuous EEG monitoring (can be useful in some circumstances)

Acute surgical interventions vary, depending upon the etiology of the hemorrhagic stroke. They include hematoma evacuation, ventriculostomy, aneurysm clipping/coiling, and AVM resection/embolization.

Frequent evaluation of the patient's neurological status is required. The goals of all treatment are prevention of hematoma expansion, control of ICP, and reduction of secondary complications such as acute hydrocephalus, vasospasm, and seizures, while maintaining sufficient cerebral blood flow and minimizing cerebral metabolic demands (such as by preventing fever and seizures).

Rehabilitation

There are about 5.8 million stroke survivors in the US.[3] Regardless of the etiologies of their strokes, many patients with measurable neurological deficits will need acute and long-term rehabilitation including physical, occupational, speech, and swallowing therapy. As soon as the patient is stable and can participate, a multidisciplinary rehabilitation regimen should be initiated.

Stroke recovery takes place most rapidly in the first six months, although patients may still make additional functional recovery gradually for up to two years.[15] Besides rehabilitation of physical deficits from stroke, therapies targeting stroke patients' frequent emotional, psychiatric, and cognitive deficits, such as depression, emotional labiality, and memory decline, should be closely integrated into the treatment plan. Stroke survivor group therapy and other social support networks are critically important for stroke patients' reintegration into society and their long-term wellness.

References

1. Easton JD, Saver JL, Albers GW, *et al.* (2009) Definition and evaluation of transient ischemic attack: A scientific statement for healthcare professionals from the American Heart Association/American Stroke Association Stroke Council; Council on Cardiovascular Surgery and Anesthesia; Council on Cardiovascular Radiology and Intervention; Council on Cardiovascular Nursing; and the Interdisciplinary Council on Peripheral Vascular Disease. The American Academy of Neurology affirms the value of this statement as an educational tool for neurologists. *Stroke* **40**: 2276–2293.
2. Albers GW, Caplan LR, Easton JD, *et al.* (2002) Transient ischemic attack — proposal for a new definition. *N Engl J Med* **347**: 1713–1716.

3. Lloyd-Jones D, Adams RJ, Brown TM, *et al.* (2010) Heart disease and stroke statistics — 2010 update: A report from the American Heart Association, *Circulation* **121**: e46–e215.
4. O'Donnell MJ, Xavier D, Liu L, *et al.* (2010) Risk factors for ischaemic and intracerebral haemorrhagic stroke in 22 countries (the INTERSTROKE study): A case-control study. *Lancet* **376**: 112–123.
5. Giles MF, Rothwell PM. (2010) Systematic review and pooled analysis of published and unpublished validations of the ABCD and ABCD2 transient ischemic attack risk scores. *Stroke* **41**: 667–673.
6. Fuster V, Ryden LE, Cannom DS, *et al.* (2006) ACC/AHA/ESC 2006 Guidelines for the Management of Patients with Atrial Fibrillation: A report of the American College of Cardiology/American Heart Association Task Force on Practice Guidelines and the European Society of Cardiology Committee for Practice Guidelines (Writing Committee to Revise the 2001 Guidelines for the Management of Patients with Atrial Fibrillation): Developed in collaboration with the European Heart Rhythm Association and the Heart Rhythm Society. *Circulation* **114**: e257–e354.
7. Garwood CL, Corbett TL. (2008) Use of anticoagulation in elderly patients with atrial fibrillation who are at risk for falls. *Ann Pharmacother* **42**: 523–532.
8. Adams HP Jr, del Zoppo G, Alberts MJ, *et al.* (2007) Guidelines for the early management of adults with ischemic stroke: A guideline from the American Heart Association/American Stroke Association Stroke Council, Clinical Cardiology Council, Cardiovascular Radiology and Intervention Council, and the Atherosclerotic Peripheral Vascular Disease and Quality of Care Outcomes in Research Interdisciplinary Working Groups: The American Academy of Neurology affirms the value of this guideline as an educational tool for neurologists. *Stroke* **38**: 1655–1711.
9. National Institute of Neurological Disorders and Stroke rt-PA Stroke Study Group. (1995) Tissue plasminogen activator for acute ischemic stroke. *N Engl J Med* **333**: 1581–1587.

10. Kwiatkowski TG, Libman RB, Frankel M, *et al*. (1999) Effects of tissue plasminogen activator for acute ischemic stroke at one year. National Institute of Neurological Disorders and Stroke Recombinant Tissue Plasminogen Activator Stroke Study Group. *N Engl J Med* **340**: 1781–1787.
11. Hacke W, Kaste M, Bluhmki E, *et al*. (2008) Thrombolysis with alteplase 3 to 4.5 h after acute ischemic stroke. *N Engl J Med* **359**: 1317–1329.
12. Bluhmki E, Chamorro A, Davalos A, *et al*. (2009) Stroke treatment with alteplase given 3.0–4.5 hr after onset of acute ischaemic stroke (ECASS III): Additional outcomes and subgroup analysis of a randomised controlled trial. *Lancet Neurol* **8**: 1095–1102.
13. Vahedi K, Hofmeijer J, Juettler E, *et al*. (2007) Early decompressive surgery in malignant infarction of the middle cerebral artery: A pooled analysis of three randomised controlled trials. *Lancet Neurol* **6**: 215–222.
14. Delcourt C, Huang Y, Wang J, *et al*. (2010) The second (main) phase of an open, randomised, multicentre study to investigate the effectiveness of an intensive blood pressure reduction in acute cerebral haemorrhage trial (INTERACT2). *Int J Stroke* **5**: 110–116.
15. Hankey GJ, Spiesser J, Hakimi Z, *et al*. (2007) Rate, degree, and predictors of recovery from disability following ischemic stroke. *Neurology* **68**: 1583–1587.

Chapter 76

Epilepsy

Lara V. Marcuse and Madeline C. Fields**

Key Pearls

- A single antiepileptic drug (AED) will render 70% of people with epilepsy seizure-free. The remaining 30% are considered refractory.
- In adults, the most common type of epilepsy is focal epilepsy of the medial temporal lobe.
- The goal of treatment is to have no seizures and no unwanted side effects of medication.
- Convulsive status epilepticus is a neurological emergency with high morbidity and mortality that requires immediate care. Nonconvulsive status epilepticus should be on the differential for any patient with an altered mental status of unknown etiology.
- If an individual has a witnessed seizure, nothing should be put into his or her mouth. When the shaking stops, the person should be rolled onto his or her side to help protect the airway.

Introduction

A seizure is defined as a transient occurrence of signs and/or symptoms due to abnormal, excessive or synchronous neuronal activity in the brain.[1] Seizures can have motor, sensory, cognitive and/or emotional manifestations. They can be caused by genetic defects, head trauma, strokes, brain tumors or intracranial hemorrhages. Metabolic derangements and infections can cause seizures as well.

*Mount Sinai School of Medicine, New York, NY, USA.

Epilepsy is typically defined as two or more seizures that are not provoked. A seizure is considered provoked if it is in close temporal relationship with an acute central nervous system insult, which may be metabolic, structural, infectious or inflammatory in nature. For example, if someone has a seizure the hour after being hit on the head by a brick, this seizure is considered provoked. If the same individual develops recurrent seizures weeks after the accident, he or she would be considered to have epilepsy.

Common Seizure Types

Seizures can start on both sides of the brain in a large distributed bilateral network (generalized onsets) or can have an onset in one part of one hemisphere (focal onsets).

Tonic Clonic Seizures

These are also known as "grand mal" seizures and are the most commonly imagined and portrayed seizures. A seizure of this type begins with loss of consciousness, falling and whole body stiffening. This may be accompanied by a loud cry, as air gets pressed out of the individual by a stiffening diaphragm. The stiff or tonic phase is followed by rhythmic body jerking in the clonic phase. A generalized tonic clonic seizure can appear identical to a tonic clonic seizure that began as a partial seizure.

Absence Seizures

These usually begin in childhood and consist of a short period (usually less then 10 s) of staring, at times with blinking. During this time, the person cannot speak or understand what is being said. This is a generalized seizure, and the EEG shows generalized spike and wave activity.

Myoclonic Seizures

Many people experience a few jerks while falling asleep. This is normal myoclonus and not seizure activity. Myoclonic seizures are a jerk or a series of jerks that occur while the person is awake and may involve a single limb, or both sides of the body at the same time. Myoclonic jerks are often most frequent in the morning. These are usually generalized seizures, and EEG shows generalized polyspike and wave.

Focal Seizures

During a focal seizure, an individual may remain aware and alert. Such small seizures without loss of awareness are sometimes called "auras" or "warnings." The symptoms depend on the brain region: a small focal seizure from the occipital lobe will cause a visual hallucination, while a seizure from the temporal lobe may cause a feeling of *déjà vu* or a rising sensation in the stomach.

A larger focal seizure can spread and cause impairment in awareness. At this point, an individual may not respond to questions, and can exhibit very odd behavior and movements. A person having a focal seizure with loss of awareness can sometimes be mistaken for someone taking illicit drugs or having a mental illness.

Secondarily Generalized Tonic Clonic Seizures

Focal seizures can spread to involve the whole brain, causing a tonic clonic seizure. These seizures can appear identical to a seizure that is generalized at the onset (see above).

Epilepsy Classification

The International League Against Epilepsy (ILAE) recently developed a new classification system dividing the underlying causes of epilepsy into three categories: genetic, structural/metabolic, and unknown. Juvenile myoclonic epilepsy and childhood absence epilepsy would both fall into the genetic category. These types of epilepsies are thought to be the result of ion channel mutations. A child with epilepsy secondary to tuberous sclerosis or nonketotic hyperglycinemia would fall into the structural/metabolic category.

Diagnosis

The key to the diagnosis of epilepsy is an in-depth history and physical exam. The history should include details about:

- Perinatal trauma
- Prematurity
- Head trauma
- Family history
- Previous CNS infections
- Toxic exposure including drugs and alcohol
- Prior seizures (which may have been subtle, and even unrecognized by the patient)

Imaging, particularly MRI, is important after any seizure of unknown etiology. This will help diagnose mesial temporal sclerosis, brain tumors, infarcts, or other structural lesions. A CT scan is often appropriately performed in an emergency room, but is not adequate for diagnosing some of the more subtle causes.

Basic chemistries and a CBC are important. A lumbar puncture may be indicated. EEG is crucial for the diagnosis. Patients are now routinely admitted to the hospital for EEG with video to capture their episodes. This is particularly useful for distinguishing events that mimic seizures, such as transient ischemic attacks, polysomnias, paroxysmal movement disorders, subcortical myoclonus, and syncope.

Treatment

Antiepileptic Medications

There are multiple medications used for the treatment of epilepsy (see Table 1). No one agent is preferred to all others. Carbamazepine, oxcarbazepine, gabapentin, pregabalin, and phenytoin are all approved for the treatment of focal epilepsy and may worsen some seizures with a generalized onset.

Table 1. Seizure Medications

Drug	Seizure Indication	Alternative Indication	Mechanism of Action	Important Side Effects
Phenobarbital	Partial and generalized seizures	Sedative, hypnotic, preanesthetic	GABA	Fatigue, cognitive difficulties, osteoporosis
Phenytoin	Partial and generalized tonic clonic seizures	*Anxiety control and mood stabilization	Sodium channels	Gingival hyperplasia, rash, cerebellar atrophy, bone marrow suppression
Carbamazepine	Partial seizures	Trigeminal neuralgia, mania	Sodium channels, GABA	Fatigue, rash, bone marrow suppression, osteoporosis
Valproate	Partial and generalized seizures, LGS, infantile spasms, neonatal seizures, febrile seizures	Mania, migraine headaches	GABA, sodium channels, calcium channels	Weight gain, PCOS, hepatotoxicity, pancreatitis, teratogenicity, hyperammonemia
Felbatol	Refractory partial seizures, LGS, *generalized seizures	None	NMDA receptors, calcium channels, sodium channels	Aplastic anemia, hepatotoxicity. Currently restricted to patients with refractory epilepsy.
Gabapentin	Partial seizures	Postherpetic neuralgia, *neuropathy, *anxiety	Calcium channels, GABA	Fatigue, lower extremity edema
Lamotrigine	Partial and generalized seizures, LGS	Bipolar disorder	Blocks voltage-dependent sodium channels	Rash, SJS, insomnia
Zonisamide	Partial and *generalized seizures	None	Sodium channel blockade	Fatigue, mood changes, nephrolithiasis

(Continued)

Table 1. (*Continued*)

Drug	Seizure Indication	Alternative Indication	Mechanism of Action	Important Side Effects
Oxcarbazepine	Partial seizures	*Bipolar disorder	Sodium channel	Hyponatremia, dizziness
Levetiracetam	Partial and generalized seizures, myoclonic seizures	*Tremor	Unknown	Irritability, depression, fatigue
Pregabalin	Partial seizures	Neuropathy, fibromyalgia, post herpetic neuralgia *anxiety	Calcium channels, GABA	Fatigue, weight gain
Topiramate	Partial and generalized seizures, LGS	Migraines, *movement disorders, *impulse control, *weight loss	Sodium channels, GABA, AMPA, carbonic anhydrase inhibitor	Weight loss, expressive aphasia, nephrolithiasis, parasthesias
Rufinamide	LGS, *partial seizures	None	Sodium channels	Nausea, vomiting, dizziness
Lacasamide	Partial seizures	Diabetic peripheral neuropathy	Sodium channels	Dizziness
Vigabatrin	Refractory complex partial seizures, infantile spasms	None	GABA	Irreversible visual field loss, mood difficulties

LGS — Lennox–Gastaut syndrome; PCOS — polycystic ovarian syndrome; SJS — Stevens–Johnson syndrome.
*Not FDA approved but commonly used.

Often, the choice of an antiepileptic drug depends on the seizure type and comorbidites of the patient. For example, an elderly man with partial epilepsy and a painful sensory neuropathy might do very well on gabapentin, as this medication can both address his seizure disorder and potentially improve his neuropathic pain syndrome. The goal for every patient is to have no seizures and no unwanted side effects from the medication.

A single AED will render 70% of people with epilepsy seizure-free. Polytherapy adds increasingly small benefits and often multiplies side effects.

Diet

The ketogenic diet — a high fat/protein, very low carbohydrate diet — can be a remarkably effective treatment for epilepsy, especially in children with refractory epilepsy. It requires strict adherence and supervision but can reduce seizures that have been refractory to multiple medications.[2]

Lifestyle Issues

Adequate sleep and avoidance of excessive alcohol intake are the mainstays of epilepsy treatment. Very often, epilepsy emerges in susceptible individuals when they are fatigued. Exercise, yoga, and biofeedback can all be a complementary part of the treatment of epilepsy.

Surgery

Any patient with refractory focal epilepsy should be considered for resective epilepsy surgery. Anterior temporal lobectomy is curative for many people with medial temporal lobe epilepsy. The risks of brain surgery must be weighed against the potential benefits of the surgery. Neuropsychological testing, the intracarotid amobarbital procedure (WADA), recording seizures both extracranially and — in some circumstances — intracranially, and intracranial brain mapping can all help define the risks and benefits.

Other Treatments

Vagal nerve stimulation can be helpful in refractory epilepsy regardless of the etiology. Newer techniques like deep brain stimulation, responsive intracranial stimulation, and intracranial focal cooling are currently under investigation.

Status Epilepticus

Status epilepticus is defined as more than 5 min of continuous seizure activity or two or more seizures between which there is incomplete recovery of consciousness.[3] This revised definition came about because a typical seizure rarely lasts longer than 5 min; seizures for longer can be detrimental and earlier treatment is more effective.

For individuals with epilepsy, virtually any seizure type or epilepsy syndrome can become status epilepticus. Status epilepticus is also seen as the result of structural insults, like CNS hemorrhage, stroke, brain tumor, or anoxia, as well as metabolic derangements and infections.

Status epilepticus can manifest as obvious convulsive activity or can be very subtle and nonconvulsive. Nonconvulsive status epilepticus is frequently found in medically ill hospitalized patients with a poor mental status.[4]

Convulsive and nonconvulsive status epilepticus have high morbidity and mortality, and are neurological emergencies. Initial management of individuals with convulsive status epilepticus starts with management of their airway, breathing, and circulation (ABC). Serum glucose via a fingerstick, CBC, electrolytes (including magnesium, calcium, and phosphorus), urine toxicology, and AED levels (for people with known epilepsy) should be measured immediately.

The cornerstone of treatment for the ongoing seizure is rapid administration of AEDs. Lorazepam is the first line agent, given at a dose of 0.1 mg/kg, at a rate not to exceed 2 mg/min. The standard maximum for lorazepam is 8 mg. If convulsive activity has not stopped, then fosphenytoin should be infused at a dose of 20 mg/kg, at a rate not to exceed 150 mg/min.

If this is not successful, other AED infusions are often given, like phenobarbital 20 mg/kg or valproic acid 20–40 mg/kg.

If convulsive activity continues, intubation should be rapidly performed so that an IV sedative can be started, such as midazolam, proprofol, or pentobarbital. These drugs should initially be titrated to the cessation of any clinical seizure activity. It is then important to connect the patient to VEEG monitoring and ideally titrate the infusions to the cessation of any epileptiform activity and/or seizures. Subclinical seizures are very common after convulsive status epilepticus.

If there is concern about meningitis or encephalitis, empiric antibiotic and antiviral treatment should be initiated. Imaging should be performed if there is any concern about a focal neurological emergency causing the seizures. If infection is suspected, a lumbar puncture is required. If there is an underlying cause of that status epilepticus, correction of the underlying cause (when possible) is as important to the patient's prognosis as stopping the seizures.

Women and Epilepsy

Hormones can affect epilepsy, as some women with epilepsy report worsened seizures around their menses. If a catamenial pattern emerges with accurate logging of seizures and menses, timed antiepileptic drugs can be tried, though there is no FDA-approved treatment for catamenial epilepsy.

Many of the AEDs interfere with the efficacy of oral contraception. This is particularly true of carbamazepine, phenytoin, phenobarbital, primidone, topiramate, and oxcarbazepine. A second barrier method may be needed to prevent unwanted pregnancy. Any woman of childbearing age taking antiepileptic medication should receive folic acid supplementation to prevent neural tube defects.

Women with epilepsy will need counseling regarding pregnancy and epilepsy. While many of the AEDs have known teratogenic effects, the vast majority of women with epilepsy have healthy babies. Newer prospective data are redefining which drugs are more teratogenic. Lamotrigine and carbamazepine have relatively safe profiles. Valproic acid has a higher incidence of major malformations and subsequent detriment to cognitive development. Whenever possible, monotherapy should be used instead of polytherapy.

There are some conceivable risks of breastfeeding while women are on antiepileptic medications. The older, more protein-bound medications are transmitted less into the breast milk than newer, less protein-bound medications. Despite the possible risks, the proven benefits of breastfeeding, including reduced risk of immunologically mediated disorders and enhanced cognitive abilities, are compelling. The American Academy of Neurology recommends encouraging breastfeeding in women with epilepsy.[5]

Driving and Epilepsy

Restrictions on driving are often cited by people with epilepsy as one of the most difficult parts of their condition. Every state has different guidelines regarding epilepsy and driving, and it is the role of the physician to inform patients about those guidelines. No physician in the United States has the authority to tell a patient that they may drive, as this decision is made by each state's driving authority.

References

1. Fisher RS, Boas W, Blume W, *et al.* (2005) Epileptic seizures and epilepsy: Definitions proposed by the Internations League Against Epilepsy (ILAE) and the International Bureau for Epilepsy (IBE) *Epilepsia* **46**: 470–472.
2. Cross JH. (2010) Dietary therapies — an old idea with a new lease of life. *Seizure*: *Eur J Epilepsy* [doi:10.1016/j.seizure.2010.10.021].
3. Lowenstein DH, Alldredge BK. (1998) Status epilepticus. *New Engl J Med* **338**: 970–976.
4. Oddo M, Carrera E, Claassen J, *et al.* (2009) Continuous electroencephalography in the medical intensive care unit. *Crit Care Med* **37**(6): 2051–2056.

5. Harden CL, Pennell PB, Koppel BS, *et al*. (2009) Practice Parameter update: Management issues for women with epilepsy — focus on pregnancy (an evidence-based review): Vitamin K, folic acid, blood levels, and breastfeed Practice Parameter update: Management issues for women with epilepsy — focus on pregnancy (an evidence-based review): Vitamin K, folic acid, blood levels, and breastfeeding. *Neurology* **73**: 142–149.

Psychiatric Illness

Chapter 77

Assessment of Capacity

Teresa Lim and Deborah B. Marin**

Key Pearls

- Physicians overestimate decisional capacity.
- Decisional capacity is situational-decision-specific.
- The four components of capacity are expression of a choice, understanding the information that is presented about the proposed treatment, appreciation of the situation, and rational manipulation of information.
- The use of a semistructured evaluation of capacity can structure the evaluation, decrease inconsistencies, and ensure that key points are covered in the assessment.
- Decisional capacity is situation and decision-specific. Patients who have impaired capacity to make decisions regarding a medical treatment do not necessarily lack capacity to make decisions regarding other aspects of their care.

Introduction

Hospitalists are often faced with the task of assessing patients' capacity for many decisions, including the ability to (1) accept or refuse treatment, (2) complete advance directives, (3) handle one's finances, and (4) live independently. Impaired capacity in hospitalized patients is as high as

*Mount Sinai School of Medicine, New York, New York, NY, USA.

31%[1] and can be caused by a variety of medical conditions, including but not limited to delirium, dementia, stroke, and psychosis. The prevalence of delirium at the time of hospital admission ranges from 10% to 31% and the incidence of delirium in hospitalized patients ranges from 3% to 29%. Intact decisional capacity is a criterion for valid informed consent, and given that patients are likely to undergo invasive medical procedures,[3] the ability of physicians to accurately determine capacity is of great importance.

Clinicians have a tendency to overestimate the decisional capacity of patients.[4–6] One study demonstrated that 28% of elderly, medically ill hospitalized patients were not identified by their physicians as having compromised decisional capacity.[4] Another study found that medical residents' clinical impressions of capacity status were inaccurate — 29% of patients with impaired capacity were identified as having intact capacity by medical residents.[6] Physicians' interrater agreement on decisional capacity has been shown to be only 56%.[7] Inaccurate assessment of capacity can also be the result of misconceptions about decisional capacity, including the following assumptions: (1) patients have capacity unless they refuse treatment, (2) capacity status is not situation specific, and (3) patients with dementia or mental illness lack capacity.[8]

The Four Components of Capacity

Capacity is conceptualized as having four components: (1) expression of a choice, (2) understanding the information that is presented about the proposed treatment, (3) appreciation of the situation, and (4) rational manipulation of information.[9] The ability to communicate a choice requires that a patient reach a decision and express his or her choice. Patients who are either comatose or in a vegetative state are considered to not have met this criterion. The ability to understand is evident when a patient exhibits an understanding of the information that was presented to him or her regarding the proposed treatment. Understanding can be demonstrated by the patient's ability to paraphrase what has been told to him or her regarding the diagnosis, the recommended treatment, and the benefits, risks, and alternatives to the treatment. Appreciation of a situation requires that the patient relate the clinical information to his or her circumstances, which involves the patient having insight into and acceptance of the illness. Refusing treatment does not necessarily indicate that a patient lacks capacity if he or she demonstrates awareness of the consequences of refusing treatment. The ability to rationally manipulate information takes into account the thought process involved in the decision-making. Patients who exhibit adequate understanding and appreciation can be considered to have impaired capacity if they did not follow a logical thought process to arrive at their decision. On the other hand, patients who make a choice that may not be considered "reasonable" can have capacity if they demonstrated that they employed a logical thought process to arrive at their decision.

Sliding Scale Model of Capacity

The stringency of the standards employed in the determination of capacity determines the probability of either of the following errors occurring: (1) incorrectly identifying a capable patient as lacking capacity and (2) incorrectly identifying an incapable patient as having capacity. One approach to avoiding such errors is to recognize that determination of capacity is specific to a situation and decision. It has been proposed that the stringency of criteria used to assess capacity should vary according to the situation i.e. the more serious the consequences of the decision, the more stringent the criteria for intact capacity.[10,11] A model utilizing the four components of capacity has been proposed, and it includes three different standards, each corresponding to varying severity of the consequences of the treatment decision.[10] The first and least stringent standard is applicable to clinical scenarios in which the proposed treatment is effective, carries minimal risk, and there are few or no alternatives to this treatment. The only stipulation that is required to be considered capable of giving consent is that the patient has a general sense of orientation of the situation.[10] The second and more stringent standard would be applied in a clinical setting that has the following characteristics: (1) the proposed treatment carries a greater-than-minimal risk, (2) the proposed treatment has less definitive benefit, and (3) there are alternatives to the proposed treatment. In this situation, the patient must exhibit an understanding of the proposed treatment, and the risk, benefits, and alternatives to the treatment. The third and most stringent standard is applied in clinical situations where an effective and life-saving treatment is available and refusal of treatment could result in severe morbidity and mortality. In such a situation, the patient must satisfy the most rigorous standard of capacity in that he or she exhibits an appreciation of the nature and consequences of his or her decision as it pertains to the situation, and a demonstration of the ability to rationally manipulate the information.

Instruments to Aid in the Assessment of Capacity

The under recognition of impaired decisional capacity status in patients and poor interrater agreement could be in part due to the use of idiosyncratic criteria for capacity assessment. A more structured approach to capacity assessment can lessen such problems. The use of a semistructured evaluation of capacity has been shown to decrease the inconsistencies of a clinician's evaluation of capacity, and to improve interrater agreement amongst physicians.[12,13] These instruments have been studied in various patient populations. The use of an instrument not only helps to structure the evaluation but also ensures that the key points are covered in the assessment. Some instruments that have been most frequently studied in the medically ill population are summarized in Table 1.

In the event that the use of a capacity instrument is not feasible, one could structure the evaluation to include questions that assess the four components. Appelbaum has outlined the questions to address in the assessment of the four-component capacity,[14] and alternative questions to those suggested by him are included in Table 2.

Table 1. Capacity Instruments

Instrument	Elements Measured	Length of Adminstration	Patient Population	Reliability	Comments
MacArthur Competence Assessment Tool for Treatment (MacCAT-T)	Expression of a choice, understanding, appreciation, reasoning	15–20 min	Medical inpatients, schizophrenia, dementia, depression, psychosis, anorexia nervosa, normal controls	High interrater reliability; intraclass correlation coefficient = 0.75–0.99	• Semistructured interview. • Individualize instrument to each patient.
Hopkins Competency Assessment Test (HCAT)	Understanding	10 min	Medical inpatients, Alzheimer's disease, nursing home residents, psychotic patients in outpatient setting, normal controls	High interrater reliability; Pearson's product–moment correlation coefficient = 95%	• Semistructured interview. • Unable to be individualized to each patient.
Aid to Capacity Evaluation (ACE)	Expression of a choice, understanding, appreciation	15 min	Medical inpatients	High interrater reliability; interrater agreement of 93% (k = 0.79)	• Semistructured interview. • Individualize instrument to each patient.

Table 2. Questions to Assess the Four Components of Capacity

Component of Capacity	Possible Questions
Expression of a choice	Were you able to give some thought to what we had talked about (i.e. proposed treatment, risks, benefits, and alternatives)? Have you come to a decision? What is your decision?
Understanding of the information regarding treatment	Are you aware of your diagnosis? What have you been told about your diagnosis? Could you please tell me what treatment was recommended and what is your understanding as to how this treatment can improve the condition? What are the benefits of getting this treatment? What are the risks involved in getting this treatment? Are there alternatives to the treatment that was recommended and if so what are the alternatives?
Appreciation of the situation as it pertains to the patient	What are your thoughts about what is wrong with your health? Do you think that you require treatment for your current condition? How do you think the recommended treatment can help you? If you decide to not receive treatment, how will this decision affect you?
Rational manipulation of the information	What are your thoughts regarding your decision? How is it that you arrived at your decision? What helped you to come to your decision? Are there any beliefs that affected your decision to accept/reject your decision (to assess for delusions and hallucinations)?

Issues to Consider when Assessing Capacity

The Folstein Mini Mental Status Exam (MMSE) was developed in a psychiatric setting to measure general cognitive abilities and is often used as part of the capacity assessment because it can be easily and rapidly administered. Despite its advantages and widespread use, it has been shown that patients had significantly greater deficits in their understanding and cognitive abilities compared to healthy controls despite having normal scores on the MMSE.[4,15] These results suggest that the MMSE might not be a sensitive instrument in detecting specific cognitive dysfunction related to impaired capacity.

Decisional capacity is situation- and decision-specific. Patients who have impaired capacity to make decisions regarding their medical treatment do not necessarily lack capacity to make decisions regarding other aspects of their lives. In addition, capacity status is not permanent and could change over time. For example, a patient with delirium might lack capacity during his or her acute episode of illness but might regain capacity when the underlying medical condition is treated. It is also important to keep in mind that a patient's understanding of the proposed treatment is dependent on the information that is presented to him or her by the treatment team. Dunn *et al.* showed that information presented in a brief and organized manner improved patients' understanding.[16]

Assessment of capacity can sometimes be challenging and it would be appropriate for the treatment team to ask for a psychiatry consult to aid in the evaluation of the patient's capacity status. In the event that a patient has been deemed to lack capacity, decisions regarding medical treatment should be directed to his or her agent as determined in a healthcare proxy.

The standard clinical practice of obtaining informed consent requires that patients have the capacity to make decisions regarding their medical care. Thus, the ability to accurately and reliably assess capacity is critical given that many disease states cause impaired capacity. The current practice of assessing capacity through clinical judgment may result in inaccurate estimation of intact capacity and poor interrater reliability. Structuring one's evaluation through the use of either an instrument or questions as described above can help to improve the accuracy and reliability of the assessment.

References

1. Raymont V, Bingley W, Buchanan A, *et al.* (2004) Prevalence of mental incapacity in medical inpatients and associated risk factors: Cross-sectional study. *Lancet* **364**: 1421–1427.

2. Siddiqui N, House A, Holmes J. (2006) Occurrence and outcome of delirium in medical in patients: A systematic literature review. *Age Ageing* **35**: 350–362.
3. Tu J, Pashos C, Naylor D, *et al.* (1997) Use of cardiac procedures and outcomes in elderly patients with myocardial infarction in the United States and Canada. *N Engl J Med* **336**: 1500–1505.
4. Fitten L, Waite M. (1990) Impact of medical hospitalization in treatment decision-making capacity in the elderly. *Arch Intern Med* **150**: 1717–1721.
5. Barton C Jr, Mallik H, Orr W, *et al.* (1996) Clinician's judgment of capacity of nursing home patients to give informed consent. *Psychiatr Serv* **47**(9): 956–960.
6. Etchells E, Katz M, Schuchman M, *et al.* (1997) Accuracy of clinical impressions and mini–mental state exam scores for assessing capacity to consent to major medical treatment. Comparison with criterion-stand psychiatric assessment. *Psychosomatics* **38**: 239–245.
7. Marson D, McInturff B, Hawkins L, *et al.* (1997) Consistency of physician judgments of capacity to consent in mild Alzheimer's disease. *J Am Geriatr Soci* **45**(4): 453–457.
8. Ganzini L, Volicer L, Nelson W, *et al.* (2003) Pitfalls in assessment of decision making capacity. *Psychosomatics* **44**: 237–243.
9. Appelbaum P, Grisso T. (1988) Assessing patients' capacities to consent to treatment. *N Eng J Med* **319**: 1635–1638.
10. Drane J. (1984) Competency to give and informed consent: A model for making clinical assessment. *JAMA* **252**: 925–927.
11. Tancredi L. (1982) Competency for informed consent. *Int J Law Psychiatr* **5**: 51–63.
12. Marson D, Earnst K, Jamil F. (2000) Consistency of physicians' legal standard and personal judgments of competency in patients with Alzheimer's disease. *J Am Geriatr Soci* **48**(8): 911–918.
13. Etchells E, Darzins P, Silberfeld M, *et al.* (1999) Assessment of patient capacity to consent to treatment. *J Gen Intern Med* **14**: 27–34.
14. Appelbaum P. (2007) Assessment of patients' competence to consent to treatment. *New Eng J Med* **357**: 1834–1840.

15. Cassell E, Leon A, Kaufman S. (2001) Preliminary evidence of impaired thinking in sick patients. *Ann Intern Med* **134**(12): 1120–1123.
16. Dunn L, Jeste D. (2001) Enhancing informed consent for research and treatment. *Neuropsychopharmacology* **24**: 595–607.

Chapter 78

Substance Use Disorders

Sanjay H. Patel, Niru S. Nahar[†] and Evaristo O. Akerele**

Key Pearls

- Nicotine gum is ineffective if the patient is consuming acidic fluids such as coffee and orange juice.
- Lorazepam (Ativan) is the medication of choice in patients with impaired liver function.
- Patients can die from alcohol or barbiturate withdrawal.
- Activated charcoal has no role in a benzodiazepine overdose and increases the risk of aspiration.
- In pregnant women, never use Suboxone® (buprenorphine/naloxone); always use Subutex® (buprenorphine).
- Tactile hallucinations are characteristic of cocaine intoxication.

Introduction

Substance use disorder is a significant public health issue, with an estimated cost of US$180.9 billion in 2002.[1] Alcohol and tobacco are the most commonly abused substances; prescription drugs (particularly painkillers) are an increasingly common reason for presentation. The most effective pharmacologic treatments to date have been developed for alcohol, sedative, and opioid use disorders. The primary treatment for stimulants and hallucinogens is symptomatic and supportive. Psychotherapy as a treatment modality

*Mount Sinai School of Medicine, New York, NY, USA.
[†]Haslem Hospital Center New York, NY, USA.

enhances treatment efficacy for all drugs. Principles such as brief interventions and evaluation of the patient's present stage of change allow for simple interventions that are effective. Substance use affects 40%–60% of individuals with mental illness, but all populations should be screened in the initial interview.[2] The following sections will address the major substances of abuse, including diagnosis and key treatment modalities.

Alcohol

From simple intoxication to severe withdrawal, the prevalence of alcohol-related problems in hospitalized patients ranges from 12.5% to 30%.[3] Patients should be screened with validated instruments such as the CAGE Questionnaire, which consists of the following questions:

- Have you felt the need to **C**ut down on your drinking?
- Have people **A**nnoyed you by criticizing your drinking?
- Have you ever felt **G**uilty about drinking?
- Have you ever felt that you needed a drink first thing in the morning (**E**ye-opener)?

Other key elements of the history include: frequency of drinking; typical quantity; frequency of heavy drinking; impaired control over drinking; increased salience of drinking; morning drinking; guilt after drinking; blackouts; alcohol-related injuries; and others concerned with drinking.

Alcohol Intoxication

The patient may present with slurred speech, incoordination, unsteady gait, nystagmus, impairment of attention or memory, stupor or coma. The condition is usually diagnosed with the positive breath test and blood alcohol level (varying greatly, depending on tolerance).

Management

This should be supportive, such as thiamine prior to food or glucose administration and a nonconfrontational approach.

Alcohol Withdrawal

Alcohol withdrawal can be complicated by seizures or delirium, and it is one of the most potentially life-threatening conditions. Without medication, withdrawal symptoms peak at about three days from the last use of alcohol. Early identification and prevention are essential. A careful history can elicit previous alcohol-related symptoms, including blackouts, delirium tremens, and alcohol-related seizures. Validated instruments, such as the Clinical Institute Withdrawal Assessment for Alcohol (CIWA-Ar), can help assess the degree of withdrawal through the following categories: agitation, anxiety, sweating, nausea or vomiting, tremor, disorientation, headache, and hallucinations (auditory, visual, or tactile). Medications should be started on presentation for any patient who has a history of alcohol withdrawal seizures or who shows clear signs of withdrawal.

Management

Benzodiazepines are recommended as the primary treatment for alcohol withdrawal. Longer-acting agents (e.g., chlordiazepoxide and diazepam) may be more effective in preventing seizures and generally contribute to a smoother withdrawal, with fewer rebound symptoms. Shorter-acting agents (e.g., lorazepam and oxazepam), in contrast, may have a lower risk of oversedation. Chlordiazepoxide should be avoided in patients with liver impairment, due to the risk of hepatic encephalopathy. No single medication schedule can be applied to all patients. Frequent assessment allows individualized dosing. The three strategies of dosing involve loading-dose, fixed-schedule, and symptom-triggered, as seen in Table 1.

Other Complications of Alcohol and Their Management

Other dangerous complications of alcohol include delirium tremens and the Wernicke–Korsakoff syndrome (Table 2).

Table 1. Dosing Strategies for Alcohol Withdrawal

Dosing Strategy	Sample Medications	Notes
Loading-dose	Diazepam 20 mg orally, 1 dose	• Gives a moderate-to-high dose to provide sedation. • Drug tapers off through self-metabolism.
Fixed-schedule	• Chlordiazepoxide 50 mg po q 6 hr for 4 doses, then 25 mg po q 6 hr for 8 doses • Lorazepam 2 mg q 6 hr for 4 doses, then 1 mg q 6 hr for 8 doses	• Useful for patients with a history of severe withdrawal or at high risk for withdrawal. • Additional medications must be available for when symptoms are not well controlled (CIWA-Ar >8–10 or elevated vital signs).
Symptom-triggered	• Chlordiazepoxide 50–100 mg q 4 hr until vital signs stabilize • Lorazepam 2–4 mg q 1 hr until vital signs stabilize	• Patients are assessed every 4 hr with a CIWA-Ar (more sensitive than vital signs) and vital signs and medications are given as needed. • Always hold for sedation.

Other Commonly Abused Substances

The other commonly abused drugs are sedatives/hypnotics, opioids, and nicotine.

Sedatives and Hypnotics

This category includes benzodiazepines, barbiturates, and other hypnotics. A sedative reduces excitement and can calm anxious patients; a hypnotic induces sleep.

Intoxicated patients can present with reduced anxiety; a feeling of well-being; lowered inhibitions; slowed pulse and breathing; lowered

Table 2. Complications of Alcohol

Complication	Timeline	Signs/Symptoms	Treatment
Alcoholic hallucinations	12–48 hr to weeks	Vivid AH with clear sensorium; frequently threatening; occasionally seen with tinnitus; risk of violence and suicide	No specific treatment; generally clears within 30–60 days. Protect patient in safe environment.
Alcohol withdrawal delirium (DTs). CIWA-Ar score >20 is a strong risk for DT.	Typically 24–78 hr after last drink; up to 7 days after last drink	Confusion, disorientation, tremor, hyperactivity, fever, elevated vital signs, hallucinations (generally visual and frightening)	Prevention is key. Rule out other causes of delirium; give thiamine. Monitor patient on 1:1 observation to prevent harm to self or others.
Wernicke's encephalopathy (WE) Korsakoff's psychosis (KP)	Seen in chronic alcoholics WE: abrupt onset KP: slow to start and may be late sequela of long-standing alcohol use	WE: appears suddenly with ophthalmoplegia and ataxia, followed by altered mental status (global confusion). KP: anterograde amnesia (nonreversible) is more common than confabulation; hallucinations are rare.	Thiamine, IM or IV, immediately, can present advancement of the syndrome; also folic acid for anemia and peripheral neuropathy, and multivitamins with minerals, including zinc.

blood pressure; poor concentration, fatigue; confusion; impaired coordination, memory, judgment; addiction; respiratory depression and arrest. Additionally, patients intoxicated with barbiturates may present with sedation, drowsiness, depression, unusual excitement, fever, irritability, poor judgment, slurred speech, and dizziness. For patients intoxicated with benzodiazepines, there is sedation, drowsiness, or dizziness.

Management of Intoxication

The initial treatment for a patient who has taken an overdose of a sedative or hypnotic is like any other patient with drug intoxication. Benzodiazepines produce less respiratory depression than barbiturates.

In addition to supportive measures, an *overdose of benzodiazepine* can be treated with flumazenil, a benzodiazepine antagonist. Flumazenil should be administered in an initial IV dose of 0.2 mg given over 30 s, followed by another 0.2 mg IV dose if there is no response after 45 s. This procedure can be repeated at 1 min intervals up to a cumulative dose of 5 mg. Observe patients for at least 2 hr after recovery from flumazenil for late respiratory depression or resedation. Flumazenil is contraindicated in patients with increased intracranial pressure (ICP) or closed-head injury (CHI), those with a history of epilepsy, and those known to have ingested a tricyclic antidepressant (TCA) agent.[4]

An *overdose of barbiturates* is treated with intravenous sodium bicarbonate to alkalinize the urine, which increases the rate of barbiturate excretion. The dose of the bicarbonate varies, depending on the patient's metabolic state. Urine pH should be monitored and maintained at 7.5. Dialysis may be required, depending on the severity of the patient's condition.

Withdrawal. The most frequent symptoms are insomnia, gastric problems, tremors, agitation, fearfulness, muscle spasms, increased blood pressure, and increased heart rate and body temperature. Less frequent effects are irritability, sweating, depersonalization, derealization, hypersensitivity to stimuli, depression, suicidal behavior, psychosis, hallucinations, seizures, and delirium tremens. Severe symptoms usually occur as a result of abrupt or overrapid withdrawal.

Management of withdrawal. Treatment of withdrawal syndromes is identical for withdrawal from all sedatives–hypnotics, because all drugs in this category, including barbiturates, sleeping pills, benzodiazepines, and alcohol, exhibit cross-dependence. The basic principle is to withdraw the addicting agent slowly to avoid convulsions. Patients who have mild dependence on benzodiazepines can be managed by a slow taper of the drug in an outpatient setting. The alternative is to replace short-acting benzodiazepines (e.g. alprazolam) with equivalent dosing of a longer-acting drug (e.g. clonazepam), which may provide for a milder withdrawal syndrome during the taper.[5] The weekly tapering dose can be calculated by dividing the total dose by 5 and reducing the dose by this amount weekly. The dose for most patients can be reduced to zero in 4–8 weeks. Anticonvulsant carbamazepine, gabapentin, and topiramate can be used in the treatment of benzodiazepine detoxification; they lack addiction potential.[6]

In the case of barbiturates, establishment of the patient's approximate drug tolerance level is the most important step. In severe cases of withdrawal, the level of tolerance is determined by giving pentobarbital, 200 mg by mouth, and wait 1 hr to look for signs of nystagmus, ataxia, drowsiness, dysarthria, decreased blood pressure, and decreased pulse. If two or more signs are present, pentobarbital has to be converted to phenobarbital (phenobarbital 30 mg for every 100 mg of pentobarbital given); if not, pentobarbital is given (100 mg by mouth) every hour until two or more signs are present or a total of 600 mg pentobarbital has been given. Phenobarbital could be decreased by 10% of the initial dose per day. For patients with severe hepatic failure and for hemodynamically unstable patients who require very rapid medication titration to control withdrawal symptoms, short-acting medications should be used, such as midazolam, diazepam, or lorazepam, depending on the rapidity of reversal of the effects required. After adjusting the frequency of administration to the duration of action, the medication could be reduced to 10% of the total daily dose per day.[5]

Narcotics (Opioids)

There has been a steady increase in opioid-related visits to emergency rooms over the past ten years, including a doubling of the number of visits for narcotic pain relief between 2004 and 2008.[7] Injection drug use predisposes individuals to hepatitis B and C as well as acquired immune deficiency syndrome; there is also increased risk of endocarditis, septicemia, and pulmonary emboli.

Acute intoxication causes pain relief, euphoria, drowsiness/nausea, constipation, confusion, sedation, respiratory depression and arrest, unconsciousness, coma, and even death.

Overdose

An opiate overdose is treated with naloxone, typically at repeating doses of 0.4 mg/mL IV or IM every 2 min as needed for a total dose of 1–2 mg. Because of the long half-life of methadone, a patient who overdoses on methadone may require an IV naloxone drip.

Withdrawal

Opiate withdrawal begins 8–12 hr after the last use, with more severe signs occurring 24–36 hr later, and the withdrawal syndrome subsiding in 5–10 days if untreated. For patients sustained on methadone, withdrawal symptoms have a delayed time course: beginning after 24–30 hr and concluding after 2-4 weeks. The Clinical Opiate Withdrawal Scale (COWS) summed score of the 11 items can be used to assess a patient's level of opiate withdrawal and to make inferences about his or her level of physical dependence on opioids: 5–12, mild withdrawal; 13–24, moderate; 26–36, moderately severe; more than 36, severe withdrawal. The signs and symptoms of withdrawal are summarized below:

Signs and Symptoms of Opiate Withdrawal[8]:

- Dysphoria, anxiety, irritability
- Restlessness
- Rhinorrhea and lacrimation
- Muscle and bone aches
- Yawning
- Nausea, vomiting
- Diarrhea, increased bowel sounds
- Dilated pupils

- Elevated heart rate
- Sweating
- Tremor

Management of Opioid Withdrawal

Medications for opioid withdrawal can be divided into opioid agonists and nonopioid medications. Opioid treatments involve the substitution of a long-acting opioid such as methadone or buprenorphine.

When methadone is used, patients get an initial dose of 10–20 mg. If vital signs do not stabilize, the patient can receive additional doses of 5–10 mg of methadone every 2 hr, with a limit of 40 mg per 24 hr period. The patient is then tapered off methadone over a 10-day period. Patients may sometimes need more less methadone due to induction/inhibition of the hepatic enzymes, especially individuals undergoing HIV treatment.[12]

Buprenorphine is preferable as the first line in opioid detoxification where indicated. After a mandatory 12 hr (short-acting opioids such as heroin) or 24 hr (long-acting opioids such as methadone) abstinence, the patient is started on a 2 mg buprenorphine every 1–2 hr, maximum of 8 mg on day 1. Over the next two days, the dose of buprenorphine/naloxone (Suboxone) should be increased to 12–16 mg per day. The objectives of induction should be to stabilize the patient as rapidly as possible, to minimize any withdrawal symptoms, and to eliminate further use of illicit opioids. The Clinical Opioid Withdrawal Scale is used to assess need.

Clonidine is used along with other symptom relief medications for opioid withdrawal, and is given at 0.1–0.2 mg every 4 hr as needed for withdrawal symptoms. Blood pressure must by monitored for hypotension after the first dose. In addition to clonidine, antiemetics (ondansetron), nonopiod pain medications (such as ketorolac), and antidiarrheal medications should be given as needed. Opioid-dependent patients who present with pain should always receive adequate medication to relieve the pain. The assumption must not be made that they are medication-seeking. Methadone, buprenorphine, and naltrexone may also be used for maintenance treatment along with psychotherapy and behavioral therapy.

Stimulants (Cocaine and Amphetamines)

The signs and symptoms of intoxication are similar for cocaine and amphetamines. Crack cocaine is a short-acting form of cocaine that is sold in crystals that can be smoked. Users will frequently experience euphoria and increased sexual desire, along with anorexia, insomnia, anxiety, hyperactivity, and rapid speech and thought process. Cocaine-induced psychosis can entail hallucinations, including formication, the unpleasant feeling of insects crawling under the skin. Patients must be monitored for potential serious medical complications, such as myocardial infarction, stroke, and seizure. Less severe consequences include perforation of the nasal septum or bronchitis from smoking cocaine.

Cocaine users will frequently follow a pattern of a 2–3-day binge followed by a "crash," which entails sleeping off the high feeling depressed, and potentially suicidal.

Occasional stimulant use does not require any specific medical treatment, except in the case of a life-threatening overdose. Stimulants can be withdrawn abruptly and, in fact, a gradual reduction in usage can be very difficult. Mild intoxication can be treated by "talking down" the patient.

Hallucinogens and Other Substances

Supportive care is the primary treatment for the substances below, along with psychotherapeutic treatments such as brief interventions and referral to outpatient rehabilitation.

Marijuana. Over 34% of Americans use marijuana. An episode of marijuana-induced psychosis, while usually short-lived, led to subsequent psychotic episodes in 77% and a diagnosis of a schizophrenia spectrum disorder in 45%, usually within three years.[9] Early exposure to marijuana increased the likelihood of years of subsequent drug problems. A study of over 300 fraternal and identical twin pairs found that early marijuana users had elevated rates of other drug use and drug problems later on. The odds of other drug use ranged from 2.1 to 5.2 times higher.[10] Marijuana withdrawal symptoms include: irritability, anger, aggression, depressed mood, headaches, restlessness, trouble with sleeping and strange dreams, decreased appetite and weight loss; tobacco withdrawal is similar except for opposite effects on appetite and weight.

Management. Dronabinol (Marinol — synthetic THC) is the most promising drug to date.[11] Sativex (an aerosol combining THC and cannabidiol) may be useful when available.

Ecstacy (3,4-methylenedioxy-methamphetamine, MDMA). Symptoms include reduced inhibitions and euphoric mood; can be co-ingested with other substances. Immediate concerns are for dehydration and hyperthermia, which in extreme cases may cause death by cardiac arrhythmias. Excess water intake to avoid this can lead to hyponatrenia, seizures, and death; symptoms may be compared to those of both the serotonin syndrome and the neuroleptic malignant syndrome.

GHB (gamma hydroxybutyrate, date rape drug). Acutely users may experience confusion, agitation, hallucinations, loss of consciousness, and coma. Management of GHB ingestion in a breathing patient includes oxygen supplementation intravenous access, and comprehensive physiological and cardiac monitoring. If clinically well in 6 hr, the patient is discharged.

PCP (phencyclidine — "angel dust"). Usually smoked; can be snorted, injected, or taken orally. Patients can become agitated, aggressive, and display great strength. Hypertension, nystagmus, tachycardia, flushing, profuse sweating, generalized numbness of extremities, blurred vision, dysarthria, ataxia, muscular incoordination, marked analgesia, and anesthesia. Self-mutilation (Van Gogh's syndrome), such as blinding one self or biting one's own arm, is not uncommon. "Talking down" is inadvisable due to risk of aggression. Benzodiazepines and haldol are helpful. Monitor CPK levels serially.

LSD (D-lysergic acid diethylamide). *Psychologically*: hallucinations, increased color perception, altered mental state, thought disorders, delusions, body image changes, and impaired depth, time, and space perceptions. *Physiologically*: tachycardia, hypertension, dilated pupils, sweating, loss of appetite, sleeplessness, dry mouth, tremors, speech difficulties, and piloerection. "Talking down" and supportive therapy are the main treatment.

Table 3. Criteria for Different Levels of Care

Key Placement Levels	Criteria
Level I: outpatient (non-intensive)	Minimal risk in all domains: intoxication/ withdrawal, biomedical, emotional-behavioral, treatment readiness, relapse/continued use potential, recovery environment; and with no significant medical, psychological, or social concerns.
Level II: intensive outpatient /partial hospitalization service	Does not meet the criteria for inpatient rehabilitation, intensive residential rehabilitation, methadone treatment services; however, the client has a moderate-to-severe dependence condition or there is a substantial risk of relapse.
Level II: medically monitored intensive ***outpatient***	Moderately severe risk in intoxication/ withdrawal or biomedical or emotional domains plus high risk in any other domain, lack of support for early abstinence, or when the individual is experiencing a situational crisis or is unable to abstain without admission to a supervised setting.
Level III: residential/inpatient treatment rehabilitation service (long-term care)	Unable to participate in and comply with treatment outside a 24 hr structured treatment setting or there is an imminent health risk from continued drug use, and there are no complications or comorbidities requiring medical management/ monitoring daily, but has substantial deficits in functional skills in areas of activities of daily living, interpersonal skills, vocational/ educational, or maladaptive social behavior.
Level IV: medically managed intensive ***inpatient*** (detoxification and residential medically supervised withdrawal)	Severe risk due to intoxication/ withdrawal or biomedical or emotional/ behavioral signs/symptoms; significant risk due to complications or comorbidities; or incapacitated by substances and there is substantial risk of physical harm to the individual or others or there is lack of support for early abstinence. CIWA score greater than 10; COWS score greater than 24.

Source of information: American Society of Addiction Medicine (ASAM), New York State Office of Alcoholism and Substance Abuse Services (OASAS).

Ketamine ("special K"). A dissociative anesthetic and hallucinogen, with intoxication marked by amnesia, moderate dilation of pupils, increased muscle tone, and seizure.

Nitrates, inhalants, solvents. Users may exhibit nausea or vomiting, cramps, muscle weakness, loss of motor function, and damage to the cardiac or neurologic systems.

Nicotine. Replacement therapies include nicotine patch, gum, and inhaler. Use the following dosing for the nicotine patch: 21 mg if 10+ cigarettes daily; 14 mg if 5–10 cigarettes; 7mg if <5 cigarettes. For nicotine gum, use 4 mg every 2 hr if smoking one pack daily, or 2 mg if less than one pack. Nicotine gum is ineffective if the patient is consuming acidic fluids such as coffee and orange juice. Bupropion is effective for smoking cessation. Varenicline is also effective.

Level of Care and Referral

The provider should make an appropriate placement to ensure that an individual in need of substance abuse services is placed in the least restrictive but most clinically appropriate level of care available (Table 3).

Conclusion

In view of the health, societal, and economic consequences, it behooves us to develop modalities for reducing substance use disorders. Prevention is probably most cost-effective. Rapid and effective treatment of the complications of substance abuse saves lives and improves prognosis, especially in individuals with comorbid illnesses. Significant progress has been made in the treatment of substance use disorders, especially for alcohol and opioids. Furthermore, the role of psychotherapeutic interventions is increasingly important.

References

1. *The Economic Costs of Drug Abuse in the United States,* 1992–2002. Publication No. 207303 (2004), Office of National Drug Control Policy. Executive Office of the President, Washington, DC.
2. Kessler RC. (2004) The epidemiology of dual diagnosis. *Biol Psychiatry* **56**(10): 730–737.
3. Moore RD, *et al.* (1989) Prevalence, detection, and treatment of alcoholism in hospitalized patients. *JAMA* **261**(3): 403–407.
4. Weinbroum AA, *et al.* (1997) A risk-benefit assessment of flumazenil in the management of benzodiazepine overdose. *Drug Saf* **17**(3): 181–196.
5. Stern T, (ed), (2004) Drug-addicted patients. In: *Massachusetts General Hospital Handbook of General Hospital Psychiatry*, 5th ed. Mosby Press.
6. Zullino D. (2004) Anticonvulsant drugs in the treatment of substance withdrawal. *Drugs Today (Barc)* **40**(7): 603–619.
7. SAMHSA US Department of Health and Human Services, Office of Applied Studies (ed). (2010) The DAWN Report: Trends in Emergency Department Visits Involving Nonmedical Use of Narcotic Pain Relievers, Rockville.
8. Wesson DR, and Ling W. (2003) The Clinical Opiate Withdrawal Scale (COWS). *J Psychoactive Drugs* **35**(2): 253–259.
9. Arendt M, *et al.* (2005) Cannabis-induced psychosis and subsequent schizophrenia-spectrum disorders: Follow-up study of 535 incident cases. *Br J Psychiatry* **187**: 510–515.
10. Lynskey MT, *et al.* (2003) Escalation of drug use in early-onset cannabis users vs co-twin controls. *JAMA* **289**(4): 427–433.
11. Haney M, *et al.* Marijuana withdrawal in humans: Effects of oral THC or divalproex. *Neuropsychopharmacology* **29**(1): 158–170.
12. Akerele, *et al.* (2002) Effects of HIV triple therapy on methadone levels. *Am J Addict* **11**(4): 308–314.

Chapter 79

Depression: Diagnosis and Treatment

Kyle Lapidus, Laili Soleimani* and Dan V. Iosifescu**

Key Pearls

- Major depressive disorder is relatively common, with a prevalence of 22%–33% in medically ill patients.
- Patients with major depressive disorder have a 20-fold increase in the risk of suicide compared to the general population.
- The key to the diagnosis of depression is a high index of clinical suspicion when facing a constellation of vague, nonspecific physical symptoms and/or in the context of significant psychosocial distress.
- While a series of antidepressant medications could be useful, the single most important factor for success is ensuring adherence to treatment for at least 6–8 weeks.
- After a successful course of treatment, patients should continue their medications for at least six more months to avoid early relapse. Patients with a history of chronic or highly relapsing depression will need to continue treatment for a significantly longer period.

Introduction

Depression encompasses a large number of psychobiological syndromes with the core features of depressed mood and/or loss of interest associated with cognitive and somatic disturbances, which cause significant functional impairment.

*Mount Sinai Medical Center, New York, NY, USA.

Table 1. Criteria for an Acute Episode of Major Depressive Episode

- At least five of the following symptoms must be present continuously for two weeks, and at least one should be either depressed mood or anhedonia.
  - Depressed mood (or irritability in children and adolescents)
  - Anhedonia
  - Appetite change or weight change
  - Insomnia or hypersomnia
  - Psychomotor agitation or retardation
  - Fatigue or loss of energy
  - Feelings of worthlessness or guilt
  - Decreased concentration
  - Recurrent thoughts of death and suicidal ideation
  - No history of manic or hypomanic episode
- Symptoms should cause clinically significant functional impairment.
- Symptoms should not be secondary to a substance (e.g. a drug of abuse or, a medication) or a general medical condition (e.g. hypothyroidism).
- Symptoms are not better accounted for by bereavement.

Depressive disorders are classified as mood disorders and are distinguished from bipolar disorders by the absence of a manic episode. Depressive disorders include major depressive disorder (MDD — Table 1[1]), dysthymic disorder ("low grade" chronic depression occurring more than 50% of the days over at least two years) and minor depression (a minimum of two depressive symptoms present for at least two weeks).

MDD is relatively common, with a prevalence of more than 10% in the primary health setting (female: male ratio of 2), 15%–20% among the nursing home population and 22%–33% in medically ill patients. Depression is frequently underrecognized; epidemiological studies suggest that less than half (47%) of the cases are identified by physicians.

Important factors in the etiology of depression include genetic vulnerability, changes in the neurotransmitter levels (e.g. catecholaminergic and serotonergic), altered neuroendocrine function, and psychosocial stressors/trauma.

Evaluation

Diagnostic Evaluation

The key to diagnosis is clinical suspicion: always ask about depressed mood and anhedonia when you notice nonspecific symptoms suggestive of depression (Table 2), then obtain more details about the onset, duration, accompanying psychological symptoms, possible psychosocial precipitating factors (e.g. relationship problems, work-related stressors, or living conditions), and the impact of these symptoms on the daily life of the patient.

Common symptoms of depression include:

- Depressed mood
- Anxiety, excessive worrying
- Panic attacks
- Irritable mood
- Anger attacks
- Crying spells
- Loss of interest or pleasure
- Distractability
- Change in appetite
- Change in sleep
- Fatigue
- Pain (e.g. headaches, back pain)
- Muscle tension
- Heart palpitation
- Guilt
- Sense of worthlessness
- Recurrent thoughts of death or suicide

Inquire about a history of past depressive episodes and treatments, other psychiatric disorders (including mania), and possible use of alcohol and other substances that can inform your diagnostic and treatment decisions.

Asking about the physical symptoms, medical and medication history, as well as performing a physical exam will help to rule out the possibility of depressive disorders secondary to medical conditions or medications (Table 2).

Table 2. Examples of Medical Conditions Causing Depressive Symptoms

- Autoimmune disorders (e.g. SLE, rhumatoid arthritis)
- Neurological disease (e.g. stroke, Parkinson's disease, seizure disorder, Alzheimer's disease, Huntington's disease, multiple sclerosis, traumatic brain injury)
- Endocrine disorders (e.g. hypercalcemia, hypercortisolism, hyperparathyroidism, hyperthyroidism, hypocortisolism, hypoparathyroidism, hypothyroidism)
- Malignancies (e.g. gastrointestinal cancer, pancreatic cancer)
- Infectious disease (e.g. hepatitis, human immunodeficiency virus, mononucleosis)
- Medications or substances: antihypertensive medications (e.g. propranolol, thiazides, clonidine), anticholinergic agents, anticonvulsant agents, oral contraceptives, sedatives (e.g. barbiturates, benzodiazepines), anti-Parkinsonian medications (e.g. methyldopa, amantadine), alcohol

Requesting routine and specific (e.g. thyroid function, vitamin B12 and folate levels) laboratory tests can aid in diagnosing specific abnormalities in a subset of patients who do not respond to standard antidepressant treatments.

Standardized scales (clinician-administered and self-administered) can help to quantify depressive symptoms and to improve depression detection and treatment monitoring. Scales can be chosen based on the patient population and practice setting. For example, self-administered measures (such as the Quick Inventory of Depressive Symptomatology, QIDS-SR; http://www.ids-qids.org) can be quickly completed and scored, although other time-intensive, interviewer-administered measures (e.g. the Hamilton Depression Rating Scale, (HAM-D) may be necessary for cognitively impaired patients.

Safety Evaluation

Always ask (and document) thoughts of death, suicide and homicide, as patients suffering from MDD have a 20-fold higher risk of suicide than the general population. Positive responses should be followed by assessment of the content of the thoughts (plans or intent), working with patient and family to limit access to lethal means (e.g. firearms and large amounts of medications), a psychiatry consult, and/or possible hospitalization.

Differential Diagnosis

Depression is a common symptom among a number of psychiatric conditions. Table 3[2] lists the most common psychiatric differential diagnoses of MDD.

Table 3. Psychiatric Differential Diagnoses of Major Depression

Differential Diagnoses	Characteristic Features
Nonpathological periods of sadness	Short duration, few associated symptoms, and lack of significant functional impairment or distress.
Bereavement	In response to the loss of a loved one, usually ameliorating over 2 months and not lasting more than 6 months.
Adjustment disorder with depressed mood	In response to an immediate stressor; does not meet full criteria for a major depressive episode.
Seasonal depression	Recurrent episodes with a clear seasonal pattern (onset in fall or winter and full remission usually by spring).
Premenstrual dysphoric disorder (PMDD)	Significant depressed mood, anxiety, and irritability during the 1–2 weeks before menses and resolving with menses.
Postpartum depressive disorder	Full depressive episode with an onset within a few months of delivery. To be differentiated from postpartum blues (fewer symptoms, onset shortly after delivery and usually subsides within 3 weeks).
Bipolar I or bipolar II disorder	History of one or more manic, mixed, or hypomanic episodes.
Mood disorder due to a general medical condition	Direct physiological effect of a general medical condition.
Substance-induced mood disorder	Caused by the direct physiological effect of a substance (including medication); symptoms develop within a month of substance use.
Dysthymic disorder	Depressed mood present on more than 50% of days over a 2-year period, in the absence of major depressive episodes.

(*Continued*)

Table 3. (*Continued*)

Differential Diagnoses	Characteristic feature
Schizoaffective disorder	Recurrent periods of at least 2 weeks of delusions or hallucinations; at least some of these periods occur in the absence of prominent mood symptoms.
Schizophrenia, delusional disorder, psychotic disorder not otherwise specified	Depressive symptoms are brief relative to the total duration of the psychotic disturbance (e.g. delusions, hallucinations).
Posttraumatic stress disorder (PTSD)	Occurs within 6 months of a stressful event; hyperarousal, episodes of flashbacks, nightmares, detachment, "numbness," maladaptive coping responses, and excessive use of alcohol and drugs.
Dementia	Progressive history of declining cognitive functioning (usually before depressive symptoms). Low scores (usually less than 23) on the mini–mental status examination (MMSE).

Depression in Patients with General Medical Conditions

Depression is more prevalent among the patients with medical conditions (including cardiovascular disease, diabetes, and other conditions listed in Table 3) and has been suggested to increase the mortality rate by as many as 4.3 times. Depression itself is harder to treat in medically ill patients. It is very important to treat both medical and depressive symptoms in these patients; this can improve the outcome of medical treatment and adherence to medical therapy and rehabilitation. Atypical depressive symptoms and associated positive laboratory findings for a nonprimary depressive disorder should warrant a full medical workup.

Treatment

Useful treatments for depression include pharmacotherapy, focused psychotherapies, somatic treatments, and lifestyle changes.[3]

Pharmacotherapy

Commonly used antidepressants and doses are listed in Table 4.[4] While several pharmacological agents are FDA-approved, none are clearly superior in efficacy. They differ in the pharmacological and side effect profile (Table 5).[5] For all, the beginning of antidepressant efficacy may be delayed for several weeks. As a general rule, antidepressant side effects can be minimized by slowly increasing the dosage (especially in the elderly), although this strategy may also delay the beginning of efficacy.

Selective serotonin reuptake inhibitors (SSRIs) are frequently used as a *first-line treatment* of depressive disorders, because their specificity results in safety in an overdose and a favorable side effect profile. They also effectively treat anxiety disorders and other psychiatric comorbidities.

Serotonin–norepinephrine reuptake inhibitors (SNRIs) may be useful in SSRI nonresponders and in specific chronic pain conditions; they tend to be more expensive.

Tricyclic antidepressants (TCAs) are older, inexpensive agents that also act primarily by inhibiting serotonin and norepinephrine reuptake, are effective as antidepressants, and effectively treat chronic pain. They also interact with many other receptors, which may contribute to their efficacy, but results in side effects that may limit tolerability and compliance. TCAs block muscarinic acetylcholine receptors, leading to *anticholinergic side effects* (Table 5). The risk of confusion and disorientation is most significant in elderly patients. TCAs also antagonize histamine H1 receptors and α_1 adrenergic receptors; caution is advised in patients with narrow angle glaucoma, prostatic hypertrophy, or low blood pressure. The most dangerous side effect of TCA treatment is *QT_C prolongation*, which makes TCAs potentially *lethal in an overdose*; an EKG is advisable before and four weeks after initiating TCA treatment. Plasma levels can help guide dosage adjustments.

Monoamine oxidase inhibitors (MAOIs) are most often used in patients with atypical depression or in treatment-resistant patients who fail trials of other medications. They act by inhibiting MAO A and B, enzymes that break down monoamines, including serotonin, dopamine, and norepinephrine. These enzymes are found in neurons and glia, throughout the GI tract and

Table 4. Recommended Dosages for Approved Antidepressants

Drug	Usual Dose (mg/day)	Initial Dose (mg/day)	Notes
Selective Serotonin Reuptake Inhibitors (SSRIs)			
Citalopram (Celexa)	20–60	10–20	Few drug interactions
Escitalopram (Lexapro)	10–20	10	Few drug interactions
Paroxetine (Paxil)	10–50	10–20	Short half-life
Sertraline (Zoloft)	25–200	25–50	
Fluvoxamine (Luvox)	50–300	25–50	
Fluoxetine (Prozac)	10–60	10–20	Longest half-life
Serotonin–Norepinephrine Reuptake Inhibitors (SNRIs)			
Venlafaxine (Effexor)	75–225	37.5	
Venlafaxine XR (Effexor XR)	75–375	37.5	
Duloxetine (Cymbalta)	40–60	20–40	
Tricyclic/Tetracyclic Antidepressants (TCAs)			
Amitriptyline (Elavil)	100–300	10–50	
Clomipramine (Anafranil)	100–250	25	
Doxepin (Adapin)	100–300	25–50	
Imipramine (Tofranil)	100–300	10–25	
Trimipramine (Surmontil)	100–300	25–50	
Desipramine (Norpramin)	100–300	25–50	Favorable tolerability
Nortriptyline (Pamelor)	50–150	10–25	Favorable safety, tolerability
Protriptyline (Vivactil)	15–60	10	Activating
Amoxapine (Asendin)	100–400	50	
Maprotiline (Ludiomil)	100–225	50	
Monoamine Oxidase Inhibitors (MAOIs)			
Phenelzine (Nardil)	45–90	15	
Tranylcypromine (Parnate)	30–60	10	
Isocarboxazid (Marplan)	30–60	20	
Selegiline (Eldepryl)	30–40	10	Selective MAO-B inhibitor
Other Antidepressants			
Bupropion (Wellbutrin)	300–450	100–150	Available as SR and XL/XR
Mirtazapine (Remeron)	15–45	15	

Table 5. Important Side Effects of Antidepressants

Drug Class	Important Side Effects
Selective serotonin and serotonin–norepinephrine reuptake inhibitors (SSRIs and SNRIs)	Nausea, decreased appetite, weight loss, diaphoresis, insomnia, sedation, nervousness, sexual dysfunction, headache, dizziness
Tricyclic/tetracyclic antidepressants (TCAs)	*Anticholinergic*: dry mouth, constipation, hyperthermia, sinus tachycardia, blurred vision, urinary retention, cognitive/memory impairment *Antihistaminic*: sedation, increased appetite, weight gain, hypotension *Antiadrenergic*: postural hypotension, dizziness, tachycardia, reduced seizure threshold, sexual dysfunction *Cardiac conduction effects similar to those of class 1A antiarrhythmics* Cardiotoxicity in overdose
Monoamine oxidase inhibitors (MAOIs)	Insomnia, sedation, weight gain, orthostatic hypotension, sexual dysfunction Less common: pyridoxine deficiency with parasthesias, tremor, anticholinergic effects *Hypertensive crisis*: occurs with tyramine ingestion (e.g. aged cheese and meats, fava beans, soy sauce) *Serotonin syndrome — life-threatening*, with rapid onset of hyperthermia, hypertension, tachycardia, shock
Bupropion (Wellbutrin)	Agitation, dry mouth, insomnia, nausea, constipation, tremor, headache Increased seizure risk
Mirtazapine (Remeron)	*Antihistaminic*: sedation, increased appetite, weight gain, hypotension, dry mouth, constipation, dizziness

liver, and in platelets. MAOIs available in the US *irreversibly inhibit MAOs*, so their effects persist through several drug-free days until enzyme stores are regenerated. Intake of *foods containing* the sympathomimetic amine *tyramine* can result in potentially *lethal hypertensive crises. Tryptophan-containing foods* also pose a risk of *serotonin syndrome*. Other medications that may react with MAOIs to cause these syndromes include meperidine, tramadol, dextromethorphan, and SSRIs. To avoid serotonin syndrome, a washout period of at least two weeks (five weeks from fluoxetine) is recommended when one is switching to or from an MAOI.

Additional agents, including bupropion and mirtazapine, are relatively safe in an overdose. *Bupropion* has dopaminergic properties and energizing effects; it is also used as an aid in smoking cessation, and has few sexual side effects. Because of increased seizure risk, bupropion is contraindicated in seizure disorder or bulimia. *Mirtazapine*, a more sedating antidepressant, is well used in combination with other agents due to limited drug–drug interactions. Its side effects result mainly from histamine H1 receptor blockade.

Augmentation with *atypical antipsychotics, thyroid hormone, lithium, psychostimulants*, and *nutritional supplements* may be used in cases of partial or nonresponse to an antidepressant agent.

Psychotherapy

Cognitive behavioral therapy and *interpersonal therapy* are effective treatments for depressed patients. Although *short-term dynamic psychotherapy* may also be used, less evidence supports this approach. Patients with moderate or severe depression may benefit more from a combination of pharmacotherapy and psychotherapy.

Somatic Treatments

Electroconvulsive therapy (ECT) is *well established* and *highly effective* in resistant depression. Electrical stimulation is applied bilaterally or unilaterally to the head to induce a seizure. ECT requires anesthesia and can cause cognitive side effects and transient amnesia along with hypertension and arrhythmias, and is generally used after patients have failed pharmacological trials and/or in very severe forms of depression. Relative contraindications include coronary artery disease, arrhythmia, and increased intracranial pressure or lesions.

Other options include *phototherapy*, which involves the application of bright light and may be particularly *useful in seasonal depression. Vagus nerve stimulation* (which consists in a surgically implanted device sending electrical impulses via ascending fibers of the vagus nerve) and *transcranial magnetic stimulation* (involving a noninvasive brain depolarization induced by a magnetic field) are also FDA-approved for the treatment of major depression.

Other Treatments

Other interventions with some efficacy in the treatment of depression include *lifestyle changes* (e.g. physical exercise) and some *dietary supplements* (e.g. omega-3 fatty acids, S-adenosyne methionine, l-methylfolate, St. John's wort).

Phases of Treatment

Acute Phase Treatment

- The choice of treatment is based on the severity of the symptoms, the history of prior positive responses, the presence of other psychiatric symptoms, the side effect profile of the medication, and the patient's preference (e.g. psychotherapy without/with psychotherapy for the mild/moderate symptoms, ECT for severe depression, and presence of psychotic features or catatonia).
- In cases of failure after 4–8 weeks of treatment, for subjects with no improvement, consider raising the dose to the optimal tolerable level (optimization) before switching to another drug within the class or another class of drugs. For partial responders, a combination of

antidepressant medications (adding buproprion, low dose TCA, mirtazapine, or buspirone) or augmentation strategies (with atypical antipsychotics, lithium, tri-odothyronine (T3), psychostimulants, or dopaminergic agents) can be used prior to switching medications.

Continuation of Treatment

After sustained remission, continue treatment for 6–9 months with a full antidepressant dose to decrease the risk of relapse.

In general, it is important to explain depression as an illness associated with neurochemical dysregulation in the brain, rather than a personal weakness or fault. Patients should also be educated about the anticipated side effects of the medications; this will improve patient compliance. More than 60% of MDD patients are at risk for recurrence. Patients with recurrent depression should be educated about the early signs of depression; some may require lifelong antidepressant therapy.

When to Refer to a Psychiatrist

- Significant risk of suicide or homicide
- Current pregnancy or planning for future pregnancy
- Poor social support
- Disability caused by depression
- Suboptimal response to one or two adequate treatments
- Comorbid psychiatric problems (psychosis, mania, severe anxiety, substance abuse, panic attacks, PTSD, dementia)
- Need for alcohol or illicit drug detoxification

References

1. American Psychiatric Association. (2000) *Diagnostic and Statistical Manual of Mental Disorders DSM-IV-TR*, 4th ed.
2. First MB, Frances A, Pincus HA. *DSM-IV-TR® Handbook of Differential Diagnosis* (DOI: 10.1176/appi.books.9781585622658.119311).

3. *American Psychiatric Association Guidelines for Treatment of Patients with Major Depressive Disorder*, 2nd ed. (DOI: 10.1176/appi.books.9780890423370.109668).
4. Schatzberg AF, Nemeroff CB. (2009) *The American Psychiatric Publishing Textbook of Psychopharmacology*, American Psychiatric, Washington, D.C: (DOI: 10.1176/appi.books.9781585623860).
5. Stahl SM. (2008) *Depression and Bipolar Disorder: Stahl's Essential Psychopharmacology*. Cambridge University Press.

Chapter 80

Schizophrenia

Joseph M. Cerimele, Alejandra Durango* and Vladan Novakovic*,†*

Key Pearls

- Schizophrenia carries a risk of significant morbidity and mortality from chronic medical disorders, and from suicide which occurs in 10% of patients.
- Approximately 50% of patients have a non-nicotine substance use disorder, and nicotine dependence occurs in 80%–90% of patients.
- Patients with schizophrenia are more likely to experience complications when hospitalized than patients without schizophrenia, including decubitus ulcers, nosocomial infection, and venous thromboembolism.
- Except for management of an emergency, such as neuroleptic malignant syndrome, abrupt discontinuation of antipsychotic agents should not be done without consultation with a psychiatrist.
- All antipsychotics can cause acute movement disorders, including akathisia and dystonia, and chronically these agents can cause tardive dyskinesia.

*Mount Sinai School of Medicine, New York, NY, USA.
†James J. Peters Veterans Affairs Hospital, Bronx, NY, USA.

Clinical Syndrome

Schizophrenia is a chronic, disabling, heterogeneous psychiatric syndrome characterized by core disturbances in cognition (e.g. impairment of attention, verbal fluency, working memory), positive symptoms (e.g. hallucinations, delusions, disorganized speech), and negative symptoms (e.g. affective flattening, inability to logically link thoughts, amotivation).[1,2] The onset is generally in late adolescence to early adulthood, with a natural history of progressively worsening symptoms and impairment. The illness is often recognized at the first onset of positive symptoms, which are usually treatment-responsive, resulting in persistent negative and cognitive symptoms, although positive symptoms may recur or even be chronic. The disorder's prevalence is between 0.5% and 1.5%, with an incidence of 0.5–5.0 per 10,000.[1] After the illness onset, patients with schizophrenia may have few or no social relationships, and may be homeless or unemployed. This illness carries significant morbidity and mortality, with 10% of patients completing suicide.[2] The familial pattern of schizophrenia is well studied; first-degree relatives of patients with schizophrenia have a risk of developing the disorder that is 10 times greater than that of the general population.[1]

Co-occurring Disorders

Substance Use Disorders

Substance use disorders are common in patients with schizophrenia, with most studies suggesting that 50% of patients have a co-occurring substance (other than nicotine) use disorder.[4] In this population, nicotine dependence occurs in 80%–90% of patients.[1] Patients have reported improvements in attention and have demonstrated improved working memory with nicotine use. The subjective experience of improved cognition may partly explain the high prevalence of tobacco use. Alcohol and cannabis are the most commonly used nonnicotine substances among patients with schizophrenia.[4] Because of the high prevalence of substance use disorders in these patients, screening for substance use should be done, and appropriate toxicological and infectious disease testing should be performed.

General Medical Disorders

For decades, physicians have reported that many disorders of nonbrain organ systems occur more often in patients with schizophrenia than in the general population. Leucht *et al.* reviewed this topic in 2007.[5] They found that cardiovascular diseases, obesity, diabetes mellitus, HIV infection, hepatitis, osteoporosis, and other disorders have higher prevalence in patients with schizophrenia compared to controls. While it is likely that numerous factors account for this, the authors described contributions from behavioral (e.g. avolition and impaired communication skills), iatrogenic (adverse effects of medications), and system-related factors (patients less likely to receive primary care). It is also possible that an unknown pathophysiological process of schizophrenia contributes to the development of these co-occurring disorders.

In addition to behavioral and social contributions, these co-occurring disorders, may account for the shortened lifespan seen in patients with schizophrenia. Saha *et al.* performed a systematic review of population-based studies (37 studies from 25 countries) reporting mortality in patients with schizophrenia.[6] The primary outcome of this study was measured with a standardized mortality ratio (SMR) for all-cause mortality. Patients with schizophrenia demonstrated an elevated SMR of 2.58, which translated into an overall reduced lifespan by 20–25 years. While the authors suggested that second-generation antipsychotics may contribute to this increased risk of death, a population-based cohort study from 2009 showed that in schizophrenia patients, receiving long-term treatment with antipsychotic agents was associated with lower mortality compared to not receiving antipsychotic agents.[7] This suggests that the 20–25-year shortened lifespan in these patients is not due to adverse effects of antipsychotic treatment.[8]

Frequently Untreated Disorders

As noted above, patients with schizophrenia generally have co-occurring chronic disorders. Some chronic conditions, such as diabetes mellitus, hypertension, and dyslipidemia, may frequently go untreated. One report from the large National Institute of Mental Health–funded clinical study, the CATIE trial (a multicenter study examining the effectiveness of antipsychotic therapy in schizophrenia), showed that the rates of non-treatment for diabetes, hypertension, and dyslipidemia were 30.2%, 62.4%, and 88.0% respectively.[9] These untreated disorders likely contribute to the high mortality in this population. Furthermore, untreated co-occurring disorders may worsen the clinical progression of schizophrenia. Friedman *et al.* used a series of cognitive tests to compare patient groups with schizophrenia, schizophrenia and hypertension, and schizophrenia and obesity to comparison subjects without hypertension, obesity, or schizophrenia, patients with obesity only, and patients with hypertension only.[10] The researchers found that hypertension worsened the cognitive symptoms of patients with schizophrenia, and that obesity was associated with negative effects on delayed memory in the schizophrenia group and the control group. They concluded that treating co-occurring chronic disorders (specifically hypertension and other vascular risk factors) would improve cognition, and could reduce mortality, in patients with schizophrenia.

Hospital Complications

As noted above, these patients infrequently receive primary care services, and may be at risk of developing acute exacerbations or long-term manifestations of chronically untreated disorders. Furthermore, once in the hospital, patients with schizophrenia may be unable to accurately communicate complaints to the hospital staff, may be avoided by staff, and may experience in-house complications.[11] One study of hospital discharges from 2002 to 2007 used the Nationwide Inpatient Sample to test whether hospital adverse events occurred more frequently for those with schizophrenia.[12] The authors found that during a nonpsychiatric hospitalization, patients with schizophrenia were more likely to experience some complications. For instance, the odds ratios in those with schizophrenia for more commonly occurring complications were: decubitus ulcers (1.43), nosocomial infection (1.19), postoperative respiratory failure (1.96), sepsis (1.59), and pulmonary embolism/deep venous thrombosis (1.23). Hospital physicians should consider the overall increased risk of complications when managing these patients.

Antipsychotic Agents

Mechanisms

All effective antipsychotic agents are thought to work at least in part through antagonism of the dopamine D2 receptor in the striatum. The conventional, or first-generation, antipsychotic agents vary based on the potency with which the D2 receptor is antagonized, and the degree of anticholinergic effects. In general, higher-potency medications (haloperidol, fluphenazine) have higher risk of extrapyramidal symptoms (e.g. akathisia, dystonia) and fewer anticholinergic effects, while lower-potency medications (chlorpromazine) have more anticholinergic effects. The atypical, or second-generation, antipsychotic agents are commonly used, and generally act through D2 and serotonin (5-HT2A) antagonism or partial agonism. Except for management of an emergency (e.g. neuroleptic malignant syndrome, or agranulocytosis due to clozapine dosing), abrupt discontinuation of antipsychotic agents should not be done without consultation with a psychiatrist. This point is critical for clozapine, as reinitiating dosing occurs slowly, and reaching the target dose may take weeks. Treatment with clozapine is generally reserved for the most treatment-refractory patients, and often represents a severe course of schizophrenia.

Adverse Effects

Adverse effects of antipsychotic agents are generally divided into acute and chronic. All antipsychotics can cause acute movement disorders, including akathisia (restlessness) and dystonia (stiffness); akathisia may improve with benzodiazepine dosing, while dystonia responds to dosing of an anticholinergic agent. Chronically, these agents can cause tardive dyskinesia, a hyperkinetic choreoathetotic movement disorder most prominent in the face, neck, and upper extremities. While all antipsychotic agents can cause weight gain, the second-generation antipsychotic agents (particularly olanzapine and clozapine) can severely impact several metabolic parameters, including weight, lipid levels, and insulin sensitivity.[13] A severe, life-threatening complication of antipsychotic dosing is neuroleptic malignant syndrome (NMS).[14] This syndrome should be considered in any patient taking dopamine antagonists who develops fever, stiffness, or delirium. Supportive measures and cessation of the offending agent should be implemented promptly in confirmed cases of NMS.

Other adverse effects of antipsychotics include sedation, elevated prolactin, hypotension, and cardiac conduction delays. Discontinuation of antipsychotics could be considered (in consultation with a psychiatrist) if any of these adverse effects have contributed to the reason for hospitalization. Otherwise, antipsychotic medications should be continued as prescribed by the outpatient psychiatry team.

Discharge Preparation

In many ways, discharge preparation for patients with schizophrenia resembles preparation for patients without schizophrenia. However, because of this disorder's impact on cognitive function, it is necessary to assess the patient's understanding of the reasons for hospitalization, and to determine the patient's ability to perform postdischarge care. The importance of followup primary and specialty care should be stressed. Some patients have case managers through community mental health centers. Hospital staff should communicate all followup care plans with the case manager, and transportation and home care services should be considered. Some patients may have lived in a shelter prior to hospitalization, and might plan to return to the shelter postdischarge. This living arrangement should be considered in discharge preparation. Functional status in schizophrenia can be measured using patient self-report, physician clinical assessment, or performance-based measures. Standardized ratings are rarely used in discharge preparation, but can be found in a recent review by Mausbach *et al.*[15]

Antipsychotic medications that were discontinued during the hospitalization should probably be reinitiated prior to discharge. Communication with the patient's outpatient psychiatrist or consultation with the in-house psychiatry service could be considered in determining appropriate dosing.

References

1. American Psychiatric Association. (2000) *Diagnostic and Statistical Manual of Mental Disorders*, 4th ed. text revision: DSM-IV-TR. American Psychiatric Publishing Inc., Washington, DC.
2. Freedman R. (2003) Schizophrenia. *N Engl J Med* **349**: 1738–1749.
3. Sadock BJ, Sadock VA. (2007) Schizophrenia. In: *Kaplan & Sadock's Synopsis of Psychiatry*, 10th ed., Lippincott Williams & Wilkins, Philadelphia, pp. 467–497.
4. Green AI, Drake RE, Brunette MF, Noordsy DL. (2007) Schizophrenia and co-occurring substance use disorder. *Am J Psychiatry* **164**: 402–408.
5. Leucht S, Burkard T, Henderson J, *et al.* (2007) Physical illness and schizophrenia: A review of the literature. *Acta Psychiatr Scand* **116**: 317–333.
6. Saha S, Chant D, McGrath J. (2007) A systematic review of mortality in schizophrenia. *Arch Gen Psychiatry* **64**: 1123–1131.
7. Tihonen J, Lonnqvist J, Wahlbeck K, *et al.* (2009) 11-year follow-up of mortality in patients with schizophrenia: A population-based cohort study (FIN11study). *Lancet* **374**: 620–627.
8. Chwastiak LA. (2009) The unchanging mortality gap for people with schizophrenia. *Lancet* **374**: 590–592.
9. Nasrallah HA, Meyer JM, Goff DC, *et al.* (2006) Low rates of treatment for hypertension, dyslipidemia and diabetes in schizophrenia: Data

from the CATIE schizophrenia trial sample at baseline. *Schizophr Res* **86**: 15–22.

10. Friedman JI, Wallenstein S, Moshier E, *et al.* (2010) The effects of hypertension and body mass index on cognition in schizophrenia. *Am J Psychiatry* [doi:10.1176/appi.ajp.2010.09091328].
11. Freudenreich O, Stern TA. (2003) Clinical experience with the management of schizophrenia in the general hospital. *Psychosomatics* **44**: 12–23.
12. Khaykin E, Ford DE, Pronovost PJ, *et al.* (2010) National estimates of adverse events during nonpsychiatric hospitalizations for persons with schizophrenia. *Gen Hosp Psychiatry* **32**: 419–425.
13. Lindenmayer JP, Czobor P, Volavka J, *et al.* (2003) Changes in glucose and cholesterol levels in patients with schizophrenia treated with typical and atypical antipsychotics. *Am J Psychiatry* **160**: 290–296.
14. Strawn JR, Keck PE, Caroff SN. (2007) Neuroleptic malignant syndrome. *Am J Psychiatry* **164**: 870–876.
15. Mausbach BT, Moore R, Bowie C, *et al.* (2009) A review of instruments for measuring functional recovery in those diagnosed with psychosis. *Schizophr Bull* **35**: 307–318.

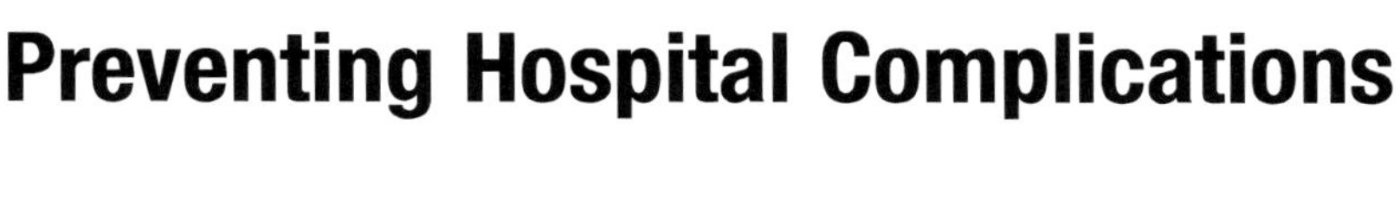

Preventing Hospital Complications

Chapter 81

Fall Prevention

Erin Rule and Brian Markoff **

Key Pearls

- In-hospital falls are a major contributor to patient morbidity and mortality.
- In-hospital falls increase length of stay as well as healthcare costs.
- Risk factors for falls are especially common in hospitalized patients.
- Fall risk can be minimized using a multidisciplinary approach.
- Avoid centrally acting sedative hypnotics.

Consequences of Falls

Inpatient falls are extremely common and have high potential for harm to patients. It is estimated that between 2% and 15% of inpatients will experience at least one fall during a hospitalization. Approximately 30% of inpatient falls result in injury, and between 4% and 6% result in serious injury.[1] Common injuries associated with falls include cranial trauma, soft tissue injury and fractures.[2] There are also psychological effects of falling, including anxiety and fear of falling, which can result in further decrease in mobility and decline in function.[2]

These complications increase the cost to patients and to hospitals. Case control studies indicate that patients who fell during hospitalization

*Mount Sinai School of Medicine, New York, NY, USA.

had a length of stay (LOS) between 4.4 and 12.3 days longer than for control subjects.[2,3] However, the fall itself may not be completely responsible for this increased LOS, as the propensity to fall may be a marker for severity of illness. Another study found that the cost of hospitalization for fallers was double the cost of hospitalization for nonfallers within the same diagnosis related group (DRG).[2] Even if a fall does not result in serious injury, costs and LOS increase due to diagnostic procedures such as X-rays and CT scans needed to rule out injury. There are also likely to be additional, ongoing healthcare costs associated with treating a serious injury sustained from a fall, including rehabilitation or long-term care facility placement.

In addition, falls are now considered to be a preventable complication of hospitalization by the Centers for Medicare of Medicaid Services (CMS), and hospitals are no longer reimbursed for the costs associated with diagnosing or treating complications of a fall.[4] It is in the best interest of patients, healthcare providers and hospitals to prevent falls.

Risk Factors for Falls

There have been many fall risk factors identified, most of which are common in hospitalized patients (see Table 1). Some of these risk factors are specific to the hospital setting, while others may be due to chronic medical conditions that are present at the time of hospital admission. Age >75 has been associated with increased risk for falling.[5] Gait instability and lower extremity weakness are also among the most common risk factors for a fall. Patients with neurological impairment, including a prior history of stroke, Parkinson's disease or peripheral neuropathy, commonly have gait abnormalities that increase their risk of falling. These patients may not have their usual assistive devices, such as canes or walkers, with them in the hospital. However, gait abnormalities that are new to the patient after admission may also contribute to falls. These include recent knee or hip surgery. Another chronic medical condition that can contribute to a patient's risk for falling is visual impairment. This can be exacerbated during hospitalization if a patient does not have his or her glasses with

Table 1. Fall Risk Factors

Risk Factors	Potential Physician/Staff Interventions
Intrinsic Risk Factors	
Gait instability / lower limb weakness	• Assess functional status with physical therapy • Use assistive devices as needed
Urinary / stool incontinence or frequency or need for assisted toileting	• Bedside commode • Frequent checks to ask patient if they need to be assisted to commode or bathroom
Agitation / confusion or cognitive impairment (dementia or delirium)	• Avoid medications that may contribute • Frequent reorientation
Visual / auditory impairment	• Provide glasses and hearing aids from home
Orthostatic hypotension	• Check orthostatic BP and HR • Consider reducing antihypertensive doses • Ensure oral fluids available at patient's bedside
Previous fall history	• Document prior fall history • Post sign / alert so all staff are aware of risk
Extrinsic Risk Factors	
Medications / polypharmacy	• Review medications daily • Limit sedative medications including anticholinergics, psychoactive medications
Lack of / inappropriate use of assistive devices	• Provide canes and walkers when appropriate • Provide bedside commodes when appropriate
Condition of floor / poor lighting	• Clear pathway to bathroom for patients • Turn lights on during day • Show patients how to control lights
Height of bed or chairs	• Always place bed at lowest height when leaving room
Tethers: catheters, IV tubing, oxygen	• Minimize use of urinary catheters and continuous IV medications/fluids • Avoid using restraints if possible
High patient to nurse ratio	• Consider closer monitoring with frequent checks or 1:1 staffing

them or in the setting of an unfamiliar environment. Activities that require a patient to get out of bed, such as increased urinary or stool frequency and incontinence or the need for assisted toileting, also increase the risk of falling.

Once a patient is admitted to the hospital, perhaps the most common risk factor for falling is confusion, as seen in patients with dementia or delirium.[6]

While most of the above risk factors are intrinsic to the patient, many risk factors are related to the patient's physical environment and are considered to be extrinsic to the patient. These include factors such as flooring, poor illumination, inappropriate footwear, inadequate assistive devices (e.g. lifting devices, walkers and wheelchairs), and improper use of devices such as bedside rails.[7] Poor design of furnishings such as beds and chairs, and lack of support equipment near toilets and baths, also contribute to falls.[7] In addition, staffing issues can impact the patient's risk of falling. Increased nurse-to-patient ratios have also been shown to lower fall risk.[1]

Many medications have been implicated in falls during hospitalization, but the main class is centrally acting sedative hypnotics. These medications can contribute to fall risk in any age group, but the effect is more pronounced in elderly patients, especially those with underlying dementia. Other studies have found that having diabetes or using diabetes medications is also a risk factor.[1]

Finally, any patient who has fallen in the past is at high risk for falling in the future.

Prevention of Falls

Many studies have been performed to evaluate interventions to prevent falls, but results are inconsistent (Table 1). Fall research is difficult to perform and many trials are case controls rather than randomized, controlled trials. The best results have been achieved with a multidisciplinary team approach including physicians, nurses, physical therapists and pharmacists. However, one meta-analysis showed that even with a multitargeted intervention the rate of falls was reduced only by 18%.[8] This indicates that despite the controlled circumstances of a clinical trial, most in-hospital falls are not preventable.

Single Interventions

Exercise Programs

There is mixed evidence from meta-analyses for using exercise to prevent falls as a single intervention.[8,9] However, exercise is a component of several successful multifaceted interventions.

Vitamin D Supplementation

There is mixed evidence regarding vitamin D supplementation. A meta-analysis of double-blinded, randomized trials of vitamin D supplementation found that supplementation with 700–1000 IU of Vitamin D daily reduced falls by 19%.[10] This effect reached statistical significance only after 2–5 months of supplementation, so the supplements would not impact fall rates during a single hospitalization.

Medication Review

There is evidence that a medication review by a pharmacist is effective in reducing the rate of falls in nursing home patients. This evidence does not extend to acute care hospitals.[9] The goal of a medication review is to avoid sedative medications or medications that may cause dizziness or orthostatic hypotension. It is also important to keep in mind that elderly patients with underlying cognitive impairment are at the highest risk for these side effects.

Restraints and Bedrails

There is conflicting evidence regarding the use of restraints and bedrails to prevent falls. Many studies have shown that the use of these devices can increase the rate of fall-related injury as patients try to overcome their restraints.[15] Cases of serious injury and even death have been reported with bedrail and restraint use, and both The Joint Commission and the FDA have issued safety alerts for the use of bedrails.[1] However, other studies have found that bedrail use does decrease the rate of falls.[1] This data is difficult to interpret because patients who are restrained are more likely to suffer cognitive impairment, confusion and gait abnormalities and therefore increased fall risk. Restraint and bedrail use should be limited and combined with other risk reduction methods.

Environmental Factors/Furniture

In one study, the implementation of "low–low" beds for patients thought to be at highest risk for falls did not reduce the rate of falls or the rate of injury from falls.[11] Providing bedside commodes and assistive devices such as walkers or canes for patients who are cognitively intact but have an unsteady gait is a common practice with little evidence to support it.

Staffing

Studies have shown that the rate of falls is reduced with improved nurse-to-patient ratios.[1] One study showed that fall rates were reduced with a nursing education initiative regarding fall prevention strategies, including the use of toileting schedules and discussion of high-risk medications.[12] The use of sitters for constant patient supervision or moving a patient to a room more easily observed by nurses is common practice, but little evidence exists to support this.

Multifaceted Interventions

Several trials of multifaceted interventions in hospitals have had modest success in reducing fall rates. Some of the most promising data are from a meta-analysis which showed an 18% reduction in the fall rate with a multifaceted intervention.[8] However, many of these trials include patients in subacute care hospitals, which have longer LOSs than typical acute care hospitals. There is some evidence to suggest that only patients with longer lengths of stay (greater than three weeks) benefit from these interventions.[9] Other studies have not shown any significant difference in fall rates with hospital fall prevention programs.[13,14]

Minimizing the Impact of Falls

Although it is not possible to prevent all falls, we can try to minimize the severity of injuries from falls. Calcium and vitamin D supplementation has been shown to reduce the incidence of hip fracture after a fall.[8] In addition, there is modest evidence that hip protectors reduce the rate of hip fracture after a fall in nursing home patients.[8]

Conclusion

In-hospital fall risk factors are difficult to modify. There is mixed evidence that any fall intervention program reduces fall rates. Additional research and innovative approaches are necessary in order to reduce falls and the resulting injuries.

References

1. Krauss MJ, Evanoff B, Hitcho E, *et al*. (2005) A case-control study of patient, medication, and care-related risk factors for inpatient falls. *J Gen Int Med* **20**(2): 116–122.
2. Hill KD, Vu M, Walsh W. (2007) Falls in the acute hospital setting — Impact on resource utilisation. *Aust Health Rev* **31**(3): 471–477.
3. Bates DW, Pruess K, Souney P. (1995) Serious falls in hospitalized patients: Correlates and resource utilization. *Am J Med* **99**(2): 137–143: [doi: 10.1016/S0002-9343(99)80133-8].
4. Inouye SK, Brown CJ, Tinetti ME. (2009) Medicare nonpayment, hospital falls, and unintended consequences. *New Engl J Med* **360**(23): 2390–2393.
5. Fischer ID, Krauss MJ, Dunagan WC, *et al*. (2005) Patterns and predictors of inpatient falls and fall-related injuries in a large academic

hospital. *Infect Contr Hosp Epidemiol*: **26**(10): 822–827 [doi:10.1086/502500].

6. Lakatos BE, Capasso V, Mitchell MT, *et al.* (2009) Falls in the general hospital: Association with delirium, advanced age, and specific surgical procedures. *Psychosomatics* **50**(3): 218–226.
7. Tzeng HM, Yin CY. (2008) The extrinsic risk factors for inpatient falls in hospital patient rooms. *J Nurs Care Qual* **23**(3): 233–241.
8. Oliver D, Connelly JB, Victor CR *et al.* (2007) Strategies to prevent falls and fractures in hospitals and care homes and effect of cognitive impairment: Systematic review and meta-analyses. *BMJ (Clin Res Ed)*, **334**(7584): 82. [doi:10.1136/bmj.39049.706493.55].
9. Cameron ID, Murray GR, Gillespie LD, *et al.* (2010) Interventions for preventing falls in older people in nursing care facilities and hospitals. *Cochrane Database Syst Rev (Online)* **1**(1): CD005465.
10. Bischoff-Ferrari HA, Dawson-Hughes B, Staehelin HB, *et al.* (2009) Fall prevention with supplemental and active forms of vitamin D: A meta-analysis of randomised controlled trials. *BMJ (Clin Res Ed)*, **339**: b3692.
11. Haines TP, Bell RA, Varghese PN. (2010) Pragmatic, cluster randomized trial of a policy to introduce low–low beds to hospital wards for the prevention of falls and fall injuries. *J Am Geriatr Soc* **58**(3): 435–441.
12. Krauss MJ, Tutlam N, Costantinou E, *et al.* (2008) Intervention to prevent falls on the medical service in a teaching hospital. *Infect Contr Hos Epidemiol* **29**(6): 539–545.
13. Cumming RG, Sherrington C, Lord SR, *et al.* (2008) Cluster randomised trial of a targeted multifactorial intervention to prevent falls among older people in hospital. *BMJ (Clin Res Ed)*, **336**(7647): 758–760.
14. Coussement J, De Paepe L, Schwendimann R, *et al.* (2008) Interventions for preventing falls in acute- and chronic-care hospitals: A systematic review and meta-analysis. *J Am Geriatr Soc* **56**(1): 29–36.
15. Tan KM, Austin B, Shaughnassy M, *et al.* (2005) Falls in an acute hospital and their relationship to restraint use. *Ir J Med Sci* **174**(3): 28–31.

Chapter 82

Prevention and Management of Pressure Ulcers

*Kathy Navid**

Key Pearls

- Prevention of pressure ulcers involves identifying high risk patients and optimizing their support surface, nutrition, hydration, repositioning and general skin care.
- Treatment of pressure ulcers should focus on staging and reassessment of healing, optimizing wound care based on the wound condition, debridement for devitalized tissue, pain control, and identifying and treating superimposed infection.
- Dressings are selected based on the wound environment, with no evidence-based recommendations of standard dressings over advanced dressings.
- Optimal nutrition in both prevention and treatment involves adequate caloric and protein intake. Vitamin and mineral supplementation are recommended only in suspected or confirmed deficiencies.
- Treatment of stage I ulcers involves intensifying preventive strategies and a protective transparent film dressing, stage II ulcers are treated with occlusive or permeable dressings, and stage III/IV ulcers with appropriate dressings, treatment of infection and debridement if necrotic tissue is present.

*Mount Sinai Queens Hospital, Long Island City, NY, USA.

Introduction

Pressure ulcers are common, debilitating and costly complications for hospitalized patients. They are defined as soft tissue ischemic injury from prolonged pressure on skin, especially over bony prominences, often with other contributing factors such as shear and frictional forces. The prevalence of pressure ulcers varies widely by institution. In hospitalized patients, the prevalence is approximately 15%, and nosocomial ulcer formation occurs in approximately 5%.[1] Those at greatest risk are elderly patients, neurologically impaired patients, those with prolonged surgical procedures and intensive care unit patients.

Etiology/Pathogenesis

Understanding the etiology of pressure ulcers is important for targeting preventive strategies. Immobility causing prolonged pressure over several hours leads to tissue hypoxia and ischemia. Shear and frictional forces also contribute to pressure ulcer formation. Shearing forces result from skin remaining stagnant while gravity pulls down muscle and subcutaneous tissue, and this most commonly happens in patients on an incline. Frictional forces occur when the skin is pulled across a surface, such as when a patient is dragged across bedlinen. Poor nutrition also predisposes to pressure ulcer formation. The role of moisture and urinary incontinence leading to skin maceration has not been proven; however, fecal contamination has been implicated in accelerating pressure ulcer formation.[2]

Prevention of Pressure Ulcers

Efforts to prevent pressure ulcers include protocols designed to assess high risk patients, minimize pressure with repositioning and support surfaces, optimize skin health and nutrition, and minimize shear and friction forces.

Risk Assessment

Immobility is the most important risk for pressure ulcers. Other important factors include altered level of consciousness, age, comorbidities and malnutrition. Several risk assessments exist but the most commonly used are the Norton[3] and Braden[4] scales, both of which have been validated. The Norton scale assesses five domains: activity, incontinence, mental status, mobility and physical condition, while the Braden scale identifies at-risk individuals based on activity, dietary intake, friction, mobility, sensory perception and skin moisture. A risk assessment tool such as the Braden or Norton scale and clinical judgment are recommended to identify high risk patients.

Repositioning and Bed Positioning

The theoretical benefit of repositioning lies in the fact that permanent damage to skeletal muscle occurs after more than 2 hr of ischemia in animal models[5] and based on data suggesting that erythema occurs in healthy adult skin after 2 hr on a standard mattress.[6] Though the paucity of reliable data on repositioning was recently illustrated in a Cochrane review that was unable to identify any studies that met inclusion criteria to assess the benefit of repositioning,[7] repositioning every 2 hr is a potentially beneficial practice and remains recommended.

To minimize shear forces, the bed should be maintained at the lowest incline possible (less than 30°) that is appropriate to the patient's medical conditions. Foam wedges should be used to avoid direct contact between bony prominences. To minimize friction forces, lifting devices such as a trapeze or bedlinen should be used to move rather than drag patients who cannot assist with position change or transfers. Special heel protectors or elevation of the heels should be employed. Finally, physical therapy with range of motion and maintaining mobility should be pursued if consistent with the goals of care.[8]

Support Surfaces

Nonpowered (static) or powered (dynamic) mattresses and overlays are available for patients at high risk of pressure ulcers. Nonpowered mattresses and overlays that are applied to the top of a mattress are filled with air, foam, gel, water or a combination of these. Powered mattresses mechanically vary the pressure beneath the patient and are more costly. The advantage of support surfaces in preventing pressure ulcers over standard hospital mattresses was demonstrated in a study where patients undergoing elective surgery who received a foam overlay had a reduced incidence of pressure ulcers.[9] No difference between the incidence of pressure ulcers in powered and nonpowered mattresses or overlays has been shown.[10]

Nutrition and Skin Health

Adequate hydration and nutrition are important in both the prevention and the treatment of pressure ulcers. An association exists between malnutrition and development of pressure ulcers. Assessment for caloric needs should be made and adequate caloric intake provided. Protein supplementation is recommended if no contraindications exist for both prevention and treatment. The optimal nutritional vitamin and mineral supplements are uncertain, with clinical trials not showing benefit from routine supplementation. Confirmed or suspected deficiencies should be supplemented, while routine replacement with micronutrients is not recommended. Dry sacral skin is a risk factor for pressure ulcers; therefore, moisturizing skin is considered a reasonable strategy.[10] The advantage of one topical moisturizing lotion over another is unclear. In addition, mild cleansing agents at regular intervals and avoiding both vigorous massage and hot water are recommended for general skin care.

Treatment of Pressure Ulcers

Treatment of pressure ulcers involves using the same strategies described for prevention, including optimizing nutrition, repositioning and using support surfaces. In addition, treatment involves local wound care, debridement, assessment for healing, pain control and treatment in the cases of superimposed infection. Select patients may be candidates for surgical closure. Adjunctive therapies such as negative pressure (vacuum), electric current, ultrasound, laser and light have not shown clear benefit in high-quality randomized control trials.

Staging and Treatment Based on Stage of Ulcer

The most commonly used staging system for pressure ulcers originated from the National and European Pressure Ulcer Advisory Panel (NPUAP and EPUAP), which classifies ulcers based on the depth of tissue loss[11] (Table 1).

Wound Care

Several dressings are available for pressure ulcers, each of which has different properties of hydration, debridement and absorbency. Of note is that no particular dressing has been shown to be superior to another in clinical trials.[12] Therefore, dressings are chosen based on the condition of the wound, availability and cost. The general principles of wound care

Table 1. Staging and Treatment of Pressure Ulcers

	Characteristics	Treatment
Stage 1	Skin intact Nonblanchable erythema	Intensify preventive strategies Cover with transparent film
Stage 2	Partial loss of dermis Shallow open ulcers	Occlusive or permeable dressing
Stage 3	Full thickness skin loss exposed fat	Appropriate dressings and debridement if necrotic tissue is present
Stage 4	Full thickness skin loss Exposed bone, muscle or tendon	Same as stage 3
Deep tissue injury	Purplish/maroon skin discoloration with intact skin Potential for deeper tissue damage	Intensify preventive strategies

Table 2. Recommended Dressing by Wound Type

Wound Condition	Desired Wound Environment	Specific Dressings
Dry	Hydrating	Hydrogel or hydrocolloid
Moderate-to-heavy exudate	Absorbent	Calcium alginate, hydrofiber, foams
Necrotic tissue	Debridement	*Enzymatic*: collagenase, dexoyribonuclease, fibrinolysin
		Mechanical: saline-moistened gauze
		Autolytic: hydrogel, hydrocolloid
		Biologic: sterile maggot larvae
Infected	Antimicrobial*	Silver dressings
		Topical antibiotics
		Topical antiseptics
Pain	Moist	Silicone
		Topical Opioids with debridement
		Avoid Gauze Dressings
Nonhealing	Granulating	Collagen

* use only during active infection.

consist in maintaining a moist environment that promotes granulation. However, wounds with excess exudate lead to maceration, in which case absorptive dressings are preferable (Table 2).

Debridement to remove necrotic tissue so as to promote granulation and reduce bacterial growth has been performed for decades; however, it has not been studied in randomized trials. Sharp debridement is performed if there is evidence of heavy eschar or necrotic tissue.

If sharp debridement cannot be performed or is not urgent, mechanical, enzymatic, autolytic or biologic debridement may be effective. Each of these modalities has potential benefits and harms:

- Mechanical debridement involves using saline-moistened gauze to remove necrotic tissue but can remove viable tissue as well.

- Enzymatic debridement degrades necrotic tissue with proteolytic enzymes (collagenase, fibrinolysin, deoxyribonuclease) and can cause irritation to healthy skin.
- Autolytic debridement involves using occlusive dressings to promote degradation of dead tissue by physiologic enzymes and should be avoided in infected ulcers.
- Biologic debridement involves the use of sterile larvae of maggots to remove dead tissue, and aesthetics and pain are limitations on its use.

Assessment for Healing

The most commonly used validated tool for assessing healing in pressure ulcers is the PUSH (Pressure Ulcer Scale for Healing) tool, developed by the NPUAP. This tool documents changes in size, exudate, necrosis and presence of granulation tissue. Healing should be expected over a two-week time period. Nonhealing ulcers after this time should prompt consideration of superimposed infection.

Pain Control

Pain management is essential for treatment of ulcer pain, coordination of pain medications with painful dressing changes, and debridement. Gauze dressings require more frequent changes and may be more painful, so alternate dressings may be considered (see Table 2).

Infection

Pressure ulcers are initially colonized with skin flora and later colonized with fecal and urogenital organisms. Data suggest that pressure ulcer wound cultures with greater than or equal to 10(5) CFU/g of tissue have impaired healing and the only manifestation of infection may be failure to heal over a two-week period despite optimal care. Swab cultures are not recommended, as they often reflect colonization rather than true infection. If clinical infection is suspected, deep tissue biopsy for culture should be performed, which is the gold standard for diagnosis of an infected ulcer. Superficial infection can be treated with local wound care and topical antibiotics. Deep infections should be treated with systemic antimicrobials and debridement. The antimicrobial treatment of skin and soft tissue infections is covered in another chapter. Secondary bacteremia and osteomyelitis from infected ulcers are associated with increased mortality.

Conclusion

The implementation of pressure ulcer prevention has reduced the incidence of pressure ulcers in hospitalized patients. Many questions remain as to the optimal approach to prevention and treatment, as systematic reviews of powered support surfaces, adjunctive therapies and advanced wound dressings have not shown clear benefit. Regulatory and financial forces, such as decreased reimbursement for hospital-acquired complications, will hopefully intensify efforts in prevention and research for this common condition.

References

1. VanGilder C, Amlung S, Harrison P, Meyer S. (2009) Results of the 2008–2009 International Pressure Ulcer Prevalence Survey and a 3-year, acute care, unit-specific analysis. *Ostomy/Wound Manage* **11**: 39–45.
2. Brandeis GH, Ooi WL, Hossain M *et al*. (1994) A longitudinal study of risk factors associated with the formation of pressure ulcers in nursing homes. *J Am Geriatr Soc* **42**: 388.
3. Pressure ulcers prevalence, cost and risk assessment : consensus development conference statement — The National Pressure Ulcer Advisory Panel *Decubitus* **2**: 24.
4. Bergstrom N, Braden BJ, Laguzza A, Holman V. (1987) The Braden scale for predicting pressure sore risk. *Nurse Res* **36**: 205.
5. Harris AG, Leiderer R, Peer F, Messmer K. (1996) Skeletal muscle microvascular and tissue injury after varying durations of ischemia. *Am J Physiol* H2388–H2398.

6. Knox DM, Anderson TM, Anderson PS. (1994) Effects of different turn intervals on skin of healthy older adults. *Adv Wound Care* **7**: 48.
7. Moore ZEH, Cowman S. (2010) Repositioning for the treating of pressure ulcers. *Cochrane Lib* **5**: 1–11.
8. Agency for Health Care Policy and Research. *Pressure Ulcer in Adults: Prediction and Prevention. Clinical Practice Guideline, Number 3*. Public Health Service, US Department of Health and Human Services.
9. Nixon J, McElvenny D, Mason S, *et al*. (1998) A sequential randomized controlled trial comparomg a dry visco-elastic polymer pad and standard operating table mattress in the prevention of postoperative pressure sores. *Int J Nurs Stud* **35**: 193–203.
10. Reddy M, Gill S, Rochon P. (2006) Preventing pressure ulcers: A systematic review. *JAMA* **8**: 974–984.
11. European Pressure Ulcer Advisory Panel and National Pressure Ulcer Advisory Panel. (2009) Treatment of pressure ulcers: Quick reference guide. National Pressure Ulcer Advisory Panel, Washington DC.
12. Reddy, Madhuri, Gill, Sudeep, Kalkar, Sunila, *et al*. (2008) Treatment of pressure ulcers: A systematic review *JAMA* **300**: 22647–2662.

Consultation and Peri-Operative Medicine

Chapter 83

The Essentials of Medical Consultation

Eva Flores and Salvatore Cilmi**

Key Pearls

- Hospitalist physicians now perform the great majority of inpatient, and, in some cases, outpatient medical consultations for non-medical specialty services.
- A national survey reveals that most hospitalists believe the practice of perioperative medicine to be an important part of their careers currently underemphasized during residency training. There are may opportunities for hospitalist physicians to institute educational goals and principles around medical consultation in contemporary hospital environments.
- ASK GMC is a simple mnemonic that encapsulates the essence and key principles of medical counsultation: Ascertain the question; Specify the urgency; Keep it simple, brief and specific; Get to appreciate your role; Mind your business and your manners; and Communicate directly.

Medical consultations can represent medicine at its best…and its worst. The comfort of being an internist and yet also being considered a "specialist consultant" is often a welcome delight for an internist. As in all of medicine, there are a wide variety of practice skill sets and quality of consultations, but there are a number of guidelines and a fair body

*New York Presbyterian Hospital-Weill Cornell Medical Center, New York, NY, USA.

of literature to guide some of the most important questions asked of us, mainly the preoperative evaluation (the inappropriately labeled "medical clearance") and questions surrounding diabetes, hypertension and anticoagulation. With about 42 million noncardiac inpatient surgeries performed annually and a significant portion of those patients having risk factors for heart disease, the topic of how to perform a medical consultation efficiently and effectively becomes quite important.[1]

Interestingly, a national survey revealed that hospitalists rated perioperative consultations as an important part of their careers, but underemphasized in residency training, with the educational mismatch correlating directly with time spent training in medical consultation (<1 month versus >3 months).[2]

What makes for an efficient and effective consultation that benefits the patient and gives both the requester and the consultant a positive experience? First, to define what a good consultation includes, it must be understood what is expected by the requester and from the consultant. In 1983, Goldman *et al.* summarized the "Ten Commandments for Effective Consultation," giving attending physicians, for the first time, a concrete guide to follow in consultative medicine that holds true today.[3] These include:

1. Determine the question.
2. Establish urgency.
3. Look for yourself.
4. Be as brief as appropriate.
5. Be specific.
6. Provide contingency plans.
7. Thou shalt not covet thy neighbor's turf.
8. Teach with tact.
9. Talk is cheap and effective.
10. Provide appropriate follow-up.

These principles provide invaluable advice on professionalism, especially when consulting for surgical services, and role-modeling of good behavior when training house officers in performing medical consultations. In 2007, Salerno *et al.* updated Goldman's principles for the 21st century and expanded upon the differences between surgical subspecialties and nonsurgical consult preferences.[4] These articles are especially helpful as guides when one is starting out in consultation medicine and for teaching residents sound consultation practices. They are also appropriate for medical and surgical co-management services, which have become more common in hospitals in the past decade. Surgical comanagement is discussed in detail in a separate chapter.

As experienced consultants in both traditional medical consultations and comanaging orthopedic patients, the essence of the commandments and the key principles of medical consultation can be summarized with the acronym ASK GMC (ASK General Medicine Consult) (see Table 1).

ASK GMC

Ascertain the Question

Without the specific question to address, it is difficult to know what you have been called upon to comment on. In a survey study of physicians with at least one postgraduate year of experience, 94% of respondents perceived clear framing of the consultation question to be the most important.[5] Not surprisingly, however, the literature demonstrates that there is a

Table 1. ASK GMC (ASK General Medicine Consult): Essentials for Medical Consultants

Ascertain the question.
Specify the urgency.
Keep it simple, brief and specific.
Get to appreciate your role.
Mind your business and your manners.
Communicate directly.

discrepancy between what surgeons perceive as the question and whether consultants think that there is an actual specific question.[6–8]

It is helpful to always ask the requester to clarify the specific question asked, for example, clarifying between a surgical request for "following the patient for medical management" and a surgical request on a patient with atrial fibrillation with the question "Does the patient need to be bridged with anticoagulation and how?" This helps to focus your interview with the patient, guides the recommendations you make and educates your caller that consults are called to address a specific question in mind. The exception is when you are doing the consultation as part of a comanagement service in which addressing the multiple medical problems that a patient may have will be not only more common and appropriate, but likely expected.

Specify the Urgency

In general, emergent calls should be seen within 60 min, urgent calls within 2–4 hr and routine consults within 24 hr. The urgency of the consult is usually specified by the caller or implied in the reason for the call (e.g. "calling for a preoperative evaluation for a patient with COPD exacerbation who needs surgery that evening" versus "calling for a preoperative evaluation for a TAH/BSO in two days"). If you are still unsure at the end of the call as to the urgency, then ask directly in order to prioritize the order of seeing consults.

In a teaching institution, it is imperative that the residents understand the need to address urgent consults in a timely fashion. The time from call to bedside for an urgent matter such as hypertensive urgency should be minutes, not hours. Timely performance of consultations is critical for good patient care, and it also contributes to amicable and trustworthy relationships with referring colleagues.

Keep It Brief, Specific and Provide Contingency Plans

Callers are not seeking vague recommendations such as "optimize HTN regimen with beta blocker or ACE inhibitor." They are looking for concise and specific drug therapy recommendations that include the name of the medication (preferably generic), dose, schedule, duration, and alternatives.[4,5] Providing a contingency plan, especially when you anticipate that the patient will not tolerate oral intake for several days, is also preferred by requesters. In general, but especially when consulting for surgeons, the smallest number of recommendations necessary (<5) is best. These should be prioritized and numbered clearly so as to communicate most effectively.[4,9]

Get to Appreciate Your Role

Consult requests may come from various services, such as psychiatry, rehab medicine or medical subspecialty services, but it is very likely that the bulk of your work will be for surgical services. To have the proper mindset makes all the difference between feeling frustrated and getting an understanding for the customers' mindset and expectations. Negotiating turf is vitally important in medicine today. In the growing era of medical and surgical comanagement services, lines are becoming blurred, but the consultant's role should be defined specifically and early. In a traditional consultation model, limiting the recommendations to the question asked is preferred. Other subspecialty services may have specific protocols for dealing with various aspects of management, such as venous thromboembolism prevention in orthopedic patients and blood pressure control parameters (e.g. for neurosurgical patients undergoing craniotomy). Thus, your routine advice on these topics may not be welcome or taken into consideration. If you are consulting within the structure of a comanaged surgical service, then shared responsibilities may include dealing with all of the patients' medical issues and probably lending your experience in discharge planning and systems knowledge in expediting the patients' hospital stay.

Mind Your Business and Your Manners

A consultant must always be courteous to a consulting service, even when faced with improper or rude behavior. Especially on a consultation service with medical residents, the medical attending should serve as a role model for professionalism, one of the core ACGME competencies required for all physicians-in-training. This professional behavior often results in improvement in communication and understanding among the various specialty services in the contemporary hospital.

Communicate Directly

A great consultation can be undermined by poor communication and follow-up. Verbally communicating recommendations, via phone or in person, is an essential adjunct to the written consultation note.[4] Direct communication ensures that your important recommendations are transmitted to the requesting team and this increases the likelihood that the suggestions will be carried out. The frequency of follow-up and thus further verbal communications is dependent on the acuity of the situation and any major changes in the plan of care. Any important new recommendations should continue to be verbally communicated. The written recommendations should be clear and concise, preferably in a numeric or bulleted format, and limited to 3–5 recommendations.

With these principles in play, medical consultation can continue to be one of the most interesting and satisfying components of a hospitalist's career.

References

1. DeFrances CJ, Lucas CA, Buie VC, Golosinskiy A. (2008) 2006 National Hospital Discharge Survey. National health statistics reports; no. 5. National Center for Health Statistics, Hyattsville, MD.
2. Association of Professors of Medicine. (2001) Hospitalists' perceptions of their residency training needs: Results of a national survey. *Am J Med* **111**: 247–254.
3. Goldman L, Lee T, Rudd P. (1983) Ten commandments for effective consultations. *Arch Intern Med* **143**: 1753–1755.

4. Salerno SM, Hurst FP, Halvorson S, Mercado DL. (2007) Principles of effective consultation: An update for the 21st-century consultant. *Arch Intern Med* **167**: 271–275.
5 Boulware DR, Dekarske AS, Filice GA. (2009) Physician preferences for elements of effective consultations. *J Gen Intern Med* **25**(1): 25–30.
6 Lee T, Pappius EM, Goldman L. (1983) Impact of inter-physician communication on the effectiveness of medical consultations. *Am J Med* **74**: 106–112.
7 Conley J, Jordan M, Ghali WA. (2009) Audit of the consultation process on general internal medicine services. *Qual Saf Health Care* **18**: 59–62.
8 PausJenssen L, Ward HA, Card SE. (2008) An internist's role in perioperative medicine: A survey of surgeons' opinions. *BMC Fam Pract* **9**(4): 1–6.
9 Cohn SL. (2003) The role of the medical consultant. *Med Clin N Am* **87**: 1–6.

Chapter 84

Developing and Implementing a Co-management Model of Care

Tomas Villanueva and Amir K. Jaffer***

Key Pearls

- Co-management is more than just medical consultation. The hospitalist must actively manage pre-existing and newly developed medical issues rather than just make recommendations for the surgical team.
- Consensus meetings should take place to determine goals, patient selection and communication protocols. These items should become part of a written document in preparation for a co-management program.
- The quality metrics that will be tracked and the financial implications for the program need to be assessed prior to implementation.
- Piloting the co-management program before full implementation is important.
- Regular meetings including the stakeholders should be held to assess the progress of the program.

Co-management is not merely medical consultation. To be successful, the role of the hospitalist in co-managing surgical or subspecialty patients

*Baptist Hospital of Miami, Baptist Health South Florida, Miami, Fl, USA.
**University of Miami School of Medicine, Miami, Fl, USA.

must be as clearly defined in advancing postoperative care as it is in assessing preoperative risk. As a co-manager, a hospitalist must actively manage pre-existing and newly developed medical issues rather than just make recommendations for the surgical team.

One of the fastest-growing aspects of hospital medicine is within the area of co-management. Even though hospitalists may not have had experience during their training in managing these types of patients. The 2005–2006 Society of Hospital Medicine (SHM)[1] survey indicated that 85% of hospital medicine groups did co-management. This was an increase of 47% of orthopedic cases seen by hospitalists between 2001 and 2006. More recently, a study indicated that inpatient physicians continue to provide more co-management of surgical patients.[2]

At least four important studies address the utility of hospitalists in the co-management of surgical patients. The HOT (Hospitalist Orthopedic Team) trial was a randomized controlled trial assessing the effect of hospitalists on the management of patients undergoing elective hip and knee arthroplasty.[3] There was no effect on length of stay or patient outcomes, though the co-management model did decrease minor postoperative medical complications and improve physician and nurse satisfaction. Macpherson *et al.* conducted a retrospective trial where an internist joined a cardiothoracic surgery service at a tertiary care center.[4] They found a decrease in overall mortality and resource utilization such as lab testing and consultations. There was significant reduction in the length of stay and the number of X-rays performed. The third study, by Jaffer *et al.*[5] showed that an outpatient, preoperative evaluation clinic staffed by hospitalists followed by inpatient postoperative management at a large tertiary care center provides a practical model for managing preoperative patients and may be associated with a low rate of postoperative pulmonary complications. Finally, Simon *et al.*[6] described pediatric hospitalist co-management of patients undergoing spinal fusion surgery. In this retrospective cohort study, 14 of 115 patients were comanaged by a pediatric hospitalist. When compared to a historical control of patients with similar medical complexity but not comanaged by hospitalists, the length of stay was reduced by 2.4 days (8.6 vs. 6.2 days).

There is no consensus on the exact definition of co-management, but the SHM Task Force on Co-management and its subsequent Advisory Panel[1] define it as "shared responsibility, authority and accountability for the care of a hospitalized patient." In the case of co-managed surgical patients, the patient's surgeon manages the surgery-related treatments and a hospitalist manages the patient's medical conditions. The success of any program is based on thorough communication among all stakeholders, to establish goals and expectations, in addition to measuring intentional or nonintentional consequences. The Advisory Panel[1] suggests the following steps to ensure success:

1. Indentify champions and stakeholders at your institution.
2. Schedule consensus meetings between the key stakeholders and additional groups such as nursing, information technology and finance.
3. Determine goals:
    a. Patient selection;
    b. Communication protocols;
    c. Develop a service agreement.
4. Define key metrics for the program.
5. Predetermine financial considerations.
6. Pilot the program.

Identifying Champions and Stakeholders

Historically, most programs are initiated via informal conversations among interested parties. It is highly recommended that a formal meeting be scheduled to identify leaders among all stakeholders to function as champions and build support among the staff and administration. Champions are individuals who innovate, are committed, lead program development and communicate. They help with negotiation and resolve conflict when stakeholders have different agendas, help get buy-in from the leadership of the hospital and help the team utilize a quality improvement approach to patient care.

Stakeholders include the hospital leadership — specifically, leaders of divisions or departments interested in the co-management model of care and leadership of the hospital medicine group or division. Having representatives from nursing, case management, finance and billing involved is also essential.

Consensus Meetings

Once all stakeholders and champions are identified, it is vital to arrange consensus meetings to determine in advance the "rules of engagement" for the program. Legal risks related to hospitalists handling problems which ordinarily are handled by surgeons should be identified and predetermined.[7] Clear and concise communication is paramount for agreement among all stakeholders.

Once verbal agreement has been reached, a written agreement should be completed, which should clearly define the roles, responsibilities and program expectations among all stakeholders in order to resolve conflict when issues arise.[7]

It should be clear how the following issues will be handled:

- Patient selection;
- The hospitalist's specific role (e.g. preoperative evaluation, postop-management of hyperglycemia, anticoagulation management);
- Postoperative complications;
- Writing orders;
- Ordering consults.

Other questions that need to be addressed include:

- Will there be midlevel provider support for the hospitalists?
- Who will the nurse call (specialist or hospitalist?) when problems arise?
- What will the hospitalist's role be in the discharge process? Who will dictate the discharge summary?
- Who will be responsible for communicating discharge information to the community physician?

- Who is responsible for medication reconciliation?
- Will the hospitalist bill as a consultant or as an attending physician?
- What will be the expectations for communication between the hospitalist and the specialist?
- Will there be a defined multidisciplinary team for co-management?
- If so, what clinicians will be members of the team?
- Will there be multidisciplinary team rounds?
- Can the hospitalist consult an additional physician to the team?
- Will there be a process for resolving issues/conflicts regarding the design or operation of the co-management program?
- Will there be any tools, protocols, pathways or guidelines to support the co-management program?

By identifying the goals and issues upfront, services involved in the co-management model of care are less likely to encounter unmet expectations and dissatisfaction due to changing roles and expectations after the service is implemented.

Define Key Metrics for the Program

Measuring performance is vital to determining success in all quality improvement initiatives. These metrics should be the product of a program's goal, and should be measured continuously and reported frequently among stakeholders. Dashboards are an excellent communication tool for informing clinicians and displaying outcomes to administrators. IT should be involved to ensure that reports are readily available for analysis and acceptance from the team. Metrics that may have value in tracking performance include: number of admissions, risk-adjusted average length of stay, risk-adjusted mortality, unplanned transfers to ICU, rates of venous thromboembolism (VTE), prophylaxis rates, hospital-acquired infections (including pneumonia and wound infections) and catheter-related infections (including sepsis). Patient satisfaction, provider satisfaction, readmission rates and financial metrics such as cost of hospitalization are also worth tracking. Occupancy rate and bed turnover, as well as discharge process measures, may also be tracked.[7]

Clinical outcome measures such as patient safety and quality metrics, glycemic control, "never" events, acute renal failure, myocardial infarction, pulmonary embolism, stroke and delirium may also be worth tracking.

Financial Considerations

It is essential to ensure that all financial issues pertaining to revenue and expenses are addressed prior to initiating a program in addition to a frank discussion on deficit funding should expenses related to staffing exceed revenues. Physician stakeholders should analyze how they will be compensated and avoid burdening the patient with additional expenses. Once these financial issues are resolved, they should also be outlined in the written agreement.

Financial considerations include[7]:

- Determining whether the hospitalist will bill as a consultant or as an attending physician;
- Determining who bills what (surgeon/specialist, hospitalist, midlevel), and periodic review of collection rates;
- Rejected claims and writeoffs;
- Considerating key assumptions and expenses related to patient volume, coverage workload per hospitalist and use of midlevel staff;
- Monitoring billing to ensure that bills are submitted in a timely manner;
- Identifying the contractual issues of involved providers;
- Understanding the documentation, coding and billing practices within your institution.

Piloting the Program

Piloting gives the opportunity for stakeholders to iron out the kinks and enlighten the team on issues, whether expected or not, that may arise.

It also allows the team to examine and revise the written agreement if needed. It is suggested that the hospitalist should pilot with a small sample of patients or work with one surgeon/specialist only. Only when the pilot program is seen as functioning smoothly among the team should one implement the program fully.

Conclusion

In less than a decade, the focus of hospital-based medical care has shifted from staffing a shift to improving the quality of healthcare delivery in a system through which patients move. The lessons which hospitalists have learned in quality improvement and in improving systems of care are perfectly suited for application to surgical and subspecialty services. Co-management may offer improvement in a surgical or a subspecialty patient's medical care, but it is for us to prudently study the care of these patients and go about co-management in an organized manner. This can be done by collecting data on these patients and their care that will allow us to show more definitely that the co-management model of care is indeed superior to some of our established models of care.

References

1. Medicine SoH. 2005–2006 SHM Survey: The Authoritative Source on the State of Hospital Medicine Highlights/Executive Summary, pp. 1–5.
2. Kuo YF, Sharma G, Freeman JL, Goodwin JS. (2009) Growth in the care of older patients by hospitalists in the United States. *N Engl J Med* **360**(11): 1102–1112.
3. Huddleston JM, Long KH, Naessens JM, *et al.* (2004) Medical and surgical comanagement after elective hip and knee arthroplasty: A randomized, controlled trial. *Ann Intern Med* **141**(1): 28–38.
4. Macpherson DS, Parenti C, Nee J, *et al.* (1994) An internist joins the surgery service: Does comanagement make a difference? *J Gen Intern Med* **9**(8): 440–444.

5. Jaffer A, Brotman DJ, Sridharan ST, *et al.* (2005) Postoperative pulmonary complications: Experience with an outpatient preoperative assessment program. *J Clin Outcomes Manag* **12**: 505–510.
6. Simon TD, Eilert R, Dickinson LM, *et al.* (2007) Pediatric hospitalist comanagement of spinal fusion surgery patients. *J Hosp Med* **2**(1): 23–30.
7. *A White Paper on "A Guide to Hospitalist/Orthopedic Surgery Comanagement."* Society of Hospital Medicine, Philadelphia, pp. 1–12 (2009).

Chapter 85

Preoperative Cardiac Assessment

*Dennis Chang**

Key Pearls

- Patients having emergency surgery are two times more likely to have a perioperative cardiovascular event than patients having nonemergency surgery.
- The six components of the Revised Cardiac Risk Index are: high risk surgery, coronary artery disease, congestive heart failure, cerebrovascular accident, creatinine greater than 2 mg/dL, and diabetes mellitus on insulin.
- Stress tests have a low positive predictive value for perioperative cardiovascular events.
- Beta blockers and HMG-CoA reductase inhibitors decrease perioperative cardiovascular events in high-risk populations.
- Stress tests and cardiac revascularization should be obtained when based on the patient's clinical symptoms; testing would have been indicated regardless of whether the patient was having surgery.

Introduction

Significant advances in medical therapy for patients with chronic disease have allowed them to live longer, and consequently more patients with

*Mount Sinai School of Medicine, New York, NY, USA.

higher acuity are having surgery. It is estimated that annually[1] more than 100 million patients worldwide undergo noncardiac surgery and 900,000 patients worldwide experience a major perioperative cardiac event.[1] The consequences of these events can be severe. Patients with postoperative myocardial infarctions have a 15%–25% increase in hospital mortality[1] and a hazard ratio of 18 for nonfatal myocardial infarction and cardiovascular death in the six months after surgery.[2]

Role as Preoperative Consultant

Due to the morbidity and mortality associated with perioperative cardiac events, it has become common practice for patients to be evaluated by a hospitalist, internist or cardiologist prior to noncardiac surgery. This chapter will discuss how to:

- Estimate a patient's cardiac risk for noncardiac surgery;
- Determine whether a patient requires further evaluation to assess their cardiac risk;
- Develop a plan to optimally manage and minimize their perioperative risk.

Initial Assessment for Cardiac Risk Using the ACC/AHA Guidelines

In 2007, the ACC/AHA revised their guidelines for assessing cardiac risk prior to noncardiac surgery (Fig. 1). The guidelines are based on the five questions below:

1. What is the urgency of the surgery?
2. Is the patient having active cardiac symptoms?
3. Is the surgery low-, intermediate-, or high-risk for perioperative cardiovascular complications?
4. What is the patient's functional capacity?
5. How many Revised Cardiac Risk Index[3] factors does the patient have?

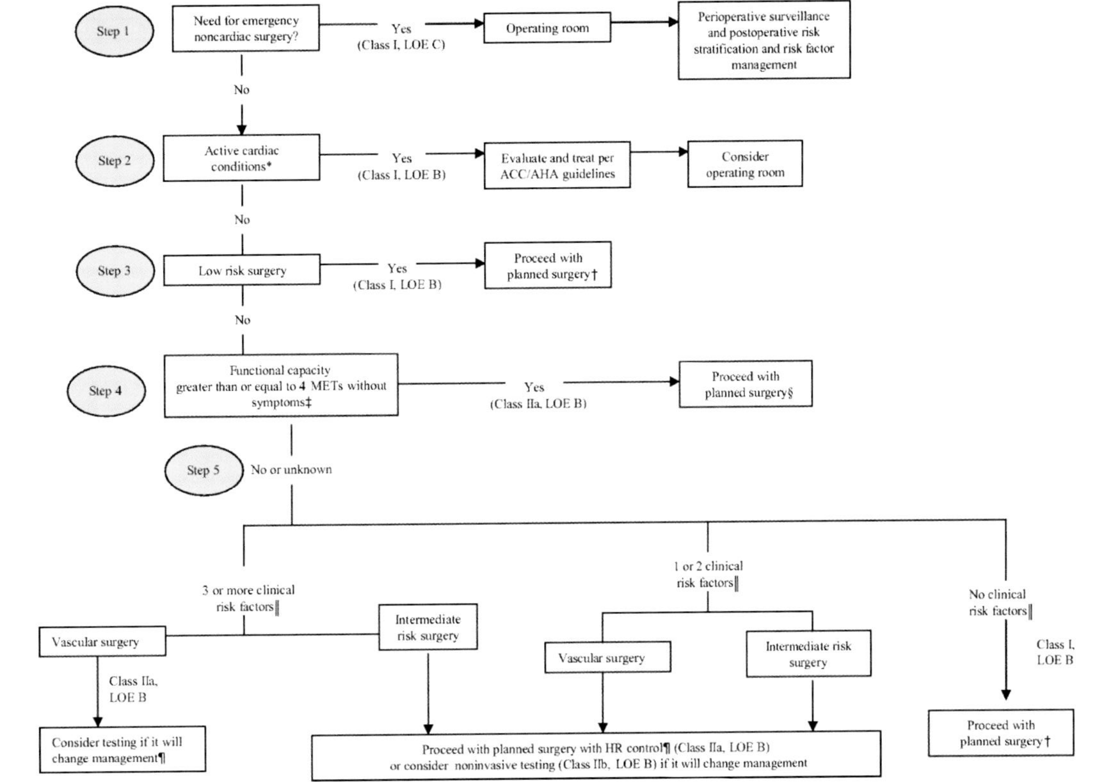

Fig. 1. Cardiac evaluation and care algorithm for noncardiac surgery based on active clinical conditions, known cardiovascular disease, or cardiac risk factors for patients 50 years of age or more.[4] (Reprinted with permission from the American Heart Association.)

Urgency of Surgery

Patients having emergency surgery are twice as likely to have a cardiovascular complication compared to patients having the same procedure electively.[1] Since by definition emergency surgery must be done in order to prevent imminent mortality or morbidity, all patients needing emergency surgery may proceed to the operating room.

The role of the perioperative physician is to make sure appropriate medications are continued or adjusted. Since some patients cannot take oral medications postoperatively, medications must be switched to their equivalent parenteral forms. Medications that require special attention are antihypertensives, cardiac medications (especially β-blockers), and diabetic medications.

Unstable and Severe Cardiac Conditions

A thorough history and exam should be performed to look for any severe or unstable cardiac conditions (Table 1). Surgeries should be delayed until the unstable cardiac conditions are treated appropriately.

Surgical Risk

Surgeries have an inherent cardiac risk that can be categorized into three groups: low-risk, intermediate-risk, and high-risk (Table 2).

Low-risk surgeries have an overall risk for perioperative cardiovascular complications of less than 1% and any clinically stable patient without active cardiac conditions (see Table 1) under-going low-risk surgery may proceed to the operating room regardless of their cardiovascular risk factors or functional status.

Functional Capacity

Functional capacity is defined as the number of metabolic equivalents a patient can achieve. One metabolic equivalent is defined as the energy expended by a 70 kg, 40-year-old male at rest for 1 min. Patients who are

Table 1. Unstable and Severe Cardiac Conditions*

Unstable coronary syndromes	1. Unstable angina
	2. Severe angina = Canadian Cardiovascular Society (CCS) class III or IV CCS Class III: angina with minimal activity (<2 blocks; <1 flight of stairs) CCS Class IV: angina at rest and with any physical activity
	3. Recent myocardial infarction: within 30 days
	4. Recent cardiac stent placement: within 30 days
Decompensated heart failure	1. Worsening heart failure
	2. New onset heart failure
	3. New York Heart Association functional class IV: symptoms at rest
Arrhythmias	1. High-grade atrioventricular (AV) block
	a. Mobitz II AV block
	b. 3rd degree AV block
	2. Symptomatic ventricular arrhythmias
	3. Uncontrolled supraventricular arrhythmias (include atrial fibrillation with HR >100 bpm at rest)
	4. Symptomatic bradycardia
	5. New ventricular tachycardia
Severe valvular disease	1. Aortic stenosis (severe)
	a. Symptomatic or
	b. Mean pressure gradient >40 mmHg or
	c. Valve area <1.0cm^2
	2. Mitral stenosis (symptomatic)

* Adapted from ACC/AHA 2007 Guidelines on Perioperative Cardiovascular Evaluation and Care for Noncardiac Surgery.[47]

able to achieve four or more metabolic equivalents without symptoms have a low rate of perioperative cardiovascular complications (Table 3), and management will rarely be changed with cardiovascular testing.[4] Therefore, most patients who can achieve four metabolic equivalents may proceed to surgery.

Revised Cardiac Risk Index

Based on the ACC/AHA algorithm (Fig. 1), if a patient is not able to achieve 4 METs, is undergoing a moderate or high-risk surgery, and is not

Table 2. Cardiac Risk Stratification for Noncardiac Surgery[4]

Low risk surgery (<1%)	Intermediate risk surgery (1%–5%)	High risk surgery (>5%)
Endoscopic procedures	Carotid Endarterectomy	Open aortic repair
Superficial procedures	Intraperitoneal surgery	Peripheral vascular repair
Ophthalmologic	Intrathoracic surgery	
Breast surgery	Laproscopic intrathoracic or -peritoneal surgery	
Dental	Percutaneous transluminal angioplasty (PTA)	
Gynecologic	EVAR (Endovascular aneurysm repair)	
	Neurologic surgery	
	Transplantation	
	Urologic surgery (cystoscopy is low-risk)	
	Head and neck surgery	
	Orthopedic surgery	
	Prostate surgery	

Table 3. Metabolic Equivalent Activity Table

Number of METs	Activity
1 MET	Watching TV
	Sitting at a desk
4 METS	2 flights of stairs
	5 blocks at a normal pace (4 mph)
	Light housework (dusting/dishwashing)
	Walking a golf course
>4 METS	Jogging
	Tennis

having severe or unstable cardiac symptoms, a more thorough assessment of the cardiac risk factors must be done. Lee's revised cardiac risk index (RCRI) is the most validated tool for assessing perioperative cardiovascular risk[3] (Table 3). The ACC/AHA guidelines derive their clinical risk factors from the RCRI, except that high-risk or intermediate-risk surgery is not a clinical risk factor in the guidelines.

Patients are divided into three perioperative cardiovascular risk groups: low-risk (RCRI 0), intermediate risk (RCRI 1–2), and high risk (RCRI ≥3):

Low-risk group: perioperative cardiovascular risk <1%
Patients without any risk factors have a perioperative risk of <1% and may proceed to surgery without further cardiac workup.[4] Stress-testing these individuals may actually be associated with harm.[5]

Intermediate-risk group: perioperative cardiovascular risk 1%–5%

High-risk group: perioperative cardiovascular risk >5%

Current data suggest that stress tests and even cardiovascular catheterization of intermediate and high-risk groups are warranted only when patients are having active or concerning cardiac symptoms.

Table 4. Revised Cardiac Risk Index (RCRI)[4]

	RCRI points*	Rate of Perioperative CV Complications†
1. Intermediate, or high-risk surgeries	0	0.4%
2. Coronary artery disease	1	1.1%
3. Congestive heart failure	2	4.6%
4. Cerebrovascular disease	≥3	9.7%
5. Diabetes mellitus (on insulin)		
6. Chronic renal insufficiency (creatinine >2.0 mg/dL)		

* Each risk factor equals one point.
† Cardiovascular complications: myocardial infarction, pulmonary edema, ventricular fibrillation, primary cardiac arrest, complete heart block.

Stress tests are poor at identifying patients at risk for perioperative cardiovascular complications. A meta-analysis of over 35 studies found a positive predictive value (PPV) of 13% and a negative predictive value

(NPV) of 98% for dobutamine stress echocardiography (DSE), and a PPV of 11% and an NPV of 97% for myocardial perfusion stress scintigraphy (MPS).[6] Although the NPV is high for stress tests, in a high-risk patient a stress test's NPV lowers their post-test probability of cardiovascular events to the level of a moderate-risk patient and typically does not change perioperative management.

Two randomized controlled trials, CARP and DECREASE-V, have shown that cardiac revascularization does not decrease perioperative cardiovascular complications compared to medical management. The CARP trial randomized patients going for vascular surgery to coronary revascularization and medical management. There was no difference in overall mortality or cardiac mortality between the two groups.[7] The DECREASE-V trial took high-risk patients (RCRI ≥3) with >5 ischemic segments on stress testing and randomized them to revascularization and no revascularization, with all patients receiving beta blockers titrated to a goal heart rate of 60–65 beats per minute. Again, there was no difference in overall mortality or cardiac mortality between the two groups.[8]

The available evidence suggests that stress testing and cardiac revascularization should not be obtained routinely or based purely on the RCRI score. Stress tests and cardiac revascularization should be obtained when based on their clinical symptoms; testing would have been indicated regardless of whether the patients were having surgery. In general, this includes patients having unstable angina, unexplained chest pain, or shortness of breath with minimal or no exertion.

Medical Management

Beta Blockers

There continues to be much debate about which cardiovascular risk groups would benefit from β-blockers. Negative trials such as MaVS[9] and POISE[10] have shown that β-blockers do not reduce perioperative cardiovascular complications. However, these trials were on low-risk patients or β-blockers were started on the day of surgery and not titrated to a goal heart rate. This is in contrast to the trials which showed a benefit for β-blockers perioperatively, such as DECREASE[11] and DECREASE IV,[12] which started β-blockers at a median of 30 days prior to surgery and titrated them to a goal heart rate between 50 and 70 beats per minute. A retrospective database analysis of 782,000 patients showed that perioperative β-blockers improved outcomes in patients with an RCRI greater than 2 but were detrimental in low-risk patients with an RCRI of 0.[13] Although there is conflicting evidence, perioperative β-blockers should be administered in the following patients:

- Patients already taking β-blockers;
- Patients with other indications for β-blockers (i.e. coronary artery disease, congestive heart failure);
- Patients with an RCRI ≥3.

β-blockers should be titrated to a goal heart rate of 50–70 beats per minute over a period of at least 7 days, but preferably started 30 days prior to surgery.[11]

Statins

Statins have shown great promise in reducing perioperative cardiovascular complications in recent trials on high-risk patients. In the randomized trial DECREASE III, 500 high-risk patients undergoing vascular surgery were given fluvastatin or a placebo. Myocardial infarctions within 30 days of surgery occurred in 19% of the placebo group, compared to 10.8% in the fluvastatin group.[14] In the largest retrospective trial to date, Lindenauer reviewed 780,091 patients undergoing both intermediate- and high-risk surgeries, and found an overall 1% reduction in perioperative cardiovascular complications in patients taking statins compared to non-statin patients.[15] The odds ratios in this study were 2.60, 4.50, 7.07, and 9.34 for patients with an RCRI of 1, 2, 3, and ≥4, respectively. Statins also appear to be safe in the perioperative period, with no increased myopathy or rhabdomyolysis.[16]

However, in intermediate-risk patients, the evidence is not as clear. DECREASE IV did not show any statistical benefit for statins in intermediate risk patients undergoing noncardiac surgery.[12]

Statins should be administered perioperatively for most patients in the following situations:

1. Patients already on a statin prior to surgery;
2. Patients eligible based on the National Cholesterol Education Program (NCEP) Guidelines;
3. High-risk patients (RCRI ≥3) undergoing vascular surgery.

Statins can be considered perioperatively for:

1. Intermediate-risk patients (RCRI 1–2) having vascular surgery;
2. High-risk patients (RCRI ≥3) undergoing nonvascular surgery.

Though the optimal timing and dose is unclear, it is reasonable to start a statin at a low-to-moderate dose 2–4 weeks prior to surgery. Starting statins in the immediate preoperative period is probably safe but their efficacy is unclear.

Postoperative monitoring

The benefits of obtaining an electrocardiogram (ECG) and serial troponins postoperatively are not well studied. However, 53% of patients experiencing perioperative myocardial infarction (MI) do not have clinical signs or symptoms of MI[17] and patients who experience perioperative MIs have a hazard ratio of 18 for nonfatal MI and cardiovascular death in the six months after surgery.[2] Because of this evidence, it is reasonable to check postoperative ECGs and troponins on postoperative days 1 and 2 in patients who are at high-risk for perioperative cardiovascular events (RCRI ≥3).

References

1. Devereaux PJ, Goldman L, Cook DJ, *et al.* (2005) Perioperative cardiac events in patients undergoing noncardiac surgery: A review of the

magnitude of the problem, the pathophysiology of the events and methods to estimate and communicate risk. *CMAJ* **173**: 627–634.
2. Mangano DT, Browner WS, Hollenberg M, *et al.* (1992) Long-term cardiac prognosis following noncardiac surgery. The Study of Perioperative Ischemia Research Group. *JAMA* **268**: 233–239.
3. Lee TH, Marcantonio ER, Mangione CM, *et al.* (1999) Derivation and prospective validation of a simple index for prediction of cardiac risk of major noncardiac surgery. *Circulation* **100**: 1043–1049.
4. Fleisher LA, Beckman JA, Brown KA, *et al.* (2007) ACC/AHA 2007 guidelines on perioperative cardiovascular evaluation and care for noncardiac surgery: A report of the American College of Cardiology/American Association Task Force on Practice Guidelines (writing committee to revise the 2002 guidelines on perioperative cardiovascular evaluation for noncardiac surgery) — developed in collaboration with the American Society of Echocardiography, American Society of Nuclear Cardiology, Heart Rhythm Society, Society of Cardiovascular Anesthesiologists, Society of Cardiovascular Angiography and Interventions, Society for Vascular Medicine and Biology, and Society for Vascular Surgery. *Circulation* **116**: 1971–1996.
5. Wijeysundera DN, Beattie WS, Elliot RF, *et al.* (2010) Non-invasive cardiac stress testing before elective major non-cardiac surgery: Population based cohort study. *BMJ* **340**: b5526.
6. Kertai MD, Boersma E, Bax JJ, *et al.* (2003) A meta-analysis comparing accuracy of six diagnostic tests for predicting perioperative cardiac risk in patients undergoing major vascular surgery. *Heart* **89**: 1327–1334.
7. McFalls EO, Ward HB, Moritz TE, *et al.* (2004) Coronary-artery revascularization before elective major vascular surgery. *N Eng J Med* **351**: 2795–2804.
8. Poldermans D, Schouten O, Vidakovic R, *et al.* (2007) A clinical randomized trial to evaluate the safety of a noninvasive approach in high-risk patients undergoing major vascular surgery: The DECREASE-V Pilot Study. *J Am Coll Cardiol* **49**: 1763–1769.

9. Yang H, Raymer K, Butler R, *et al*. (2006) The effects of perioperative beta-blockage: Results of the Metoprolol after Vascular Surgery (MaVS) study: A randomized controlled trial. *Am Heart J* **152**(5): 983–990.
10. POISE Study Group. (2008) Effect of extended-release metoprolol succinate in patients undergoing non-cardiac surgery (POISE trial): A randomized controlled trial. *Lancet* **371**: 1839–1847.
11. Poldermans D, Bax JJ, Kertai, MD. (1999) Dutch Echocardiographic Risk Evaluation Applying Stress Echocardiography Study Group. The effect of bisoprolol on perioperative mortality and myocardial infarction in high-risk patients undergoing vascular surgery. *N Eng J Med* **341**: 1789–1994.
12. Dunkelgrun M, Boersma E, Schouten O, *et al*. (2009) Bisoprolol and fluvastatin for the reduction of perioperative cardiac mortality and myocardial infarction in intermediate-risk patients undergoing noncardiovascular surgery: A randomized controlled trial (DECREASE IV). *Ann Surg* **249**: 921–926.
13. Lindenauer PK, Pekow P, Wang K, *et al*. (2005) Perioperative beta blocker therapy and mortality after major noncardiac surgery. *N Eng J Med* **353**: 349–361.
14. Schouten O, Boersma E, Hoeks SE, *et al*. (2009) Fluvastatin and perioperative events in patients undergoing vascular surgery. *N Eng J Med* **361**: 980–999.
15. Lindenauer PK, Pekow P, Wang K, *et al*. (2004) Lipid-lowering therapy and in-hospital mortality following major noncardiac surgery. *JAMA* **291**: 2092–2099.
16. Schouten O, Kertai MD, Bax JJ, *et al*. (2005) Safety of perioperative statin use in high-risk patients undergoing major vascular surgery. *Am J Cardiol* **95**: 658–660.
17. Devereaux PJ, Goldman L, Cook DJ, *et al*. (2005) Surveillance and prevention of major perioperative ischemic cardiac events in patients undergoing noncardiac surgery: A review. *CMAJ* **173**: 779–788.

Chapter 86

Perioperative Management of Diabetes

*Maria Skamagas**

Key Pearls

- The glucose goal perioperatively is 100–180 mg/dL.
- Type 1 diabetics require basal insulin at all times, even when taking "nothing by mouth" (NPO).
- Oral diabetes medications should be held on the day of surgery.
- Adjust the dose of basal insulin perioperatively, depending on whether the patient has type 1 or type 2 DM and the degree of outpatient glycemic control at baseline.
- Intraoperatively, blood glucose should be checked every 1–2 hr.

Hyperglycemia is associated with worse outcomes in surgical patients, including wound infection, poor wound healing, sepsis, and mortality.[1–5] Glycemic control before and after surgery may help reduce these complications. In patients undergoing cardiothoracic surgery[6,7] and possibly in other critically ill surgical patients,[8] postoperative glycemic control using intravenous insulin infusions reduces wound infection and mortality. However, subsequent trials have not confirmed the finding of reduced mortality, and the NICE-SUGAR[9] study found increased mortality in post-surgical critically ill patients treated with intravenous insulin to tight glycemic goals. Despite the lack of definitive data from randomized trials, recommendations for management of surgical ward patients can be made

*Mount Sinai School of Medicine, New York, NY, USA.

Table 1. Glucose Goals in the Surgical Patient[10]

Population	BG Goals (mg/dL)
General surgical patient	Premeal: 100–140 Random: 100–180
Critically ill surgical patient	140–180

based on extrapolation from other settings, consensus statement,[10] and expert review.[11,12] Prior to surgery, it is prudent to consult with the physician overseeing the patient's outpatient diabetes care in those requiring insulin, and in all patients with diabetes who are undergoing major surgery.

Glucose Goals

Key Questions

When managing glucose in a diabetic patient undergoing surgery or a procedure requiring NPO status, several key aspects of the patient's diabetes and its management need to be assessed. These include:

1. Does the patient have type 1 or type 2 diabetes?
2. What diabetes medications is the patient taking at home?
    - Insulin (types and doses)
    - Oral medications
    - Injectable endocrine hormones
3. Is glycemic control at home good or poor, based on:
    - HbA1c
    - Blood glucose range
    - Hypoglycemic events

Type 1 and Type 2 Diabetes

Individuals with type 1 diabetes (DM1) do not make insulin, and thus require basal insulin injections (long-acting insulin) to avoid diabetic ketoacidosis (DKA) and hyperglycemia even when NPO. Basal insulin provides 24 hr of blood insulin levels which suppress hepatic glucose production and lipolysis, thus preventing hyperglycemia in the fasting state and ketoacid formation (DKA). Examples of basal insulin are glargine once daily, detemir twice daily, and NPH twice daily. Surgery and general anesthesia result in increased circulating catecholamines, cortisol, and other counter-regulatory hormones[13] which increase blood glucose and lipolysis, and increase the risk of DKA if the patient has not received basal insulin. When type 1 diabetics eat carbohydrates, rapid-acting insulin is required to control blood glucose elevations after the meal.

The characteristics of individuals with DM1 include: diagnosis in youth (usually less than 30 years of age), initial presentation with DKA or symptomatic hyperglycemia and insulinopenia (weight loss, polyuria, polydipsia, polyphagia), lean body mass at diagnosis, and requiring insulin since diagnosis. Occasionally, individuals are diagnosed with DM1 at an advanced age. Type 1 diabetics can also be overweight/obese if they lead an unhealthy lifestyle; this may translate to increased insulin resistance.

Individuals with type 2 diabetes (DM2) suffer from both reduced insulin secretion and increased insulin resistance (difficulty in using the insulin that is made by beta cells). DM2 is managed with diet, physical activity, oral medications, and/or insulin. For type 2 diabetics who require insulin injections, some need only basal insulin to control glucose and others require both basal and mealtime insulin. The majority of people with DM2 produce enough endogenous insulin to avoid DKA. However, some have little capacity for insulin secretion (i.e. long-standing diabetes requiring multiple insulin injections), and in the setting of severe stress or illness are vulnerable to DKA. Prolonged NPO status results in reduced basal insulin requirements. This is likely related to a reduction in hepatic glycogen stores,[14] and possibly improved insulin action[15] and insulin secretion. It is important to keep this in mind when adjusting insulin perioperatively.

The characteristics of individuals with DM2 include overweight/obesity or increased abdominal adiposity/waist circumference, family history of diabetes, high risk ethnicity (non-Caucasians), and acanthosis nigricans. Although DM2 is more common with advancing age, it is increasingly diagnosed in obese younger individuals, including children and teenagers.

Diabetes Medications

It is crucial to know the names and doses of diabetes medications that a patient is taking at home, and whether the patient is adherent (always, sometimes, infrequently) to the regimen. These include insulins, oral medications, and injectable endocrine hormones (non-insulin). Insulin is used to control perioperative blood glucose. Oral medications are discontinued on the day of surgery or when the patient commences NPO (see Chapter 46, Table 3, "Oral Diabetes Medications and Injectable Endocrine Hormones").

Patients who have good glycemic control on only oral medications may only need a correction insulin scale (see Chapter 46, Table 4, "Correction Insulin Scales") on the day of surgery, and gradual resumption of oral medications postoperatively as PO intake returns to baseline. If sulfonylureas (e.g. glimepiride, glipizide, glyburide) or short-acting insulin secretagogues (e.g. repaglinide, nateglinide) are given to a patient with poor PO intake or NPO status, the patient will be at high risk for hypoglycemia. Patients with poor glycemic control on oral medications may benefit from initiation of basal insulin prior to surgery (see Chapter 46, Figure 2, "Management of Type 2 Diabetes in Hospitalized Patients").

Patients who have good glycemic control on insulin usually require reduction in basal insulin doses (e.g. glargine, detemir, NPH) preoperatively to provide a margin of safety in avoiding hypoglycemia (see Table 2). Those with poor control require adjustment of insulin doses and adherence to the regimen to meet outpatient goals prior to elective surgery. If surgery is urgent and glycemic control is poor, then adjustments to the regimen must be made based on insulin doses, adherence, and home glucoses.

A correction insulin scale may be used to reduce elevated blood glucose (see Chapter 46, Table 4, "Correction Insulin Scales"). Standing mealtime insulin (e.g. lispro, aspart, glulisine, regular) should be held in

Table 2. Basal Insulin: Preoperative Dosing

Type 1 DM: Give 80%–100% of basal insulin (glargine or detemir).

If the patient has tightly controlled glucose levels at home (i.e. fasting glucose 70–130 mg/dL), one may give only 80% of basal insulin to reduce the risk of hypoglycemia, especially if there will be prolonged fasting.

Typical doses of basal insulin in DM1 = 0.25–0.3 units/kg/day. In obese type 1 DM with insulin resistance, the dose may be higher.

Ex.: At home, the patient injects glargine 20 units at bedtime. Give 16–20 units on the night before surgery.

***Type 2 DM*:** Give 50%–80% of home basal insulin dose (glargine or detemir).
If NPO >24 hr, give only 50% basal insulin.

Ex.: At home, the patient injects glargine 40 units at bedtime. Give 20 units on the night before surgery.

If NPH insulin is used at home, then:

- Reduce the dose of NPH: Give 80%–100% NPH bedtime dose, 50% NPH morning dose

or

- Convert to glargine/detemir — add up the total daily dose of NPH. Give ~50%–60% as glargine or detemir.

If mixed insulin (ex.: 70/30 mix or 75/25 mix) is used at home:
- *Do not use mixed insulin* in a patient who is NPO (increased risk of hypoglycemia due to rapid-acting insulin component)
- Give ~40%–50% of the total dose as glargine or detemir.

Major surgery and type 1 DM (ex.: cardiothoracic, vascular, CNS, extensive abdominal surgery)

The absorption of subcutaneous (SC) insulin and glucose control during a prolonged surgery may be variable. Consider IV insulin drip at 0.5–1 units per hour, and D51/2NS at 100 mL/hr. Check the glucose every hour. Goal glucose: 100–180 mg/dL.

Major surgery and uncontrolled type 2 DM — consider IV insulin drip.

patients who are NPO. Postoperatively, as patients resume PO intake, mealtime insulin may be gradually resumed.

It is important to recognize that mealtime carbohydrate and caloric portions in a hospital are controlled and may be less than what a patient eats at home. Therefore, a patient may require less prandial medication to control mealtime glucose excursions in the hospital. This should be factored into the titration of mealtime insulin and prandial medications in order to avoid hypoglycemia.

Baseline Glucose Control

Chronic hyperglycemia (glucose >200 mg/dL, HbA1c >8%–9%) or frequent hypoglycemia (glucose <70 mg/dL) at home warrants adjustment of diabetes medications and diet with an aim for better glucose control prior to surgery. There is an association with increased postoperative infections (pneumonia, wound infection, sepsis) in diabetic patients with a preoperative HbA1c >7%,[5] and an increased risk of deep sternal wound infections in diabetics undergoing coronary artery bypass grafting and with a preoperative blood glucose >200 mg/dL.[16]

Pre-op Management

- Schedule surgery/procedure early in the morning to avoid prolonged NPO.
- Hold oral diabetes medications on the day of surgery (or when NPO status commences). Extended release metformin is held on the day before *and* the day of surgery.
- Insulin used in the preoperative period includes:

1. **Basal insulin** = long-acting insulin daily or intermediate-acting insulin twice daily (see Table 3)
   Glargine once daily
   Detemir divided twice daily
   NPH divided twice daily.
2. **Correction insulin scale**: may use every 4–6 hr to correct high blood glucose (see Chapter 46, Table 4, "Correction Insulin Scales").
   Rapid-acting insulins are preferred. Examples: lispro, aspart, glulisine.

Intra-op Management

- Check blood glucose every 1–2 hr, to ensure that there is no hypoglycemia or severe hyperglycemia.
- Correction insulin scale may be used to correct high blood glucose.
  Duration of action of IV regular insulin: 1 hr.
  Duration of action of SC aspart, lispro, glulisine insulin: 4–6 hr.
- Avoid stacking insulin doses (using more frequently than the duration of action), as this may cause hypoglycemia.

Post-op Management

Type 1 DM

- Continue basal insulin.
- Resume prior mealtime insulin doses gradually as PO intake returns to baseline.
- If the patient is eating less than usual, give smaller doses with meals after the patient eats his or her meal (e.g. 50% of the usual dose after he or she eats 50% meal).
- If the patient is able to count carbohydrates, one may use the insulin-to-carbohydrate ratio before meals.
- Use a correction insulin scale before meals.

Type 2 DM

- Restart oral medications postop day 1–2, if the patient is clinically stable and eating meals.
- Metformin — confirm normal kidney function before restarting metformin.
- Sulfonylureas (i.e. glimepiride, glipizide, glyburide) and meglitinides (e.g. repaglinide, nateglinide) — restart at ≤ half of the home dose and titrate up as the PO intake returns to baseline.
- Resume basal insulin.

- Resume prior mealtime insulin doses gradually as PO intake returns to baseline.
- Use a correction insulin scale before meals.

For management of critically ill surgical patients, see Chapter 33 on "Glycemic Management in Critically Ill Patients."

References

1. Umpierrez GE, Isaacs SD, Bazargan N, *et al.* (2002) Hyperglycemia: An independent marker of in-hospital mortality in patients with undiagnosed diabetes. *J Clin Endocrinol Metab* **87**: 978–982.
2. Pomposelli JJ, Baxter JK 3rd, Babineau TJ, *et al.* (1998) Early postoperative glucose control predicts nosocomial infection rate in diabetic patients. *J Parenter Enteral Nutr* **22**: 77–81.
3. Noordzij PG, Boersma E, Schreiner F, *et al.* (2007) Increased preoperative glucose levels are associated with perioperative mortality in patients undergoing noncardiac, nonvascular surgery. *Eur J Endocrinol* **156**: 137–42.
4. Ata A, Lee J, Bestle SL, *et al.* (2010) Postoperative hyperglycemia and surgical site infection in general surgery patients. *Arch Surg* **145**: 858–64.
5. Dronge AS, Perkal MF, Kancir S, *et al.* (2006) Long-term glycemic control and postoperative infectious complications. *Arch Surg* **141**: 375–380.
6. Furnary AP, Zerr KJ, Grunkemeier GL, Starr A. (1999) Continuous intravenous insulin infusion reduces the incidence of deep sternal wound infection in diabetic patients after cardiac surgical procedures. *Ann Thorac Surg* **67**: 352–360.
7. Furnary AP, Gao G, Grunkemeier GL, *et al.* (2003) Continuous insulin infusion reduces mortality in patients with diabetes undergoing coronary artery bypass grafting. *J Thorac Cardiovasc Surg* **125**: 1007–1021.
8. van den Berghe G, Wouters P, Weekers F, *et al.* (2001) Intensive insulin therapy in the critically ill patients. *N Engl J Med* **345**: 1359–1367.

9. The NICE-SUGAR Study Investigators. (2009) Intensive versus conventional glucose control in critically ill patients. *N Engl J Med* **360**: 1283–1297.
10. Moghissi ES, Korytkowski MT, DiNardo M, *et al.* (2009) American Association of Clinical Endocrinologists and American Diabetes Association consensus statement on inpatient glycemic control. *Endocr Pract* **15**: 353–369.
11. Meneghini LF. (2009) Perioperative management of diabetes: Translating evidence into practice. *Cleve Clin J Med* **76** (Suppl 4): S53–S59.
12. Tridgell DM, Tridgell AH, Hirsch IB. (2010) Inpatient management of adults and children with type 1 diabetes. *Endocrinol Metab Clin North Am* **39**: 595–608.
13. Kennedy DJ, Butterworth JF. (1994) Endocrine function during and after cardiopulmonary bypass: Recent observations. *J Clin Endocrinol Metab* **78**: 997–1002.
14. Exton JH, Corbin JG, Harper SC. (1972) Control of gluconeogenesis in liver. V. Effects of fasting, diabetes, and glucagon in lactate and endogenous metabolism in the perfused rat liver. *J Biol Chem* **247**: 4996–5003.
15. Halberg N, Henriksen M, Söderhamn N, *et al.* (2005) Effect of intermittent fasting and refeeding on insulin action in healthy men. *J Appl Physiol* **99**: 2128–2136.
16. Trick WE, Scheckler WE, Tokars JI, *et al.* (2000) Modifiable risk factors associated with deep sternal site infection after coronary artery bypass grafting. *J Thorac Cardiovasc Surg* **119**: 108–114.
17. Bailon RM, Partlow BJ, Miller-Cage V, *et al.* (2009) Continuous subcutaneous insulin infusion (insulin pump) therapy can be safely used in the hospital in select patients. *Endocr Pract* **15**: 24–29.

Chapter 87

Preoperative Pulmonary Assessment

*Adam S. Morgenthau**

Key Pearls

- Major postoperative pulmonary complications include pneumonia, respiratory failure, prolonged mechanical ventilation, bronchospasm, atelectasis, pulmonary embolism and exacerbations of underlying chronic lung disease.
- The rate of postoperative pulmonary complications is strongly associated with procedure proximity to the diaphragm.
- Patient factors most strongly associated with postoperative risk are age, ASA class, CHF, general health status, COPD and smoking.
- The routine use of spirometry and chest radiography for preoperative assessment is not recommended.
- Postoperative pulmonary complications prolong the hospital stay by an average of 1–2 weeks.

Introduction

Every hospitalist should be familiar with the preoperative evaluation of patients with pulmonary disease. Postoperative pulmonary complications (PPCs) prolong the hospital stay by an average of 7–14 days.[1] Elderly patients who develop PPCs have reduced long-term survival.[2] In one review, the incidence of PPCs in patients undergoing noncardiothoracic

*Mount Sinai School of Medicine, New York, NY 10029, USA.

surgery varied widely, from 2%–19%.[3] In patients undergoing cardiothoracic surgery, the incidence ranged from 8%–39%.[4] The wide variation can be attributed to the heterogeneity among patients selected for study and the differing definitions of PPCs within studies.

In more recent studies, however, only PPCs known to prolong the hospital stay or contribute to morbidity or mortality are examined.[5,6] PPC are precisely classified as major or minor, depending upon severity and adverse impact on patients. Risk factors are categorized as either patient-related or procedure-related. Consistent terminology has simplified epidemiologic analysis and facilitated the development of evidence-based guidelines for the preoperative evaluation of patients with pulmonary disease.[7] This chapter provides a practical approach to the preoperative assessment of patients with pulmonary disease.

Definition of PPCs

The major PPCs include:

- Pneumonia
- Respiratory failure
- Prolonged mechanical ventilation
- Bronchospasm
- Atelectasis
- Pulmonary embolism
- Exacerbations of underlying chronic lung disease

The minor PPCs include but are not limited to laryngospasm and requirements for supplemental oxygen.

Procedure-related and Patient-related Risk Factors

Risk factors may be related to the procedure or to the patient (Table 1). Surgical factors that may affect risk are the site and duration of surgery, the type of sedation and whether the surgery is emergent. The rate of postoperative complications is strongly associated with procedure proximity to

Table 1. Summary Strength of the Evidence for the Association of Patient, Procedure, and Laboratory Factors with Postoperative Pulmonary Complications*

Factor	Strength of Recommendation†	Odds Ratio‡
Potential patient-related risk factor		
Advanced age	A	2.09–3.04
ASA class ≥ II	A	2.55–4.87
CHF	A	2.93
Functionally dependent	A	1.66–2 51
COPD	A	1.79
Weight loss	B	1.62
Impaired sensorium	B	1.39
Cigarette use	B	1.26
Alcohol use	B	1.21
Abnormal findings on chest examination	B	NA
Diabetes	C	
Obesity	D	
Asthma	D	
Obstructive sleep apnea	I	
Corticosteroid use	I	
HIV infection	I	
Arrhythmia	I	
Poor exercise capacity	I	
Potential procedure-related risk factor		
Aortic aneurysm repair	A	6.90
Thoracic surgery	A	4.24
Abdominal surgery	A	3.01
Upper abdominal surgery	A	2.91
Neurosurgery	A	2.53
Prolonged surgery	A	2.26
Head and neck surgery	A	2.21
Emergency surgery	A	2.21
Vascular surgery	A	2.10
General anesthesia	A	1.83
Perioperative transfusion	B	1.47
Hip surgery	D	
Gynecologic or urologic surgery	D	
Esophageal surgery	I	

(*Continued*)

Table 1. (*Continued*)

Factor	Strength of Recommendation	Odds Ratio
Laboratory tests		
Albumin level <35 g/L	A	2.53
Chest radiography	B	4.81
BUN level >7.5 mmol/L (>21 mg/dL)	B	NA
Spirometry	I	

*ASA — American Society of Anesthesiologists; BUN - blood urea nitrogen; CHF — congestive heart failure; COPD - chronic obstructive pulmonary disease; NA — not available.

†Recommendations: A — good evidence to support the particular risk factor or laboratory predictor: B — at least fair evidence to support the particular risk factor or laboratory predictor; C — at least fair evidence to suggest that the particular factor is not a risk factor or that the laboratory test does not predict risk; D – good evidence to suggest that the particular factor is not a risk factor or that the laboratory test does not predict risk; I — insufficient evidence to determine whether the factor increases risk or whether the laboratory lest predicts risk, and evidence is lacking, is of poor quality, or is conflicting. From reference 12.

‡For Factors with A or B ratings. Odds ratios are trim-and-fill estimates. When these estimates were not possible, we provide the pooled estimate.

Reproduced with permission from Semtana *et al.* (2006) *Ann Intern Med* **144**(8): 581–595.

the diaphragm.[8] Major abdominal, thoracic and open abdominal aortic aneurysm repair have the greatest risk.[9] Procedures lasting longer than 3 hr are also high-risk. Head and neck surgeries, neurosurgery and emergent procedures are higher-risk than peripheral and/or elective operations.[10] Although laparoscopic surgery results in reduced pain, smaller reductions in vital capacity after surgery and minimal recovery time compared to standard open operations, the technique does not appear to lower PPC rates.[10]

General anesthesia is modestly associated with PPC risk.[11] Peripheral nerve conduction blocks confer very little risk. The risk associated with spinal or epidural anesthesia is controversial.[7]

Patient factors most strongly associated with risk are[9]:

- Age
- American Society of Anesthesiologists Physical Status (ASA) Classification (Table 2)

Table 2. American Society of Anesthesiologists Classification*

ASA Class	Class Definition	Rates of PPCs by Class %
I	A normally healthy patient	1.2
II	A patient with mild systemic disease	5.4
III	A patient with systemic disease that's not incapacitating	11.4
IV	A patient with an incapacitating systemic disease that is a constant threat to life	10.9
V	A moribund patient who is not expected to survive for 24 hours with or without operation	NA

*Information is from reference 9. ASA — American Society of Anesthesiologists; NA — not applicable; PPC — postoperative pulmonary complication.
Reproduced with permission from Qaseem *et al.* (2006) *Ann Intern Med* **144**: 575–580.

- Congestive heart failure (CHF)
- General health status
- COPD
- Smoking

According to the American College of Physicians (ACP) evidence-based review, age is an independent risk factor for PPCs. Patients greater than or equal to 80 years of age demonstrate an odds ratio of 5.63 for developing PPCs. Functional status and ASA class strongly influence PPC risk. Patients with mild systemic disease (ASA class II) have a 2.55 odds ratio for developing PPCs compared to patients in ASA class I. Similarly, moribund patients who are not expected to survive without surgery (ASA class V) have an odds ratio of 4.87 for developing PPCs. Functional dependency is also associated with increased risk. Total dependence, defined as the inability to perform activities of daily living, predicted PPCs with an odds ratio of 2.51. COPD, smoking history and CHF also affect risk, albeit more modestly.

Recently, Johnson and colleagues[12] published a preoperative risk index for predicting postoperative respiratory failure. New risk factors that were not identified in the ACP guidelines were sepsis, ascites, creatinine >1.5 mg/dL and dyspnea.

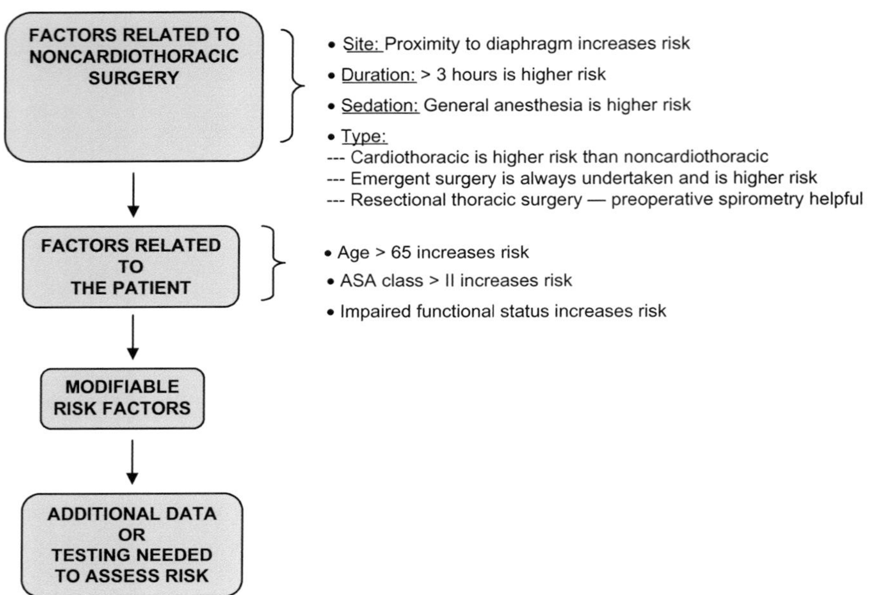

Fig. 1. Practical approach to the preoperative pulmonary evaluation

A Practical Approach to Preoperative Assessment of Patients with Pulmonary Disease

A practical approach to the preoperative assessment of patients with pulmonary disease can be undertaken by asking several logical questions about the patient who will be having surgery (Fig. 1):

1. What type of procedure will the patient be having?
2. What are the comorbid illnesses of the patient who will be going to surgery?
3. Does the patient have risk factors which can be modified to reduce postoperative risk?
4. Are additional data required to assess the patient's risk and to determine whether they will tolerate the surgery?

The Procedure

Surgical procedures may be classified into several different types. They may be elective or nonelective. They may also be classified according to the site of the procedure: cardiothoracic or noncardiothoracic surgery. The risk of postoperative complications from noncardiothoracic surgery is reduced in comparison with cardiothoracic surgery. Thoracic surgery is a type of cardiothoracic surgery, and can be further subclassified into resectional thoracic and nonresectional thoracic surgery.

Preoperative pulmonary risk assessment is not helpful for urgent nonelective surgery. Nonelective surgery, by definition, must be undertaken regardless of risk.

Preoperative spirometry can be helpful for certain subgroups of patients. Resectional thoracic surgery is precluded if the predicted postoperative lung function is too minimal to support an independent lifestyle and resumption of activities of daily living after surgery. Guidelines from the American College of Chest Physicians and the British Thoracic Society suggest that patients with a preoperative FEV1 in excess of 2 L (or >80% predicted) generally tolerate pneumonectomy, whereas those with a preoperative FEV1 greater than 1.5 L tolerate lobectomy. However, if there is either undue exertional dyspnea or coexistent interstitial lung disease, then measurement of DLCO should also be performed. Patients with preoperative results for FEV1 and DLCO that are both >80% predicted do not need further physiological testing. Preoperative spirometry does not predict PPC risk in patients undergoing nonresectional thoracic surgery.

Comorbid Illnesses

Factors such as advanced age, COPD, smoking, general health status and certain metabolic factors increase PPC risk. Risk factors should be modified to reduce the likelihood of postoperative complications. Certain patients may require preoperative testing. Only the most common conditions encountered in the preoperative evaluation will be discussed.

Modifiable Risk Factors in Patients with Specific Conditions

A complete history and physical exam are prerequisites for the preoperative evaluation of patients with pulmonary disease. Important historical features are the following: age, functional capacity, general health, smoking status and the presence of comorbid illnesses such as obstructive sleep apnea (OSA), chronic obstructive pulmonary disease (COPD), congestive heart failure (CHF) and asthma. Examination should focus on the cardiopulmonary system. Preoperative testing may be required in certain patients.

Patients with dyspnea

Dyspnea, the subjective experience of breathing discomfort, is a common symptom. Preoperative testing is necessary in certain instances. Pulmonary function testing can diagnose airflow obstruction or restrictive lung disease. Chest radiography may detect pneumonia, heart failure or interstitial lung disease. An echocardiogram may diagnose ventricular dysfunction or pulmonary hypertension. Severe anemia is a common cause of dyspnea. In complex cases where other test results are equivocal, cardiopulmonary exercise testing may distinguish between cardiac and pulmonary causes of dyspnea or whether deconditioning is present. It is important to determine the cause of dyspnea, so that patients can be given effective treatments for optimization prior to surgery.

Asthma

Poorly controlled asthma, as demonstrated by wheezing prior to surgery, may increase the risk of PPCs.[13,14] One study showed that the use of asthma medications and emergency room visits in the 30 days prior to surgery influence PPC risk.[14]

Preoperative corticosteroids and inhaled beta agonists markedly decrease the incidence of bronchospasm after tracheal intubation.[13,14.] But whether corticosteroids reduce PPC risk is unknown. The risk of PPCs is low in asthmatic patients undergoing surgery and may be comparably low to that of the general surgical population.[15] Several studies have demonstrated that preoperative corticosteroids do not increase the risk of postoperative infections or delay wound healing.[15,16] Regardless, asthmatics should be free of wheezes or be at their baseline lung exam, have no cough or dyspnea, and have peak expiratory flow rates greater than 80% of baseline prior to surgery.

Chronic obstructive pulmonary disease

Chronic obstructive pulmonary disease (COPD) increases the risk of PPCs.[9] The more severe the COPD, the more severe the risk. However, the severity of COPD and, therefore, postoperative risk cannot be correlated directly with the reduction in FEV1 and/or DLCO. While spirometry may be useful for assessing disease severity and adequacy of bronchodilator therapy, the stratification of patients according to risk is primarily determined by history and physical examination. There is little or no role for preoperative pulmonary function testing.

Preoperative antibiotics do not reduce PPC risk in COPD patients. Inhaled anticholintergics, long-acting beta agonists and inhaled corticosteroids may ameliorate symptoms and improve certain aspects of lung function in symptomatic patients.[17]

Patients with COPD can improve exercise tolerance and reduce dyspnea and fatigue by participating in exercise training programs.[18] Preoperative chest physiotherapy with inspiratory muscle training decreases PPC rates.[19]

Obstructive sleep apnea

It is estimated that 26% of adults are at high risk for obstructive sleep apnea (OSA).[20] The signs and symptoms of OSA are relatively obvious. The Epworth Sleepiness Scale can be used to measure sleepiness and has been validated primarily in OSA,[21] but only the STOP Bang questionnaire has been validated in the preoperative population (Table 3).[22] OSA has implications for anesthesia management and may increase PPC risk.

Table 3. STOP-Bang Questionnaire to Screen for Obstructive Sleep Apnea

1. Snoring
   Do you snore loudly (loud enough to be heard through closed doors}?
2. Tired
   Do you often feel tired, fatigued, or sleepy during daytime?
3. Observed
   Has anyone observed you stop breathing during your sleep?
4. Blood pressure
   Do you have or are you being treated for high blood pressure?
5. BMI
   BMI more than 35 kg/m^2?
6. Age
   Age greater than 50 years?
7. Neck circumference
   Neck circumference greater than 40 cm?
8. Gender
   Gender male?

High risk of OSA: answering YES to 3 or more items, *Low risk of OSA:* answering YES to less than 3 items.
From Chung F, Yegneswaran B, Liao P, *et al.* STOP questionnaire. A tool to screen patients for obstructive sleep apnea. Anesthesiology 2008:108:812; with permssion.
Reproduced with permission from Sweitzer *et al.* (2009) *Med Clin N Am* **93**: 1017–1030.

In addition, patients with OSA may be at increased risk due to a high prevalence of comorbid illnesses, including diabetes, hypertension, atrial fibrillation, bradyarrhythmias, ventricular ectopy, stroke, heart failure, pulmonary hypertension, cardiomyopathy, coronary artery disease and myocardial infarction.[23] They are also prone to several postoperative complications, such as airway obstruction, tachyarrhythmias, hypoxemia, atelectasis, ischemia, pneumonia and prolonged hospitalization.[24]

Patients with OSA should be risk-stratified for surgery, and comorbid conditions should be optimized. Echocardiography may be indicated if CHF or pulmonary hypertension is suspected; however, no data demonstrate that the echocardiogram improves postoperative outcomes. Patients should be encouraged to lose weight. Whether noninvasive positive pressure ventilation improves postoperative outcomes is controversial.[25]

Pulmonary hypertension

Exercise tolerance is strongly associated with PPC risk in patients with pulmonary hypertension. Pulmonary hypertension patients who had a New York Heart Association functional class greater than 2 demonstrated an increased risk of developing PPCs.[26] Similarly, patients who were unable to walk more than 332 m during a 6 min walk test had a higher mortality rate than those who were able to walk the same distance.[27] Echocardiographic findings such as pericardial effusion, the amount and presence of septal shift or an enlarged right atrium were predictors of worse postoperative prognosis. Finally, patients should be vasodilator tested preoperatively, because knowing the response to therapy can help guide management of postoperative complications.

Cigarette use

Smokers are at increased risk for pulmonary and nonpulmonary postoperative complications,[28] and a smoking history of more than 20 pack years predicts greater risk than lesser amounts of smoking.[29] Smokers are more likely than nonsmokers to develop wound infections, oxygen desaturation, laryngospasm and severe coughing with anesthesia.[30]

Cessation of smoking prior to surgery reduces PPC risk but the duration of preoperative abstinence remains controversial. Most experts agree that patients must refrain from smoking two months prior to surgery in order to maximally reduce PPC risk.

Conclusions

The primary objective of the preoperative evaluation of patients with pulmonary disease is to stratify patients according to risk so as to reduce the likelihood of PPCs. Although the routine use of preoperative spirometry and chest radiography is not recommended, patients with certain pulmonary illnesses may require preoperative testing to assess postoperative risk. Certain patients with asthma or COPD may benefit from preoperative corticosteroids. Those with OSA should be encouraged to lose weight prior to surgery. Smokers should refrain from smoking at least two months before surgery to maximally reduce PPC risk.

References

1. Lawrence VA, *et al.* (1996) Risk of pulmonary complications after elective abdominal surgery. *Chest* **110**(3): 744–750.
2. Khuri SF, *et al.* (2005) Determinants of long-term survival after major surgery and the adverse effect of postoperative complications. *Ann Surg* **242**(3): 326–341; discussion 341–343.
3. Fisher BW, Majumdar SR, McAlister FA. (2002) Predicting pulmonary complications after nonthoracic surgery: A systematic review of blinded studies. *Am J Med* **112**(3): 219–225.
4. Gatti G, *et al.* (2002) Predictors of postoperative complications in high-risk octogenarians undergoing cardiac operations. *Ann Thorac Surg* **74**(3): 671–677.
5. Kroenke K, *et al.* (1992) Operative risk in patients with severe obstructive pulmonary disease. *Arch Intern Med* **152**(5): 967–971.
6. Pedersen T, Eliasen K, Henriksen E. (1990) A prospective study of mortality associated with anaesthesia and surgery: Risk indicators of mortality in hospital. *Acta Anaesthesiol Scand* **34**(3): 176–182.
7. Lawrence VA, Cornell JE, Smetana GW. (2006) Strategies to reduce postoperative pulmonary complications after noncardiothoracic surgery: Systematic review for the American College of Physicians. *Ann Intern Med* **144**(8): 596–608.
8. Cook MW, Lisco SJ. (2009) Prevention of postoperative pulmonary complications. *Int Anesthesiol Clin* **47**(4): 65–88.
9. Sweitzer BJ, Smetana GW. (2009) Identification and evaluation of the patient with lung disease. *Med Clin North Am* **93**(5): 1017–1030.

10. Smetana GW, Lawrence VA, Cornell JE. (2006) Preoperative pulmonary risk stratification for noncardiothoracic surgery: Systematic review for the American College of Physicians. *Ann Intern Med* **144**(8): 581–595.
11. Ballantyne JC, *et al.* (1998) The comparative effects of postoperative analgesic therapies on pulmonary outcome: Cumulative meta-analyses of randomized, controlled trials. *Anesth Analg* **86**(3): 598–612.
12. Johnson RG, *et al.* (2007) Multivariable predictors of postoperative respiratory failure after general and vascular surgery: Results from the patient safety in surgery study. *J Am Coll Surg* **204**(6): 1188–1198.
13. Silvanus MT, Groeben H, Peters J. (2004) Corticosteroids and inhaled salbutamol in patients with reversible airway obstruction markedly decrease the incidence of bronchospasm after tracheal intubation. *Anesthesiology* **100**(5): 1052–1057.
14. Warner DO, *et al.* (1996) Perioperative respiratory complications in patients with asthma. *Anesthesiology* **85**(3): 460–467.
15. Su FW, *et al.* (2004) Low incidence of complications in asthmatic patients treated with preoperative corticosteroids. *Allergy Asthma Proc* **25**(5): 327–333.
16. Kabalin CS, Yarnold PR, Grammer LC. (1995) Low complication rate of corticosteroid-treated asthmatics undergoing surgical procedures. *Arch Intern Med* **155**(13): 1379–1384.
17. Qaseem A, *et al.* (2007) Diagnosis and management of stable chronic obstructive pulmonary disease: A clinical practice guideline from the American College of Physicians. *Ann Intern Med* **147**(9): 633–638.
18. Celli B, *et al.* (2006) Improving the care of COPD patients — suggested action points by the COPD exacerbations taskforce for reducing the burden of exacerbations of COPD. *Prim Care Respir J* **15**(3): 139–142.
19. Warner DO. (2000) Preventing postoperative pulmonary complications: The role of the anesthesiologist. *Anesthesiology* **92**(5): 1467–1472.
20. Punjabi, NM. (2008) The epidemiology of adult obstructive sleep apnea. *Proc Am Thorac Soc* **5**(2): 136–143.

21. Sangal RB, Sangal JM, Belisle C. (1999) Subjective and objective indices of sleepiness (ESS and MWT) are not equally useful in patients with sleep apnea. *Clin Electroencephalogr* **30**(2): 73–75.
22. Chung F, *et al.* (2008) STOP questionnaire: A tool to screen patients for obstructive sleep apnea. *Anesthesiology* **108**(5): 812–821.
23. Caples SM, Gami AS, Somers VK. (2005) Obstructive sleep apnea. *Ann Intern Med* **142**(3): 187–197.
24. Hwang D, *et al.* (2008) Association of sleep-disordered breathing with postoperative complications. *Chest* **133**(5): 1128–1134.
25. Crummy F, Piper AJ, Naughton MT. (2008) Obesity and the lung: 2. Obesity and sleep-disordered breathing. *Thorax* **63**(8): 738–746.
26. Ramakrishna G, *et al.* (2005) Impact of pulmonary hypertension on the outcomes of noncardiac surgery: Predictors of perioperative morbidity and mortality. *J Am Coll Cardiol* **45**(10): 1691–1699.
27. Raymond RJ, *et al.* (2002) Echocardiographic predictors of adverse outcomes in primary pulmonary hypertension. *J Am Coll Cardiol* **39**(7): 1214–1219.
28. Warner DO, (2006) Perioperative abstinence from cigarettes: Physiologic and clinical consequences. *Anesthesiology* **104**(2): 356–367.
29. Warner MA, Divertie MB, Tinker JH. (1984) Preoperative cessation of smoking and pulmonary complications in coronary artery bypass patients. *Anesthesiology* **60**(4): 380–383.
30. Myles PS, *et al.* (2002) Risk of respiratory complications and wound infection in patients undergoing ambulatory surgery: Smokers versus nonsmokers. *Anesthesiology* **97**(4): 842–847.

Chapter 88

Perioperative Management of Oral Anticoagulants and Antiplatelet Agents

Ramiro Jervis and Andrew Dunn**

Key Pearls

- Vitamin K antagonist therapy does not need to be interrupted for most patients undergoing cataract, dental, and cutaneous surgeries.
- Patients at low risk for thromboembolic events are unlikely to benefit from perioperative bridging therapy.
- The benefits of perioperative bridging anticoagulation are unlikely to outweigh the risks for most patients at intermediate risk, particularly patients undergoing major surgery.
- For patients at high risk of thromboembolism, full-dose bridging anticoagulation should be started 48–72 hr after major surgery, due to a high risk of bleeding.
- Patients with recently implanted drug eluting or bare metal stents should continue dual antiplatelet therapy uninterrupted for 12 months and 6 weeks, respectively.

Introduction

The perioperative management of patients taking vitamin K antagonists (VKAs) or antiplatelet agents is a common clinical scenario. Continuation of these agents may lead to unnecessary bleeding but interruption may

*Mount Sinai School of Medicine, New York, NY, USA.

lead to a preventable stroke or other thromboembolic complications. Presented below is a rational strategy for weighing the risks and benefits of anticoagulation and antiplatelet therapy perioperatively.

Perioperative Use of Vitamin K Antagonists

VKAs are used for three major indications: atrial fibrillation, mechanical heart valves, and venous thromboembolism. Prior to deciding on a strategy to withhold VKAs, an estimate of the risk of a venous or arterial event must be determined. Extrapolating patients' annual risk of thromboembolic events to their daily risk of post operative complications can be misleading, as patients may be hypercoagulable perioperatively. Perioperative hypercoagulability increases the risk of postoperative venous complications as much as 100-fold. Nonetheless, yearly risk may be used as a guide to determine perioperative risk.

Atrial Fibrillation

The CHADS scoring system assigns one point each for CHF, hypertension, age greater than 75 years, diabetes, and two points for a history of stroke or TIA.[1] This simple tool can predict the yearly risk of arterial thromboembolic events and help stratify the risk of an event perioperatively:

- *Low risk*: CHADS score of 0–2
- *Intermediate risk*: CHADS score of 3–4
- *High risk*: CHADS score of 5–6 or arterial thromboembolic event within three months

Mechanical Heart Valves

The estimated annual risk of stroke for mechanical heart valves without anticoagulation has been estimated to be as low as 3% and as high as 15%. Several factors influence the likelihood of a thromboembolic event, including valve position, valve type, and a history of atrial fibrillation or a previous stroke. Though the data vary widely, the best evidence supports the following risk stratification scheme:

- *Low risk*: bileaflet or tilting disk aortic valve without a history of atrial fibrillation, CHF, or stroke
- *Intermediate risk*: bileaflet or tilting disk aortic valve with a history of atrial fibrillation, CHF, or stroke
- *High risk*: any mitral valve, caged ball aortic valve, multiple valves

Venous Thromboembolism

The risk of serious morbidity or mortality from a venous thromboembolic event is substantially lower than for patients at risk for a stroke or other arterial thromboembolic event. In addition, the risk of recurrent DVT or PE can be ameliorated by prophylaxis-dose anticoagulation, which has no proven benefit for arterial events. Patients on VKAs at risk for another DVT or PE may be categorized as follows:

- *Low risk*: single VTE >3 months earlier, less potent thrombophilia (e.g. factor V Leiden mutation or prothrombin gene mutation)
- *Intermediate risk*: recurrent VTE, VTE and history of cancer, VTE and potent thrombophilia (e.g. antithrombin III deficiency or lupus anticoagulant)
- *High risk*: VTE within three months

Bleeding Risk

Postoperative bleeding can lead to serious consequences, including reoperation and death. In addition, patients aggressively bridged to reduce the risk of thromboembolism may have a bleeding event that requires withholding anticoagulation for a longer period of time than would have occurred had a nonbridging strategy been used.

Dental procedures, skin biopsies, ENT and ocular procedures, simple breast surgery, as well as cardiac catheterization and radio frequency ablation, are low risk for perioperative bleeding. In fact, the risk is low (≤1%) even in the presence of therapeutic anticoagulation for dental, cataract, and minor dermatologic procedures. VKA therapy can be continued for these procedures.

In contrast, all major surgeries, which can be defined as surgeries expected to last ≥60 min, have a higher rate of bleeding (as high as 20%) when anticoagulation is restarted soon after surgery.[2] Due to this risk, it is best to delay restarting full-dose anticoagulation for 48–72 hr after major surgery.

Some minor procedures involve highly vascular tissue and are thus at higher risk of bleeding. They include urologic procedures, such as transurethral resection of the prostate or bladder resection, and pacemaker or implantable cardioversion device implantation. When perioperative anticoagulation is required due to a high risk of thromboembolism, these procedures require a bridging strategy similar for patients after major surgery, including cessation of warfarin five days prior to surgery and delaying restarting full-dose parenteral anticoagulation for 48–72 hr after the procedure.

Optimal Strategies for Bridging: Recommendations

For minor procedures with low bleeding risk (i.e. dental extraction, superficial dermatologic procedures, cataracts), patients may continue with their usual full-dose VKA therapy as the risk of bleeding is low.

Patients at lowest thromboembolic risk groups do not require bridging anticoagulation; the VKA should be stopped five days prior to the procedure and restarted on the night of surgery.

The optimal strategy is less clear for patients at intermediate risk for thromboembolic events. Given the lack of randomized trials proving a benefit and the potential harm of full-dose anticoagulation perioperatively, particularly for patients undergoing major surgery, full-dose bridging is not recommended for most patients in this subgroup. Intermediate risk patients on long-term VKA due to prior venous events may benefit from prophylaxis-dose anticoagulation, which has been shown in other settings to substantially reduce the risk of events and carries a low bleeding risk, and will cause less bleeding than therapeutic dose regimens.

Bridging with heparin or LMWH should be offered to patients at the highest risk for venous or arterial thromboembolic events (see Table 1).

Optimal Bridging Therapy: Logistics

The VKA should be held five days prior to the date of the procedure or surgery. VKAs may be restarted on the night of surgery, provided that hemostasis is adequate.

Bridging with unfractionated heparin (UFH) or LMWH is started two days prior to surgery. As the half-life of intravenous UFH is short, this medication can be discontinued 4 hr prior to the procedure.[3] The elimination

Table 1. Perioperative Management of Vitamin K Antagonists

Thromboembolictic Risk	Management Strategy
Low	*No bridging.* Hold anticoagulation 5 days prior.
Intermediate	*Minor Surgery or Low Bleeding Risk:* No bridging suggested for most patients. Given low risk of major bleeding, bridging can be reasonable for select patients. *Major or High Bleeding Risk Surgery:* Bridging not recommended for most patients given risk of bleeding. Strategy should be tailored to individual risk factors and patient preference. Consider prophylaxis dose bridging for patients with VTE history.
High	*Minor Surgery or Low Bleeding Risk:* Bridging recommended *Major or High Bleeding Risk Surgery:* Bridging recommended. Post-operative full-dose anticoagulation should be delayed 48–72 hr after major surgery due to the risk of major bleeding.

*BMS — bare metal stent; DES — drug-eluting stent.

half-life of LMWH is such that its effect may persist up to 24 hr; hence the last preoperative LMWH dose should be administered no later than the morning of the day before surgery. If a once-daily therapeutic dose is being utilized, then the final preoperative dose should be one-half the daily dose to decrease the risk of an anticoagulant effect being present when surgery begins.

For minor surgery, IV UFH or full-dose LMWH can be restarted 12–24 hr after surgery, which often is the morning after surgery. Following major surgery, postoperative bridging may lead to significant bleeding risk when restarted in that timeframe. For these patients, full-dose UFH or LMWH should be delayed for at least 48–72 hr to minimize the risk.

Antiplatelet Therapy

Risk Stratification

Patients should be stratified by their risk of cardiac or cerebrovascular events. This risk stratification is summarized as follows:

- *Low risk*: patients on antiplatelet medications for primary prophylaxis
- *Intermediate risk*: patients on antiplatelet medications after a prior vascular event or with known atherosclerotic disease
- *High risk*: patients with a bare metal stent (BMS) placed within 6 weeks or a drug-eluting stent (DES) within 12 months.

Risks of Antiplatelet Interruption

Patients on aspirin for primary prophylaxis are at low annual and low perioperative risk for an acute coronary event. Patients with a history of vascular disease or a prior event, however, are at higher risk, particularly when aspirin is discontinued.[4] One randomized study suggested a nearly five-fold greater risk of a cardiac event when aspirin therapy was interrupted.[5]

Patients with a recent BMS or DES are at the highest risk for a cardiac event. For these patients, interruption of aspirin and thienopyridine prior to stent endotheliazation at 6 weeks or 12 months for BMS or DES, respectively leads to poor outcomes.[6–8] The potentially catastrophic outcomes of in-stent thrombosis include myocardial infarction and death. Interruption of dual antiplatelet therapy (DAPT) after a duration of 6 months may be safe in patients with third generation stents and without unstable disease or extensive/complex CAD; a prospective cohort suggests that everolimus coronary stents carry a low risk of stent thrombosis with DAPT interruption after 6 months.[9] Discussion with the patient's cardiologist will be essential to properly weigh the benefits and risks when considering discontinuing DAPT at a duration of less than 12 months for patients with a DES.

Perioperative Bleeding Risk

The risk of major bleeding is low for certain superficial and minor surgeries, including dental, dermatologic, and cataract procedures.[10–14] The perioperative bleeding risk of thienopyridines is unclear, but is likely not dramatically different than the risk of aspirin monotherapy. The bleeding risk of dual therapy is clearly higher.

The risk of bleeding perioperatively for major surgery with aspirin monotherapy is also low.[15] The Pulmonary Embolism Prevention (PEP) trial examined the use of aspirin to prevent venous thromboembolism for patients undergoing hip fracture or hip or knee replacement surgery. Patients receiving aspirin had no increase in fatal or wound-related bleeding but had more gastrointestinal bleeding and were more likely to require transfusion (2.4% vs. 2.9%).[16] Overall, the majority of evidence suggests an increased risk of bleeding of questionable clinical significance with perioperative antiplatelet therapy.

Recommendations for Perioperative Management of Antiplatelet Therapy

Patients on aspirin for primary prophylaxis are at low risk for an acute coronary event and can have the antiplatelet agent held for seven days prior to surgery.

Table 2. Perioperative antiplatelet Management

Ischemic Risk	Examples	Strategy
Low	Primary prevention (no history of vascular disease)	Hold aspirin 7 days prior
Intermediate	History of atherosclerosis; (cardiovascular, peripheral vascular or cerebrovascular disease)	*Low bleeding risk*: Continue aspirin and/or thienopyridine. *Moderate or high bleeding risk:* Hold aspirin and thienopyridine agent at least 7 and 5 days prior, respectively. Consider continuing aspirin if bleeding risk not excessive
High	Recent coronary stent placement (BMS within 6 weeks or DES within 12 months)*	Delay surgery until 6 weeks after BMS or 12 months after DES implantation. Consider continuing aspirin and thienopyridine if surgery cannot be delayed and bleeding risk not prohibitive. Consultation with cardiologist if considering withholding dual anti-platelet therapy prior to 12 months for patients with a DES.

*BMS — bare metal stent; DES — drug-eluting stent.

For patients at intermediate risk of an ischemic event, aspirin or thienopyridines may be continued during procedures with low bleeding risk (i.e. dental extraction, superficial dermatologic procedures, cataracts). Patients on both antiplatelet agents undergoing minor procedures who have not had a recent DES or BMS placed can have the thienopyridine agent held and undergo the procedure while continuing with aspirin.

For patients at intermediate risk for an ischemic event who are undergoing major surgery, clinicians can consider continuing aspirin perioperatively. The risks and benefits should be individualized, though the overall risk of bleeding is likely to be low for most surgeries.

Patients at the highest risk for ischemic events (recent DES or BMS) should remain on dual antiplatelet therapy for at least 12 months and

6 weeks, respectively, and elective surgery delayed until antiplatelet therapy can be withheld safely.[6] Whenever DAPT is interrupted in patients at high risk for ischemic events, aspirin should continue perioperatively unless bleeding risk is considered excessive. If surgery cannot be delayed, DAPT should be continued when possible as the risk of in-stent thrombosis outweights the increased risk of bleeding for most patients. The period of time in which DAPT should be continued can potentially be decreased in patients with certain 3rd generation stents in consultation with the patient's cardiologist.

References

1. Gage BF, Waterman AD, Shannon W, *et al.* (2001) Validation of clinical classification schemes for predicting stroke: Results from the National Registry of Atrial Fibrillation. *Jama* **285**(22): 2864–2870.
2. Dunn AS, Spyropoulos AC and Turpie AG. (2007) Bridging therapy in patients on long-term oral anticoagulants who require surgery: The Prospective Peri-operative Enoxaparin Cohort Trial (PROSPECT). *J Thromb Haemost* **5**(11): 2211–2218.
3. Douketis JD, Berger PB, Dunn AS, *et al.* (2008) The perioperative management of antithrombotic therapy: American College of Chest Physicians Evidence-Based Clinical Practice Guidelines (8th Edition). *Chest* **133**(6 Suppl): 299S–339S.
4. Burger W, Chemnitius JM, Kneissl GD and Rucker G. (2005) Low-dose aspirin for secondary cardiovascular prevention: Cardiovascular risks after its perioperative withdrawal versus bleeding risks with its continuation — review and meta-analysis. *J Intern Med* **257**(5): 399–414.
5. Oscarsson A, Gupta A, Fredrikson M, *et al.* To continue or discontinue aspirin in the perioperative period: A randomized, controlled clinical trial. *Br J Anaesth* **104**(3): 305–312.
6. Grines CL, Bonow RO, Casey DE Jr, *et al.* (2007) Prevention of premature discontinuation of dual antiplatelet therapy in patients with coronary artery stents: A science advisory from the American

Heart Association, American College of Cardiology, Society for Cardiovascular Angiography and Interventions, American College of Surgeons, and American Dental Association, with representation from the American College of Physicians. *Circulation* **115**(6): 813–818.

7. Kaluza GL, Joseph J, Lee JR, *et al.* (2000) Catastrophic outcomes of noncardiac surgery soon after coronary stenting. *J Am Coll Cardiol* **35**(5): 1288–1294.
8. Sharma AK, Ajani AE, Hamwi SM, *et al.* (2004) Major noncardiac surgery following coronary stenting: When is it safe to operate? *Catheter Cardiovasc Interv* **63**(2): 141–145.
9. Krucoff MW, Rutledge DR, Gruberg L, *et al.* (2011) A new era of prospective real-world saftey evaluation: Primary Report of XIENCE v USA. JACC: *Cardiovas Intervent* **4**(12): 1298–1309.
10. Madan GA, Madan SG, Madan G and Madan AD. (2005) Minor oral surgery without stopping daily low-dose aspirin therapy: A study of 51 patients. *J Oral Maxillofac Surg* **63**(9): 1262–1265.
11. Brennan MT, Valerin MA, Noll JL, *et al.* (2008) Aspirin use and post-operative bleeding from dental extractions. *J Dent Res* **87**(8): 740–744.
12. Napenas JJ, Hong CH, Brennan MT, *et al.* (2009) The frequency of bleeding complications after invasive dental treatment in patients receiving single and dual antiplatelet therapy. *J Am Dent Assoc* **140**(6): 690–695.
13. Krishnan B, Shenoy NA, Alexander M. (2008) Exodontia and antiplatelet therapy. *J Oral Maxillofac Surg* **66**(10): 2063–2066.
14. Bartlett GR. (1999) Does aspirin affect the outcome of minor cutaneous surgery? *Br J Plast Surg* **52**(3): 214–216.
15. Belisle S, Hardy JF. (1996) Hemorrhage and the use of blood products after adult cardiac operations: Myths and realities. *Ann Thorac Surg* **62**(6): 1908–1917.
16. Prevention of pulmonary embolism and deep vein thrombosis with low dose aspirin: Pulmonary Embolism Prevention (PEP) trial. *Lancet* **355**(9212): 1295–1302.

Chapter 89

Postoperative Fever

*Dennis Chang**

Key Pearls

- The majority of postoperative fevers that occur in the first 72 hr are benign.
- There have been no studies correlating atelectasis with postoperative fever.
- The most common infectious causes of postoperative fever are surgical site infections, urinary tract infections and hospital-acquired or ventilator-associated pneumonia.
- A useful mnemonic for postoperative fever is the "four Ws": Wind (pulmonary); Water (urine); Wound; What did we do?
- Not all postoperative fevers are due to infectious causes. Do not forget about gout, pulmonary embolism, drug fever and alcohol withdrawal.

Background

Postoperative fever is a common event after surgery, with published incidence rates ranging from 14% to 91%.[1] The majority of fevers that occur in the first several days postoperatively are benign, and workups for these early fevers are often expensive and unnecessary. In one study of gynecologic-surgical patients, routine infectious workups cost a total

*Mount Sinai School of Medicine, New York, NY, USA.

of US$2201 per serious infection diagnosed, and in another study the cost was US$3946 per bloodstream infection diagnosed.[2,3] Therefore, it is critical to understand the infectious and noninfectious causes of postoperative fever and how these causes change depending on the timing of the fever.

Timing of Fever

The timing of a postoperative fever is essential to diagnosing the cause of fever and can be organized into four categories:

- Immediate 0–4 hr postoperatively
- Acute 4 hr to 1 week postoperatively
- Subacute 1–4 weeks postoperatively
- Delayed >1 month postoperatively

Immediate

Fevers in the immediate postoperative period are typically noted by the anesthesiologist and the surgical team, and include:

- Infection present prior to surgery
- Reaction to medications or blood transfusions
- Inflammation secondary to the trauma of surgery itself
- Malignant hyperthermia

Malignant Hyperthermia

The most common triggering agents for malignant hyperthermia are succinylcholine and inhaled anesthetics (halothane, isoflurane, enflurane, sevoflurane, desflurane). The onset of symptoms usually begins within 30 min of administration but has also been reported after the cessation of anesthesia. The clinical signs are masseter muscle rigidity or spasm, and hyperthermia. The acute treatment is discontinuation of the offending agent, and treatment of hyperthermia with cooling measures and dantrolene.

Acute Postoperative Fever

Acute postoperative fever is typically defined as any fever within the first week postoperatively. However, a more practical approach is to think of early postoperative fever and late postoperative fever.

Early Postoperative Fever (First 72 hr Postoperatively)

The majority of postoperative fevers that occur within the first 72 hrs postoperatively are benign and resolve without any treatment. In a study by Lesperance *et al.* 245 out of 1032 post surgical patients had an early postoperative fever of greater than 100.4°F. Only 18 (7%) of these 245 patients had an infectious cause of their fever, and in 9 of these patients the physical exam and clinical picture would have accurately diagnosed the infection without further testing.[4] In a study by de la Torre *et al.* 29% of postoperative patients had an early postoperative fever and only 11% of these had an infectious cause of their fever.[2] Ward *et al.* evaluated 1100 patients undergoing total joint arthroplasty, and out of the 161 patients who had a fever only 13% had a positive fever evaluation. They found the following independent predictors of a positive workup: fever occurring after postoperative day 3 [odds ratio (OR), 23.3], multiple febrile days (OR 8.6) and maximum fever greater than 39.0°C (OR 2.4).[5]

Based on the above studies, the following approach should be taken in the early postoperative period. First, a thorough history and physical should be obtained to look for signs and symptoms of infection. Special attention should be paid to the following:

- Preoperative course:
    - Any signs of infection prior to the operation
- Operative course
    - Perioperative drug administration
    - Perioperative blood product transfusions
    - Any complications during surgery

- Physical examination:
  - Surgical site
  - Extremities — look for signs of deep vein thrombosis or gout
  - Skin — any rashes which may be a sign of drug reaction or cellulitis
  - Foreign bodies — urinary catheters, intravascular catheters, nasogastric tubes

Appropriate workup should be undertaken based on the history, symptoms and exam findings. If no infectious signs and symptoms are present, there is no need to pursue further diagnostic workup and the patient may be observed. The majority of these early postoperative fevers will resolve on their own without intervention. However, certain groups have a higher incidence of infection postoperatively. High risk patients in one study were patients with preoperative infection, immunodeficiency, indwelling vascular access, mechanical heart valves, bowel operation and admission to an intensive care unit.[6]

Although the majority of early postoperative fevers are benign, approximately 10% have an infectious cause (Table 1). The most common infectious causes of early postoperative fever are surgical site infection, urinary tract infection and pneumonia. In the landmark study by Garibaldi, 42%, 33% and 21% of postoperative infections were caused by surgical site infection, urinary tract infection and pneumonia, respectively.[9] A useful mneumonic is the "four Ws":

- Wind: pulmonary causes — pneumonia, pulmonary embolism, aspiration
- Water: urinary tract infection
- Wound: surgical site infection
- "What did we do?": drug fever, blood product reaction, catheter infections

It is also important to note that not all fevers are infectious. For example, fever is often seen in gout and acute venous thrombosis. It is important to consider the noninfectious causes of postoperative fever listed in Table 1.

Table 1. Causes of Postoperative Fever

Infectious Causes	**Comments**
Surgical site infection (SSI)	• Most dangerous is myonecrosis, which is caused by *Clostridium perfringens* or group A streptococci; this is a surgical emergency requiring immediate debridement. • Typically seen on postoperative day 4 or later.
Urinary tract infection	• Foley catheters should be removed as soon as possible.
Catheter-related infections	
Pneumonia	• Aspiration • Hospital-acquired • Ventilator associated
Clostridium difficile	• Community acquired (present prior to surgery) • Even a few doses of prophylactic antiobiotics prior to surgery can cause *C. difficile*.
Acalculous cholecystitis	• Surgery is the 2nd-most-common cause of acalculous cholecystitis. No. 1 is trauma.[7]
Intra-abdominal abscess / anastomotic leak	• Patients with nasogastric tubes are at high risk.
Sinusitis	
Infection present prior to surgery	
Parotitis	• Secondary to dehydration and poor food intake.
Viral infections from blood products	• Delayed fever period (>1 month after surgery) • Cytomegalovirus (CMV), hepatitis viruses, human immunodeficiency virus (HIV) • Rarely, parasitic infections (toxoplasmosis, babesiosis, malaria)
Infective endocarditis	• Subacute to delayed fever period (weeks to months postoperatively)
Noninfectious Causes	
Acute gout	• >90% postsurgical gout occurs in the lower extremities.[8]
Pulmonary embolism / Deep vein thrombosis	• Surgical patients are at high risk for thrombosis.

(*Continued*)

Table 1. *(Continued)*

Infectious Causes	Comments
Myocardial infarction	
Alcohol or illicit drug withdrawal	
Pancreatitis	• Especially after abdominal surgery
Drug fever	• Most commonly antibiotics (β-lactams, sulfa), H2 blockers, phenytoin, heparin (see also Table 2) • Neuroleptic malignant syndrome • Serotonin syndrome
Thrombophlebitis	
Cerebral infarction / hemorrhage	
Subarachnoid hemorrhage	
Adrenal insufficiency	

Atelectasis

Contrary to popular belief, there have been no studies correlating atelectasis with postoperative fever. In a study by Engoren, 100 postoperative cardiac surgery patients had daily chest radiographs and had continous temperature measurements via a bladder thermometry. The number of patients with fever decreased over time, while the incidence of atelectasis increased over time.[10] Postoperative fever should not be ascribed to atelectasis.

Late Postoperative Fever (72 hr to 1 Week Postoperatively)

The most common causes of a late postoperative fever are surgical site infections, urinary tract infections and hospital-acquired or ventilator-associated pneumonia. Fevers that begin in this period are much less likely to be benign and a thorough search for both infectious and noninfectious causes of postoperative fever should be undertaken (Table 1).

Table 2. Drug-induced Fever

Category	Common Drugs
Antimicrobials	*Penicillins*: ampicillin, cloxacillin, nafcillin, oxacillin, penicillin, piperacillin, ticarcillin *Cephalosporins*: cefazolin, cefotaxime, ceftazidime, cephalexin, *Antiviral*: acyclovir *Antifungal*: amphotericin B *Urinary tract agents*: trimethoprim-sulfamethoxazole, nitrofurantoin *Miscellaneous*: declomycin, erythromycin, furadantin, isoniazid, minocycline, novobiocin, rifampin, streptomycin, terramycin, tetracycline, vancomycin
Antineoplastic agents	Mercaptopurine, bleomycin, chlorambucil, cisplatin, cytosine arabinoside, daunorubicin, hydroxyurea, interferon, L-asparaginase, procarbazine, streptozocin, vincristine, azathioprine, cyclophophamide, cytarabine
Cardiovascular agents	Clofibrate, diltiazem, dobutamine, furosemide, heparin, hydrochlorothiazide, methyldopa, procainamide, quinidine, triameterene, hydralazine, nifedipine, labetalol
Immunosuppressant	Azathioprine, mycophenolate mofetil, sirolimus
Symphathomimetic and hallucinogenic agents	Amphetamine, lysergic acid, methamphetamine
Antiseizure	Carbamazepine, phenytoin
Antidepressants	Fluoxetine
Other	NSAIDS, allopurinol, cimetidine, folate, iodide, mebendazole, metoclopramide, propylthiouracil, prostaglandin, ritodrine, sulfasalazine, theophylline, theophylline, thyroxine

Subacute Fever (1–4 Weeks Postoperatively)

During this time period, bacterial infections continue to be the most likely cause of fever. The most common infectious causes are surgical site infections, intravascular catheter infections and *Clostridium difficile*. Febrile drug reactions and deep vein thrombosis are the most common noninfectious causes of subacute postoperative fever.

Table 3. Common Causes of Postoperative Fever for Specific Surgeries

Surgery	Infection	Comments
Cardiothoracic surgery	• Pneumonia	• >5% of post-cardiac-surgery patients develop pneumonia.[11]
	• Mediastinitis	• Incidence 1–5%. • *S. aureus* positive blood cultures should raise the possibility of mediastinitis. • Cultures may be positive prior to wounds showing signs of infection.
	• Postpericardiotomy syndrome	• Days to weeks after surgery • Similar to postmyocardial infarction pericarditis
Neurosurgery	• Meningitis	• Infectious or chemical
	• Thermoregulation disruption	• After hypothalamic surgery
Transplant	• Reactivation of viral or protozoan infection • Organ rejection	
Vascular surgery	• Graft infection	• Usually immediately after • Rarely can be months/years later
	• Postimplantation syndrome	• Severe inflammatory response syndrome (SIRS) after endovascular aortic stent placement • Can occur days after implantation[12] • Usually self-limited
Obstetric/gynecologic Surgery	• Postpartum endometritis • Pelvic thrombophlebitis	
Urologic surgery	• Lumbar spine infection	• Rare • Post–lower urinary tract infection • Infection spreads through Baston's venous plexus to lumbar spine

Delayed (>1 Month Postoperatively)

Delayed postoperative fevers are also usually caused by infection but the infections tend to be from indolent organisms, including:

- Viral infections from blood products
  - Cytomegalovirus (CMV)
  - Hepatitis viruses
  - Human immunodeficiency virus (HIV)
  - Rarely, parasitic infections (toxoplasmosis, babesiosis, malaria)
- Surgical site infections
- Infective endocarditis

Postoperative Fever in Specific Surgeries

Besides the infectious and noninfectious causes of postoperative fever, there are specific causes of postoperative fever unique to each surgery. Listed in Table 3 are common surgeries and their associated infections.

Summary

Postoperative fever can be benign or a sign of a life-threatening infection. The key to deciding the significance of a postoperative fever is a thorough history and physical, a thorough understanding of the infectious and non-infectious causes of postoperative fevers and knowing how long after surgery the fever occurs.

References

1. Dellinger EP. (2004) Approach to the patient with postoperative fever. In: SL Gorbach, JG Bartlett, NR Blacklow (eds). *Infectious Diseases*, 3rd ed. Lippincott Williams & Wilkins, Philadelphia, PA, pp. 817–822.
2. de la Torre SH, Mandel L, Goff BA. (2003) Evaulation of postoperative fever: Usefulness and cost-effectiveness of routine work-up. *Am J Obstet Gynecol* **188**: 1642–1647.

3. Lee JJ, Martin DR. (2010) The efficacy of blood culture in postoperative patients. *Am Surg* **76**(10): 1172–1175.
4. Lesperance R, Lehman R, Lesperance K, et al. (2010) Early postoperative fever and the "routine" fever work-up: Results of a prospective study. *J Surg Res*. In press. Available online May 11, 2010.
5. Ward DT, Hansen EN, Takemoto SK, Bozic KJ. (2010) Cost and effectiveness of postoperative fever diagnostic evaluation in total joint arthroplasty patients. *Arthroplasty* **25**(6) (Suppl 1): 43–48.
6. Kendrick JE, Numnum TM, Estes JM, *et al.* (2008). Conservative management of postoperative fever in gynecologic patients undergoing major abdominal or vaginal operations. *J Am Coll Surg* **207**: 393–397.
7. Huffman JL, Schenker S. (2009) Acute acalculous cholecystitis: A review. *Clin Gastroenterol Hepatol* **8**: 15–22.
8. Kang EH, Lee EY, Lee YJ, *et al.* (2008) Clinical features and risk factors of postsurgical gout. *Ann Rheum Dis* **67**: 1271–1275.
9. Garibaldi RA, Brodine S, Matsumiya S, Coleman M. (1985) Evidence for the non-infectious etiology of early postoperative fever. *Infect Control* **6**(7): 273–277.
10. Engoren M. (1995) Lack of association between atelectasis and fever. *Chest* **107**: 81–84.
11. Leal-Noval SR, Rincón-Ferrari MD, García-Curiel A, *et al.* (2001) Transfusion of blood components and postoperative infection in patients undergoing cardiac surgery. *Chest* **119**: 1461–1468.
12. Arnaoutoglou E, Papas N, Milionis H, *et al.* (2010). Post-implantation syndrome after endovascular repair of aortic aneurysms: Need for postdischarge surveillance. *Interact Cardiovasc Thorac Surg* **11**: 449–454.

Pain Management

Chapter 90

Hospital-based Opioid Analgesia

*Jay R. Horton**

Key Pearls

- Pain management and appropriate diagnostic and therapeutic efforts may occur simultaneously. There is no scientific basis for leaving pain untreated to aid in diagnosis.
- There is no standard dosing regimen that will work for all patients. The treatment plan must be individualized.
- Dosing frequencies are determined by considering both the time-to-peak effect and the duration of analgesia. The minimum time between doses should allow for observation of analgesia, sedation, and respiratory depression before the next dose is administered, and the maximum time should be no greater than the average duration of analgesia.
- Patients should be reassessed frequently to monitor analgesia and adverse effects.
- Patient and family education is essential in order to address concerns and misconceptions about opioids, as these widely held beliefs can be major barriers to the successful treatment of pain.

Introduction

Pain is the leading reason for hospital visits.[1] Pain assessment and management in hospitalized patients can be challenging, as pain is a highly subjective experience with both sensory and emotional aspects. Opioids

* Mount Sinai School of Medicine, New York, NY, USA.

can be a safe and effective means of managing moderate-to-severe acute postoperative cancer pain and chronic noncancer pain in hospitalized patients when prescribed according to accepted guidelines.[2–4] Table 1 provides definitions that are important for understanding opioid analgesia.

Inadequate pain control has serious consequences, including the conversion of acute, postoperative, cancer and chronic noncancer pain,

Table 1. Definitions

Term	Definition
Acute pain	Pain caused by injury that usually ceases when the injury heals.
Addiction	A chronic disease that may include the following behaviors: impaired control of drug use, compulsive use, continued use despite harm, and craving. It does not usually occur due solely to pain management with opioids. The incidence of addiction in patients prescribed opioids for pain with no history of substance abuse is less than 1%.[9] The prevalence of addiction in patients with pain is estimated to be approximately the same as that in the general population.[9] Screening tools are available, such as the Opioid Risk Tool[5] and the Revised Screener and Opioid Assessment for Patients with Pain[6] to help identify patients who should be referred or comanaged, not to exclude patients from appropriate pain treatment.
Adjuvant analgesics	Drugs that are usually prescribed for a condition other than pain, but that have analgesic effects for particular types of pain as well.
Breakthrough pain	An increase in pain that "breaks through" otherwise well-controlled pain.
Chronic pain	Pain that persists longer than is anticipated. Often considered to be pain lasting beyond 3 months.
Modified-release opioids	Oral or transdermal opioids that are formulated to gradually release medication into the bloodstream and are sometimes referred to as sustained-release, extended-release, or controlled-release.[9] The duration of action ranges from 8 hr to 72 hr. These medications must never be crushed, cut, or chewed, as that can cause the opioid to be delivered more rapidly and result in an overdose.

(Continued)

Table 1. (*Continued*)

Term	Definition
Multimodal analgesia	The use of a combination of analgesics that target different parts of the pain pathway with the goal of improved analgesia and reduced side effects with lower doses of the individual agents.[9]
Neuropathic pain	Pain that is caused or facilitated by damage to the central or peripheral nervous system. Neuropathic pain may sometimes be treated effectively with nonopioid or opioid analgesics, but often requires adjuvant therapy.
Nociceptive pain	Pain caused by an insult to tissue that causes damage or is potentially damaging and is then transmitted normally by the peripheral and central nervous systems. Nociceptive pain often responds to nonopioid and opioid analgesics.
Nonopioid analgesics	Acetaminophen and NSAIDs.
Opioid analgesics	A class of analgesics that are mu receptor agonists.
Physical dependence	A normal response to taking regular doses of opioids that usually appears after approximately 2 weeks. Reducing, stopping, or antagonizing opioids in patients who are physically dependent on opioids may cause withdrawal, characterized by anxiety, pain, nausea, vomiting, and other symptoms, but this does not mean that the patient is addicted to opioids (see "Addiction," above).
Pseudoaddiction	Behaviors that are reminiscent of addiction, but are caused by inadequate pain treatment and disappear or diminish with more adequate analgesia.
Short-acting opioids	Oral formulations of opioids that have not been modified to be extended-, controlled-, or sustained-release. They may come as tablets, capsules, or elixirs.
Tolerance	A normal response manifested by decreased analgesic or adverse effects occurring after initiation of a new opioid or an increased dose. The time to onset of tolerance is variable but is usually a few days to 2 weeks. For practical purposes, one may assume that it occurs after approximately 7 days. Decreased analgesia may be treated with an increased dose of the opioid, but if tolerance occurs after the patient has been on a stable dose of the opioid, it may be a sign of new or worsening pathology.

anxiety, depression, isolation, cognitive and functional impairment, falls, sleep disturbance, anorexia, decreased quality of life, and increased healthcare utilization.[9,10]

Treatment Model

The World Health Organization (WHO) analgesic ladder, originally published in the 1980s, provides an overall strategy for the medical management of pain and describes the role of opioid analgesics in that strategy based on pain severity.[8,9,15] Meta-analyses have demonstrated that the WHO analgesic ladder is an effective means of controlling cancer and noncancer pain.[2,3] A description of the steps of the WHO analgesic ladder can be found in Table 2.[8,9,15]

Table 2. Pain Management Strategy Based on the WHO Analgesic Ladder

Step	Nonopioids (acetaminophen or NSAIDs)	Adjuvants	Opioids
Mild pain.	Nonopioids are the first-line agents for mild pain.	May add adjuvant agents, especially if symptoms suggest neuropathic pain.	Not part of initial treatment of mild pain.
Moderate pain or mild pain that does not respond to step 1.	May be advantageous as part of multimodal analgesia, but only if not included in a combination opioid–nonopioid formulation.	May be advantageous as part of multimodal analgesia, especially if symptoms suggest neuropathic pain.	Combination opioid–nonopioid formulations with attention to nonopioid dose limits; alternatively, pure opioids to avoid this restriction.
Severe pain or moderate pain that does not respond to step 2.	May be advantageous as part of multimodal analgesia, even for severe pain.	May be advantageous as part of multimodal analgesia, especially if symptoms suggest neuropathic pain.	Pure opioids.

Choosing an Opioid

Which Opioid Medication?

One of the first decisions to be made is the choice of a specific opioid medication. Opioid medications have some clinically important differences. Clinicians must appreciate how opioids differ from one another on the basis of potency, time-to-peak effect, duration of analgesia, metabolism, and clearance. Considerations when one is choosing a particular opioid include[9,13]:

- The patient's previous experience with particular opioids
- Pharmacokinetics
- Available formulations
- The preferred route of administration
- The patient's kidney and liver function
- The care setting and the capabilities of caregivers
- The patient's cognitive status and available support
- Patient adherence and reliability
- Cost

Table 3 provides relevant details of commonly available opioids in the United States. Table 4 contains guidance regarding the choice of opioid for patients with kidney or liver impairment.[4,16,17] Although patient and opioid characteristics should be used to choose an appropriate opioid, there are great differences between individuals, and patients may need several trials of other opioids before a final therapy is selected.[4]

Which Route of Administration?

Opioids may be administered by a variety of routes. The choice of route should be guided by safety and patient convenience.[8]

Oral

The oral route is often considered to be most preferred and is usually the goal for outpatient management of chronic or ongoing pain. Oral

Table 3. Opioid Pharmacokinetics

	Peak Minutes	Plasma Half-Life Hours	Duration of Analgesia Hours	Notes
Morphine	60–90 (SA) 90–180 (MR) 7–20 (IV)	2–4 (SA) 3–10 (MR) 2–4 (IV)	3–6 (SA) 8–24 (MR) 3–4 (IV)	Commonly the basis of comparison for equianalgesic dosing, but it is not always the first choice, depending on patient comorbidities.
Codeine	30–60 (PO)	2–4 (PO)	3–4 (PO)	Not recommended for moderate-to-severe pain. Although it is available as a short-acting single agent (without acetaminophen), it is not as effective as other pure mu agonists and is associated with more adverse effects. Must be metabolized to morphine to produce analgesia. There is wide variation in ability to transform codeine with both poor and rapid metabolizers prone to adverse effects and poor analgesia.
Fentanyl	12–48 hr (TD) 15 (TM) 15–30 (IV)	>24 (TD) 2.6–11 (TM) 3.7 (IV)	48–72 (TD) 1–5 (TM) 0.5–2 (IV)	Has high potency and high lipophilicity, which partially account for its effectiveness in transdermal and transmucosal formulations. Due to wide variation in reported equianalgesic conversion ratios, exercise caution when converting to or from fentanyl. Do not cut patches. Do not apply heat to patches, as this can cause an overdose. Do not prescribe it to patients with temperature over 39°C.

(*Continued*)

Table 3. (*Continued*)

	Peak Minutes	Plasma Half-Life Hours	Duration of Analgesia Hours	Notes
Hydrocodone	60–90 (PO)	2–4 (PO)	3–6 (PO)	Not recommended, as it is only available in combination with acetaminophen and titration is therefore limited.
Hydromorphone	30–90 (PO) 10–20 (IV)	2–3 (PO) 2–3 (IV)	2–5 (PO) 3–4 (IV)	Has greater potency than morphine, which, if not appreciated, can lead to an overdose. Not currently available in modified-release form in the United States, which limits its usefulness as opioid monotherapy.
Meperidine				Should be avoided, due to adverse effects associated with the accumulation of its metabolite, normeperidine, which can cause myoclonus, seizures, and psychomimetic adverse effects, especially in the elderly or those with reduced renal function. It has no role in pain management, as there are several safe alternatives and many hospitals have removed this from the formulary.
Methadone		12–150 (PO)	4–8 (PO)	Methadone has a complex pharmacokinetic and pharmacodynamic profile that makes equianalgesic dosing particularly difficult. Consult with an experienced clinician before initiating or adjusting the dose.

(*Continued*)

Table 3. *(Continued)*

	Peak Minutes	Plasma Half-Life Hours	Duration of Analgesia Hours	Notes
Oxycodone	60–90 (SA) 90–180 (MR)	3–4 (SA) 4.5 (MR)	3–6 (SA) 8–12 (MR)	
Oxymorphone	30–90 (SA) 60 (MR) 15–30 (IV)	7–9.5 (SA)	3–6 (SA) 12 (MR) 3–4 (IV)	
Propoxyphene				Not recommended. Has been shown to have analgesic efficacy no better than that of acetaminophen, but its metabolite may accumulate and cause neuroexcitatory side effects, ataxia, or dizziness, especially in older adults or those with reduced renal function.
Tramadol		5–8 (SA)	4–6 (SA) 24 (MR)	Has both mu opioid agonist and serotonin and norepinepherine reuptake inhibition properties. May be appropriate for patients with mild-to-moderate pain, but in most cases other options will be safer.
Mixed agonist–antagonists: buprenorphine, pentazocine, butorphanol, nalbuphine				Agonist–antagonist opioid drugs are not useful for most patients with moderate-to-severe pain, as they are limited by a ceiling dose. In addition, they should never be administered to patients who are physically dependent on opioids, as that may precipitate withdrawal.

SA = short-acting; MR = modified-release; IV = intravenous; PO = oral; TD = transdermal; TM = transmucosal.

Table 4. Guidelines for Opioids in Kidney and Liver Disease

	Kidney Disease[1]		Liver Disease	
	Renal failure	**Dialysis**	**Stable cirrhosis**	**Severe disease**
Morphine	Not recommended	Not recommended Not dialyzed	Caution ↓ dose ↓ frequency*	Not recommended
Codeine	Not recommended	Not recommended	Not recommended	Not recommended
Fentanyl	Preferred	Preferred Not dialyzed, but minimal toxicity	Preferred	Preferred
Hydrocodone	Caution ↓ dose ↓ frequency*	Caution ↓ dose ↓ frequency	Caution ↓ dose ↓ frequency*	Not recommended
Hydromorphone	Preferred ↓ dose ↓ frequency*	Preferred Not dialyzed, but minimal toxicity	Caution ↓ dose ↓ frequency*	Caution ↓ dose ↓ frequency*
Meperidine	Not recommended	Not recommended	Not recommended	Not recommended
Methadone[2]	Preferred — with consultation only	Preferred — with consultation only Not dialyzed, but minimal toxicity	Preferred — with consultation only	Preferred — with consultation only
Oxycodone	Caution ↓ dose ↓ frequency*	Caution ↓ dose ↓ frequency*	Caution ↓ dose ↓ frequency*	Caution ↓ dose ↓ frequency*

(*Continued*)

Table 4. *(Continued)*

	Kidney Disease[1]		Liver Disease	
	Renal failure	**Dialysis**	**Stable cirrhosis**	**Severe disease**
Oxymorphone	Caution ↓ dose ↓ frequency*	Caution ↓ dose ↓ frequency*	Not recommended Contraindicated in moderate-to-severe hepatic impairment	Not recommended Contraindicated in moderate-to-severe hepatic impairment
Tramadol	Caution, clearance not significantly altered in mild-to-moderate impairment	Not recommended	Caution ↓ dose ↓ frequency*	Not recommended

*↓ Dose means to reduce the dose by 25%–50%.

↓ frequency means to reduce standing orders for short-acting opioids from q 4 hr to q 6 hr for around-the-clock short-acting opioids and to q 2–3 hr for break-through doses.

1. Avoid modified-release opioids including fentanyl patches in kidney disease unless patients have stable kidney function and stable opioid doses. Note that even the "safest" opioids are not dialyzable.
2. Consult with an experienced clinician before initiating or adjusting the dose of methadone.

administration is also preferred for hospitalized patients whose pain is well-controlled, as it is the most convenient and least expensive route.[8] Short-acting opioids are most often used on an as-needed basis for acute and breakthrough pain, but also may be administered around the clock for chronic or persistent pain. Some short-acting opioids are combined with acetaminophen or an NSAID, but these combinations are not very useful, due to the dose limitations imposed by the nonopioid component. Modified-release opioids are formulated to gradually release the opioid in the gastrointestinal tract, and are appropriate for chronic and persistent pain only and may help such patients with pain relief, sleep, and adherence.[11]

Parenteral

For patients with acute pain, an exacerbation of previously well-controlled pain, or who need very high opioid doses, a parenteral route of administration is advantageous.[8] Most hospitalized patients have intravenous access and this is the preferred parenteral route. Intravenous administration via intermittent injection is helpful for acute pain, breakthrough pain, and exacerbations of chronic pain. Continuous intravenous infusion should be used only in opioid-tolerant patients for chronic or persistent pain that requires around-the-clock administration. Intravenous patient-controlled analgesia (PCA) has options for intermittent bolus injections on patient demand, continuous infusion, or both. It is useful in a variety of inpatient and (occasionally) outpatient settings, including patients with acute, postoperative, and chronic pain.

Less commonly, the subcutaneous route may be used for patients who do not have intravenous access but would benefit from parenteral administration. Intramuscular administration is not recommended, owing to unpredictable absorption and serum concentrations, and higher rates of complications, including pain, nerve injury, abscesses, and scarring.

Transdermal

The transdermal fentanyl patch is the only transdermal opioid currently available in the United States. It is appropriate only for the management of pain in opioid-tolerant patients who are on stable opioid doses, and should never be used to manage acute pain.

Transmucosal

Fentanyl is also available in several transmucosal formulations (lozenge, tablet, and film). These formulations are appropriate only for opioid-tolerant patients who require an opioid for breakthrough pain.

Initiation of Opioid Therapy in Opioid-Naïve Patients

Opioid-naïve adults with moderate-to-severe pain should start with a low dose of a short-acting opioid on an as-needed basis, as this allows for rapid and safe titration and pain relief.[13] Starting doses of short-acting oral opioids are morphine 15 mg orally, oxycodone 10 mg orally, and hydromorphone 4 mg orally. Oral doses may be given every 2–4 hr, as needed. Parenteral opioids should be considered for severe and rapidly escalating pain situations. Starting doses of intravenous opioids are morphine 5 mg intravenously, hydromorphone 0.8 mg intravenously, and fentanyl 50 mcg intravenously. Intravenous doses may be given every 15–20 min, as needed, until the pain is controlled.

Patients who are elderly or have renal or hepatic impairment often require lower starting doses, more gradual titration, and more frequent reassessment.[9,10,18] Such patients may be started at approximately 50% of the recommended adult starting doses above. Although most opioid-naïve patients should be started on short-acting opioids on an as-needed basis, some patients with cognitive impairment may not reliably ask for pain medications and may benefit from being offered short-acting opioids every 4 hr, around the clock.[9,10,18]

Pain should be reassessed 60–90 min following administration of short-acting oral opioid doses and 10–20 min following administration of parenteral opioid doses. Persistent pain should be reassessed at least 3–4 times per day if it is not well-controlled and at least twice daily if it is well-controlled.

Continuation of Opioid Therapy in Opioid-Tolerant Patients

Patients who have been regularly taking opioids for approximately seven days or more are assumed to have developed tolerance (see Table 1) and will require higher doses than opioid-naïve patients to control new or worsening pain. For patients who are opioid-tolerant and have pain that is present most of the day, opioids should be prescribed around the clock (i.e. "standing") with additional doses available, as needed for breakthrough pain.[7]

Around-the-Clock Dose

Start by calculating the total amount of opioid taken in the past 24 hr. If pain is stable and well-controlled, the 24 hr dose may then be given in divided doses using a modified-release opioid (every 8, 12, or 24 hr, depending on the formulation). If pain is *moderate* and further titration is desired, consider using a short-acting opioid equivalent to the 24 hr dose given in divided doses every 4 hr, around the clock. If pain is *severe*, consider using a parenteral opioid equivalent to the 24 hr dose given in divided doses every 4 hr, around the clock.

Breakthrough Pain Dose

The breakthrough dose is approximately 10% of the 24 hr around-the-clock opioid dose, prescribed every 1 or 2 hr, as needed. The same opioid is used if possible. For example, a patient taking modified-release oxycodone 30 mg orally every 12 hr, around-the-clock, would receive a breakthrough dose of short-acting oxycodone 5 mg (rounded down from 6 mg) orally every 1 hr, as needed. The breakthrough dose for patients on fentanyl transdermal patches is also calculated based on 10% of the 24 hr dose, but to simplify the calculation the following method may be used: The breakthrough dose of oral morphine is approximately one-third of the fentanyl patch dose (for example, if the patient is prescribed a fentanyl patch 75 mcg/hr every 72 hr, the breakthrough dose is short-acting morphine 25 mg orally every 1 hr, as needed).

Opioid Titration

Opioids have no ceiling effect and it is not possible to know beforehand the dose that will be required to control a particular patient's pain. Opioid doses should be increased until adequate analgesia is achieved or until adverse effects limit further titration.

If the patient's use of breakthrough doses is frequent or if pain control is poor, opioids should be titrated to adequate analgesia or until adverse effects limit further titration. The goal of titration is improved comfort and function with limited or well-managed adverse effects. Titrate opioids only after the steady state has been reached (every 4–5 half-lives). Most of the commonly used intravenous opioids may safely be titrated every 12 hr, most short-acting oral opioids can safely be titrated every 18–24 hr, and modified-release opioids can safely be titrated every 2–3 days.

For mild-to-moderate pain, increase the opioid dose by 25%–50%. For moderate to severe pain, increase the opioid dose by 50%–100%. Short-acting or intravenous opioids should be used during titration to control moderate-or-severe pain. Modified-release opioids should be started only after the pain has been controlled with intravenous or short-acting opioids. Increase the breakthrough dose (to 10% of the new 24 hr total) when the around-the-clock dose is titrated.

Equianalgesic Opioid Doses

Different opioids and routes have different potencies, so an equianalgesic chart (Table 5) must be used to estimate equivalent doses when changing

Table 5. Opioid Analgesic Equivalences

Opioid Agonists	IV/Subcut./IM (mg)	PO/Rectal (mg)	Ratio (IV : PO)
Morphine	10	30	1 : 3
Codeine[1]	130	200	1 : 1.5
Fentanyl[2]			
Hydrocodone[3]		30	
Hydromorphone	1.5	7.5	1 : 5
Meperidine[4]	75	300	1 : 4
Methadone[5]			
Oxycodone		20	
Oxymorphone	1	10	1 : 10

1. Not recommended for moderate-to-severe pain.
2. Convert morphine 2 mg PO/24 hr to fentanyl 1 mcg/hr transdermal patch.[9,19] Also, convert fentanyl continuous IV infusion to fentanyl transdermal patch 1:1.[14] Never prescribe transdermal fentanyl to opioid-naïve patients.
3. Not recommended for moderate-to-severe pain.
4. Not recommended.
5. Methadone has a complex pharmacokinetic and pharmacodynamic profile that makes equianalgesic dosing particularly difficult. Consult with an experienced clinician before initiating or adjusting the dose.

the drug or route.[7,9] For patients who are opioid-tolerant an additional adjustment must be made, because different opioids have different efficacies and different mu receptor subtype affinities which may lead to differing degrees of tolerance to both analgesic and adverse effects — a result referred to as incomplete cross-tolerance.[9,20]

The standard advice for patients who are tolerant to the original opioid and have well-controlled pain is to decrease the calculated dose of the new opioid by 25%–50% to allow for incomplete cross-tolerance.[8,9] When pain is poorly controlled, and in the absence of clinically significant adverse effects, one may choose not to make this adjustment for incomplete cross-tolerance. Before rotating to another opioid for poorly controlled pain, be sure that adequate titration had been conducted with the original opioid. Be prepared to increase or decrease the new dose in the first 24 hr following the rotation, as equianalgesic charts represent population means and there may be wide variation of those means.

Case Study

The following example illustrates an equianalgesic conversion with a dose reduction for incomplete cross-tolerance:

A patient, who has been taking regular doses of hydromorphone for several months, has been titrated during this admission to hydromorphone 4 mg orally every 4 hr, around the clock and hydromorphone 2 mg orally every 1 hr, as needed. In the past 24 hr she has taken all six of the around-the-clock doses and three breakthrough doses. She is comfortable and, other than constipation which is controlled by a laxative regimen, she reports no adverse effects. She would like a more convenient way to control her pain. Since there is no modified-release form of hydromorphone, a different modified-release opioid such as oxycodone extended-release may be used. The calculation is as follows:

$$\text{Total hydromorphone in 24 hr} = 24\text{ mg} + 6\text{ mg} = 30\text{ mg}.$$

As per the equianalgesic table, oral hydromorphone 7.5 mg is equivalent to oral oxycodone 20 mg. Set up an equianalgesic equation from these three pieces of data:

$$\frac{7.5\text{ mg oral hydromorphone}}{20\text{ mg oral oxycodone}} = \frac{30\text{ mg oral hydromorphone / 24 hr}}{X\text{ mg oral oxycodone / 24 hr}}$$

Cross-multiply to solve for X. $(20 \times 30)/7.5 = 80$.

This means that 80 mg of oral oxycodone is equianalgesic to 30 mg of oral hydromorphone. Because she has been taking hydromorphone for more than seven days, we will consider her to be tolerant and will reduce this calculated dose by 50% for incomplete cross-tolerance and the target dose of oral modified-release oxycodone per 24 hr will be 40 mg. This could be achieved using oxycodone extended release 20 mg orally every 12 hr, around the clock.

The breakthrough dose is 10% of the 24 hr dose of the around-the-clock opioid. In this case, the 24 hr dose we have chosen is extended-release oxycodone 40 mg, so the breakthrough dose would be short-acting oxycodone 5 mg orally every 1 hr, as needed.

Adverse Effects of Opioids

With the exception of constipation, patients typically develop tolerance to the adverse effects of opioids in the hours to days following initiation or titration of opioid therapy. Despite this, adverse effects are one of the leading reasons patients discontinue opioid therapy. A general approach to the management of adverse effects may proceed as outlined in Table 6[7,9] and specific guidance for common adverse effects is provided in Table 7.[7,8,18,19]

Opioid Antagonists

Naloxone is an opioid antagonist that should be used only for clinically significant opioid-induced respiratory depression, a rare occurrence in patients on chronic stable opioid doses.[9] In order to minimize the risk of serious adverse effects that can be associated with naloxone (seizures,

Table 6. Strategy for Managing Opioid Adverse Effects

Order in Which to Employ Strategies	Comments
Consider other etiologies.	All of the symptoms associated with opioid adverse effects may have other etiologies. It is particularly common in the case of cognitive changes to blame opioids when in fact it is almost always multifactorial. Before employing the following strategies, consider whether other medications or comorbidities may be responsible for the observed symptoms.
Reduce the opioid dose.	If pain is very well-controlled, the opioid dose may be decreased by 25%. Consider multimodal analgesia (addition of nonopioids or adjuvants) so that opioid dose reduction can be accomplished without sacrificing analgesia.

(*Continued*)

Table 6. (*Continued*)

Order in Which to Employ Strategies	Comments
Treat the adverse effect.	Most opioid adverse effects are time-limited (with the exception of constipation). Consider a 1- or 2-week trial of treatment (as described in Table 7), then discontinue and reassess for the presence of adverse effects.
Rotate to another opioid.	Patients who experience adverse effects on one opioid may not have them on another. In addition, for patients who have adverse effects on an opioid to which they have analgesic tolerance, rotation to another opioid at a decreased equianalgesic dose (due to incomplete cross-tolerance) may reduce or eliminate adverse effects.

Table 7. Treatment of Adverse Effects of Opioids

Adverse Effect	Treatment
Constipation	Common in hospitalized patients taking opioids, and tolerance develops slowly, if at all. A prophylactic bowel regimen should be prescribed at the initiation of opioid therapy. Rule out impaction with a digital rectal exam or abdominal X-ray if clinically indicated, as rectal disimpaction must occur before treating with oral laxatives. Prophylaxis: docusate plus senna. If constipated for 2 days, add lactulose. If constipated for 3 or more days, add bisacodyl suppository, docusate minienema (docusate, PEG, glycerin), fleet mineral oil retention enema, or sodium phosphate oral sol. If no results, add a high colonic tap water enema (nursing order).
Nausea and vomiting	Most common with initiation or increased dose of opioids. Tolerance develops within days to weeks for most, but not all. Slow titration of opioids may help.

(*Continued*)

Table 7. (*Continued*)

Adverse Effect	Treatment
	Consider dexamethasone, serotonin receptor antagonists (such as ondansetron), prochlorperazine, haloperidol, or benzodiazepines. If evidence of slow gastrointestinal tract, consider metoclopramide. If accompanied by vertigo, consider dimenhydrinate or transdermal scopolamine.
Pruritis	Most common in postoperative setting with intraspinal opioids. Decrease in opioid dose is the single most effective treatment. Cold compresses or topical local anesthetics may be helpful if it is localized. Ondansetron or gabapentin may be tried. Antihistamines, such as diphenhydramine, are sedating, which may explain why patients experience relief of pruritis with these agents.
Confusion	Consider other potential etiologies, especially infection, CNS malignancy, hepatic or renal impairment, electrolyte imbalance, and inadequate pain control. Treat with haloperidol. Avoid benzodiazepines, unless used in the setting of agitated delirium which does not respond to haloperidol alone.
Sedation	Sedation is most common during opioid initiation or dose increase. While sedation often lasts only a few days, it is important to remember that respiratory depression is usually preceded by sedation, so it should prompt increased vigilance and attempts to reduce the dose while preserving analgesia. For persistent sedation, psychostimulants such as caffeine or methylphenidate may be tried.
Respiratory depression	Respiratory depression due to opioids is rare when established guidelines are used for opioid administration. Sedation almost always precedes respiratory depression, and tolerance to respiratory depression develops much faster than that to analgesia. Manage by: addressing contributing causes; decreasing or stopping opioid doses while observing respiratory status; and administering naloxone to reverse opioids if the patient is unresponsive or minimally responsive or if respiratory status does not improve.

pulmonary edema) and symptoms of opioid withdrawal (anxiety, pain, nausea, vomiting, diarrhea, among others), naloxone should be started at a low dose and titrated up as needed.[7,9] Dilute one ampule (0.4 mg) in normal saline to a total volume of 10 mL and administer 0.02 mg (0.5 mL)–0.04 mg (1 mL) intravenously every 1–2 min, as needed. The half-life of naloxone (1 hr) is shorter than that of opioid agonists; therefore additional doses or a continuous infusion of naloxone may be needed for patients on modified-release opioids, fentanyl patches, or long-acting opioids such as methadone.

Tapering and Discontinuation of Opioids

Occasionally patients will need to have opioids decreased or discontinued altogether, because the reason for the pain has been diminished or resolved. In such situations, acute withdrawal may be avoided if opioids are tapered by 10% per day until a dose is reached that achieves pain control without adverse effects. If the patient does not experience a recurrence of pain during the taper, then opioids may be stopped altogether when the usual starting doses are reached. In cases where patients must be tapered off urgently, this can be accomplished more rapidly, but attempting more than a 50% decrease in dose per day is not advised unless the patient's life is in danger due to respiratory depression.

References

1. Niska R, Bhuiya F, Xu J. (2010) National Hospital Ambulatory Medical Care Survey: 2007 emergency department summary. *Natl Health Stat Rep* **26**: 1–31.
2. Azevedo Sao Leao Ferreira K, Kimura M, Jacobsen Teixeira M. (2006) The WHO analgesic ladder for cancer pain control, twenty years of use. How much pain relief does one get from using it? *Support Care Cancer* **14**: 1086–1093.
3. Furlan AD, Sandoval JA, Mailis-Gagnon A, Tunks E. (2006) Opioids for chronic noncancer pain: A meta-analysis of effectiveness and side effects. *CMAJ* **174**: 1589–1594.

4. Smith HS. (2009) Opioid metabolism. *Mayo Clin Proc* **84**: 613–624.
5. Webster LR, Webster RM. (2005) Predicting aberrant behaviors in opioid-treated patients: Preliminary validation of the Opioid Risk Tool. *Pain Med* **6**: 432–442.
6. Butler SF, Fernandez K, Benoit C, *et al.* (2008) Validation of the Revised Screener and Opioid Assessment for Patients with Pain (SOAPP-R). *J Pain* **9**: 360–372.
7. American Pain Society. (2008) *Principles of Analgesic Use in the Treatment of Acute Pain and Cancer Pain*, 6th ed. American Pain Society, Glenview, IL.
8. Nicholson B. (2003) Responsible prescribing of opioids for the management of chronic pain. *Drugs* **63**: 17–32.
9. Pasero C, McCaffery M. (2011) *Pain Assessment and Pharmacologic Management*. Mosby, St. Louis, MO.
10. American Geriatrics Society Panel on the Pharmacological Management of Persistent Pain in Older Persons. (2009) Pharmacological management of persistent pain in older persons. *J Am Geriatr Soc* **57**: 1331–1346.
11. Argoff CE, Silvershein DI. (2009) A comparison of long- and short-acting opioids for the treatment of chronic noncancer pain: Tailoring therapy to meet patient needs. *Mayo Clin Proc* **84**: 602–612.
12. Fine PG, Mahajan G, McPherson ML. (2009) Long-acting opioids and short-acting opioids: Appropriate use in chronic pain management. *Pain Med* **10**: S79–S88.
13. Fitzgibbon DR. (2007) Clinical use of opioids for cancer pain. *Curr Pain Headache Rep* **11**: 251–258.
14. Prommer E. (2009) The role of fentanyl in cancer-related pain. *J Palliat Med* **12**: 947–954.
15. World Health Organization (WHO). (1996) *Cancer Pain Relief*, 2nd ed. WHO, Geneva.
16. Dean M. (2004) Opioids in renal failure and dialysis patients. *J Pain Symptom Manage* **28**: 497–504.
17. Quigley C. (2005) The role of opioids in cancer pain. *BMJ* **331**: 825–829.

18. Chai E, Horton JR. (2010) Managing pain in the elderly population: Pearls and pitfalls. *Curr Pain Headache Rep* 28. Sep.: [Epub ahead of print].
19. Skaer TL. (2006) Transdermal opioids for cancer pain. *Health Qual Life Outcomes* **4**: 24.
20. Fine PG, Portenoy RK. (2009) Establishing "best practices" for opioid rotation: Conclusions of an expert panel. *J Pain Symptom Manage* **38**: 418–425.

Palliative Care

Chapter 91

Overview of Ethical Principles and Ethical Analysis

*Anca Dinescu**

Key Pearls

- Ethical analysis is unique to each patient and should be conducted at the bedside.
- Ethical analysis represents a systematic process that provides the reasons for one's moral value judgments and decisions.
- Ethical analysis integrates the ethical principles with the available medical knowledge, technology and principles of law, economics, spirituality and faith.
- Start by assessing patient's capacity to participate in the decision at hand.
- The four most commonly used ethical principles are autonomy, beneficence, nonmaleficence and distributive justice.

Ethics

Ethics is the branch of philosophy that studies the nature and justification of general ethical principles governing right conduct, establishing moral justifications for what is right and what is wrong in human actions. To reach the core of a classical dilemma, one must ask one question: Why?

*Washington VA Medical Center, Washington DC, USA.

Bioethics

Bioethics (from *bios*, life; *ethos*, behavior) is the study and practical application of ethical principles in the clinical setting. It was born of healthcare professionals' understanding that legal rights, ethical principles and moral reasoning are increasingly part of daily medicine. The body of scholarship that we have today in bioethics derives from the initial set of ethical principles, but also involves an interplay of knowledge about law, science, technology, communication skills, health policy, economics and various faiths. Bioethics assists the healthcare and research community in examining moral issues involved in our understanding of life and death, and in resolving ethical dilemmas in medicine and science.

Ethical analysis

This is a systematic process that provides the reasons for an individual's moral value judgments and decisions, and also will eventually serve as support for future, similar moral value judgments.

In the same way that healthcare professionals perform risk–benefit analysis when applying evidence-based medicine, ethical analysis should integrate the ethical principles and the available knowledge in science, technology, law, economics and spirituality and faith.

Autonomy

This represents the principle that independent actions and choices of the individual should not be constrained by others, and involves supporting and facilitating the capable patient in exercising self determination. Autonomy is a fundamental principle that lies at the base of most medical decisions of modern medicine. In order to be able to exert the autonomy principle in the clinical setting, the patient needs to have *the necessary information* regarding the decision at stake and to be *able to process that information*.

The pertinent information regarding the specific decision is represented by the clinical indication for the proposed intervention, detailed explanation of the intervention itself, risks and benefits, prognosis of the specific issue with and without the intervention, and alternative treatments. *Assessing patient's capacity to participate in specific decisions should be part* of any ethical analysis and ensures that the patient can truly process the information and exert his or her autonomy. Autonomy needs always to be *enhanced* by the physician's opinion and recommendation. Burdening a patient with too many options, specifically ones that are mainly theoretical options rather than viable ones for this specific patient, diminishes patient autonomy. The medical team should be comfortable about making their recommendation for that patient in the light of their medical expertise, in order to allow the patient to exert his or her autonomy.

At times, autonomy can conflict with other principles. For instance, in the case of a patient requesting withdrawal or withholding of life sustaining treatments, since life preservation is considered a legitimate interest of the patient, autonomy conflicts with the principle of beneficence. In these situations, modern ethical analysis in the United States considers that autonomy remains the first principle of medical ethics and should take precedence over all others.

Beneficence

This is the principle that one has a duty of helping others by doing what is best for them and promoting their best interest. Beneficence is usually at the basis of decisions made when autonomy is impossible to be honored (i.e. a patient without capacity, with no advanced directive and no surrogate available when we cannot really assess patient wishes).

Whenever beneficence is involved, the person performing the analysis should consider the evidence that resides at the base of the ethical decision. Usually the evidence falls into two categories: substituted judgment and the best interest standard. *Substituted judgment* gives preference to the patient's voice, how the patient, if able to fully understand his or her condition, would make the decision using the patient values. It remains the preferred evidence as relates directly to the patient values. The *best interest standard* considers what would be most likely to benefit or promote the well-being of a hypothetical reasonable patient in the same circumstances as those of the patient. In the clinical setting, the best interest standard would consider mitigating pain and suffering, restoring and enhancing comfort, maximizing the potential for independent functioning, and prolonging life. Best interest should be used if no data exist about the patient's own values.

Nonmaleficence (Do Not Harm)

This is the the principle that one has a duty to not inflict harm or risk of harm on others. Knowing all aspects of that specific patient plan of care will help the healthcare professional to adhere to the "do not harm" principle. Team meetings, where all disciplines are consulted regarding all potential harmful effects of the proposed intervention, are particularly important. At times the nonmaleficence principle will conflict with autonomy, such as in cases where patients request interventions which are considered without benefit or even potentially dangerous. In these conditions, physicians can claim the nonmaleficence principle and refrain from providing interventions which are considered to be of more harm than benefit.

Distributive Justice

This is the principle that the benefits and burdens ought to be distributed equitably, that scarce resources ought to be allocated fairly, that no person or group bears a disproportionate share of benefits or burdens. When applied to healthcare, this principle is used in analyzing the fairness of the health system. In the light of distributive justice, an ideal healthcare system should include equity in access and financing of medical care. For example, what percentage of the US budget should be allocated to Medicare, and Medicaid? The same principle should guide the health system to assure efficiency in resource management and allocation, especially the scarce one. This is of particular concern in the area of organ donation and transplant. This principle has application in triage situations where allocation of time is crucial. Distributive justice is sometimes viewed as conflicting with the autonomy principle, such as in the case of resource allocation for prolonging the dying process of a terminally ill patient rather than focusing on what is really important for that person. In the United States, the principle of autonomy should take precedence.

A practical approach to ethical analyses incorporating the necessary steps and the relevant ethical principles is presented in the Table 1.

Table 1. Practical Approach to Ethical Analyses

Step-by-Step Analysis	Process Task	Ethical Principles Served
1. Capacity assessment	The patient is: • Able to understand and weigh the benefits and risks of the specific intervention; • Consistent over time; • Able to apply his or her own values to the decision process; • Able to communicate the decision.	Autonomy
2. Review of medical data	• Premorbid functional and cognitive status *Allows the medical team to understand and place patient's current condition in context.*	Autonomy Nonmaleficence
	• History of current illness • Natural disease progression without medical intervention *Allows team to avoid unnecessary interventions, potential harmful decisions, apply best interest standard.*	Autonomy Nonmaleficence Beneficence
	• Viable curative or palliative therapeutic options • Symptom management	Autonomy Beneficence

(*Continued*)

Table 1. (*Continued*)

Step-by-Step Analysis	Process Task	Ethical Principles Served
3. Review of social data	• **Living situation** Some patient goals (e.g. to be discharged home) cannot be reached in certain living situations. • **Past social history** A history of drug dependence/ abuse can preclude certain interventions. • **Insurance** Certain therapeutic options are limited by specific insurance companies.	Autonomy Beneficence Distributive justice
4. Review of legal data	• **Existent advanced directives** • **Previous decisions/ agreements reached?** *Allows not burdening the patient by rediscussing painful decisions.*	Autonomy Beneficence
5. Review of spiritual data	• **Religious beliefs** The team can get appropriate support in negotiating goals, explaining outcomes, integrating viable options with certain religious practices. • **Existent spiritual support** *Allows not burdening the patient, enlisting spiritual support.*	Autonomy Beneficence Nonmaleficence

References

1. Dubler NN, Liebman C. (2004) *Bioethics Mediation: A Guide to Shared Solutions*. United Hospital Fund of New York.
2. Furrow BR, Greaney TL, Johnson SH, *et al*. (2001) *Bioethics: Health Care Law and Ethics*. 4th ed.
3. Post LF, Jeffrey Bluestin J, Dubler ND. (2006) *Handbook for Health Care Ethics Committees*. The John Hopkins University Press.
4. Menikoff J. (2001) *Law and Bioethics: An Introduction*. Georgetown University Press.

Chapter 92

Establishing Goals of Care for the Hospitalized Patient

*Evgenia Litrivis**

Key Pearls

- Understanding and establishing patients' goals of care can help ensure that patients do not receive unwanted medical interventions or therapies.
- Open communication through a family meeting is an established strategy for eliciting a patient's goals of care.
- The first step in establishing an informed patient's goals of care is to ensure that the patient has a clear understanding of his or her medical condition and prognosis.
- Patients often base their treatment preferences on their perceptions of their prognoses.
- It is important to review patients' goals of care periodically, as medical treatment preferences can change over the course of a patient's illness.

Introduction

A fundamental component of a physician's role in providing care for the hospitalized patient is eliciting and respecting a patient's treatment preferences or *goals of care*. Currently, the majority of Americans die in acute care hospitals, despite data revealing that most Americans' preferred site

*Mount Sinai School of Medicine, New York, NY, USA.

of death is the home.[1] Yet, as Americans live longer, recurrent hospitalizations for sequelae of chronic and life-threatening illnesses become more commonplace. Many of these hospitalizations are marked by aggressive medical and surgical interventions in the weeks to months before patients' deaths, which may not meet the patients' overall goals of care or provide benefit due to underlying poor prognoses. The SUPPORT (Study to Understand Prognoses and Preferences for Outcomes and Risks of Treatments) investigators[2] evaluated the experiences of over 9000 seriously ill hospitalized patients. SUPPORT demonstrated that many hospitalized patients receive medical treatments that are discordant with their previously stated wishes and that the majority of treating physicians are often not aware of their patients' resuscitation preferences.

With the growth of the hospital medicine movement, hospitalists have the unique opportunity to improve the overall quality of care for the hospitalized patient, by ensuring the alignment of patients' and families' treatment preferences and values with medical care plan delivery. This can be best achieved through ongoing, open communication where treating physicians elicit patients' or surrogate decision-makers' overall goals of care. This leads to enhanced quality of medical care, as well as improved resource utilization with the concomitant decreased use of potentially inappropriate, aggressive medical and surgical interventions, fewer ICU days[3,4,5] and a decreased rate of the hospital as site of death.[6]

Goals of Care

Multiple potential goals of medical care exist today. Examples of possible goals of care are:

- Prevention of disease
- Cure of disease
- Life prolongation
- Functional maintenance or improvement
- Comfort maximization
- Achievement of a good death

Some patients may have already established medical treatment preferences prior to hospital admission. As a treating physician it is important to ask about this, especially if a patient's condition is unstable or critical. Treatment preferences are often outlined in documents known as *living wills*. A living will provides written instructions about a patient's care preferences, usually under the circumstances of an irreversible illness and takes effect when the patient no longer has decision-making capacity. In addition, some patients may have a *durable power of attorney for healthcare*, otherwise known as a *healthcare proxy*. A healthcare proxy is someone the patient has appointed and entrusted to make medical decisions on the patient's behalf, under the circumstance that the patient loses decision-making capacity. Ideally, the patient has shared his or her medical treatment preferences with the appointed healthcare proxy prior to losing his or her ability to participate in the medical decision-making process.

When goals of care have not been established, open and empathic communication, often through a family meeting, is a strategy for eliciting patients' or surrogate decision-makers' treatment preferences. Below is a suggested structure for running a family meeting.[7]

Doc, How Long Have I Got to Live?

Often, goals of care are addressed or readdressed in the setting of progression of a patient's underlying illness. Providing a patient and/or appointed decision-maker with prognostic information, particularly when a prognosis is limited, can be one of the most daunting tasks in the field of medicine. Physicians will often avoid discussing prognoses with patients and their families, because many feel that they have received relatively little training in how to offer prognostic information empathetically and effectively.[8]

Yet, patients and their family members often base their treatment decisions on their perceptions of underlying prognoses. Therefore it is important that patients or appointed decision-makers have an appreciation for a patient's overall prognosis.

Table 1. Steps for a Successful Family Meeting

1. Invite the patient and all relative healthcare providers and family members to the meeting.	The legal decision-maker should be identified by the medical team prior to the meeting, and his or her presence should be assured at the meeting.
2. Meet before the meeting.	The healthcare team should meet briefly and independently of the patient and/or family to review any Advance Care Planning documentation that may exist and to come to a consensus regarding important medical facts, the patient's underlying prognosis, and medically appropriate treatment options going forth. A facilitator for the family meeting should be identified to run the meeting.
3. Select an appropriate setting.	Choose a quiet setting where everyone present for the meeting can sit, and an attempt should be made to keep interruptions to a minimum.
4. Start with introductions and an opening statement about the purpose of the meeting.	"Thank you for meeting with us today. The purpose of today's meeting is to discuss how you are doing [or how your (mother/husband/etc.) is doing] and to make some decisions regarding treatment options going forth. We'd also like to answer any questions or address any concerns you may have."
5. Prior to sharing clinical information, get a sense of the patients and/or family's current level of understanding.	"I know that you've spoken to many doctors and have received a lot of information. What have the doctors told you so far about your condition?" "What have the doctors told you is going on with your [mother/husband/etc.] so far?"
6. Provide a clear, jargon-free medical update and review, pausing frequently to ensure that the patient and/or family understand.	When sharing bad news, provide the patient and/or family with a "warning shot." Ex.: "I'm afraid I have some bad news to share with you."

(*Continued*)

Table 1. (*Continued*)

7. Explore the patient's or surrogate decision-maker's expectations and values. Discuss treatment options.	"Knowing this information, what is important for you going forth?" "What are you hoping for moving forth?" "If your [mother/husband/etc.] were present, what would he or she want?" "I recognize how stressful this is for you. I don't want you to feel like you are making treatment decisions — you are here to advocate what your [mother/husband/etc.] would have wanted given the circumstances."
8. Respond to the patients and/or family members' emotions empathetically.	"I see this is very difficult for you."
9. Wrap-up and documentation.	Summarize major points and ensure that an adequate followup plan exists.

There is inherent uncertainty about medical prognostication, so it may be helpful for clinicians, when sharing prognostic estimates, to utilize time frames, such as "On average, patients with your stage of heart disease live days to weeks."

If a patient or appointed decision-maker does not initiate a discussion on prognosis, a physician can ask, "A concern that patients often have is that of time. Is that something you've wondered about?" If the answer is "No," the subject should not be pursued at that encounter, as providing prognostic information when a patient is not ready to hear it can cause mistrust or a schism in the physician–patient relationship. If the patient or appointed decision-maker answers "Yes," an example of a prognostic statement is:

"In my experience, patients at your stage of ____ disease on average live weeks to months. That means some people live a shorter time than that, and others live longer. Let's hope you are in the 'longer' group."

Such statements makes the facts very clear while acknowledging variability and allowing hope.

Addressing Cardiopulmonary Resuscitation/Code Status Preferences

Addressing a patient's code status preference is best done in the setting of discussing the patient's overall goals of care.

Table 2. Recommended Steps for Addressing Code Status[9–11]

1. Ensure an appropriate, quiet setting where all participants can be seated.
2. Elicit the patient's understanding of his or her illness. Ex.: "I'd like to talk to you today about medical decisions you or your family will need to make in the future. It is very important that, as your doctor, I have a clear understanding of your preferences, especially while you are undergoing treatment in the hospital. I know you've seen a lot of doctors while you've been hospitalized. Based on what the doctors have told you, what is your current understanding of your condition?"

   Before proceeding, it is essential that in order for a patient to make the most-informed decision regarding code status, the patient should have a firm appreciation of his or her disease burden and prognosis. If not, it is important for that to be clarified at this time.
3. Explore the patient's future goals and priorities. Ex.: "When you think about the future, what is most important to you with the time you have left?"

   Listen carefully as the patient discusses goals for the future. You can ensure understanding by recapping his or her goals. Ex.: "What I'm understanding is that it is very important to you that you are able to be as interactive as possible with your family and friends and for you to be as comfortable as possible."
4. Explore the patient's cardiopulmonary resuscitation preferences. Ex.: "We have discussed your current health status and your goals for your future. There will come a point, unfortunately, where your_disease will continue to progress and complications eventually will cause your heart to stop beating and you will stop breathing. I want to make sure that I know how to best care for you at that time. When this happens, some patients want life support measures to be attempted — including CPR. [Depending on the health literacy level, it may be important to state the components of CPR — chest compressions and a breathing machine.] Other patients want a natural death, without CPR and with a focus on being kept as comfortable as possible at the time of their death. What are your thoughts about this?"
5. Respond to emotions as the discussion unfolds.
6. Establish a plan. Clarify orders that you will implement and ensure that you will carry out the patient's goals.

Conclusions

Goals of care often change over the span of a patient's illness. It is therefore imperative, before proposing a medical care plan, that physicians understand whether the planned medical treatments are in fact aligned with the patient's treatment goals. Complications along the patient's illness course, including increased frequency of emergency room visits and hospitalizations, increased symptom burden and decreased functionality, should act as markers to signal that the goals should be reassessed. Periodic review of patients' goals of care will help ensure that the patients do not receive unwanted medical therapies and that medical care plans meet the patients' overall goals, thus ensuring a high quality of care.

References

1. von Gunten CF, *et al.* Where Do Patients Die? (http://endoflife.stanford.edu). End of Life Curriculum Project. US Veterans Administration and SUMMIT, Stanford University Medical School.
2. SUPPORT Principal Investigators. (1995) A controlled trial to improve the care for seriously ill hospitalized patients. The study to understand prognoses and preferences for outcomes and risks of treatments (SUPPORT). *JAMA* **274**: 1591–1598.
3. Campbell ML, Guzman JA. (2003) Impact of a proactive approach to improve end-of-life care in a medical ICU. *Chest* **123**: 266–271.
4. Lautrette A, Darmon M, *et al.* (2007) A communication strategy and brochure for relatives of patients dying in the ICU. *N Engl J Med* **356**: 469–478.
5. Morrison RS, Penrod JD, *et al.* (2008) Cost savings associated with US hospital palliative care consultation programs. *Arch Int Med* **168**: 1783–1790.
6. Hanson LC, Usher B, *et al.* (2008) Clinical and economic impact of palliative care consultation. *J Pain Symptom Manag* **35**: 340–346.

7. Weissman DE, Rosielle D, *et al.* (2007) (www.eperc.mcw.edu). EPERC: Goals of Care and The Family Conference, The Medical College of Wisconsin, Inc.
8. Christakis N. (1998) Attitude and self-reported practice regarding prognostication in a national survey of internists. *Arch Inten Med* **158**: 2389–2395.
9. von Gunten CF. (2001) Discussing do-not-resuscitate status. *J Clin Oncol* **19**: 1576–1581.
10. Back A, Arnold R Tulsky J. (2009) Talking about dying: "Do not resuscitate" orders and goodbyes. In *Mastering Communication with Seriously Ill Patients: Balancing Honesty with Empathy and Hope.* Cambridge University Press, New York, pp. 121–136.
11. von Gunten CF, Weissman DE. (2005) Discussing DNR Orders — Part 1, 2nd ed. Fast Facts and Concepts #23 (http://www.mcw.edu). End of Life/Palliative Education Resource Center, Medical College of Wisconsin.

Chapter 93

Management of Common Nonpain Symptoms in Palliative Care

*Emily Chai**

Key Pearls

- Symptoms are not only common but often the primary cause of distress among patients with serious illness.
- Many symptoms, such as constipation, nausea, and secretions, can be prevented. All others can be minimized and supported.
- Symptom management involves conceptualizing and reversing treatable etiologies, discussing treatment options, assessing the symptom frequently to evaluate for treatment effectiveness and side effects, and providing support to the patient and the family.
- Pharmacological therapy for anexoria can increase appetite and weight, though not typically in the form of muscle mass, and there is no mortality impact.
- Terminal delirium refers to the restlessness, agitation, and confusion that occur in the last days to weeks of life. A reversible cause is found in 50% of cases. Haloperidol is the first-line agent, especially for older adults, in whom benzodiazepines may cause paradoxical agitation.

*Mount Sinai School of Medicine, New York, NY, USA.

Introduction: Importance of Symptom Management

Symptom management is often overwhelming for clinicians, because much of medical education has been focused on how to manage various disease states. Yet it is the manifestation of symptoms that often brings patients to the healthcare provider, and it is the physical symptoms themselves that are often the primary cause of distress in patients with serious illness.

In 1994, Searle and Cartwright noted that while pain (84%), loss of appetite (71%), and nausea and vomiting (51%) were prominent in cancer patients, noncancer patients at the end of life have similar symptom burdens, with pain (67%) and trouble with breathing (49%) as the most common symptoms.[1]

Treating the patient's symptoms can improve his or her quality of life. While this is important during active treatment because treatment tolerance may depend on whether symptoms are controlled, it is even more important for patients who may be at the end of life, where cure is no longer an option. Managing symptoms may alleviate fear and anxiety so as to allow the patient the "good" death he or she hopes for. This chapter will provide management guidelines for common nonpain symptoms encountered by hospitalists during the course of curative treatment and at the end of life.

How to Manage Common Symptoms

General Management

Symptom management begins with a general symptom assessment. This approach is similar to the process clinicians undergo when trying to diagnosis the underlying disease etiology. This involves:

- Symptom history:
  - ✓ Onset
  - ✓ Palliative/provocative factors
  - ✓ Quality
  - ✓ Radiation
  - ✓ Severity and its effect on "function"
  - ✓ Timing/temporal relationship to activities

- Physical examination
- Conceptualization of likely, treatable, and reversible causes
- Discussion of treatment options, weighing in benefits and burdens
- Assistance with decision-making
- Provision of ongoing patient and family education and support
- Involvement of the interdisciplinary team
- Frequent reassessment
- Monitoring for effectiveness
- Monitoring for side effects

While this is a process familiar to most clinicians, it is often overlooked in the course of finding a regimen that will adequately manage the patient's symptoms.

Symptom-Specific Approach

Anorexia/Cachexia

Anorexia is a lack of appetite, while *cachexia* is a complex metabolic state involving loss of appetite, weight, fat, muscle mass, and strength, often resulting in debility. *Primary cachexia* is idiopathic and is associated with increased morbidity.[2] Cachexia can also be secondary to starvation, age-related loss of muscle mass, primary depression, malabsorption, and hyperthyroidism. In the setting of serious illness, anorexia and cachexia are often signs of disease progression and not reversible. The severity of cachexia can be a predictor of survival.

Nonpharmacological interventions focus on caregiver and family education and support. Examples are:

- Help the family and the caregiver distinguish between the normal progression of disease, over which they have no control, and things they can do to make the patient feel better.
- Help the family find other ways to express care.
- Differentiate the anorexia and cachexia syndrome from starvation.
- Offer favorite foods and nutritional supplements.
- Avoid gastric irritants like spicy food and milk.

- Encourage small, frequent meals.
- Provide nutritional counseling.
- Initiate high caloric intake.
- Determine if assistance with feeding is required.

Pharmacological options (noted in Table 1) should be considered if clinicians:

- Cannot identify a reversible etiology;
- Provide education and support;
- The patient's and family's goals of care are consistent with the pursuit of all treatment options.

Table 1. Treatment Options for Anorexia and Primary Cachexia

Treatment Options	Indications & Outcomes	Dosing	Side Effects
Pharmacological			
Megestrol acetate	↑ Appetite	80–160 mg PO up to 4X/day	DVT
	↑ Weight No Δ survival	Max. daily dose 800 mg	Edema Hypogonadism
Dronabinol (FDA-approved for use only in AIDS patients)	↑ Appetite ↑ Mood Stabilize, weight	2.5 mg PO before lunch and dinner Max. daily dose 20 mg	Delirium Hypotension Tachycardia
Cyprohepatadine (non-FDA-approved indications)	↑ appetite	2–4 mg PO q8 hr	Drowsiness Constipation Not recommended for older adults.
Oral caloric and protein supplements	Can be tried but usually do not result in increased caloric intake. When tried too early, often replace routineoral intake.	Dependent on caloric need.	May not be as appetizing as regular food.

(*Continued*)

Table 1. (*Continued*)

Treatment Options	Indications & Outcomes	Dosing	Side Effects
PEG feeding	Can be used as a time-limited trial to see if this is indeed anorexia/ cachexia-related to disease progression. More often a treatment for family/ caregiver distress. No survival, quality-of-life impact. Does not improve anorexia or primary cachexia.	N/A	Not recommended for those with anorexia/ cachexia syndrome. Increased risk of aspiration. May cause diarrhea.
TPN	Alternative, temporary way of feeding those with GI obstruction. Does not change anorexia. May prolong life in selected populations, usually not those with primary cachexia.	N/A	High risk of bacterial and fungal line infection.

Most pharmacological therapy will increase appetite. Some may result in weight gain, but often not in the form of muscle mass. There is no mortality impact.

Nausea/Vomiting

Nausea is the subjective sensation caused by stimulation of the GI lining, the chemoreceptor trigger zone, the vestibular apparatus and/or the cerebral cortex that may or may not result in vomiting. *Vomiting* is the neuromuscular reflex involving abdominal and chest wall musculature to expel gastric contents in response to a stimulus.

Since the management approach to nausea and vomiting is dependent on the cause of the symptoms, the history and exam should focus on determining the likely origin of the stimulus which precipitated the nausea and vomiting reflex. Table 2 lists potential etiologies of the vomiting reflex, the neurotransmitter involved, as well as agents to consider for treatment. Table 3 lists the pharmacological agents by class with dosing and side effects.

Both nausea and vomiting have high symptom burdens that require early intervention. Interventions should be initiated simultaneously with the exploration of reversible etiologies. If nausea and/or vomiting are anticipated side effects of specific treatments, the above-discussed management strategies initiated prophylactically can enhance treatment compliance.

Constipation

Constipation can be clinically defined as uncomfortable bowel movements or bowel movements of fewer than three defecations in a week. More important than the number of defecations is establishing the norm for a particular patient.

Workup for constipation needs to include a detailed abdominal and gastrointestinal exam, including a rectal exam. If radiographic imaging is necessary, direct the radiologist to comment on the amount of stool in addition to assessing for obstruction.

While most cases of constipation can be prevented, once diagnosed it must be treated to prevent complications such as anal fissures, hemorrhoids, rectal prolapse, fecal impaction, bowel perforation and potentially death.

Nonpharmacological interventions should be considered first. They include:

- Bowel retraining, which involves emptying the bowels at the same time every day, taking advantage of the high colonic activity that occurs early in the morning, after walking and 30 min after meals.

Table 2. Etiology and Management of Nausea and Vomiting

Stimuli	Symptoms or Syndromes	Neurotransmitters Involved	Potential Agents to Use
GI tract (GIT) *Use agents that work on the GI tract and also CNS.* *GI–targeted agents to increase motility or decrease secretion.*	GI infections GI irritants GI distension GI ulcers Reflux GI compression internal or external sources Any inflammation or irritation of nearby organs	Serotonin Histamine H1	Antihistamines Dopamine antagonists Serotonergic antagonists Promotility agents
Chemoreceptor trigger zone (CTZ) *Always treat the underlying disease and the symptom simultaneously.* *If possible, remove the causative agent.*	Metabolic disorders Disease states: CHF, AMI, DKA Drugs Toxins Infections Radiation therapy Tumor-related secretions	Dopamine Serotonin	Dopamine antagonists Serotonergic antagonists
Vestibular apparatus	Drug Vestibular dysfunction	Muscurinic Cholinergic	Antimuscurinic Anticholinergic
	Tumors	Histamine H1	Antihistamine
Cerebral cortex *Treatment of underlying etiology. Meds may include benzodiazepine, dexamethasone.*	Anticipatory Anxiety Fear Increased intracranial pressure Meningitis CNS malignancies	Histamine H1	Antihistamine

Table 3. Antiemetic Agents

Treatment	Indications & Mechanism of Action	Dosing	Side Effects
Dopaminergic antagonist			
Indication: dopamine-mediated nausea — most common Mechanism of action: chemoreceptor trigger zone			
Haloperidol (Haldol —non-FDA-approved indication)	Chemically induced nausea	0.5–2 mg PO/IM/IV/SQ q 6 hr PRN	EPS (less when administered IV) QT prolongation
Prochlorperazine (Compazine)	Works on CTZ and GIT but also has effect on histamine H1 and acetylcholine and alpha-adrenergic receptors Chemically mediated nausea	5–10 mg PO q 6–8 hr or 25 mg PR q 12 hr or 5–10 mg IV q 6 hr PRN Max. daily dose 40 mg.	EPS and effects of the other receptor sites such as sedation and hypotension
Chlorpromazine (Thorazine)	Like prochloperazine	10–25 mg PO q 4–6 hr or 25 mg IV (dilute to 1 mg/mL) or 25–50 mg IM q 3–4 hr (monitor for hypotension) or 50–100 PR q 6–8 hr PRN	EPS and sedation
Metoclopramide (Reglan)	Also has anticholinergic activity, increasing peristalsis and decreasing gastroparesis	10–20 mg PO q 6 hr 10–20 mg IV/IM q 4–6 hr PRN Decrease dose in renal failure and geriatric patients.	EPS

EPS = extrapyramidal symtoms
BBB = blood brain barner
NIV = nausea and vomiting

(Continued)

Table 3. (*Continued*)

Treatment	Indications & Mechanism of Action	Dosing	Side Effects
Antihistamines			
Act on the histamine H1 receptors in the vomiting center and vestibular afferens. Also have anticholinergic effects. All these used for nausea can cause sedation.			
Diphenhydramine (Benadryl — non-FDA-approved indication)	N/V related to elevated ICP or any vestibular etiology	25–50 mg PO/IV q 6 hr PRN Decrease for renal impairment and avoid if possible in geriatric patients.	
Meclizine (Antivert — non-FDA-approved indication except for vomiting of pregnancy)	N/V related to elevated ICP or any vestibular etiology	25–50 mg PO q 6 hr PRN	
Promethazine (Phenergan)	N/V related to elevated ICP or any vestibular etiology	12.5–25 mg IV or 25 mg PO/PR q 4–6 hr PRN	
Anticholinergics			
Opioids and anesthetics can trigger acetylcholine-mediated nausea in the vestibular apparatus. Helpful also if there is partial or complete bowel obstruction by decreasing peristalsis and secretions.			
Scopolamine	For nausea and vomiting related to gastroparesis and excessive secretions	0.6–1mg SC/IV q 4 hr or Transdermal patches: 1 behind ear 4 hr before needed, replace every 3 days if needed	Crosses BBB, so use with caution in older adults.

(*Continued*)

Table 3. (*Continued*)

Treatment	Indications & Mechanism of Action	Dosing	Side Effects
Glycopyrrolate (non-FDA-approved indication)	For GI-secretion-related nausea and vomiting in bowel obstruction	0.2 mg SC/IV q 4–6 hr	Does not cross BBB.
Metoclopramide (Reglan)	Also has dopaminergic activity	10–20 mg PO q 6 hr 10–20 mg IV/IM q 4–6 hr PRN Decrease dose in renal failure and geriatric patients.	EPS
Atropine ophtho gtts (non-FDA-approved indication)	Secretion control in GI obstruction — most appropriate at end of life, since it is cheap and easy to administer	2 gtts SL q 6 hr	Can get all the side effects that come with atropine, including tachycardia, dry skin, anxiety, and restlessness. Least-studied medication — most often used at the very end of life for secretion control.
Serotonin antagonist			
Acts on 5HT3 in the CTZ, and the vagal nerves and enterochromaffin in the gut wall. Can be used for refractory nausea of different types. Use with caution in those with prolonged QT and electrolyte abnormality. Constipation, headache, hypotension. Check for drug interactions.			

(*Continued*)

Table 3. (*Continued*)

Treatment	Indications & Mechanism of Action	Dosing	Side Effects
Ondansetron (Zofran)	For prevention and treatment of chemotherapy- and radiation-induced nausea and vomiting	8 mg PO/IV q 8–12 hr or 8–24 mg as a single daily dose can be as effective	Use dissolvable tabs with precaution in PKU patients.
Granisetron (Kytril)	For prevention of chemotherapy- and radiation-induced and postoperative nausea and vomiting	2 mg PO daily or 1 mg BID or 10 mcg/kg/dose IV over 30 min prior to therapy (max. daily: 1 mg/dose)	Not for breakthrough nausea and vomiting
Dolansetron (Anzemet)	For prevention and treatment of chemotherapy- and radiation-induced nausea and vomiting	100 mg PO/IV q 24 hr (1.8 mg/kg 30 min prior to therapy)	In Canada, its use is contraindicated as a breakthrough medication.
Palonosetron (Aloxi)	For prevention of chemotherapy- and radiation-induced nausea and vomiting	0.25 mg IV 30 min prior to therapy	Good for prevention and not effective for terminating nausea and vomiting once it occurs

(*Continued*)

Table 3. (*Continued*)

Treatment	Indications & Mechanism of Action	Dosing	Side Effects
GI acting agents			
Prokinetic agents are good for impaired GI motility of any kind.			
Metoclopramide (Reglan)	Prokinetic agent Dopamine antagonist (CTZ and GIT)	For prevention of diabetic gastroparesis: 10 mg PO or SC q 4 hr PRN (30 min before meals or food)	Use of this together with an anticholinergic agent may eliminate the prokinetic effect.[3]
	Serotonin antagonist (GIT)	For breakthrough (non-FDA-approved use): 10–40 mg PO/IV q 4–6 hr PRN	EPS esp. in Geri population[3] — can use domperidone, which does not cross BBB but is not available in US. Contraindicated in complete GI obstruction.
Erythromycin (non-FDA approved use)	Gastric prokinetic agent Good for peristalsis-related problems	200 mg PO initially, then 250 mg 3 times a day premeals	Use with caution in older adults and those with impaired renal and hepatic dysfunction.
Antacids, H2 blockers, PPI	Nausea-associated hyperacidity or excessive gastric secretion	Doses will vary, depending on the medications chosen	

(*Continued*)

Table 3. *(Continued)*

Treatment	Indications & Mechanism of Action	Dosing	Side Effects
Misoprostol	Cytoprotective agent effective for nausea caused by NSAID-associated mucosal erosions	100–200 mcg PO q 6 hr with food	Use with caution in older adults and those with impaired renal and hepatic dysfunction.
Others			
Dexamethasone	Synergistic effect with other antiemetic agents nausea caused by ICP and tumor-related edema	4–20 mg PO 1–2 times per day	Adverse effects with long term use
Lorazepam	Helpful in anticipatory nausea	0.5–2 mg PO/IV q 4–6 hr PRN	Sedation may be of concern.
Octreotide (non-FDA-approved use)	Selectively inhibit secretion of fluids and electrolytes into the gut lumen. Helpful in complete GI obstruction.	150–300 mcg SQ twice a day	Be familiar with GI, endocrine, and cardiac side effects of the medication.
Acupuncture and acupressure	Postoperative and chemotherapy-induced nausea and vomiting		
Surgical decompression or diversion	GI-obstruction-related nausea and vomiting		

Table 4. Pharmacological Treatment Options for Constipation

Treatment	Indications & Mechanism of Action	Dosing of Meds Used in Palliative Care	Side Effects
Bulk laxatives *Examples:* *Citrucel* *Fibercon* *Metamucil*	Prevent constipation in patients who are capable of adequate fluid intake. Normalize stool but not a good laxative.	Not recommended in palliative care	Can cause bloating and excessive gas production. Need to use with lots of water; avoid in those <1 L per day. May ppt obstruction in debilitated patient by forming a viscous mass. Avoid in debilitated pt.
Stimulant laxatives *Examples:* *Bisacodyl* *Senna* *Cascara castor oil* *Lubiprostone (prune juice)*	Induce semiformed BM in 6–8 hr through stimulating peristalsis. Prevent opioid/ medication-induced constipation. Lubiprostone can be used for chronic constipation and IBS constipation.	*Bisacodyl*: 5–15 mg PO daily or 10 mg PR daily *Senna:* 2–4 tabs PO QHS *Lubiprostone*: Chronic constipation — 24 mcg PO twice/day IBS — 8 mcg PO twice a day	Can cause abdominal cramping. Those with anthraquinones can cause *Melanosis coli* and colonic inertia. Do not use in those you suspect have intestinal obstruction (unless available in suppository

IBS = irritable bowel syndrome

(*Continued*)

Table 4. (*Continued*)

Treatment	Indications & Mechanism of Action	Dosing of Meds Used in Palliative Care	Side Effects
			form, which acts within 1 hr).
Osmotic laxatives *Examples:* *Lactulose* *Sorbitol* *Polyethylene glycol 3350 (PEG)* *Magnesium hydroxide (MOM)* *Magnesium citrate*	Hyperosmolar agents that cause secretion of water into the intestinal lumen by osmosis distenstion of the colonic wall lead to peristalsis. Work in about 3–4 hr. Often used before GI procedures.	*Lactulose*: 15–30 mL PO daily (max. 60 mL/day) *Sorbitol:* 70% solution 2–3 tablespoonfuls (27–40 g sorbitol) PO/daily *PEG*: 17 g PO (about one heaping tablespoon) per day dissolved in 4–8 oz. of fluid for up to 6 months *Magnesium citrate*: (rarely used except in preprocedure)—150–300 mL (1.745 g/30 mL solution) PO as needed	Associated with electrolyte abnormalities due to high salt content and may ppt hypokalemia, fluid and salt overload, and diarrhea. Use with caution in patients with renal insufficiency and CHF. Avoid Mg and PO_4 in those with renal insufficiency.
Stool softeners/ lubricants/ detergent laxatives *Examples:* *Docusate* *Mineral oils* *Glycerin suppository*	Soften and lubricate the stool. Ineffective in chronically ill. Helpful in those with fissures or hemorrhoids.	*Docusate*: 100–500 mg PO in 2–3 divided doses	Mineral oils may deplete fat-soluble vitamins (A, D, E) and increase risks of aspiration if in gel or liquid form.

(*Continued*)

Table 4. (*Continued*)

Treatment	Indications & Mechanism of Action	Dosing of Meds Used in Palliative Care	Side Effects
Prokinetic agents *Examples:* *Metoclopramide*		10–20 PO/IV q 6 hr (adjust for renal patients)	EPS, restlessness, dizziness, nausea
Erythromycin		250–500 mg PO/IV q 6 hr	Nausea, vomiting abdominal pain
Large-volume enemas *Examples:* *Tap water enemas* *Soap suds* *Polyethylene glycol–electrolyte solution*	Soften stool by increasing its water content. Distend and induce peristasis. Soap suds also irritate the colon.	*Tap water enema*: room temperature water of 5–10 oz. PR (150–300 cc) *Soap suds*: can be added to tap water *Polyethylene glycol–electrolyte solution*: usually prepackaged	Avoid very-large-volume enemas.
Peripherallyacting μ-opioid antagonists *Example:* *Methylnaltrexone (Relistor)*	Treatment of opioid-induced constipation in patients with advanced disease receiving palliative care with failed laxative treatment.	One dose SUBQ every other day as needed; max. of one dose /24 hr Weight-based dosing: <38 kg or >114 kg, 0.15 mg/kg/dose 38 kg to <62 kg, 8 mg/dose (0.4 mL) 62 kg to 114 kg, 12 mg/dose (0.6 mL)	Abdominal pain, flatulence, nausea, dizziness. Contraindicated in mechanical gastrointestinal obstruction, known or suspected.

- Diet modifications, i.e. increasing fluid intake, ingesting prunes or prune juice, and adding fiber to the diet in those with adequate fluid intake.
- Regular exercise, which is associated with a lower risk of constipation. In the hospitalized patient, this intervention entails getting him or her out of bed and mobilized as soon as possible.[4]

Malignant Bowel Obstruction

Patients with metastatic abdominal or pelvic cancer can have mechanical and/or functional causes of obstruction. If the mechanism underlying the malignant bowel obstruction is due to external compression, internal occlusion, or a motility disorder, consider palliative surgery, colonic stenting, and decompressive gastrostomy as options for alleviating the symptom.

If patients are not candidates for an intervention, if patients' goals are not consistent with intervention, or if patients decline intervention, medical management would be the best alternative option.

Medical management of partial bowel obstruction

Steroids should be considered to help decrease tumor-related edema which may be worsening the obstruction. Prokinetic agents like metoclopromide may move secretions past the area of obstruction and alleviate symptoms. This class of medications is contraindicated in those with complete obstruction and high obstructions, as it can worsen the symptom burden in both of these situations.

Medical management of complete bowel obstruction

Symptom management is the treatment focus for patients who are not candidates for an interventional procedure. Symptoms that will need to be addressed include abdominal pain, colic pain, and nausea with or without vomiting.

Nausea with vomiting in complete bowel obstruction is acutely managed with the placement of a nasogastric tube. Stop intravenous fluids, restrict oral fluid intake, provide aggressive oral care, and use antiemetic agents such as haloperidol or ondansetron to eliminate nausea and to decrease emesis to 1–2 times per day.

Clinicians may consider octreotide to decrease GI secretion and increase peristalsis, but it is very expensive. Once symptoms are better-controlled, consider removing the nasogastric tube. However, in patients with high complete obstruction and high volume vomiting, a nasogastric tube may be the best or only option.

Abdominal pain and colic are typically managed with opioids and antispasmodic agents. Opioids are effective in controlling continuous abdominal pain. While colic can be managed with antispasmodic agents, it is more difficult to completely eradicate.

Fatigue/weakness

Fatigue is a subjective feeling of tiredness, weakness, or lack of energy.[5] *Primary fatigue* refers to the state where inflammatory cytokines induce a catabolic state, while *secondary fatigue* is the term used when other disease processes and comorbidities are the underlying causes.[5]

Fatigue is very subjective and relies on the patient report. As such, any patient who reports fatigue should receive a full evaluation to identify and treat reversible underlying medical conditions.

For those palliative care patients who are not able to report fatigue, screening with the question "*Do you feel unusually tired or weak*?" will address the physical and the cognitive dimensions which appear to be most clinically relevant.[5] Anyone with a numerical rating scale (NRS) reading of greater than or equal to 5 out of a total of 10 should receive a full evaluation.

The goal of treating fatigue is to improve the patient's sense of well-being and decrease the fatigue intensity so as to allow normal functioning. Treatment plans should be tailored to address individual needs.

For patients with good performance status, this may mean aerobic physical training for fatigue related to cancer treatment.[5] For those with poor performance function, consider energy conservation, energy restoration, fluid and electrolyte optimization, and a thorough medication review, and stop or

Table 5. Pharmacological Management of Fatigue

Treatment	Indications Evidence	Dosing	Side Effects
Methylphenidate (psychostimulant — non-FDA-approved use)	Studied mainly in opioid-related sedation, cancer-related fatigue; antidepressant in patients with limited life expectancy.	2.5–10 mg PO at 8 am and 12 noon Max. daily: 40–60 mg	Nervousness, tremulousness, tachycardia, insomnia, arrhythmias
Modafinil (psychostimulant — non-FDA-approved use)	Studied mainly in fatigue patients with AIDS and advanced neurological diseases (MS, ALS, PD). May be useful in cancer-related fatigue.	200 mg PO/day Max. daily: 400 mg/day Start lower in those with liver impairments.	Nervousness, tremulousness, insomnia, nausea, diarrhea
Corticosteroids (low doses)[5]	Fatigue patients with advanced disease and multiple symptoms. Limited evidence. Helpful for short duration (1–2 wk) to reach a well-defineed goal.	*Prednisone*: 2–20 mg PO/day	Effect may wane after a few weeks.

MS = multiple sclerosis
ALS = amyotrophic lateral sclerosis
PD = Parkinson's disease

replace medications that may be contributing to fatigue. All these measures can be used together with the pharmacological treatments listed in Table 5.

While fatigue may be distressing for the patient and family at the end of life, fatigue may play a protective role. Treatment of fatigue may hinder the body's protective mechanism to alleviate the suffering that occurs when the patient is dying.[5] Instead of offering treatment, clinicians may want to educate patients, family, and caregivers about the role of the underlying illness and provide the patients with the permission to rest at the end of life.

Dyspnea

Dyspnea is defined by the American Thoracic Society as the "subjective experience of breathing discomfort that consists of qualitatively distinct sensations that vary in intensity".[6]

Since dyspnea is a subjective experience, the only reliable measure is the patient's self-report. The respiratory rate, oxygen saturation, and arterial blood gases do not correlate with the feeling of breathlessness.

Both the numeric rating scale (NRS) and the visual analog scale are probably appropriate for the palliative care setting. The NRS, which is a numerical intensity rating from 0 to 5 or 0 to 10, has been evaluated in both COPD and cancer patients and may be easier to use for a seriously ill population across settings.[7,8] "For cognitively impaired patients, the Respiratory Distress Observation Scale (RDOS) is an emerging behaviorally based instrument that may be used to measure the presence and intensity of respiratory distress in patients unable to self-report to guide management".[8]

Table 6 summarizes the pharmacological management of dyspnea. Nonpharmacological interventions for breathlessness include:

- Providing reassurance;
- Cognitive/behavioral techniques — relaxation, distraction, hypnosis;
- Opening the window and allowing the patient to see outside;
- Eliminating environmental irritants such as smoke;
- Reducing the room temperature;
- Introducing humidity with a humidifier or wet towel;
- Faning or opening the window for cool air or air flow;
- Repositioning — elevating the head of the bed and moving the patient from one side to the other;
- Educating and supporting the family.

Table 6. Pharmacological Management of Dyspnea

Treatment	
Oxygen	• Potent symbol of medical care. • Fans directed at the face reduce the sensation of breathlessness as well. • Expensive • Humidified oxygen delivered via nasal cannula is better tolerated. • Avoid the use of a face mask — it often adds to the sense of suffocation. • For patients whose goals are comfort focused, clinicians should give the patient, family, and caregiver permission to discontinue oxygen and focus care on other treatments to alleviate dyspnea.
Opioids	• Relief is NOT related to respiratory rate. • No ethical or professional barriers when used with the intent of relieving suffering. • Only small oral doses are needed (in opioid-naïve patients). • Can cause nausea, lethargy and constipation

Mild dyspnea:
(1) Hydrocodone 5 mg PO q 4 h and 5 mg PO q 2 hr prn
(2) Acetaminophen with Codeine (325/30 mg) 1 tab PO q 4 h and 1 tab PO q 2 hr prn
(3) *For those who cannot take pills*:
hydrocodone/acetaminophen syrup 1–3 mL q 4 hr and 1–3 mL q 2 hr prn

Severe dyspnea:
(1) Morphine 5–15 mg q 4 hr with prn
(2) Oxycodone 5–10 mg q 4 hr with prn
(3) Hydromorphone 0.5–2 mg q 4 hr with prn

For patients on opioids:
Those on a fixed schedule of opioids can have an additional dose of a short acting opioid equivalent to 30%–50% of the baseline opioid that is taken over 4 hours every 1 hour, as needed.

Nebulized opioids are not better than nebulized saline and can lead to bronchospasm by releasing histamine — not recommended.

Anxiolytics	• Not effective when used alone for dyspnea. • Not recommended as a first line agent. • Helpful in patients in whom anxiety is prominent. • Safe in combination with opioids, however, dose may need to be decreased in patients on opioids, CNS depressants.

(*Continued*)

Table 6. (*Continued*)

Midazolam (*non-FDA-approved use*) : 0.5 mg IV q 15 min until settled, then by continuous IV or SQ infusion
Lorazepam: 0.5 mg to 2 mg PO/SL q 1 hour until settled, then dose routinely every 4–6 hours.
Diazepam: 2–10 mg PO/IV q 1 hr until settled, THEN q 6–8 hr
Clonazepam: 0.25–2 mg PO q 12 hr

Neuroleptics
Buspar: 10–15 mg/day in divided doses, increase in increments of 5 mg/day to max. of 60 mg/day

Table adapted from Ref. 9.

Delirium and Terminal Delirium

Delirium is a syndrome characterized by an acute change in attention and cognition that fluctuates in its course. In the frail patient population, it may be a sign of underlying physiological change. It can be characterized by hyperactivity, hypoactivity or a mix of the two. The hypoactive form is often unrecognized and is associated with an overall poorer prognosis.

The diagnosis of delirium may be facilitated by the use of the Confusion Assessment Method (CAM).[10] The CAM criteria require the presence of acute onset and fluctuating course *and* inattention, *plus either* disorganized thinking *or* altered level of consciousness.

Delirium should be treated as a medical emergency, since it increases mortality, morbidity, medical cost, and posthospitalization institutionalization. Treatment should be initiated for every patient identified to be delirious.

Diagnosis and management can occur simultaneously. Initiating nonpharmacological interventions[11,12] while managing precipitating factors has been shown to decrease the intensity and improve delirium symptoms. Some effective nonpharmacological interventions are:

- Reorienting (using orientation boards, clocks, calendars, encouraging the presence of family members, and providing clear and simple instructions);

- Reducing sensory deprivation (providing eyeglasses and hearing aids when available);
- Avoiding overstimulation and sleep deprivation (providing a private room close to the nurse's station for increased supervision if the patient is agitated, and providing a quiet patient care setting with low-level lighting);
- Encouraging the patient's mobility and independence, and decreasing the use of devices that may tether the patient to the bed, such as catheters, intravenous lines, and restraints.

Pharmacological treatment (Table 7) should be performed only if patients pose a risk to themselves, other patients, or staff. The only exception may be in patients at the end of life, where reversal of the underlying etiology may not be possible and delirium management is aimed at decreasing the symptom burden to prevent bereavement-related complications.

Insomnia

Insomnia, common in palliative care patients, is a subjective reference to poor sleep quality or quantity. It is often multifactorial and affects physical and emotional well-being, as well as one's ability to concentrate, cope with stress, and carry out routine activities. Complaints of insomnia warrant a thorough evaluation for individualized management strategies focused on addressing reversible etiologies such as pain, nocturia, dyspnea, environmental and emotional issues, as well as medication concerns.

While a thorough evaluation usually entails polysomnography, it is often too burdensome for seriously ill palliative care patients to undergo. Thus, nonpharmacological interventions are often tried in the home. Such interventions have clinically relevant limitations in the hospitalized setting.[13] As such, most clinicians resort to some of the pharmacological options listed in Table 8. Usually more than one modality is necessary for assisting patients with insomnia.

Table 7. Pharmacological Options for Delirium*

Class and Medication	Dose	Comments
Antipsychotics — Black box warning on all antipsychotics Side effects: • Extrapyramidal symptoms (EPSs) • Tardive dyskinesia • Neuroleptic malignant syndrome • Prolonged QTc (monitoring may not apply in patients at the very end of life) • Anticholinergic effects		
Haloperidol (Haldol)	0.5–2 mg PO q 12 hr with q 4 hr, as needed 0.5–1 mg IV q 12 hr	Available formulations: PO, IV, IM SQ. Ratio of IV to PO is 1:2. First-line agent for terminal delirium[11] and delirium in general except for hepatic encephalopathy and delirium tremens. Effective in hypoactive and hyperactive delirium.[11] IV route has faster onset but also shorter duration of action.
Chlorpromazine (Thorazine)	10–25 mg PO q 4–6 hr or 50–100 mg PR q 6–8 hr or 25–50 mg q 4–6 hr PRN	Available formulations: PO — tab and liquid, PR, IV, IM. Ratio of IV to PO is 1:1. Second-line agent to haloperidol. Preferred in hyperactive delirium (more sedating). Increased photosensitivity.
Risperidone (Risperidal)	0.5–4 mg PO q 12 hr	Available formulations: PO — tab, rapidly dissolving tab, liquid concentrate), IM. May be preferred for hyperactive delirium with psychotic features. Associated with mortality in older adults with dementia.

(*Continued*)

Table 7. (*Continued*)

Class and Medication	Dose	Comments
Olanzapine (Zyprexa, Zydis)	2.5–5 mg PO daily	Available formulations: PO — tab, rapidly dissolving tab, liquid concentrate), IM. May want to avoid in hypoactive delirium, pre-existing dementia, older age due to poor response.[11] Associated with mortality in older adults with dementia. Increased risk of CVA and hyperglycemia.
Quetiapine (Seroquel)	25–100 mg PO q 12 hr	Available formulations: PO — tab. Preferred in those with Parkinson's disease or Lewy body dementia due to lower risk of EPSs. Increased risk of hyperglycemia.
Aripiprazole (Abilify)	5–15 mg PO daily	Available formulations: PO — tab, rapidly dissolving tab, liquid concentrate), IM. May be better in those with hypoactive delirium. No adjustments needed for age, renal and hepatic impairments. Risk of CVA, hyperglycemia, and weight gain.
Benzodiazepine • May have a role in selected delirious etiologies. • Usually does not improve the delirium but may decrease the intensity by sedation. • Probably more appropriate in management of terminal delirium than potentially reversible delirious etiologies. • Side effects: ○ Oversedation ○ Paradoxical agitation		

(*Continued*)

Table 7. (*Continued*)

Class and Medication	Dose	Comments
Lorazepam (non-FDA-approved use)	0.5–1 mg PO/IV/IM 2–4 times a day and every 4 hr PRN	Available formulations: PO, IV, IM. May worsen and prolong delirium. Paradoxical agitation. Consider use in patients whose delirium is related to alcohol, sedative withdrawal. May be an option for those with Parkinson's disease and malignant neuroleptic syndrome.

These are non-FDA approved recommendations for treatment of delirium.
*Table adapted with information from Ref. 11.

The Dying Process

There are many physiological changes at the last hours of life. The most obvious may be the increasing lethargy, somnolence, agitation (terminal delirium), or coma. This may be accompanied by decreased appetite and oral intake, and decreased output. Once the actively dying process begins, there will be decreased perfusion, hypotension, and skin mottling, together with increased weakness and stiffness, loss of ability to close the eyes (loss in periorbital fat pads), and loss of ability to swallow, resulting in the "death rattle." As patients are minutes to hours from death, they experience irregular respirations, intermittent apnea, Cheyne–Stokes respirations, and last reflex breaths.

General Management

Medications should be reviewed, weighing the benefit and burden of each. Medications that will decrease the symptom burden should be initiated and those that increase the symptom burden with little or no medical value

Table 8. Pharmacological Options for Insomnia*

Class	Examples	Comments
Benzodiazepines[14]	Intermediate-acting ones are preferred:	Undergo hepatic metabolism, and flurazepam has active metabolites.
	Temazepam 7.5 mg Flurazepam 15 mg Estazolam 0.5 mg	High incidence of amnesia and rebound insomnia. May cause paradoxical agitation. Tolerance and dependence. CNS and respiratory side effects.
Benzodiazepine-like medications[14]	Zolpidem 5–10 mg Zaleplon 10–20 mg	Restore sleep in patients with nocturnal awakenings. Hepatic metabolism but no active metabolites. Low abuse potential.
Sedating antidepressants (non-FDA-approved use)	Trazadone 25–100 mg PO Doxepin 10–75 mg PO Mirtazepine 7.5–45 mg PO	
Sedating antihistamines	Diphenhydramine 25–100 mg PO	Avoid in the elderly, due to anticholinergic properties.
Melatonin	0.5–10 mg PO at night	For circadian rhythm sleep disorders.

*There are no guidelines on the use of any of these agents in patients with serious illness and life-limiting diseases who may frequently need help with sleep for several weeks or months as their condition deteriorates.
Table created with content from Refs. 14 and 15.

should be discontinued. Both the patient and the family should be offered information about the expected disease course and the symptoms of the dying process. Families should be encouraged to communicate among themselves and with the patient even if the patient is unable to respond. (Tell the family to assume that the patient can still hear them.) Suggest to the family things that they can say to their loved one, such as[16]: “I forgive you,” “Please forgive me,” “Thank you,” “I love you,” and “Goodbye.” Assess for spiritual or religious needs while being present and compassionate with the patient and the family. Clinicians should be attentive to the patient's clinical needs, which include eye, lip, and oral care, as well as skin care and turning periodically. The patient does not need to be turned every 2 hr. The interdisciplinary team should be mobilized to provide support for the family and caregiver during the actively dying period and provide grief and bereavement followup once death occurs.

Management of the Three Common Symptoms During the Last Few Days of Life

*Xerostomia (*dry mouth) increases near the end of life. Patients who do not receive artificial hydration nutrition do not have increased symptom burdens.[17] Thus, management is focused on patient/family education and support as well as aggressive oral care from caregivers. Artificial saliva in patients who are unable to swallow is not helpful.

The "Death rattle" and oral secretions result from the patient's inability to swallow, leading to pooling of saliva in the oropharynx. It is important to explain to the family that what the patient experiences is not what onlookers see. It is often a sign that death is imminent.

Management options include repositioning the patient and/or pharmacological management (Table 9). Anticholinergic agents are very effective for nonexpectorated secretions. Bronchial secretions from pulmonary pathology patients are poorly responsive.[18] If a decision has been made to treat with medication, give it early! Once secretions are present, medications decrease the rate of production rather than remove them.

Terminal delirium is the restlessness, agitation, and confusion that occur in the last days to weeks of life. It is often multifactorial. While 50% may be reversible, the other half is not.[19] It may be frightening to patients and be a "premature separation" for the family.[20]

For terminal delirium, it is particularly important to educate the family and caregivers about the nature and cause of the behavior they are seeing. Informing the family of things to expect may alleviate their fear and distress over the changes in their loved one.

Table 9. Pharmacological Options for Oral Secretions

Medication	Dosing	
Scopolamine (non-FDA-approved use)	0.6–1 mg SC/IV q 4 hr or Transdermal patches: 1 behind ear 4 hr before needed; replace every 3 days if needed	Cross blood–brain barrier.
Glycopyrrolate	0.2 mg SC/IV q 4–6 hr	Does not cross blood–brain barrier.
Atropine eye drops (non-FDA-approved use)	2 gtts SL q 6 hr	Readily available.
Hyoscyamine (non-FDA-approved use)	0.125–0.25 PO q 4 hr PRN or 0.25–0.5 mg IV/SubQ/IM q 4 hr up to 4 times a day Daily max.: 1.5 mg/day	Not appropriate for geriatric patients.

Pharmacological treatment most commonly includes antipsychotics and benzodiazepines. Haloperidol is the first-line agent for terminal delirium, especially for older adults, in whom benzodiazepines may cause paradoxical agitation. Chlorpromazine is preferred for very agitated patients, since it has the benefit of causing sedation. Benzodiazepine options for terminal delirium are mainly lorazepam and diazepam. Barbiturates such as phenobarbital are usually the last resort, when symptoms cannot be relieved with other agents.

Conclusion

While there are many symptoms that clinicians will encounter, the approach to all symptom management is similar. The process involves the conceptualization of likely etiologies, determining whether the precipitating etiology can be reversed, establishing available treatment options, weighing benefits and burdens, assisting with decision-making, supporting and educating the patient and family and, lastly, reassessing symptoms frequently for both effectiveness and side effects. With these skill sets, clinicians will be prepared to manage any symptom, regardless of whether the underlying etiology can be reversed or cured.

References

1. Seale C, Cartwright, A. (1994) *The Year Before Death*. Cambridge University Press, UK.
2. Evans WJ, Morley JE, Argilés J, *et al.* (2008) Cachexia: A new definition. *Clin Nutr* **27**(6): 793–799.
3. Davis MP, Walsh D. (2000) Treatment of nausea and vomiting in advanced cancer. *Support Care Cancer* **8**: 444–452.
4. Dukas L, Willett WC, Giovannucci EL. (2003) Association between physical activity, fiber intake, and other lifestyle variables and constipation in a study of women. *Am J Gastroenterol* **98**: 1790–1796.
5. Radbruch L, Strasser F, Elsner F, *et al.* (2008) Fatigue in palliative care patients — an EAPC approach. *Palliat Med* **22**: 13–32.
6. American Thoracic Society. (1999) Dyspnea mechanisms, assessment, and management: A consensus statement. *Am Rev Resp Crit Care Med* **159**: 321–340.
7. Dorman S, Byrne A, Edwards A. (2007) Which measurement scales should we use to measure breathlessness in palliative care? A systematic review. *Palliat Med* **3**: 177–191.
8. Mularski RA, Campbell ML, Asch SM, *et al.* (2010) A review of quality of care evaluation for the palliation of dyspnea. *Am J Respir Crit Care Med* **181**: 534–538.
9. Thomas JR, von Gunten, CF. (2003) Management of dyspnea. *J Support Oncol* **1**: 23–34.
10. Inouye SK, Vandyck CH, Alessi CA, *et al.* (1990) Clarifying confusion: The Confusion Assessment Method — a new method for detection of delirium. *Ann Intern Med* **113**: 941–948.
11. Breitbart B, Alici Y. (2008) Agitation and delirium at the end of life: "We couldn't manage him." *JAMA* **300**(24): 2898–2910.
12. Heino H, John E, Lucy C, *et al.* (2004) The prevalence, key causes and management of insomnia in palliative care patients. *J Pain Symptom Manag* **27**(4): 316–321.
13. Morin CM, Culbert JP, Schwartz SM. (1994) Nonpharmacological interventions for insomnia: A meta-analysis of treatment efficacy. *Am J Psychiatry* **151**(8): 1172–1180.

14. Hirst A, Sloan R. (2002) Benzodiazepines and related drugs for insomnia in palliative care. *Cochrane Database Syst Rev* 4: Art. No. CD003346.
15. Schenck CH, Mahowald MW, Sack RL. (2003) Assessment and management of insomnia. *JAMA* **289**: 2475–2479.
16. Byock I. (2004) *The Four Things that Matter Most: A Book About Living*. Free Press, New York.
17. Ganzini L, Goy ER, Miller LL, *et al*. (2003) Nurses' experience with hospice patients who refuse food and fluids to hasten death. *N Engl J Med* **349**: 359–365.
18. Wilders H, Menten J. (2002) Death rattle: Prevalence, prevention and treatment. *J Pain Symptom Manag* **23**: 310–317.
19. Leonard M, Raju B, Conroy M, *et al*. (2008) Reversibility of delirium in terminally ill patients and the predictors of mortality. *Palliat Med* **22**(7): 848–854.
20. Lawlor PG, Gagnon B, Mancini IL, *et al*. (2000) Occurrence, causes, and outcome of delirium in advanced cancer patients: A prospective study. *Arch Intern Med* **160**: 786–794.

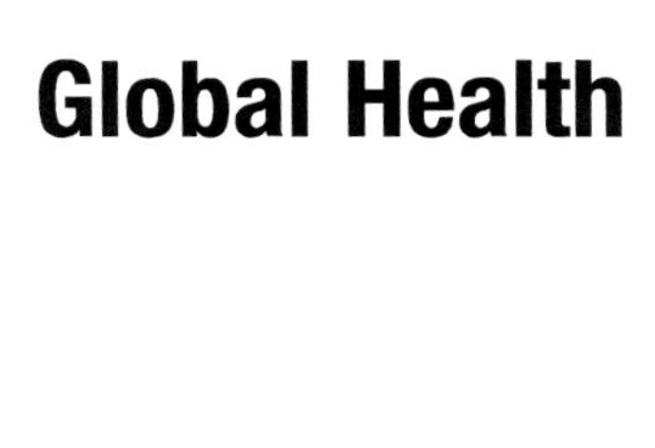
Global Health

Chapter 94

Travel Medicine for Hospitalists

*Daniel Caplivski**

Key Pearls

- Malaria should be considered early in the evaluation of all patients who have returned from endemic areas.
- Patients who have taken incomplete malaria prophylaxis are still at risk for malaria and may present with a delayed onset of symptoms.
- Incubation periods can be an important clue in distinguishing various causes of fever.
- Local causes of fever should also be considered when evaluating travelers, as symptoms may be unrelated to travel.
- Emerging fluoroquinolone resistance among *Salmonella* isolates requires careful communication with the laboratory in order to ensure that appropriate antibiotics are selected for patients with typhoid.

Introduction

The hospitalized patient with a history of foreign travel requires special attention, as the number of possible etiologies for a given set of symptoms is vastly expanded after a patient has traveled to developing countries. Illnesses such as typhoid and malaria, which are rare in the United States, must be considered rapidly in the differential diagnosis, as they may be fatal if untreated. Special diagnostic tests such as the manual examination

*Mount Sinai School of Medicine, New York, NY, USA.

of peripheral blood smears may not be part of routine evaluations for many patients, but are essential for the returned traveler with fever. The following case illustrates the importance of geography and incubation periods in differentiating possible causes of fever in returned travelers.

Case Presentation

A 23-year-old woman without an antecedent medical history presented to the emergency department with fevers, shaking chills, sweats, nausea, and joint aches. Five weeks before her presentation, she had returned from a month of volunteering in rural villages in Ghana. Approximately five days prior to her return home, she had two similar episodes of fevers, chills, and joint aches, but they had resolved. She had taken doxycycline 100 mg daily as her anti-malarial prophylaxis, but had missed some doses and discontinued the medication one week after her return instead of continuing for the full 28 days of post-travel prophylaxis. In addition to her presenting symptoms, she had been experiencing extreme fatigue, headache, diarrhea, and palpitations for two days. She noted that her fevers were occurring nightly, but during the day she had been able to attend class. Her pretravel vaccinations included vaccinations against hepatitis A virus, typhoid, yellow fever, tetanus–diphtheria, and meningococcus.

On physical examination, she was febrile to 39°C, but in no acute distress and without signs of icterus or jaundice. There were no signs of meningismus; her cardiopulmonary examination was normal, and there was no palpable hepatosplenomegaly. Laboratory values were significant for thrombocytopenia (platelet count $120 \times 10^3/\mu L$) and mild hyperbilirubinemia (total bilirubin 1.6 g/dL, with direct bilirubin 0.4 g/dL), but the creatinine and leukocyte count were both normal. Chest radiography revealed no pathology, and blood cultures were sterile. The peripheral blood smear showed numerous intracellular ring forms with double chromatin dots. The infected cells were equivalent in size to noninfected cells, and several cells were infected by more than one ring. The presence of appliqué forms (rings pressed against the membrane of the erythrocyte) was also characteristic of this type of infection (see Fig. 1).

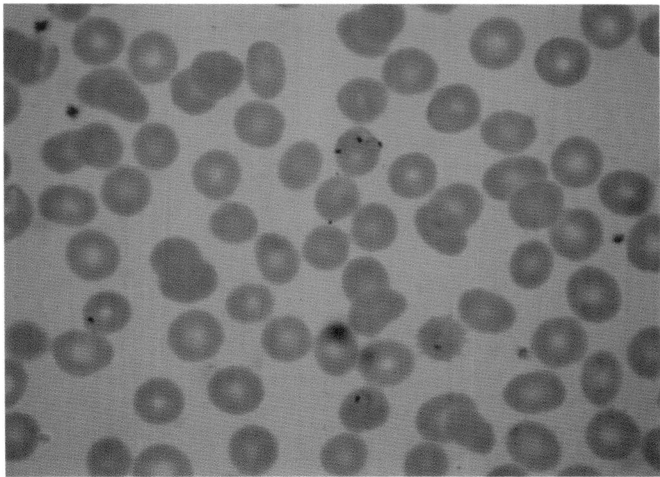

Fig. 1. Peripheral blood smear revealing intraerythrocytic ring forms with double chromatin dots, appliqué forms, and multiply infected cells.

The patient was diagnosed with *Plasmodium falciparum* malaria with an estimated parasitemia of 5%. She was treated with atovaquone/proguanil, four adult tablets orally per day for three days. She tolerated the antimalarial treatment without nausea and was discharged on the third hospital day with complete resolution of her symptoms. A peripheral blood smear collected one day after discharge showed no ring forms, but did reveal numerous gametocytes (Fig. 2).

Plasmodium falciparum Malaria

Epidemiology

Malaria is an essential diagnostic consideration in patients returning from travel in endemic areas. It can be fatal if undiagnosed and is not routinely detected by automated peripheral blood smear analyzers. It is endemic in many parts of the tropics, including South America, South Asia, Southeast Asia, and parts of the Caribbean. The greatest risk of malaria for travelers, however, is in sub-Sarahan Africa.[1,2] *Plasmodium falciparum* is largely

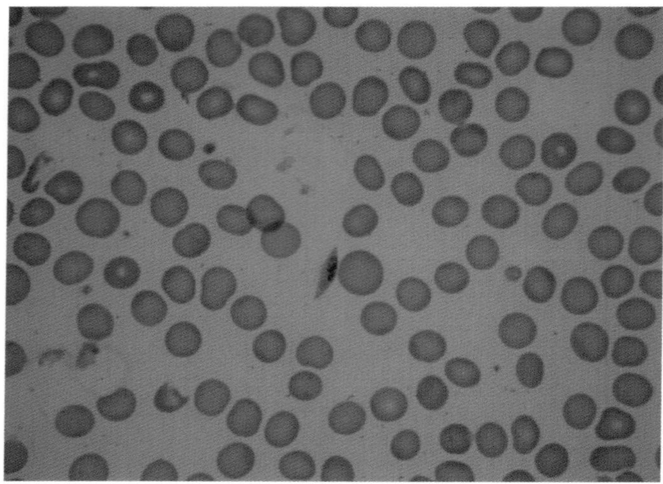

Fig. 2. Peripheral blood smear revealing banana-shaped gametocytes.

resistant to chloroquine in most of the world, with the exception of parts of Central America west of the Panama Canal and Caribbean countries such as Haiti.[4,5]

Lifecycle and Incubation Periods

An understanding of the malaria parasite's lifecycle is important to the diagnosis and treatment of the five species of *Plasmodium* that are recognized to infect humans:

- *Plasmodium falciparum*
- *Plasmodium vivax*
- *Plasmodium ovale*
- *Plasmodium malariae*
- *Plasmodium knowlesi*

Figure 3 shows the lifecycle in humans as well as within the *Anopheles* mosquito vector. All species of malaria pass through the liver, but *Plasmodium vivax* and *Plasmodium ovale* also form a hepatic hypnozoite

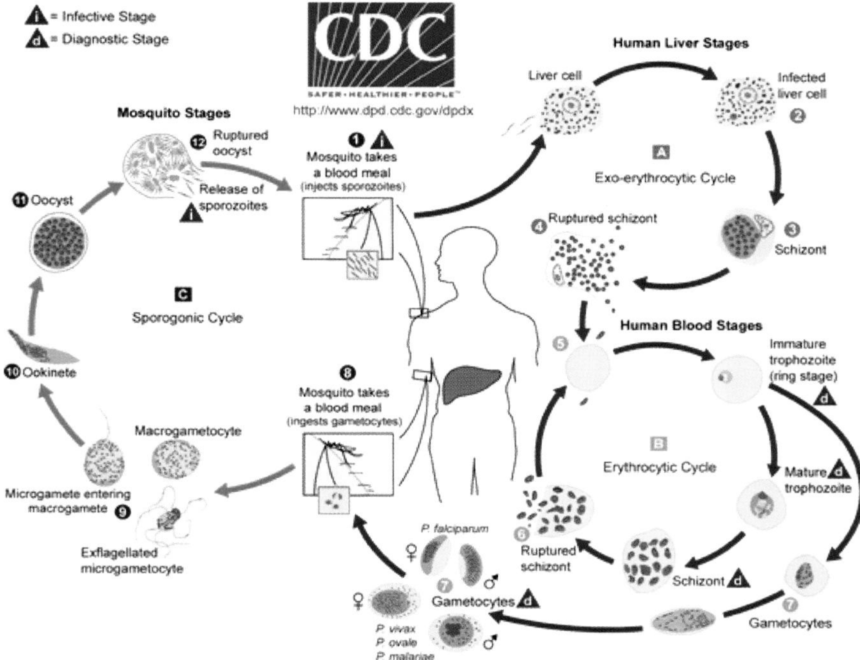

Fig. 3. Lifecycle of *Plasmodium* species.

Source: http://www.dpd.cdc.gov/dpdx/HTML/Malaria.htmf

stage that may lead to relapsing malaria. The antimalarials most commonly used for prophylaxis (atovaquone/proguanil, mefloquine, and doxycycline) are effective only against the erythrocytic schizont phase.[5,6]

Plasmodium falciparum is the most important of all species, as it may cause the most severe manifestations of malaria, including cerebral malaria and death. *Plasmodium vivax* and *Plasmodium ovale* are species that form a dormant hypnozoite stage in the liver that is not eliminated unless the patients are treated with primaquine in addition to the antimalarials that treat the erythrocytic phase. Patients with these relapsing forms of malaria may not manifest symptoms until many months after travel — even patients who take antimalarial prophylaxis correctly.[1] Patients with *Plasmodium falciparum* malaria typically present within 10–12 days of their return from travel to an endemic area, but the onset of symptoms may be delayed when antimalarials are discontinued prematurely. *Plasmodium malariae* is a less common form of malaria that generally is not as severe. An emerging primate parasite, *Plasmodium knowlesi*, has a similar appearance and has been known to cause severe infections in humans in Southeast Asia.[1,3]

Clinical Manifestations

As shown in the case above, the clinical manifestations of malaria may be diverse and nonspecific. Fever and chills are accompanied by body aches, joint pains, headache, and sweats. Fever patterns may be cyclical, as the rupture of erythrocytic schizonts may be synchronous. The older designations of quotidian, tertian, or quartan malaria refer to the cyclical nature of the fevers every 24, 48, or 72 hr. Altered mental status, renal failure, and high parasitemia (>20%) are signs of severe malaria that should be managed in an intensive care unit setting.[3] Cerebral malaria is the result of the tendency of *Plasmodium falciparum* erythrocytic schizonts to adhere to endothelial surfaces, including the small capillaries of the brain. Malaria in patients who have no baseline immunity, such as young children and travelers from nonendemic countries, is more likely to be severe and complicated by end-organ damage. Physical examination findings on patients with malaria may include extreme prostration, scleral icterus, or splenomegaly. Laboratory abnormalities such as thrombocytopenia, anemia, elevated lactate dehydrogenase, and indirect bilirubin levels may be helpful clues, though they are not specific to malaria.[1,3]

Diagnosis

Malaria diagnosis is best achieved through examination of thick and thin peripheral blood smears for the presence of intraerythrocytic parasites. As some expertise is required for the differentiation among the major species of malaria, the presence of ring forms alone should trigger the assumption that *Plasmodium falciparum* is the culprit, since it is most likely to be resistant to older antimalarials and most likely to cause severe malaria. A banana-shaped gametocyte is diagnostic of *Plasmodium falciparum*.[6] The schizont forms of

Plasmodium falciparum are generally sequestered away from the peripheral circulation, while circulating schizonts and oval or circular gametocytes are more likely to be seen in non-*falciparum* malaria. Rapid diagnostic tests are increasingly available, but should be confirmed with light microscopy.[3]

Treatment

Treatment of malaria varies by geographic region and severity of illness (see CDC tables for a full description: http://www.cdc.gov/malaria/diagnosis_treatment/index.html). Patients with signs of severe malaria (altered mental status, high parasitemia, end-organ damage such as renal failure) should be treated with intravenous agents such as intravenous quinidine and doxycycline, and monitored in an intensive care unit. The toxicity of intravenous quinidine (a pro-arrhythmic which requires intensive care unit monitoring) has led to an increased interest in intravenous artesunate. This agent is available through the Center for Disease Control Parasitic Drug Service on an emergency basis through an investigational new drug protocol. Patients with uncomplicated *falciparum* malaria may be treated with combinations of oral agents such as atovaquone/proguanil, artemether–lumefantrine, quinine and doxycycline or clindamycin, or mefloquine. Infections with *Plasmodium vivax* and *Plasmodium ovale* in travelers from most parts of the world can be treated for the blood phase of the parasite with chloroquine, but also require treatment with primaquine to eliminate the dormant hypnozoite phase in the liver. Patients should be evaluated for G6PD deficiency prior to treatment with primaquine, as it can trigger hemolytic anemia in patients who are G6PD-deficient.[1,5]

Numerous other causes of fever produce similar manifestations and separating them in the returned traveler can be challenging.

Dengue fever

Dengue is a mosquito-borne virus that is present in many parts of the world where malaria is also endemic. Dengue fever will often be accompanied by severe muscle aches and headache (often retro-orbital), as well as a

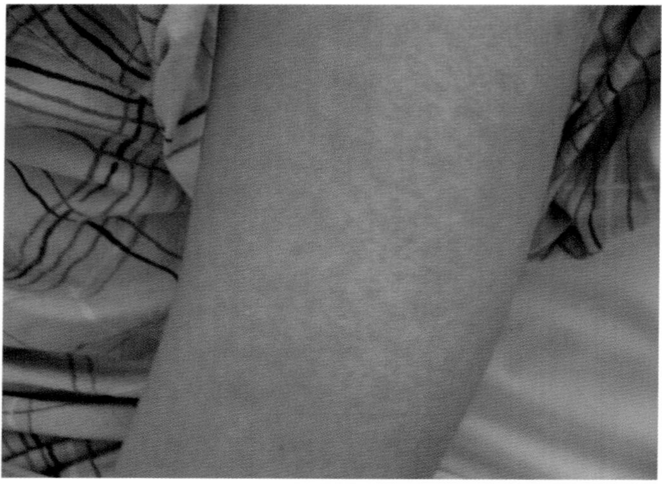

Fig. 4. Rash on the arm of a patient with dengue fever.

blanching erythematous rash (see Fig. 4). As dengue has a short incubation period, patients will often begin to have symptoms while still abroad or within five days of returning from travel. Simple dengue fever is generally self-limited and patients can be managed with supportive care, but more severe forms such as dengue shock syndrome or dengue hemorrhagic fever may be fatal.[1,2]

Typhoid fever

Typhoid fever is an infection that has a longer incubation period than dengue, and is often accompanied by high, persistent fevers and abdominal pain. Typhoid has an intermediate incubation period and patients may experience symptoms several weeks after returning from travel. Typhoid fever is caused by ingestion of the bacterium *Salmonella enterica* serovar Typhi, often in contaminated food or water in countries with lower levels of food hygiene. The diagnosis is established on routine blood cultures with recovery of gram-negative bacilli that can be distinguished from other enteric organisms when inoculated onto a triple sugar iron slant (see Figs. 5 and 6). Emerging antibiotic resistance to agents such as

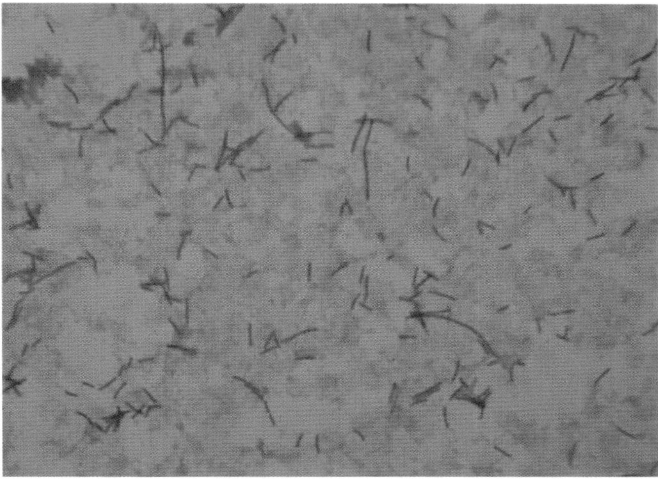

Fig. 5. Gram stain of a blood culture isolate revealing gram-negative bacilli.

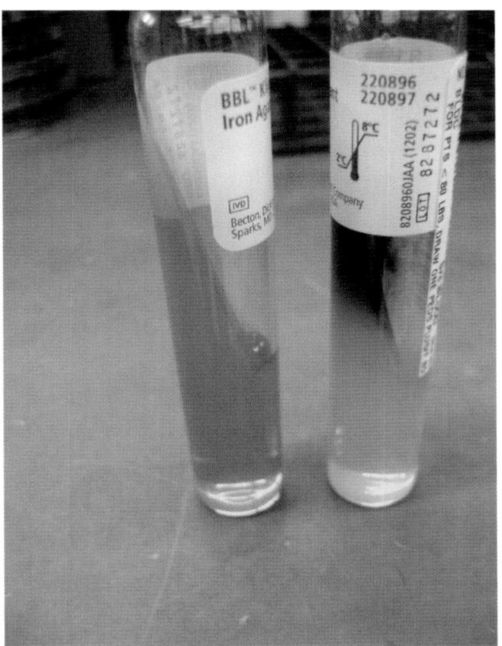

Fig. 6. Triple sugar iron slant showing an inoculated specimen on the right with yellow color indicator change and black slant in a patient with *Salmonella enterica* serovar Typhi bacteremia.

trimethoprim sulfamethoxazole and fluorquinolones has made the treatment of typhoid fever more complicated. Communication with the microbiology laboratory is especially important, since some isolates will initially appear susceptible to fluoroquinolones, but upon further testing will be discovered to be resistant. Third generation cephalosporins such as ceftriaxone are generally still effective, and oral antibiotic courses may be completed with azithromycin in many cases.

Local causes

In addition to tropical causes of fever such as malaria, dengue, and typhoid fever, local causes of fever should also be considered. Influenza, infectious mononucleosis, pneumonia, and urinary tract infection should be investigated where appropriate, as the patient's symptoms may be unrelated to exposures during travel.[1,3]

Summary

Returned travelers with fever require prompt evaluation, with consideration of both the local causes of fever and those potentially acquired abroad. Malaria, dengue, and typhoid should be considered early for all patients returning from endemic countries and appropriate treatment should be initiated as diagnostic studies are performed. Variable incubation periods may help to distinguish the various causes of fever among returned travelers.

References

1. Freedman DO. (2010) Infections in returning travelers. In: Mandell G, Bennet J, Dolin R, (eds). *Principles and Practice of Infectious Diseases*, 7th ed. Elsevier, New York, pp. 4019–4028.
2. Freedman DO, Weld LH, Kozarsky PE, *et al.* GeoSentinel Surveillance Network. (2006) Spectrum of disease and relation to

place of exposure among ill returned travelers. *N Engl J Med* **354**(2): 119–130. Erratum: *N Engl J Med* **355**(9): 967 (2006).
3. Hill DR, Ericsson CD, Pearson RD, *et al*. Infectious Diseases Society of America. (2006) The practice of travel medicine: Guidelines by the Infectious Diseases Society of America. *Clin Infect Dis* **43**(12): 1499–1539. Epub Nov. 8, 2006.
4. Mali S, Steele S, Slutsker L, Arguin PM; Centers for Disease Control and Prevention (CDC). (2010) Malaria surveillance–United States, 2008. *MMWR Surveill Summ* **59**(7): 1–15. Erratum: *MMWR Surveill Summ* **59**(29): 914 (2010).
5. CDC malaria treatment tables: http://www.cdc.gov/malaria/diagnosis_treatment/index.html
6. CDC malaria diagnosis: http://www.dpd.cdc.gov/dpdx/HTML/Malaria.htmf

Chapter 95

Cultural Competence in the Hospital Setting

Carol R. Horowitz, Alexander Green*[†]
and Joseph Betancourt[†]

Key Pearls

- Assess the patient's comfort level of communicating in English and have a very low threshold for working with professional (in-person or telephone) interpreters.
- Ask patients who need to be involved in decision-making and arrange for these key individuals to be present to discuss plans of care.
- Be honest with patients about what is happening and explore their preferences. Mistrust can lead patients to request aggressive rather than palliative care for fear that doctors are giving up, or restricting access to expensive care.
- Understand your perspectives and priorities, those of your patients, and how these differ. Be flexible and negotiate with patients when it is reasonable to do so.
- Explore the cultural, religious and spiritual practices that might impact patients' healthcare, especially when involving serious illnesses and end-of-life care.

*Mount Sinai School of Medicine, New York, NY, USA.
[†]The Disparities solutions Center, Massachusetts General Hospital, Boston, MA, USA.

Overview

Hospitalists routinely see patients who present varied perspectives, values, beliefs, and behaviors regarding health and well-being, in part influenced by their social, economic, and cultural (sociocultural) backgrounds. These include variations in recognition and communication of symptoms, thresholds for seeking care, expectations of care, and preferences regarding procedures and therapies. Sociocultural differences between patients and providers influence communication and decision-making, and are clearly linked to patient satisfaction and health. When these differences are not appreciated, explored, or addressed, patient dissatisfaction, disagreements about care, and poorer health outcomes may result.[1]

Definition and Importance

Cultural competence is the ability to communicate effectively and provide quality healthcare to patients from diverse backgrounds. This includes expanding patient-centered care (compassion, empathy, and responding to patient needs, values, and preferences) to cover useful skills in cross-cultural interactions. When seeing patients, it is important to understand that their culture, our own culture, and the culture of medicine all interact in ways that influence outcomes.

The field of cross-cultural care has emerged for three practical reasons. The US is becoming more diverse and clinicians will increasingly see patients who present differently than they expect. Effective patient–provider communication is also directly linked to improved patient satisfaction, adherence, and health outcomes.[8] Finally, providing effective cross-cultural communication is an established means of improving quality, achieving equity, and eliminating racial and ethnic disparities.

Culturally appropriate care may thwart problems commonly faced by hospitalists. Minority patients and patients with limited English proficiency have more communication difficulties, are less involved in decisions, have more difficulty understanding doctors' instructions, and are more likely to suffer from serious adverse events.[2] Communication problems (language barriers, cultural differences, and low health literacy) are the most frequent

Table 1. Resources for Hospitalists

General Cross-Cultural Issues

- National Center for Cultural Competence[11]
- Society of General Internal Medicine Disparities Task Force's Train the Trainer Guide on Health Disparities and Cross-Cultural Care[12]
- Cross-Cultural Health Care Program Resource Guide[13]

Language/Interpreters

- Robert Wood Johnson Foundation. Speaking Together Toolkit[5]
- International Medical Interpreters Association[6]
- Assessing Language Access Issues in Your Practice: A Toolkit for Physicians and Their Staff[14]

cause of serious adverse events.[3] Patients with limited English proficiency have longer hospital stays for common medical and surgical conditions.[4] Minorities are more likely to be readmitted for certain chronic conditions, such as heart failure, in part due to misunderstanding of discharge instructions. Communication issues (insufficient explanations, discounting pain and suffering, failure to recognize patients' cultural or religious beliefs, and use of language suggesting abandonment) represent key components of malpractice claims filed by patients of diverse backgrounds.

Interactions between different healthcare professionals are also cross-cultural interactions among diverse people. Recognition of these differences and use of appropriate and respectful communication skills may greatly diminish tensions and miscommunications, and improve satisfaction and teamwork in the hospital setting.

Here, we describe common challenges and situations which hospitalists face when working with patients from different cultures, and provide practical tips on how to address them, as well as resources (Table 1).

Practical Strategies to Improve Cross-Cultural Care

Language Barriers and Cross-Communication

Hospitalists are keenly aware of the frustration they and their patients experience when earnestly trying to communicate with each other despite disparate languages and communication styles. Inability to communicate

Table 2. Language Barriers

- Identify the patient's comfortableness about communicating in English.
- Have a low threshold for working with professional (in-person or telephone) interpreters.
- Know how to access and work with professional interpreters.[5,6]
- Be aware of your own behaviors, how these can impact patients, and how changing your behavior can improve communication.

due to language barriers leads to obvious roadblocks, but more subtle communication tools, such as use or avoidance of eye contact and touch, are also culturally influenced. Styles of communication (i.e. patients who show deference toward physicians, and family members who are confrontational or demanding) may be culturally based. Family members, friends, and other ad hoc interpreters are not trained in skills and vocabulary necessary for medical interpretation, often leading to dangerous miscommunication. Challenges to communication include limited availability of trained interpreters and limited clinician training in cross-cultural communication. It is important to know how to access and to have a low threshold for working with professional (in-person or telephone) interpreters,[5,6] (Table 2).

Religion, Spirituality, and Traditional Healing

A wide variety of traditions may impact health and healthcare, including dietary and healing practices, traditional remedies, and religious customs. Muslim patients with diabetes may fast during Ramadan and require adjusted insulin dosing. Illness and death are among the most powerful phenomena in our existence, and people may seek meaning in these experiences through spirituality.[7] Yet, physicians undervalue the importance of addressing patients' spiritual concerns. Over one-third of Americans use non-Western therapies with, or in place of, prescribed medications.[8] Hospitals are increasingly allowing traditional healers to care for inpatients, to improve satisfaction, as a marketing tool, and because their practices are at worst benign and at best beneficial. Spiritual and traditional

Table 3. Religion, Spirituality, Traditional Healing

- Spiritual and traditional practices should be discussed respectfully, not dismissed or taken lightly.[7]
- Engage experienced clergy or patient representatives to guide patient encounters.
- Have a list of such persons available for patients.
- Compromise. Allow or encourage healing activities to take place if they are not clearly detrimental to patient safety.[8]
- Invite spiritual leaders to learn about western medicine at your hospital. This can inform their approaches and your work.

practices should be discussed respectfully, not dismissed. Engage experienced clergy to guide patient encounters, and allow healing activities if these are not clearly detrimental to patients (Table 3).

Mistrust and Trust-Building

Trust is a crucial element in the therapeutic alliance, and is directly related to patient satisfaction and adherence. Previous bad experiences, poor communication, disrespect, and the loss of control which patients experience when ill can compromise trust — public trust in healthcare is declining. This may be magnified for minority patients whose lower inherent trust due to historical mistreatment and fear of discrimination is exaggerated by misunderstandings across languages and cultures. Clinicians should be aware of patients' cues for mistrust (i.e. concern about the necessity of a test, or mentioning a bad healthcare experience), discuss mistrust openly without taking it personally, reassure patients they intend to help, avoid medical jargon, and ask for feedback (Table 4).[9]

Table 4. Trust-Building

- Communicate clearly and effectively.
- Be aware of patients' cues for mistrust.[9]
- Reassure, develop a partnership, and allow patients some control over their care.
- Respect patients' needs and concerns.
- Discuss mistrust openly. Reassure patients of your intention to help.
- Do not take mistrust personally.

Decision-Making and Family Dynamics

How patients make decisions varies widely and is strongly influenced by cultural factors. In some cultures, the family act together as a unit to do what they feel is best, but this conflicts with mainstream medicine, which values patient autonomy and the "right to know." Some families may wish to exclude the patient from decisions, looking to a specific authority figure as decision-maker based on gender, position in the family, or ability to communicate in English. In many cultures, it is typical (and important) for family members to stay with hospitalized patients at all times. A judgmental attitude will doubtfully change patients' behaviors, but may compromise clinicians' abilities to provide care. Hospitalists should find out if patients prefer families to be involved and build trust with patients and families (Table 5).

Informed Consent and Patient/Family Refusals

The many challenges to providing informed consent to patients from diverse cultures may explain doctors' beliefs that delays in consent and

Table 5. Decision-Making, Informed Consent

- Understand your perspectives/priorities, those of your patients, and how these differ.
- Listen carefully, avoid medical jargon, and ask for feedback.
- Introduce yourself to all in the patient's room and determine their relationships.
- Ask patients about their decision-making process and who needs to be involved.
- Consider allowing a patient to waive his or her right to know (legal documents can be signed in this case) when the family wants to withhold information.
- Explain risks, benefits, and forms thoroughly to ensure understanding and trust.
- Be flexible and negotiate with patients when it is reasonable to do so, using interpreters as needed.
- If possible, allow patients and families time to review documents, so that they can make informed, collective decisions.
- If patients refuse:
  - — Ask open-ended questions about their understanding and concerns;
  - — Clearly and simply explain why you think something is in their best interest;
  - — Acknowledge and accept differences in opinion in a nonjudgmental way;
  - — Create common ground — compromise;
  - — Settle on a mutually acceptable plan.

unnecessary testing are due to poor handling of cross-cultural issues. Language barriers and limited health literacy thwart understanding of complex medical terms, legalese, and concepts such as benefit probabilities. In some cultures, telling a patient the potential dangers of a procedure is viewed as having the power of causing a bad outcome to occur. Patients may have concerns about the cost or benefit of a procedure or treatment, or believe that physicians are profiting from it. Low-literacy, low-trust, and undocumented immigrant patients may have fear and suspicion of forms they are expected to sign.

When patients disagree or refuse treatment, negotiation should not be about trying to convince them to accept what we say. It is about getting beyond the notion that whatever we think as physicians is automatically right for everyone, and teaching people what we know in a way that they can understand and that values their belief system.[9] Explain risks, benefits, and forms thoroughly to ensure patient understanding and trust, and negotiate with patients when it is reasonable to do so. Follow the steps in Table 5 if patients refuse treatments.

The Critically Ill Patient and End-of-Life Care

Hospitalizations for critical illness are especially frightening and alienating for those unfamiliar with hospitals, whose native language is not English, and who have different beliefs, customs, values, and views of illness. Patients may refuse frequent blood tests, viewed as sapping strength, as blood may be considered spiritually important and limited in its ability to regenerate. Important decisions often need to be made quickly, the patient may not be fully able to consent, and family members may arrive at different points in the process and have different roles in decision-making. In many cultures, information about a life-threatening condition is expected to go through family members, and bad news is withheld, to avoid making people lose hope. Family or unskilled interpreters may censor sensitive issues or summarize information that should be fully disclosed. Mistrust can lead patients to request aggressive rather than palliative care, fearing that doctors are giving up, or restricting access to

Table 6. Critical Illness, End-of-Life Care

- Discuss issues openly with patients and families, to elucidate their perspectives.
- Avoid inappropriate assumptions based on cultural, ethnic, or religious stereotypes.
- Discuss spiritual beliefs and customs against certain procedures, such as blood transfusions, in advance.
- Make efforts to accommodate patients' customs.
- Allow prayers, last rites, chanting, and vigils at patients' bedsides.
- Be honest with patients about what is happening and explore their preferences.

expensive care. End-of-life discussions are particularly challenging, due to cultural differences and the emotional intensity involved. Some view treatments as going against God's will, while others have strong traditions to do everything possible to preserve life.[10] Hospitalists should take time to discuss preferences openly with patients and families, avoid inappropriate assumptions based on cultural, ethnic, or religious stereotypes, make efforts to accommodate patients' customs, and allow bedside prayers, rites, and vigils (Table 6).

References

1. Institute of Medicine, Committee on Understanding and Eliminating Racial and Ethnic Disparities in Health Care. (2003) In: Smedley, BD, Stith AY, Nelson AR (eds.), *Unequal Treatment: Confronting Racial and Ethnic Disparities in HealthCare*. National Academy Press, Washington.
2. Divi C, Koss RG, Schmaltz SP, Loeb JM. (2007) Language proficiency and adverse events in US hospitals: A pilot study. *Int J Qual Health Care* **19**: 60–67.
3. Schyve PM. (2007) Language differences as a barrier to quality and safety in health care: The Joint Commission perspective. *J Gen Intern Med* **22**(Suppl 2): 360–361.

4. John-Baptiste A, Naglie G, Tomlinson G, *et al.* (2004) The effect of English language proficiency on length of stay and in-hospital mortality. *J Gen Intern Med* **19**: 221–228.
5. Robert Wood Johnson Foundation. (2008) Speaking Together Toolkit. Available at http://www.rwjf.org
6. International Medical Interpreters Association. (2010) Leading the Advancement of Professional Interpreters. Available at http://www.imiaweb.org/default.asp
7. Post S, Puchalski C, Larson D. (2000) Physicians and patient spirituality: Professional boundaries, competency, and ethics. *Ann Intern Med* **132**: 578–583.
8. *Complementary and Alternative Medicine in the United States.* Washington, DC. Institute of Medicine.
9. Betancourt JR, Green AR, Carrillo JE. (2000) The challenges of cross-cultural healthcare: Perspectives on diversity, ethics, and the medical encounter. *Bioeth Forum* **16**: 27–32.
10. Kagawa-Singer M, Blackhall LJ. (2001) Negotiating cross-cultural issues at the end of life. *JAMA* **286**: 2993–3001.
11. National Center for Cultural Competence. http://www11.georgetown.edu/research/gucchd/nccc/ (accessed Nov. 2010).
12. Society of General Internal Medicine Disparities Task Force's Train the Trainer Guide on Health Disparities and Cross-Cultural Care. www.sgim.org (accessed Nov. 2010).
13. Cross Cultural Health Care Program Resource Guide. www.xculture.org (accessed Nov. 2010).
14. California Endowment's Assessing Language Access Issues in Your Practice: A Toolkit for Physicians and their Staff. www.calendow.org/ (accessed Nov. 2010).

Index